GLENCOE
Medical Terminology
LANGUAGE FOR HEALTH CARE

Joanne Becker

Sarah Galewick

Nina Thierer

Janette B. Thomas

 Glencoe
McGraw-Hill

New York, New York   Columbus, Ohio   Woodland Hills, California   Peoria, Illinois

GLENCOE

Medical Terminology
LANGUAGE FOR HEALTH CARE

Joanne Becker, ART
Kirkwood Community College
Cedar Rapids, Iowa

Sarah E. Galewick, RN, BSN
Redding, California

Nina Thierer, CMA, BS
Associate Professor, Medical Assistant Program
Ivy Tech State College
Fort Wayne, Indiana

Janette B. Thomas, MPS, RHIA
Professor
State University of New York
College of Technology at Alfred

Library of Congress Cataloging-in-Publication Data
Glencoe's medical terminology: language for health care / Joanne Becker... [et al.].
   p.cm.
   Includes index.
   ISBN 0-02-801289-5
   1. Medicine–Terminology. I. Title: Medical terminology. II. Becker, Joanne.
     [DNLM: 1. Terminology, W 15 G558 2002]
   R123.G56 2000
   610'.1'4–dc21   00-045469

Glencoe/McGraw-Hill
A Division of The McGraw·Hill Companies
New York, New York   Columbus, Ohio   Woodland Hills, California   Peoria, Illinois

Co-developed by
Glencoe/McGraw-Hill and Chestnut Hill Enterprises, Inc.
Woodbury, CT

Glencoe **Medical Terminology: *Language for Health Care***

Send all inquiries to:
The McGraw-Hill Companies, Inc.
8787 Orion Place
Columbus, OH 43240-4027
ISBN: 0-02-801289-5

1 2 3 4 5 6 7 8 9 071 06 05 04 03 02 01 00

Brief Table of Contents

Preface

Glencoe's *Medical Terminology—Language for Health Care* was designed for you, the students in the health care curriculum, who need to be familiar with medical terms. Its purpose is to help you succeed in your chosen health care careers by familiarizing you with how medical words are formed and by providing a systematic learning structure.

Each chapter starts with a set of objectives that outline the goals each student should be able to achieve by the end of that chapter. By studying each section of the chapter, completing the exercises, and performing the chapter review at the end, you should be able to achieve the objectives in a structured manner. The majority of the chapters cover one body system and the overall effect of the book is to build knowledge of all the body systems and applicable medical terms.

FORMING MEDICAL TERMS

The first three chapters of the book introduce how most medical terms are formed. Most medical terms are built from word parts, often derived from Latin and Greek terms. These three chapters introduce many of the major word parts used in the formation of medical terms.

Chapter 2 provides the majority of general prefixes, suffixes, and combining forms needed to form the medical terminology that students in the health care curriculum will encounter. This chapter excludes those word parts that relate specifically to each body system. Chapter 3 covers word parts related to specific body systems. The most commonly used system word parts are then repeated in the individual body system chapters. This concentrated repetition is designed to reinforce the body system approach to medical word building.

USING THE SYSTEMATIC LEARNING APPROACH

Chapters 4 through 16 are the body systems chapters. The format of these chapters are designed to acquaint students with an overview of each body system while at the same time teaching them specific terms and word parts used in the appropriate medical terminology. Each body system chapter is presented in the following format:

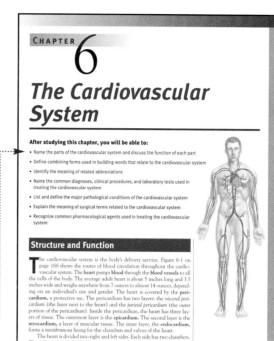

A. The **Objectives** alert you to the major concepts to learn. As you read the chapter, look for the text that helps you master each objective. Complete the exercises in each section of the chapter to check your knowledge at each stage. Answers to the exercises appear at the end of the chapter.

B. The **Structure and Function** section provides an overview of the body system and introduces **key terms**, those terms that you should memorize and understand. Key terms are set in bold type and are also listed in the vocabulary review at the end of each chapter section. Make sure to study the vocabulary review sections before doing the exercises and before moving on to the next section of the chapter. The structure and function exercises test your knowledge of the material studied in that section, emphasizing knowledge of the key terms.

C. The **Combining Forms and Abbreviations** section introduces the combining forms and abbreviations relating specifically to the body system that is the subject of the chapter. Each combining form is followed by an example. Exercises at the end of this section are designed to increase your familiarity with word building using those specific combining forms.

Combining Form	Meaning	Example
bronchiol(o)	bronchiole	*bronchiolitis* [brŏng-kē-ō-LĪ-tĭs], inflammation of the bronchioles
capn(o)	carbon dioxide	*capnogram* [KĂP-nō-grăm], a continuous recording of the carbon dioxide in expired air
epiglott(o)	epiglottis	*epiglottitis* [ĔP-ĭ-GLŎT-ī-tĭs], inflammation of the epiglottis
laryng(o)	larynx	*laryngoscope* [lă-RĬNG-gō-skōp], device used to examine the larynx through the mouth
lob(o)	lobe of the lung	*lobectomy* [lō-BĔK-tō-mē], removal of a lobe
mediastin(o)	mediastinum	*mediastinitis* [MĒ-dē-ăs-tĭ-NĪ-tĭs], inflammation of the tissue of the mediastinum
nas(o)	nose	*nasogastric* [nā-zō-GĂS-trĭk], of the nasal passages and the stomach
or(o)	mouth	*oropharynx* [ŌR-ō-FĂR-ĭngks], the part of the pharynx that lies behind the mouth
ox(o), oxi-, oxy	oxygen	*oximeter* [ŏk-SĬM-ĕ-tĕr], instrument for measuring oxygen saturation of blood
pharyng(o)	pharynx	*pharyngitis* [făr-ĭn-JĪ-tĭs], inflammation in the pharynx
phon(o)	voice, sound	*phonometer* [fō-NŎM-ĕ-tĕr], instrument for measuring sounds
phren(o)	diaphragm	*phrenitis* [frĕn-Ĭ-tĭs], inflammation in the diaphragm
pleur(o)	pleura	*pleuritis* [plū-RĪ-tĭs], inflammation of the pleura
pneum(o), pneumon(o)	air, lung	*pneumolith* [NŪ-mō-lĭth], calculus in the lungs
rhin(o)	nose	*rhinitis* [rī-NĪ-tĭs], inflammation of the nose
spir(o)	breathing	*spirometer* [spī-RŎM-ĕ-tĕr], instrument used to measure respiratory gases
steth(o)	chest	*stethoscope* [STĔTH-ō-skōp], instrument for listening to sounds in the chest
thorac(o)	thorax, chest	*thoracotomy* [thōr-ă-KŎT-ō-mē], incision into the chest wall

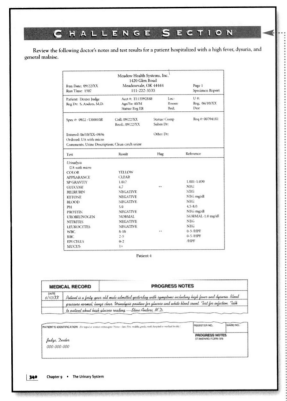

D. Diagnostic, Procedural, and Laboratory Terms introduce medical terms used in ordering and receiving laboratory reports, making diagnoses, and performing medical procedures. This section is followed by exercises based on the key terms and concepts in the section.

E. Pathological Terms cover a range of diseases for each body system. Diseases that affect or originate from several body systems are interconnected. The exercises test your familiarity with what you have just learned.

F. Surgical Terms provide an overview of common surgical procedures performed for each body system.

G. Pharmacological Terms cover the drug classes used to treat illnesses of the system being discussed and provide examples of both generic and trade name medications. (In addition, Chapter 22 provides an overview of pharmacology. Some instructors may choose to have students read Chapter 22 before proceeding to each body system chapter.)

H. The **Challenge Section** is an additional opportunity for critical thinking. This section requires students to pull answers from knowledge already learned or from an unfamiliar medical record presented within the section.

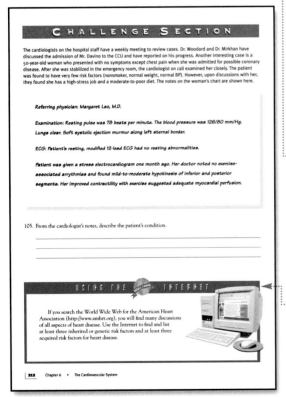

I. Using the Internet offers students an opportunity to explore medical sites to gather information, familiarize themselves with medical offerings on the Internet, and study any subjects of particular interest on their own.

J. The Chapter Review gives a complete listing of the key terms, combining forms, and abbreviations. This section serves both as a study and review tool and as a self-study check to determine how much the student has learned from the chapter. Definitions can be checked against the vocabulary review lists throughout the chapter.

K. Answers to Chapter Exercises allow self-study and instant feedback for the students to determine how well they are learning the material.

SPECIAL FEATURES

Each chapter contains some special features that reinforce learning, provide additional information, or expose students to realistic situations they may encounter in their chosen allied health professions.

A. Word Analysis—The vocabulary review sections contain a word analysis column of pronunciations and selected word analyses. The word analyses show how certain terms are formed from word parts as well as the etymologies of some words or word parts. The analysis reinforces understanding of how medical terms are built.

B. Case Studies—Throughout the text, case studies present realistic health care situations. Students are exposed to actual medical case histories, some laboratory tests, real diagnoses, health care forms, and medical decision-making. Information in the case studies shows terminology and abbreviations being used in a realistic context.

C. Critical Thinking—Following each case study, students are asked critical thinking questions relating to the case study material and to material learned in the text. Critical thinking skills are essential to the development of valuable decision-making skills.

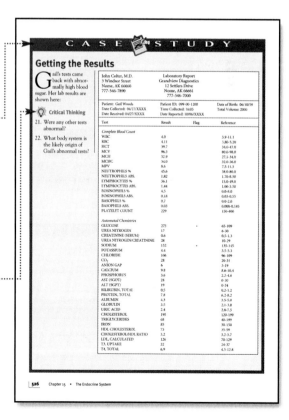

Central Nervous System

The **central nervous system** consists of the brain and spinal cord. The word *central* is the key to the purpose of this subsystem. It is the center of control, receiving and interpreting all stimuli and sending nerve impulses to instruct muscles and glands to take or respond to certain actions. Designated actions throughout the body include both voluntary and involuntary movement, sight, hearing, thinking, secretion of hormones, memory, and responses to outside stimuli. The meninges (described later) are a covering crucial to the protection of the brain and spinal cord.

Brain

The human adult **brain** weighs about three pounds, is 75 percent water, has the consistency of gelatin, contains over 100 billion neurons, and is responsible for controlling the body's many functions and interactions with the outside world. The brain has four major divisions—the brainstem, the cerebellum, the cerebrum, and the diencephalon. Figure 8-4 illustrates the brain.

MORE ABOUT...
the Blood-Brain Barrier

For many years, pharmaceutical researchers have known that the key to curing some brain ailments is to be able to deliver medication to the site of a specific disorder. The goal is to overcome the defenses of the blood-brain barrier without opening it to potentially harmful substances. Penetrating the blood-brain barrier will allow safer, nonsurgical treatment of some brain disorders.

Water-soluble substances are held back by the blood-brain barrier, while fat-soluble substances are generally allowed to pass through. Penicillin is water soluble and cannot get through easily, whereas fat-soluble substances such as alcohol, nicotine, and caffeine pass through easily. Two surgical approaches have been refined to penetrate the barrier. The first one involves two injections: one to cause the brain's capillaries to shrink temporarily, followed by a second injection of a drug that can pass between the shrunken capillaries. The other approach is to implant a disk into the brain that releases chemotherapeutic drugs near the site of a tumor. Both surgical methods are high-risk and costly. Now scientists are exploring substances that pass normally through the barrier. They can sometimes piggyback certain drug molecules to a fat-soluble substance that passes through the barrier and trick the capillaries into letting them through. Some combinations of synthetic substances are also able to penetrate the barrier. This is hopeful news for people with inoperable brain tumors, severe neurological conditions, and certain other diseases.

Figure 8-4 Parts of the brain.

Meninges — Convolutions (gyri)
Skull — Fissures
Cerebrum — Corpus callosum
Diencephalon
Midbrain
Brainstem — Pons — Cerebellum
Medulla oblongata
Spinal cord

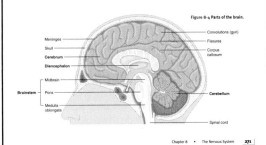

Figure 8-1 (a). The nervous system directs the function of all the human body systems. (b). The chart illustrates the functions controlled by the various parts of the nervous system.

Brain
Spinal cord
Nerves

Nervous system
Central nervous system — Brain — Spinal cord
Peripheral nervous system — 12 Cranial nerve pairs — 31 Spinal nerve pairs
Somatic system
Autonomic division
Sensory neurons — Sensory information from skin, skeletal muscles, and joints to CNS.
Motor neurons — Motor impulses from CNS to skeletal muscles
Sensory neurons — Sensory information from organs to CNS
Motor neurons — Motor impulses from CNS to smooth muscles, cardiac muscle, and glands

(a)   (b)

Table 8-1 Some Common Neurotransmitters

Neurotransmitter Group	Compounds in Neurotransmitter	Probable Nervous System Functions
acetylcholine	acetylcholine (ACh)	excites and inhibits muscular and glandular activity; affects memory
amino acids	gamma-aminobutyric acid (GABA)	inhibits certain brain activity
	glutamic acid	excites certain brain activity
	aspartic acid	excites certain brain activity
	glycine	inhibits certain spin cord activity
monoamines	dopamine	involved in brain and motor activity
	histamine	involved in brain activity
	norepinephrine (NE)	involved in heat regulation, arousal, motor activity, reproduction; acts as hormone in bloodstream
	serotonin	involved in sleep, mood, appetite, and pain
neuropeptides	somatostatin	involved in secretion of growth hormone
	endorphins	has pain-relieving properties

D. More About boxes appear throughout the book and provide some interesting medical information that would not normally appear within a medical terminology text. Such information adds interest to the study of a subject that requires much repetitive learning. These boxes may be used to stimulate class discussion.

E. Flowcharts—In most body systems chapters at least one flowchart provides a diagrammatic overview of some of the anatomical information. These flowcharts provide a picture of some of the material presented.

Specialized Chapters

Chapters 17 through 22 cover general and special areas of health care. Chapter 17, Human Development, presents the stages of the lifespan and the medical terms relating to each stage. Chapter 18 covers oncology in depth. Although cancer of each body system is presented within each body system chapter, students need to learn about the overall structure, causes, treatments, and current understanding of oncology. Specific terminology related to cancer is learned in this chapter. Chapter 19 delves into diagnostic imaging and surgery. As with oncology, imaging and surgery are also covered in each body system chapter. This chapter is an overview of these two subjects as they relate to the terminology needed by today's health care professionals. Chapter 20 covers terms in psychiatry. Chapter 21 provides an overview of terminology in dental practice. Chapter 22 is an overview of basic pharmacology for the health care student.

Additional Study Resources

In addition to the textbook, Glencoe includes an interactive CD-ROM program. The next section, "How to Use This Program," gives instructions about using the CD-ROM. Audiotapes are also available to aid students in developing proper spelling and pronunciation.

The audiotapes provide pronunciations for all key terms. Instructors who have study labs may make these tapes available for self-study. Students who wish to learn proper pronunciations at home or in their cars may purchase these cassettes for their own use.

HOW TO USE THIS PROGRAM

Medical terminology forms the basis of the knowledge needed to be successful in a health care career. Learning medical terminology requires following a structured study plan whether you are in a classroom setting or in a self-study or distance learning program. Glencoe's *Medical Terminology—Language for Health Care* provides a structure that enables students to follow an organized path to retaining and understanding medical terms.

Setting Up A Study Plan

Each body system chapter is divided into sections. Each section covers one aspect of the body system, setting off all key terms in boldface. These terms are then repeated in the vocabulary review of each section. Follow these important study steps:

- **Read the Section:** Read the section noting the key terms and their definitions.

- **Scan the Vocabulary Review:** Look at the vocabulary review section, pronounce each word, and review its definition.

- **Perform the Exercises:** Do the exercises for the section.

- **Check Your Work:** Check the answers at the end of the chapter.

- **Review Exercises You Did Not Understand:** Review the material in the section that covers the exercises you did not answer correctly. Do not go on to new material until you are sure you understand each key term.

- **Fill in the Chapter Review:** At the end of each chapter, pronounce and define each key term listed in the chapter review. Go back to the chapter to study any terms you do not understand.

USING THE CD-ROM

The Glencoe Medical Terminology CD-ROM is an interactive tutorial designed to complement the student textbook. In it you will find key terms, flash cards, drag and drop word building and labeling exercises, and games designed to challenge you such as Hangman and That's Epidemic.

System Requirements

To run this product, your computer must meet the following *minimum* specifications:

1. Pentium processor
2. Windows 95 or Windows 98
3. 32 MB RAM (64 recommended)
4. Desktop screen area set to 800 x 600 or higher
5. Desktop colors set to 16 bit (high color) or higher
6. 16-bit sound card with speakers or headphones (optional)
7. Microphone (optional)
8. Internet Explorer 5.0 or appropriate system files installed. This product does not use Internet Explorer, but it depends on many of the same system files that Internet Explorer uses.

Installation

The installation program checks your computer to confirm that it meets the minimum specifications to run this program. If you do not have Microsoft Internet Explorer 5.0 or higher installed, the setup program should detect this and direct you to the Internet Explorer setup located on the CD-ROM. If you need to run the Internet Explorer setup, go to the **IEsetup** folder and run the "setup.exe" file. Once Internet Explorer setup is complete, you will need to re-run setup for this program.

To run the setup program:

1. Insert the CD-ROM in your CD-ROM drive.
2. If your CD-ROM drive has Auto Insert Notification active, a dialog box will appear automatically, asking if you would like to install this program. Click OK to begin installation.
3. If your CD-ROM drive does not have Auto Insert Notification active, go to your windows Start menu, select "Run" and type D:\setup.exe in the dialog box (where D: is the letter of your CD-ROM drive). Click OK and follow the instructions that appear.
4. The installation program will create a Windows program group called Glencoe Medical Terminology. In that program group you will find a program icon and an uninstall icon. To start the program, go to the Windows Start Menu > Programs > Glencoe Medical Terminology > Glencoe Medical Terminology (program icon).

Changing The Desktop Setting

If your desktop screen area is 640 x 480, you must reset it to 800 x 600 or higher. You can do this yourself by opening the Windows Control Panel and double-clicking the "Display" icon. (A shortcut to this dialog is to right-mouse click anywhere on the desktop and select "Properties" from the pop-up dialog.)

From the "Display Properties" dialog that appears, select the "Settings" tab. Move the "Screen Area" slider to select the "800 x 600" option, and click "OK" to accept this change. You may have to restart your computer for the new settings to take effect.

Changing the Color Setting

For best graphics performance, your computer's colors setting should be set to high color (16-bit). To change your colors setting, go the the "Display Properties" dialog (from the Windows Control Panel, or by right-clicking the Desktop and selecting "Properties"). From the "Colors" drop-down box, select "High Color (16 bit)" and click OK. You may have to restart your computer for the new settings to take effect.

The Help Section

Once you have installed the software, you are strongly encouraged to read and review the Help section of this software. The Help section will explain in detail all of the features and activities of this software. It will also discuss frequently asked questions and offer troubleshooting tips. To access help, click on the **?** icon found on the top right of your computer screen.

MAKING PERSONAL STUDY MATERIALS

As you go through each chapter, make flash cards for combining forms, especially those that are not currently familiar to you. Your instructor will show you how to make useful flash cards to be used in studying. Appendix A is a list of all the combining forms in this textbook. Refer to it as needed.

EXPANDING YOUR KNOWLEDGE

Read all the special material as you study the chapters. Try critical thinking questions after you read the case studies and read all the margin notes and More About boxes. If you are particularly interested in any one subject, pursue it by going to the library or searching the Internet for more information.

LOCATING KEY TERMS

The Index on pages **697-720** has boldfaced entries for all key terms. Whenever you need to look up a key term, refer to the index to locate its place in the book.

Acknowledgments

Medical Art

WC Brown McGraw-Hill

Essentials of Human Anatomy and Physiology, 6th Edition

Reviewers

Jerri Adler
Lane Community College
Eugene, Oregon

Phyllis Broughton
Pitt Community College
Greenville, North Carolina

Annette Campbell
ATI Enterprises
Dallas, Texas

Patty Celani
ICM School of Business and
Medical Careers
Pittsburgh, Pennsylvania

Lisa L. Cook
Eton Technical Institute
Port Orchard, Washington

Kabir Bello, M.D.
Transworld Academy
Houston, Texas

Linda Dezern
Thomas Nelson Community College
Hampton, Virginia

Connie Dempsey
Stark State Technical College
Canton, Ohio

Walter English
Akron Medical and Dental Institute
Cuyahoga Falls, Ohio

Barbara Ensley
Haywood Community College
Clyde, North Carolina

Judith Ehninger
Lehigh Carbon Community College
Schnecksville, Pennsylvania

Monika Hollars
Indiana Business College
Marion, Indiana

Glenn Grady
Guilford Technical Community College
Jamestown, North Carolina

Trudi James-Park
Lorain County Community College
Elyria, Ohio

Jan Krueger
Empire College
Santa Rosa, California

Gwynne Mangiore
Missouri Schools for Doctor's Assistants
St. Louis, Missouri

Cornelia Mutts
Bryant and Stratton College
Virginia Beach, Virginia

Deborah Newton
Montana State University
College of Technology
Great Falls, Montana

Virginia Opitz
Northwestern Business College
Chicago, Illinois

Barbara Ramutkowski
Pima Medical Institute
Tucson, Arizona

Fran Stanley
J. Sargent Reynolds Community College
Richmond, Virginia

Patricia Stang
Medix School
Towson, Maryland

Michelle Watson
Indiana Business College
Vincennes, Indiana

Leesa Whicker
Central Piedmont Community College
Charlotte, North Carolina

Table of Contents

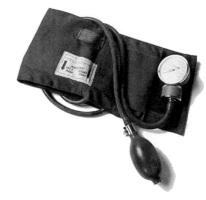

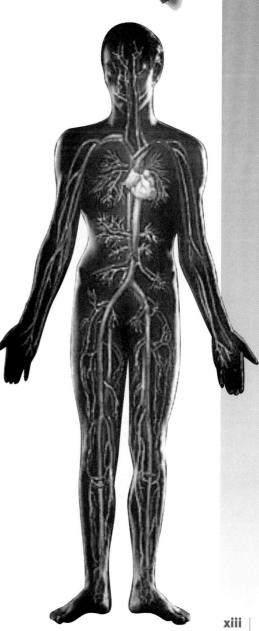

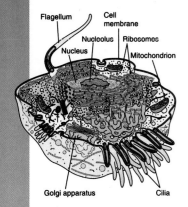

CHAPTER 4
INTEGUMENTARY SYSTEM

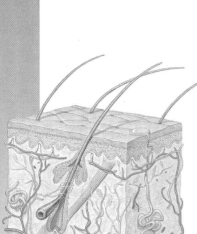

CHAPTER 5
MUSCULOSKELETAL SYSTEM

CHAPTER 6

THE CARDIOVASCULAR SYSTEM

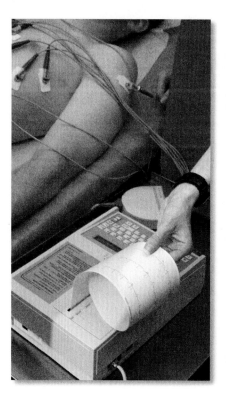

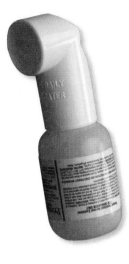

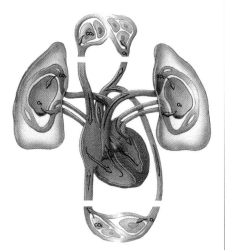

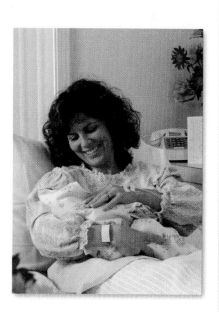

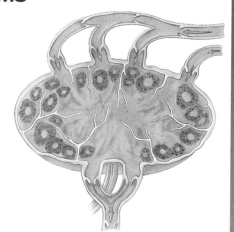

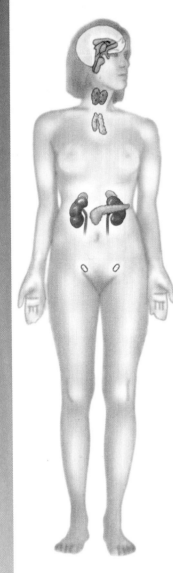

CHAPTER 17
HUMAN DEVELOPMENT

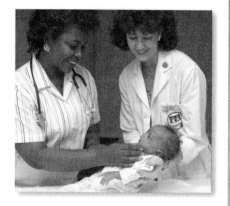

CHAPTER 18
TERMS IN ONCOLOGY–CANCER AND ITS CAUSES

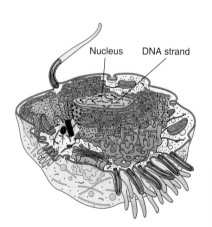

Nucleus   DNA strand

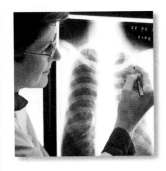

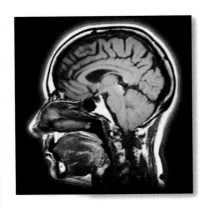

Credits

xv: Photodisc; **xvi:** Corbis Images; **xvii:** Digital Stock; **xviii:** Photodisc; **xxi:** Digital Stock; **xxii (top):** Digital Stock; **xxii (bottom):** Photodisc; **xxiii:** Photodisc; **Figure 1-1:** Dr. Jeremy Burgess/Science Photo Library; **Figures 4-6, 9-12, 14-9, 15-4, 16-5, 16-9, 18-1a and 18-1b, 18-3a and 18-3b, 19-1, 19-4:** c Carroll Weiss/Camera M.D. Studios; **Figure 4-3:** c Martin M. Rotker/Photo Researchers; **Figure 4-7:** Dr. P. Marazzi/Science Photo Library; **Figure 4-9 (right):** Biophoto Associates/Science Source; **Figures 4-9 (left), 12-10:** Nancy Wofin, M.D./Medical Images; **Figure 4-10:** c M. Abbey/Photo Researchers; **Page 73 (top):** c Frank Siteman/Stock Boston; **Page 73 (middle):** c Phil Jude/Science Photo Library; **Page 73 (bottom):** Leonard Morse, M.D./Medical Images; **Figures 5-9, 5-13, 7-6:** CNRI/Science Photo Library; **Figure 5-12:** James Stevenson/Science Photo Library; **Figure 5-14:** Joseph Lynch/Medical Images; **Figure 6-6:** c Alain Dex/Photo Researchers; **Figure 6-8:** Ken Lax/Medical Images; **Figure 6-9:** c Ouellette/Theroux/Photo Researchers; **Figures 6-13, 14-7, 19-2, 19-3:** Howard Sochurek/Medical Images; **Figure 6-18:** c Blair Seitz/Photo Researchers; **Figure 6-19:** Michael English/Medical Images; **Figure 6-21 (top):** Dr. Peter Baker/ Ohio State University; (bottom), **Figure 7-8:** Alfred Pasieka/Photo Researchers; **Figures 7-2, 17-3:** Lou Bopp; **Figure 7-5:** Damien Lovegrove/Science Photo Library; **Figures 7-10, 8-7, 17-2, 17-4, 21-5;** C. C. Duncan/Medical Images; **Figure 8-9:** Biophoto Associates/Science Source; **Figure 9-9:** c 1996 Jay Daniel/Picture Cube; **Figure 10-6:** c 1995 Kent Do Fault/Picture Cube; **Figure 12-7:** c Network Productions/The Image Works; **Figure 14-13:** c Barry Slavin, M.D./Medical Images; **Figure 16-4:** c Dan Reynolds/Medical Images/ **Figure 16-6:** c Michael English/Medical Images; **Figure 16-10:** c Ken Lax/Medical Images

The following health professionals are acknowledged for their contributions: Dr. Anan, M.D.; Dr. Jack Greenspan, D.D.S.; Dr. Taki, M. D.; Dr. Henry C. Ward, M. D.

CHAPTER 1

Learning Terminology

After studying this chapter, you will be able to:

- ◆ Explain how medical terms are developed
- ◆ Describe the process of pluralizing terms
- ◆ Describe how to interpret pronunciation marks
- ◆ List basic legal and ethical issues for health-related professionals
- ◆ Describe how medical documentation is compiled

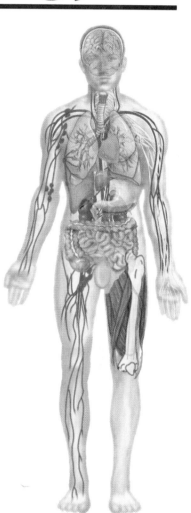

The Language of Medicine

Many everyday terms that we use to describe our health and our medical care go back to the early history of civilization. The language of medicine dates to the time when people had only spoken language, not written. Like all people who followed after them, they gave names to parts of their bodies, to illnesses, and to the cures they used. Some of these names survive in the roots and words still used today in medical terminology. For example, the ancient Greeks thought of the disease we call "cancer" as something eating at a person on the inside, and so named the condition *karkinos*, meaning both crab and cancer.

Medical terminology began to become standardized when Hippocrates (460–377 B.C.), a Greek physician (Figure 1-1), set about to organize an approach to medicine. The Hippocratic oath that is generally attributed to him has been in use for over 2,000 years.

> *I swear by Apollo the physician and Asklepios, and health, and All-Heal, and all the gods and goddesses, that, according to my ability and judgment.*
>
> *I will keep this Oath and this stipulation—to reckon him who taught me this Art equally dear to me as my parents, to share my substance with him, and relieve his necessities if required; to look upon his offspring in the same footing as my own brothers, and to teach them this*

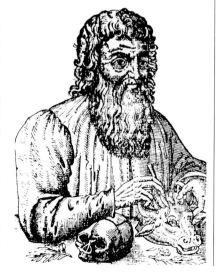

Figure 1-1 **Hippocrates, considered the founder of the practice of medicine.**

MORE ABOUT...

The Hippocratic Oath

Some aspects of the Hippocratic Oath are still debated today. For example, the phrase "I will give no deadly medicine to any one if asked" is a subject of debate now that modern medicine is capable of prolonging a life that is extremely painful and difficult. The question of whether a physician should help to end the life of a suffering patient is an extremely difficult one. Should patients have the right to choose *euthanasia,* aiding someone who chooses to die? There are many reasonable arguments on both sides of the issue. A *pessary,* a vaginal suppository used to induce abortion, was forbidden under the Hippocratic oath. Today, abortion is legally available in the United States, but the question of whether it should be legal is debated widely. Other points of the Oath, about not seducing females or males, keeping confidences, and abstaining from the deleterious (doing no harm), form the basic ethical standards of modern medicine.

Some phrases in the Oath are unfamiliar. Hippocrates was a physician only, not a surgeon, a separate profession in ancient times. The phrase "labouring under the stone" means surgery during which stones were used as weights.

Art, if they shall wish to learn it, without fee or stipulation; and that by precept, lecture, and every other mode of instruction, I will impart a knowledge of the Art to my own sons, and those of my teachers, and to disciples bound by a stipulation and oath according to the law of medicine, but to none others.

I will follow that system of regimen which, according to my ability and judgment, I consider for the benefit of my patients, and abstain from whatever is deleterious and mischievous, I will give no deadly medicine to any one if asked, nor suggest any such counsel; and in like manner I will not give to a woman a pessary to produce abortion. With purity and holiness I will pass my life and practice my Art.

I will not cut persons labouring under the stone, but will leave this to be done by men who are practitioners of this work. Into whatever houses I enter, I will go into them for the benefit of the sick, and will abstain from every voluntary act of mischief and corruption; and, further, from the seduction of females or males, of freemen and slaves. Whatever, in connection with my professional practice, or not in connection with it, I see or hear, in the life of men, which ought not to be spoken of abroad, I will not divulge, as reckoning that all such should be kept secret. While I continue to keep this Oath unviolated, may it be granted to me to enjoy life and the practice of the Art, respected by all men, in all times! But should I trespass and violate this Oath, may the reverse be my lot!

Derivation of Medical Terminology

Many medical terms originate directly from Ancient Greek or Latin terms. Table 1-1 shows a sampling of words taken directly from those languages. Notice how the terms have retained their meaning over the centuries.

Later, people of many cultures used these ancient terms in their languages. Even though the appearance of the words changed, the roots from which the words developed remained the original Greek or Latin terms. Over the ensuing centuries, people involved in medicine and the development of treatments tended to look for Greek or Latin words or roots to describe their newest discoveries. Hence, many medical terms used today are based on Ancient Greek and Latin. Word building became and remains the primary way to describe new medical discoveries. Chapters 2 and 3 introduce word parts and word building.

The word *etymology* itself is an Ancient Greek term for the study of the meaning of words.

The study of the origin of words is called *etymology.* General language terms tend to change dramatically. It takes a talented word detective to find the actual root of a word that has undergone centuries of change. Remember that most languages, up until the last 500 years, were spoken by most of the population, but were available in written form to only a few. Although books had been around for many centuries, printed material was not available to the

Table 1-1 Derivations of Terms

Modern Term	Derivation
nerve	Latin *nervus*
artery	Latin *arteria;* Greek arteria
cardi(o), the heart	Greek *kardia*
ligament	Latin *ligamentum*
cell	Latin *cella,* chamber
tendon	Latin *tendo*
vein	Latin *vena*
hernia	Latin *hernia,* rupture
gene	Greek *genos,* birth
sinus	Latin *sinus,* cavity

general population until the advent of the printing press in the sixteenth century. Even then, it took some time for large numbers of people to become readers of newspapers, journals, and books. Passing word knowledge on through only spoken communication often results in words being pronounced very differently and, ultimately, becoming changed. An example is the word *heart*. It is derived from Old English *heorte,* which ultimately comes from an early Germanic word, related to Greek *kardia,* meaning heart, and found in words like *cardiac, cardiology,* and *cardiogram*.

The change in medical terms has generally been less drastic. Most people who have studied medicine since Greek and Roman times have also studied the Latin and Greek languages as part of learning medical terminology. So, a suffix, *-tomy,* meaning "cutting," may be used in modern types of surgery (*arteriotomy,* cutting of an artery), but the basic meaning is still the original one, "cutting." Throughout this text, you will learn the parts of words that enable you to understand many medical terms.

History of Medical Terms Exercises

Fill in the Blanks

1. If a word is derived from an Old English word, it might also be related to a _____ or _____ word that means the same thing.

2. The first organized approach to medicine was formalized by _____.

3. The Hippocratic Oath forbade both _____ and _____, two issues still debated today.

4. Two languages studied throughout the history of medicine are _____ and _____.

5. When a word is passed through spoken language only, it is more likely to be altered than if it is passed through _____ language.

Pluralizing Terms

Most English plurals are formed by adding -s or -es to a word. This is also true of many medical terms (cancer, cancers; abscess, abscesses). However, medical terms derived from Ancient Greek and Latin often use the regular plural forms from those languages (bursa, bursae; embolus, emboli). Some of these ancient plural forms are eventually replaced by adding -s or -es. As you study the chapters in this text, you will learn which plurals are commonly used. Still other words have irregular plurals (foot, feet; tooth, teeth). Table 1-2 shows the formation of plurals.

Table 1-2 Formation of Plurals

Singular Words	Pluralizing Rules	Plural Words
joint, face, angioma, cancer, muscle, paraplegic	Add -s to words ending in any vowel or consonant except s, x, z, or y.	joints, faces, angiomas, cancers, muscles, paraplegics
abscess, reflex	Add -es to words ending in s, x, or z.	abscesses, reflexes
vasectomy	Remove the y and add -ies to words ending in -y preceded by a consonant. When an ending -y is preceded by a vowel, the usual plural suffix is -s.	vasectomies
appendix, radix	Remove x and add -ces to Latin words ending in x.	appendices, radices
fossa	Add -e to Latin terms ending in a.	fossae
staphylococcus	Remove -us and add -i to Latin words ending in us.	staphylococci
ganglion, datum	Remove -on from and add -a to Greek words ending in -on; remove -um from and add -a to Latin words ending in um.	ganglia, data
neurosis	Change -sis to -ses in Greek words ending in sis.	neuroses

Spelling and Pronunciation of Medical Terms

Misspellings and mispronunciations in a medical setting can result in life-threatening situations. A misspelled abbreviation for a medicine dosage was responsible for the death of several children in a cancer ward. Several new AIDS medications are close enough in sound to other drugs as to make prescribing, particularly by telephone, difficult. A physician ordered a prescription for an AIDS drug, saquinavir, for an AIDS patient. The pharmacy filled a prescription for a sedative, Sinequan, and the patient became critically ill. Aside from the possibility of written mistakes, as in a care plan, people in health care must remain vigilant in checking and rechecking verbal instructions. Misspellings that result in harm to a patient may become legal issues. Patients have the right to expect a certain standard of care. Misunderstandings caused by incorrect or misspelled words may be disastrous in certain circumstances. For example, some hospitals and doctors' offices require that written forms requesting an electrocardiogram include the abbreviation EKG instead of ECG because of the possible confusion of a written "C" with an "E" as in EEG (an electroencephalogram).

Learning how to spell and pronounce medical terms is a matter of practice. In this text, spellings and pronunciations are given in both the vocabulary review sections of each chapter and in the end-of-chapter review sections. Familiarizing yourself with correct spellings of terms is a matter of practice and of seeing the terms over and over again. Pronouncing a word out loud each time you see the pronunciation will help familiarize you with the sound of the word. (Note: Not everyone agrees on every pronunciation, and there may be regional variations. If your instructor has a particular preference, follow that preference.) Also, use your own medical dictionary as a reference when you have a question.

In this text, there are two ways we help you learn to pronounce words. First, we capitalize one syllable of all words with two or more syllables so you can tell where the heaviest accent falls. For example, the word *femoral* is pronounced FEM-or-al, with the accent on the first syllable. Next, we add marks, called *diacritical marks*, to the vowels to guide you in pronouncing them. Vowels are either long or short, as shown in Table 1-3.

Long and short vowels are just a guide to help you pronounce the words correctly. English dictionaries have much more extensive pronunciation systems, with many degrees of vowel sounds. For the purposes of learning medical terminology, long and short marks provide enough guidance.

Table 1-3 Pronunciation Guide

Vowel	Long (-) or Short (˘)	Examples of Pronunciation
a	long ā	pace, plate, atrium
e	long ē	feline, easy, beat
i	long ī	dine, line, I, bite
o	long ō	boat, wrote, rose
u	long ū	cute, cube
a	short ă	rap, cat, mar
e	short ĕ	ever, pet
i	short ĭ	pit, kitten
o	short ŏ	pot, hot
u	short ŭ	put, cut

Pronunciation Exercises

Saying What You Mean

In the following list of words, the accented syllable is shown in capital letters. The vowels need a long or short mark added. As an exercise in how familiar you already are with medical words, add the diacritical marks to the vowels. Check the answers at the end of the chapter.

6. anemia [a-NE-me-a]

7. angioplasty [AN-je-o-plas-te]

8. bursitis [ber-SI-tis]

9. disease [di-ZEZ]

10. hemoglobin [HE-mo-GLO-bin]

11. lymphoma [lim-FO-ma]

12. neuritis [nu-RI-tis]

13. osteoporosis [OS-te-o-po-RO-sis]

14. paraplegia [par-a-PLE-je-a]

15. pulse [puls]

16. radiation [ra-de-A-shun]

17. reflex [RE-fleks]

18. retina [RET-i-na]

19. rheumatism [RU-ma-tizm]

20. sciatica [si-AT-i-ka]

21. septum [SEP-tum]

22. sinus [SI-nus]

23. therapy [THAR-a-pe]

24. typhoid [TI-foyd]

25. vaccine [VAK-sen]

Legal and Ethical Issues

Health care workers share some special obligations, both legally and ethically. Many legal decisions have upheld the right of patients to privacy in the health care setting. Patients also have the right to sue over maltreatment. Ethical standards require that patients and their families are treated fairly. "Fair" may include giving the best care, keeping clear records, or respecting patients' rights. The American Hospital Association's *Patient's Bill of Rights* gives twelve guidelines for medical staff, administrative personnel, and patients. Although these are specifically meant for hospitals, most of the following guidelines provide a clear, ethical standard for patients' rights in all health care settings.

- The right to considerate and respectful care.

- The right to complete, up-to-date, and understandable information about their diagnosis, treatments, how long it will take to recover, and other possible ways to handle the condition.

- The right to make decisions about the planned care and the right to refuse care.

- The right to name someone to make health care decisions for them if they become incapacitated.

- The right to privacy in all procedures, examinations, and discussions of treatment.

- The right to confidential handling of all information and records about their care.

- The right to look over and have all records about their care explained.

- The right to suggest changes in the planned care or to transfer to another facility.

- The right to be informed about the business relationships among the hospital and other facilities that are part of the treatment and care.

- The right to decide whether to take part in experimental treatments.

- The right to understand their care options after a hospital stay.

- The right to know about the hospital's policies for settling disputes and to examine and receive an explanation of all charges.

As a worker in health care, you may be a clinical worker who provides direct care, or you may be an administrative worker who usually has access to, or responsibility for, patient records. In either case, the adherence to all legal and ethical standards is a fundamental requirement of your job. Many issues are legislated differently around the country. You must follow the rules of the state and institution for whom you work. Never take it upon yourself to make medical decisions for which you have not been trained and are not qualified.

CASE STUDY

Working in Health Care

The Crestview Walk-In Medical Center is a non-emergency clinic. It employs three doctors, four nurses, three medical assistants, and two receptionists. All twelve employees have access to the many patient records kept in the files and in the computers at Crestview. The small conference room at the back of the facility doubles as a lunchroom. Most of the staff bring their snacks and lunches to work because Crestview is in a suburban neighborhood that does not have many stores or restaurants nearby.

All the employees have one thing in common—the patients. When they gather in the conference room for meetings, the teams discuss how to handle their cases. However, when the room becomes a lunchroom, all patient discussion stops. The facility has a strict policy that allows discussion of cases only in a professional setting. Everyone observes the ethical and legal codes that forbid staff from discussing cases outside the facility and outside the domain of a work situation.

 Critical Thinking

26. Why should the facility have a policy about discussing specific cases among the staff?

27. Based on what you understand about the roles of the physicians, nurses, medical assistants, and receptionists, who do you think should have access to patient files?

Using Medical Terminology

Many careers depend on a sound knowledge of medical terminology. Written records are developed and used by many people involved in health care services. Spoken directions are used to communicate orders for health care and administrative procedures in the health care setting. The role of each health care professional usually includes the duties that each person is or is not allowed to do. For example, physicians diagnose, treat, and prescribe medications for the treatment of diseases. Nurses administer medications, track vital signs, and give care, but are not allowed to prescribe medication. Other health care employees (medical assistant, patient care technician) combine administrative and clinical duties in various health care settings. People in health information management perform many of the administrative tasks that allow facilities to get paid or reimbursed in the complicated world of health care. The systems chapters and case studies in this text will introduce you to people working in the health care environment.

From the time someone calls or visits a physician's office, that patient's medical record is involved. The medical assistant or receptionist first gathers or updates personal information about the patient, such as name, address, and insurance information, as well as learns the patient's chief complaint, or reason for the visit. The medical documentation continues to grow as the provider (the physician, nurse, nurse-practitioner, and so on) sees the patient, gathers the pertinent medical history and performs a physical examination, reaches a diagnosis, and provides procedures appropriate for the condition or illness. If a patient is hospitalized, or additional laboratory or x-ray services are needed, hospital workers, laboratory technicians, and radiologists may perform procedures, which must be documented. The patient's medical record then provides the basis for payment for these services. Coders and billing clerks then fill out the paperwork necessary to enable the provider to get paid.

Documentation of health care services must be complete for both ethical and legal reasons. Many health-care careers require an understanding of documentation. Documentation in the form of medical records typically uses many terms learned in medical terminology courses. Most health-care institutions train employees to become familiar with their own documentation formats. However, each institution may have its own format for records.

Formats for records depend on state law, the institution's responsibilities, the configuration of its computer systems, and its coding and billing practices. One plan of organization is the

Figure 1-2 The SOAP method of keeping medical records.

Name: James Westread   **Telephone:** 666–7777

Date of Birth: 3/29/XX   **Age:** 8

3/18/XX   PROBLEM 1: Tonsillitis

Chief complaint: "sore throat ×2days"

S: Sore throat, fever, difficulty swallowing
O: Temperature 101°. Pharyngitis with exudative tonsils.
A: Tonsillitis
P: 1. Throat culture
    2. 1.2 units Bactrim suspension, 5cc, 4 t.i.d.
    3. Recheck in 10 days.

3/28/XX   PROBLEM 1
S: Recheck. Feels better.
O: Temperature normal.
A: Problem 1 resolved.
P: Saline gargle if necessary.

Walk-in Medical   Physician: *Margaret Lao, M.D.*
64 Oak Street
Wellington, NY 00001
(444) 555–7777   Patient No. 89808CQ

SOAP approach. SOAP stands for *subjective, objective, assessment,* and *plan.* When first dealing with a patient, the health care practitioner receives the subjective information from the patient (how the patient feels, what the symptoms are, and so on). Next, the health care practitioner performs an examination (takes temperature, blood pressure, pulse, and so on) and orders tests (blood and urine tests, allergy tests, and so on), thereby getting the objective facts needed for a diagnosis. The assessment stage is the examination of all data and the reaching of a conclusion (the diagnosis). Finally, a plan—treatments, medications, tests, and patient education—is determined and put into action for ongoing evaluation. Figure 1-2 is an example of a SOAP medical record. Another method of documentation is *chronological,* in which patient interactions are listed in chronological order with the earliest date at the top (Figure 1-3). Figure 1-4 shows documentation for a specific procedure—with the procedure, the person performing it, and what took place.

Figure 1-3 A chronological medical record.

Patient name *Angela O'Toole*		Age *57*	Current Diagnosis *angina*
DATE/TIME			
10/10/XX	*Patient presents with increased chest pain, particularly after meals. Sent to lab*		
	for echocardiogram; BP 143/84. Leonard Glasser, M.D.		
10/14/XX	*Phone consultation with patient—echocardiogram shows status quo. Suspect*		
	acid reflux, tell patient to add Tagamet to medications. Leonard Glasser, M.D.		
10/21/XX	*Patient call—experiencing relief. Continue present medication and Tagamet.*		
	Leonard Glasser, M.D.		

PROCEDURE: *Gastroscopy*	**PATIENT:** *Holly Berger*
STAFF: *Dr. Walker*	**ID no.:** *888–22–8888*
DATE 9/28/XX	*Instrument—GIF100 video gastroscope*
	Premedication: 2% Cetacaine spray locally; Demerol 50 mg; Valium 20 mg IV;
	Atropine 0.4 mg IM.
	History: 51 year-old white female with longstanding Crohn's disease, status post
	resection of the terminal ileum and proximal colon in 1971. The patient has been
	complaining of epigastric and right-sided abdominal pain with occasional
	nausea, vomiting over the last 3 weeks. Upper GI series and small bowel follow
	through showed narrowing of the duodenal bulb and post-bulbar segment and
	then approximately 8 cm. irregular stenotic area in the right side of the abdomen,
	probably at the area of the previous anastomosis and the right proximal
	jejunal stricture.
	Procedure: The patient was brought to the endoscopy suite on a gurney. Her
	oropharynx was sprayed with 2% Cetacaine and then she was placed in the left
	lateral decubitus position.

Figure 1-4 A medical record of a gastroscopy, a surgical procedure.

Using Medical Terminology Exercises

Analyzing the Record

Write S for subjective, O for objective, A for assessment, and P for plan after each of the following phrases.

28. I feel nauseous _____

29. Allergy medicine prescribed _____

30. Has dermatitis (rash) _____

31. My arm aches _____

32. Has hypertension _____

Check Your Knowledge

Circle T for true or F for false.

33. Nurses never add to a patient's record. T F

34. A medical assistant should understand the doctor's notes. T F

35. A patient record is a confidential document. T F

36. Objective information is always given by the patient. T F

37. A plan for treatment must never be changed. T F

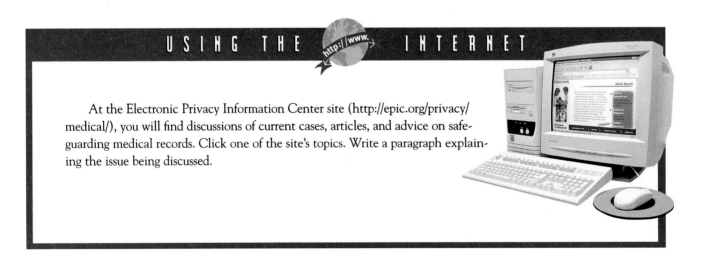

USING THE INTERNET

At the Electronic Privacy Information Center site (http://epic.org/privacy/medical/), you will find discussions of current cases, articles, and advice on safeguarding medical records. Click one of the site's topics. Write a paragraph explaining the issue being discussed.

Answers to Chapter Exercises

1. Greek, Latin
2. Hippocrates
3. euthanasia, abortion
4. Greek, Latin
5. written
6. ă-NĒ-mē-ă
7. ĂN-jē-ō-plăs-tē
8. bĕr-SĪ-tĭs
9. dĭ-ZĒZ
10. hē-mō-GLŌ-bĭn
11. lĭm-FŌ-mă
12. nū-RĪ-tĭs
13. ŎS-tē-ō-pō-RŌ-sĭs
14. păr-ă-PLĒ-jē-ă
15. pŭls
16. rā-dē-Ā-shŭn
17. RĒ-flĕks
18. RĔT-ĭ-nă
19. RŪ-mă-tĭzm
20. sĭ-ĂT-ĭ-kă
21. SĔP-tŭm
22. SĪ-nŭs
23. THĀR-ă-pē
24. TĪ-fŏyd
25. VĂK-sēn
26. Facility policy should limit discussion to case review (often supervised) and answering of specific questions. General unsupervised discussion of cases in an informal setting can lead to breaches of confidentiality.
27. Most of the staff need access to patient files. Facility policy should make the rules of access clear enough that the staff understands the legal and ethical implications of confidentiality.
28. S
29. P
30. O
31. S
32. A
33. F
34. T
35. T
36. F
37. F

2

Building Medical Terms

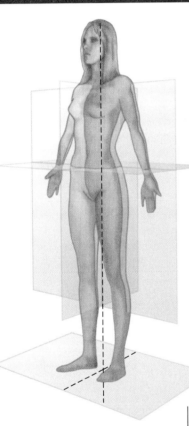

After studying this chapter, you will be able to:

- Define the four word parts used to build medical terms
- Define common medical combining forms
- Define common medical prefixes
- Define common medical suffixes
- Describe how word parts are put together to form words

Forming Medical Terms

Many medical terms are formed from two or more word parts. There are four word parts to learn about in the study of medical terminology.

- A **word root** is the fundamental portion of a word that contains the basic meaning. For example, the word root *cardi* means heart.

- **Combining forms** are the word root and a combining vowel that enable two parts to be connected. For example, the word root *cardi* + the combining vowel *-o-* can form words relating to the basic meaning "heart," such as *cardiology*, the practice that studies, diagnoses, and treats disorders of the heart.

- **Prefixes** are word parts attached to the beginning of a word or word root that modify the meaning of that word root. For example, the prefix *peri-*, meaning "around, near, surrounding," helps to form the word *pericardium*, meaning around or surrounding the heart.

- **Suffixes** are word parts attached to the end of a word or word root that modify the meaning of that word root. For example, the suffix *-oid*, meaning "like or resembling," helps to form the word *fibroid*, meaning made of fibrous tissue.

By familiarizing yourself with the word parts in Chapters 2 and 3, you will find the separate chapters about body systems easier to understand. Once you have learned the basic words and the combining forms in the systems chapters, you will be able to define many of the medical terms you will encounter as a health care professional.

Word Roots and Combining Forms

Most medical word roots come directly from Greek and Latin terms. The history of a word is called its *etymology*. The list that follows includes common medical combining forms with meanings that are not specifically part of a body system or may apply both to general terms and to specific body systems. (Body systems combining forms are discussed in Chapter 3.) Many of the combining forms in this chapter form medical terms when used with body systems terms.

Combining Forms	Meaning	Example
acanth(o)	spiny; thorny	*acanthoid* [ă-KĂN-thŏyd], spine-shaped
actin(o)	light	*actinotherapy* [ĂK-tĭn-ō-THĂR-ă-pē], ultraviolet light therapy used in dermatology
aer(o)	air; gas	*aerogen* [ĀR-ō-jĕn], gas-producing microorganism
alge, algesi, algio, algo	pain	*algospasm* [ĂL-gō-spăzm], by a spasm
amyl(o)	starch	*amylophagia* [ĂM-ĭ-lō-FĀ-jē-ă], abnormal craving for starch
andro	masculine	*androblastoma* [ĂN-drō-blăs-TŌ-mă], testicular tumor
athero	plaque; fatty substance	*atheroma* [ăth-ĕr-Ō-mă], swelling on the surface of an artery from a fatty deposit
bacill(i)	bacilli; bacteria	*bacilliform* [bă-SĬL-ĭ-fŏrm], rod-shaped like a bacterium
bacteri(o)	bacteria	*bacteriogenic* [băk-TĒR-ē-ō-JĔN-ĭk], caused by bacteria
bar(o)	weight; pressure	*barostat* [BĂR-ō-stăt], pressure-regulating device
bas(o), basi(o)	base	*basophilic* [BĀ-sō-FĬL-ĭk], having an affinity for basic dyes (said of tissue)
bio, Greek *bios,* life	life	*biopsy* [BĪ-ŏp-sē], sampling of tissue from living patients

Combining Forms	Meaning	Example
blasto	immature cells	*glioblastoma* [GLĬ-ō-blăs-TŌ-mă], growth consisting of immature neural cells
cac(o)	bad; ill	*cacomelia* [kăk-ō-MĒ-lē-ă], congenital limb deformity
calc(o), calci(o)	calcium	*calcipenia* [kăl-sĭ-PĒ-nē-ă], calcium deficiency
carcin(o)	cancer	*carcinogen* [kăr-SĬN-ō-jĕn], cancer-producing substance
chem(o)	chemical	*chemolysis* [kĕm-ŎL-ĭ-sĭs], chemical decomposition
chlor(o)	chlorine, green	*chloruresis* [klō-yū-RĒ-sĭs], excretion of chloride in urine
chondrio, chondro	cartilage, grainy, gritty	*chondrocyte* [KŎN-drō-sīt], cartilage cell
chore(o)	dance	*choreoathetosis* [KŌR-ē-ō-ăth-ĕ-TŌ-sĭs], abnormal body movements
chrom, chromat, chromo	color	*chromatogenous* [krō-mă-TŎJ-ĕ-nŭs], producing color
chrono	time	*chronometry* [krō-NŎM-ĕ-trē], measurement of time intervals
chyl(o)	chyle, a digestive juice	*chylopoiesis* [KĪ-lō-pŏy-Ē-sĭs], production of chyle in the intestine
chym(o)	chyme, semifluid present during digestion	*chymopoiesis* [KĪ-mō-pŏy-Ē-sĭs], production of chyme in the stomach
cine(o)	movement	*cineradiography* [SĬN-ĕ-rā-dē-ŎG-ră-fē], imaging of an organ in motion
coni(o)	dust	*coniometer* [kō-nē-ŎM-ĕ-tĕr], device for measuring dust
crin(o)	secrete	*crinogenic* [krĭn-ō-JĔN-ĭk], causing secretion; *endocrine* [ĔN-dō-krĭn], a gland that secretes internally into systemic circulation
cry(o)	cold	*cryocautery* [KRĪ-ō-KĂW-tĕr-ē], destruction of tissue by freezing
crypt(o)	hidden; obscure	*cryptogenic* [krĭp-tō-JĔN-ĭk], of obscure origin
cyan(o)	blue	*cyanopsia* [sī-ă-NŎP-sē-ă], condition following a cataract operation in which all objects appear blue

Combining Forms	Meaning	Example
cycl(o)	circle; cycle; ciliary body	*cyclectomy* [sī-KLĔK-tō-mē], removal of a part of a ciliary body
cyst(o), cysti	bladder, cyst, cystic duct	*cystoid* [SĬS-tŏyd], bladder-shaped
cyt(o)	cell	*cytoarchitecture* [SĪ-tō-ĂR-kĭ-tĕk-chūr], arrangement of cells in tissue
dextr(o)	right, toward the right	*dextrocardia* [DĔKS-trō-KĂR-dē-ă], displacement of the heart to the right
dips(o)	thirst	*dipsomania* [dĭp-sō-MĀ-nē-ă], alcoholism
dors(o), dorsi	back	*dorsalgia* [dōr-SĂL-jē-ă], upper back pain
dynamo	force; energy	*dynamometer* [dī-nă-MŎM-ĕ-tĕr], instrument for measuring muscular power
echo	reflected sound	*echocardiogram* [ĕk-ō-KĂR-dē-ō-grăm], ultrasound recording of the heart
electr(o)	electricity; electric	*electrocardiogram* [ē-lĕk-trō-KĂR-dē-ō-grăm], graphic record of heart's electrical currents
eosin(o)	red; rosy	*eosinophilic* [ē-ō-sĭn-ō-FĬL-ĭk], staining readily with certain dyes
ergo	work	*ergograph* [ĔR-gō-grăf], instrument for measuring work of muscular contractions
erythr(o)	red, redness	*erythroclasis* [ĕr-ĭ-THRŎK-lă-sĭs], fragmentation of red blood cells
esthesio	sensation, perception	*esthesiometry* [ĕs-thē-zē-ŎM-ĕ-trē], measurement of tactile sensibility
ethmo	ethmoid bone	*ethmonasal* [ĕth-mō-NĀ-săl], relating to the ethmoid and nasal bones
etio	cause	*etiopathology* [Ē-tē-ō-pă-THŎL-ō-jē], study of the cause of an abnormality or disease
fibr(o)	fiber	*fibroplastic* [fī-brō-PLĂS-tĭk], producing fibrous tissue
fluor(o)	light; luminous; fluorine	*fluorochrome* [FLŪR-ō-krōm], fluorescent contrast medium
fungi	fungus	*fungicide* [FŬN-jĭ-sīd], substance that destroys fungi

Combining Forms	Meaning	Example
galact(o)	milk	*galactophoritis* [gă-LĂK-tō-fō-RĪ-tĭs], inflammation of the milk ducts
gen(o)	producing; being born	*genoblast* [JĔN-ŏ-blăst], nucleus of a fertilized ovum
gero, geront(o)	old age	*gerontology* [jār-ōn-TŎL-ō-jē], study of the problems of aging
gluco	glucose	*glucogenic* [glū-kō-JĔN-ĭk], producing glucose
glyco	sugars	*glycopenia* [glī-kō-PĒ-nē-ă], sugar deficiency
gonio	angle	*goniometer* [gō-nē-ŎM-ě-tĕr], instrument for measuring angles
granulo	granular	*granuloma* [grăn-yū-LŌ-mă], small, granular lesion
gyn(o), gyne, gyneco	women	*gynopathy* [gī-NŎP-ă-thē], disease peculiar to women
home(o), homo	same; constant	*homeoplasia* [HŌ-mē-ō-PLĀ-zē-ă], formation of new, similar tissue
hydr(o)	hydrogen, water	*hydrocephaly* [hī-drō-SĔF-ă-lē], condition characterized by excessive fluid accumulation in the head
hypn(o)	sleep	*hypnogenesis* [hĭp-nō-JĔN-ě-sĭs], induction of sleep
iatr(o)	physician; treatment	*iatrogenic* [ī-ăt-rō-JĔN-ĭk], produced or caused by treatment or diagnostic procedure
ichthy(o)	dry; scaly; fish	*ichthyotoxism* [ĬK-thē-ō-TŎK-sĭzm], poisoning by fish
idio	distinct; unknown	*idiopathic* [ĬD-ē-ō-PĂTH-ĭk], of unknown origin (said of a disease)
immun(o)	safe; immune	*immunodeficient* [ĬM-yū-nō-dē-FĬSH-ěnt], lacking in some essential immune function
kal(i)	potassium	*kalemia* [kă-LĒ-mē-ă], presence of potassium in the blood
karyo	nucleus	*karyolysis* [kăr-ē-ŎL-ĭ-sĭs], destruction of a cell nucleus
ket(o), keton(o)	ketone; acetone	*ketogenesis* [kē-tō-JĔN-ě-sĭs], metabolic production of ketones
kin(o), kine	movement	*kinesthesia* [KĬN-ěs-THĒ-zē-ă], perception of movement

Combining Forms	Meaning	Example
kinesi(o), kineso	motion	*kinesiology* [kǐ-nē-sē-ŎL-ō-jē], study of movement
kyph(o)	humpback	*kyphoscoliosis* [KĪ-fō-skō-lē-Ō-sǐs], kyphosis combined with scoliosis
lact(o), lacti	milk	*lactogen* [LĂK-tō-jěn], agent that stimulates milk production
latero	lateral, to one side	*lateroduction* [LĂT-ěr-ō-DŬK-shǔn], movement to one side
lepto	light, frail, thin	*leptomeninges* [lěp-tō-mě-NĬN-jēz], two delicate layers of meninges
leuk(o)	white	*leukoblast* [LŪ-kō-blǎst], immature white blood cell
lip(o)	fat	*lipoblast* [LĬP-ō-blǎst], embryonic fat cell
lith(o)	stone	*lithotomy* [lǐ-THŎT-ō-mē], operation for removal of stones
log(o)	speech, words, thought	*logopathy* [lǒg-ŎP-ǎ-thē], speech disorder
lys(o)	dissolution	*lysemia* [lǐ-SĒ-mē-ǎ], dissolution of red blood cells
macr(o)	large; long	*macromelia* [mǎk-rō-MĒ-lē-ǎ], abnormally sized limb
medi(o)	middle; medial plane	*mediolateral* [MĒ-dē-ō-LĂT-ěr-ǎl], relating to the medial plane and one side of the body
meg(a), megal(o)	large; million	*megaloencephaly* [MĔG-ǎ-lō-ěn-SĔF-ǎ-lē], abnormally large brain
melan(o)	black; dark	*melanoderma* [MĔL-ǎ-nō-DĔR-mǎ], abnormal skin darkening
mes(o)	middle; median	*mesocephalic* [MĔZ-ō-sě-FĂL-ĭk], having a medium-sized head
micr(o)	small; one-millionth; tiny	*microorganism* [MĪ-krō-ŌR-gǎn-ĭzm], tiny organism
mio	smaller; less	*miopragia* [mī-ō-PRĀ-jē-ǎ], lessened functional activity
morph(o)	structure; shape	*morphology* [mōr-FŎL-ō-jē], study of the structure of animals and plants
narco	sleep; numbness	*narcolepsy* [NĂR-kō-lěp-sē], sleep disorder
necr(o)	death; dying	*necrology* [ně-KRŎL-ō-jē], study of the cause of death

Combining Forms	Meaning	Example
noct(i)	night	*nocturia* [nŏk-TŪ-rē-ă], urination at night
normo	normal	*normocyte* [NŎR-mō-sīt], normal red blood cell
nucle(o)	nucleus	*nucleotoxin* [NŪ-klē-ō-TŎK-sĭn], poison that acts upon a cell nucleus
nyct(o)	night	*nyctalopia* [nĭk-tă-LŌ-pē-ă], reduced ability to see at night
oncho, onco	tumor	*oncolysis* [ŏng-KŎL-ĭ-sĭs], destruction of a tumor
orth(o)	straight; normal	*orthodontics* [ōr-thō-DŎN-tĭks], dental specialty concerned with correction of tooth placement
oxy	sharp; acute; oxygen	*oxyphonia* [ŏk-sē-FŌN-nē-ă], shrillness of voice
pachy	thick	*pachyonychia* [PĂK-ē-ō-NĬK-ē-ă], abnormal thickening of the nails
path(o)	disease	*pathogen* [PĂTH-ō-jĕn], disease-causing substance
phago	eating; devouring; swallowing	*phagocyte* [FĂG-ō-sīt], cell that ingests bacteria and other particles
pharmaco	drugs; medicine	*pharmacotherapy* [FĀR-mă-kō-THĀR-ă-pē], treatment using drugs
phon(o)	sound; voice; speech	*phonometer* [fō-NŎM-ĕ-tĕr], instrument for measuring sound
phot(o)	light	*photometer* [fō-TŎM-ĕ-tĕr], instrument for measuring light
physi, physio	physical; natural	*physiotherapy* [FĬZ-ē-ō-THĀR-ă-pē], physical therapy
physo	air; gas; growing	*physocele* [FĬ-sō-sēl], swelling due to gas
phyt(o)	plant	*phytoxin* [fĭ-tō-TŎK-sĭn], substance from plants that is similar to a bacterial toxin
plasma, plasmo	formative; plasma	*plasmapheresis* [PLĂZ-mă-fĕ-RĒ-sĭs], separation of blood into parts
poikilo	varied; irregular	*poikilocyte* [PŎY-kĭ-lō-sīt], irregularly shaped red blood cell
pseud(o)	false	*pseudodiabetes* [SŪ-dō-dī-ă-BĒ-tēz], false positive test for sugar in the urine
pyo	pus	*pyocyst* [PĪ-ō-sĭst], cyst filled with pus

Combining Forms	Meaning	Example
pyreto	fever	*pyretogenous* [pī-rĕ-TŎJ-ĕ-nŭs], causing fever
pyro	fever; fire; heat	*pyrogenic* [pĭ-rŏ-JĒN-ĭk], causing fever
radio	radiation; x-ray; radius	*radiography* [RĀ-dē-ŎG-ră-fē], x-ray examination
salping(o)	tube	*salpingectomy* [săl-pĭn-JĔK-tō-mē], removal of the fallopian tube
schisto	split	*schistocytosis* [SKĬS-tō-sī-TŌ-sĭs], bladder fissure
schiz(o)	split; division	*schizonychia* [skĭz-ō-NĔK-ē-ă], splitting of the nails
scler(o)	hardness; hardening	*scleroderma* [sklēr-ō-DĔR-mā], thickening and hardness of the skin
scolio	crooked; bent	*scoliometer* [skō-lē-ŎM-ĕ-tĕr], instrument for measuring curves
scoto	darkness	*scotograph* [SKŌ-tō-grăf], appliance for helping the blind to write
sidero	iron	*sideropenia* [SĬD-ĕr-ō-PĒ-nē-ă], abnormally low level of iron in the blood
sito	food; grain	*sitotoxin* [sī-tō-TŎK-sĭn], any food poison
somat(o)	body	*somatogenic* [SŌ-mă-tō-JĔN-ĭk], originating in the body
somn(o), somni	sleep	*somnambulism* [sŏm-NĂM-byū-lĭzm], sleepwalking
sono	sound	*sonomotor* [sŏn-ō-MŌ-tĕr], relating to movements caused by sound
spasmo	spasm	*spasmolytic* [SPĂZ-mō-LĬT-ĭk], agent that relieves spasms
spher(o)	round; spherical	*spherocyte* [SFĒR-ō-sīt], spherical red blood cell
spir(o)	breath; breathe	*spiroscope* [SPĪ-rō-skōp], device for measuring lung capacity
squamo	scale; squamous	*squamofrontal* [SKWĀ-mō-FRŎN-tăl], relating to the squamous part of the frontal bone
staphyl(o)	grapelike clusters	*staphylodermatitis* [STĂF-ĭ-lō-dĕr-mă-TĪ-tĭs], skin infection caused by staphylococci
steno	narrowness	*stenocephaly* [stĕn-ō-SĔF-ă-lē], narrowness of the head

Combining Forms	Meaning	Example
stere(o)	three-dimensional	*stereology* [STĔR-ē-ŎL-ō-jē], study of three-dimensional aspects of a cell
strepto	twisted chains; streptococci	*streptodermatitis* [STRĔP-tō-dĕr-mă-TĪ-tĭs], skin inflammation caused by streptococci
styl(o)	peg-shaped	*styloid* [STĪ-lŏyd], peg-shaped; said of a bony growth
syring(o)	tube	*syringitis* [sĭ-rĭn-JĪ-tĭs], inflammation of the eustachian tube
tel(o), tele(o)	distant; end; complete	*telophase* [TĔL-ō-fāz], final stages of mitosis or meiosis
terato	monster (as a malformed fetus)	*teratogen* [TĔR-ă-tō-jĕn], agent that causes a malformed fetus
therm(o)	heat	*thermogenesis* [THĔR-mō-JĔN-ĕ-sĭs], production of heat
tono	tension; pressure	*tonometer* [tō-NŎM-ĕ-tĕr], instrument for measuring pressure
top(o)	place; topical	*topography* [tō-PŎG-ră-fē], description of a body part in terms of a specific surface area
tox(i), toxico, toxo	poison; toxin	*toxipathy* [tŏk-SĬP-ă-thē], disease due to poisoning
tropho	food; nutrition	*trophocyte* [TRŎF-ō-sīt], cell that provides nutrition
vivi	life	*viviparous* [vĭ-VĬP-ă-rŭs], giving birth to living young
xanth(o)	yellow	*xanthoderma* [zăn-thō-DĔR-mă], yellow-ish skin
xeno	stranger	*xenophobia* [zĕn-ō-FŌ-bē-ă], extreme fear of strangers or foreigners
xer(o)	dry	*xerasia* [zē-RĀ-zē-ă], dry and brittle hair condition
xiph(o)	sword; xiphoid	*xiphocostal* [ZĬF-ō-KŎS-tăl], relating to the xiphoid process and the ribs
zo(o)	life	*zooblast* [ZŌ-ō-blăst], animal cell
zym(o)	fermentation; enzyme	*zymogram* [ZĪ-mō-grăm], strips of paper for testing for location of enzymes

Prefixes

Prefixes are word parts that modify the meaning of the word or word root. They attach to the beginning of words. Prefixes tend to indicate size, quantity, position, presence of, and location. When trying to understand a word with a prefix, you can take apart the word, find the meaning of each part, and take a guess at the meaning of the original word. For example, terms for paralysis include *paraplegia, hemiplegia,* and *quadriplegia.* By taking apart the three terms, you can deduce the meaning of each word.

para- = abnormal; involving two parts   + -plegia = paralysis
hemi- = half
quadri- = four

Sometimes you need to choose the most likely definition, or you need to reason out a meaning that is not quite the prefix plus the root but makes sense. Paraplegia is paralysis of the two lower limbs; hemiplegia is paralysis of one side; and quadriplegia is paralysis of all four limbs. The meaning of limbs is not contained specifically in the prefix but it is understood from the combination of the numbers in the prefix's meaning and the root meaning paralysis—so "two paralysis" is paralysis of the two lower limbs (since you cannot have paralysis of just the upper limbs).

Prefixes	Meaning	Example
a-	without	*asepsis* [ā-SĔP-sĭs], without living organisms
ab-, abs-	away from	*abduct* [ăb-DŬKT], to draw away from a position
ad-	toward, to	*adduct* [ă-DŬKT], to draw toward the body, as a limb
ambi-	both, around	*ambidextrous* [ăm-bĭ-DĔKS-trŭs], having ability on both the right and left sides; said of the hands
an-	without	*anencephalic* [ăn-ĕn-sĕ-FĂL-ĭk], without a brain
ana-	up, toward	*anaphylactic* [ĂN-ă-fī-LĂK-tĭk], exaggerated reaction to an antigen or toxin
ante-	before	*antemortem* [ĂN-tē-mŏr-tĕm], before death
anti-	against	*antibacterial* [ĂN-tĕ-băk-TĒR-ē-ăl], preventing the growth of bacteria
apo-	derived, separate	*apobiosis* [ăp-ō-bī-Ō-sĭs], death of a part of a living organism
aut(o)-	self	*autoimmune* [ăw-tō-ĭ-MYŪN], against an individual's own tissue
bi-	twice, double	*biparous* [BĬP-ă-rŭs], bearing two young

Prefixes	Meaning	Example
brachy-	short	*brachyesophagus* [BRĂK-ē-ĕ-sŏf-ă-gŭs], abnormally short esophagus
brady-	slow	*bradycardia* [brād-ĕ-KĂR-dē-ă], abnormally slow heartbeat
cata-	down	*cataplexy* [KĂT-ă-plĕk-sē], sudden extreme muscle weakness
circum-	around	*circumoral* [sĕr-kŭm-ŌR-ăl], around the mouth
co-, col-, com-, con-, cor-	together	*codominant* [kō-DŎM-ĭ-nănt], having an equal degree of dominance; said of two genes
contra-	against	*contraindicated* [kŏn-tră-ĭn-dĭ-KĀ-tĕd], not recommended
de-	away from	*demyelination* [dē-MĪ-ĕ-lĭ-NĀ-shŭn], loss of myelin
di-, dif-, dir-, dis-,	not, separated	*disarticulation* [dĭs-ăr-tĭk-yū-LĀ-shŭn], amputation of a joint
dia-	through	*diaplacental* [dī-ă-plă-SĔN-tăl], passing through the placenta
dys-	abnormal; difficult	*dysfunctional* [dĭs-FŬNK-shŭn-ăl], functioning abnormally
ect(o)-	outside	*ectopic* [ĕk-TŎP-ĭk], occurring outside the normal place, as a pregnancy occurring outside of the uterus
end(o)-	within	*endoabdominal* [ĔN-dō-ăb-DŎM-ĭ-năl], within the abdomen
epi-	over	*epicondyle* [ĕp-ĭ-KŎN-dīl], projection over or near the condyle
eu-	well, good, normal	*eudiaphoresis* [yū-dī-ă-fō-RĒ-sĭs], normal sweating
ex-	out of, away from	*exhale* [ĔKS-hāl], breathe out
exo-	external, on the outside	*exogenous* [ĕks-ŎJ-ĕ-nŭs], produced outside of the organism
extra-	without, outside of	*extracorporeal* [ĕks-tră-kōr-PŌ-rē-ăl], outside of the body
hemi-	half	*hemiplegia* [hĕm-ĕ-PLĒ-jē-ă], paralysis on one side of the body
hyper-	above normal; overly	*hyperactive* [hī-pĕr-ĂK-tĭv], abnormally restless and inattentive
hypo-	below normal	*hypoglycemia* [Hī-pō-glī-SĒ-mē-ă], low blood sugar

Prefixes	Meaning	Example
infra-	positioned beneath	*infrasternal* [ĭn-fră-STĒR-năl], below the sternum
inter-	between	*interdental* [ĭn-tĕr-DĔN-tăl], between the teeth
intra-	within	*intramuscular* [ĬN-tră-MŬS-kyū-lăr], within the substance of the muscles
iso-	equal, same	*isometric* [ī-sō-MĔT-rĭk], of the same dimensions
mal-	bad; inadequate	*malabsorption* [măl-ăb-SŎRP-shŭn], inadequate absorption
meg(a)-, megal(o)-	large	*megacephaly* [mĕg-ă-SĔF-ă-lē], abnormal enlargement of the head
mes(o)-	middle, median	*mesomorph* [MĔZ-ō-mŏrf], body types with a balance among sizes of limbs
meta-	after	*metacarpus* [MĔT-ă-KĂR-pŭs], bones attached to the carpus
micr(o)-	small, microscopic	*microplasia* [mī-krō-PLĀ-zē-ă], stunted growth, as in dwarfism
mon(o)-	single	*monomania* [mŏn-ō-MĀ-nē-ă], obsession with a single thought or idea
multi-	many	*multiarticular* [MŬL-tē-ăr-TĬK-yū-lăr], involving many joints
olig(o)-	few; little; scanty	*oligospermia* [ŏl-ĭ-gō-SPĔR-mē-ă], low sperm count
pan-, pant(o)-	all, entire	*panarthritis* [păn-ăr-THRĪ-tĭs], arthritis involving all joints
par(a)-	beside; abnormal; involving two parts	*parakinesia* [păr-ă-kĭ-NĒ-zē-ă], motor abnormality
per-	through, intensely	*peraxillary* [pĕr-ĂK-sĭ-lār-ē], through the axilla
peri-	around, about, near	*periappendicitis* [PĔR-ē-ă-pĕn-dĭ-SĪ-tĭs], inflammation of the tissue surrounding the appendix
pluri-	several, more	*pluriglandular* [plū-rĭ-GLĂN-dū-lăr], of several glands
poly-	many	*polyarteritis* [pŏl-ē-ăr-tĕr-Ī-tĭs], inflammation of a number of arteries
post-	after, following	*postmortem* [pōst-MŌR-tĕm], after death
pre-	before	*prenatal* [prē-NĀ-tăl], before birth

Prefixes	Meaning	Example
pro-	before, forward	*prodrome* [PRŌ-drōm], to run before, as symptoms that occur before a disease
quadra-, quadri-	four	*quadriplegia* [kwăh-drĭ-PLĒ-jē-ă], paralysis of all four limbs
re-	again, backward	*reflux* [RĒ-flŭks], backward flow
retro-	behind, backward	*retroversion* [rĕ-trō-VĚR-shŭn], a turning backward, as of the uterus
semi-	half	*semicomatose* [sĕm-ē-KŌ-mă-tōs], drowsy and inactive, but not in a full coma
sub-	less than, under, inferior	*subcutaneous* [sŭb-kyū-TĀ-nē-ŭs], beneath the skin
super-	more than, above, superior	*superacute* [sū-pĕr-ă-KYŪT], more acute
supra-	above, over	*supramaxillary* [sū-pră-MĂK-sĭ-lār-ē], above the maxilla
syl-, sym-, syn-, sys-	together	*symbiosis* [sĭm-bē-Ō-sĭs], mutual interdependence
tachy-	fast	*tachycardia* [TĂK-ĭ-KĂR-dē-ă], rapid heartbeat
trans-	across, through	*transocular* [trăns-ŎK-yū-lăr], across the eye
ultra-	beyond, excessive	*ultrasonic* [ŭl-tră-SŎN-ĭk], relating to energy waves of higher frequency than sound waves
un-	not	*unconscious* [ŭn-KŎN-shŭs], not conscious
uni-	one	*uniglandular* [yū-nĭ-GLĂN-dū-lăr], involving only one gland

Suffixes

Suffixes can also be combining forms. In the section "Prefixes," the example meaning paralysis, -plegia, is both a suffix and a combining form. It both attaches to the end of the word and carries the underlying meaning of the word such as *cardioplegia*, paralysis of the heart.

Suffixes	Meaning	Example
-ad	toward	*cephalad* [SĔF-ă-lăd], toward the head
-algia	pain	*neuralgia* [nū-RĂL-jē-ă], nerve pain

Suffixes	Meaning	Example
-asthenia	weakness	*neurasthenia* [nūr-ăs-THĒ-nē-ă], condition with vague symptoms, such as weakness
-blast	immature, forming	*astroblast* [ĂS-trō-blăst], immature cell
-cele	hernia	*cystocele* [SĬS-tō-sēl], hernia of the urinary bladder
-cidal	destroying, killing	*suicidal* [sū-ĭ-SĪD-ăl], likely to kill oneself
-cide	destroying, killing	*suicide* [SŪ-ĭ-sīd], killing of oneself; *bacteriocide* [băk-TĒR-ē-ō-sīd], agent that destroys bacteria
-clasis	breaking	*osteoclasis* [ŎS-tē-ŎK-lă-sĭs], intentional breaking of a bone
-clast	breaking	*osteoclast* [ŎS-tē-ō-klăst], instrument used in osteoclasis
-crine	secreting	*endocrine* [ĔN-dō-krĭn], gland that secretes hormones into the bloodstream
-crit	separate	*hematocrit* [HĒ-mă-tō-krĭt, HĔM-ă-tō-krĭt], percentage of volume of a blood sample that is composed of cells
-cyte	cell	*thrombocyte* [THRŎM-bō-sīt], blood platelet
-cytosis	condition of cells	*erythrocytosis* [ĕ-RĬTH-rō-sī-tō-sĭs], condition with an abnormal number of red blood cells in the blood
-derma	skin	*scleroderma* [sklēr-ō-DĔR-mă], hardening of the skin
-desis	binding	*arthrodesis* [ăr-THRŎD-ĕ-sĭs, ăr-thrō-DĒ-sĭs], stiffening of a joint
-dynia	pain	*neurodynia* [nūr-ō-DĬN-ē-ă], nerve pain
-ectasia	expansion; dilation	*neurectasia* [nūr-ĕk-TĀ-zē-ă], operation with dilation of a nerve
-ectasis	expanding; dilating	*bronchiectasis* [brŏng-kē-ĔK-tă-sĭs], condition with chronic dilation of the bronchi
-ectomy	removal of	*appendectomy* [ăp-pĕn-DĔK-tō-mē], removal of the appendix
-edema	swelling	*lymphedema* [lĭmf-ĕ-DĒ-mă], swelling as a result of obstructed lymph nodes
-ema	condition	*empyema* [ĕm-pī-Ē-mă], pus in a body cavity

Suffixes	Meaning	Example
-emesis	vomiting	*hematemesis* [hē-mă-TĔM-ĕ-sĭs], vomiting of blood
-emia	blood	*uremia* [yū-RĒ-mē-ă], excess urea in the blood
-emic	relating to blood	*uremic* [yū-RĒ-mĭk], having excess urea in the blood
-esthesia	sensation	*paresthesia* [păr-ĕs-THĒ-zē-ă], abnormal sensation, such as tingling
-form	in the shape of	*uniform* [YŪ-nĭ-fŏrm], having the same shape throughout
-gen	producing, coming to be	*carcinogen* [kăr-SĬN-ō-jĕn], cancer-causing agent
-genesis	production of	*pathogenesis* [păth-ō-JĔN-ĕ-sĭs], production of disease
-genic	producing	*iatrogenic* [ī-ăt-rō-JĔN-ĭk], induced by treatment
-globin	protein	*hemoglobin* [hē-mō-GLŌ-bĭn], protein of red blood cells
-globulin	protein	*immunoglobulin* [ĭm-yū-nō-GLŎB-yū-lĭn], one of certain structurally related proteins
-gram	a recording	*encephalogram* [ĕn-SĔF-ă-lō-grăm], brain scan
-graph	recording instrument	*encephalograph* [ĕn-SĔF-ă-lō-grăf], instrument for measuring brain activity
-graphy	process of recording	*echocardiography* [ĔK-ō-kăr-dē-ŎG-ră-fē], use of ultrasound to examine the heart
-iasis	pathological condition or state	*psoriasis* [sō-RĪ-ă-sĭs], chronic skin disease
-ic	pertaining to	*gastric* [GĂS-trĭk], relating to the stomach
-ics	treatment, practice, body of knowledge	*orthopedics* [ōr-thō-PĒ-dĭks], medical practice concerned with treatment of skeletal disorders
-ism	condition, disease, doctrine	*dwarfism* [DWŌRF-ĭzm], condition including abnormally small size
-itis (pl. -itides)	inflammation	*nephritis* [nĕ-FRĪ-tĭs], kidney inflammation; *neuritides* [nū-RĪT-ĭ-dēz], inflammation of nerves

Suffixes	Meaning	Example
-kinesia	movement	*bradykinesia* [brăd-ĭ-kĭn-Ē-zē-ă], decrease in movement
-kinesis	movement	*hyperkinesis* [hī-pĕr-kĭ-NĒ-sĭs], excessive muscular movement
-lepsy	condition of	*catalepsy* [KĂT-ă-lĕp-sē], condition with having seizures seizures of extreme rigidity
-leptic	having seizures	*cataleptic* [kăt-ă-LĔP-tĭk], person with catalepsy
-logist	one who practices	*dermatologist* [dĕr-mă-TŎL-ō-jĭst], one who practices dermatology
-logy	study, practice	*dermatology* [dĕr-mă-TŎL-ō-jē], study and treatment of skin disorders
-lysis	destruction of	*electrolysis* [ē-lĕk-TRŎL-ĭ-sĭs], permanent removal of unwanted hair
-lytic	destroying	*thrombolytic* [thrŏm-bō-LĬT-ĭk], dissolving a thrombus
-malacia	softening	*osteomalacia* [ŎS-tē-ō-mă-LĀ-shē-ă], gradual softening of bone
-mania	obsession	*monomania* [mŏn-ō-MĂ-nē-ā], obsession with one idea
-megaly	enlargement	*cephalomegaly* [SĔF-ă-lō-MĔG-ă-lē], abnormal enlargement of the head
-meter	measuring device	*ophthalmometer* [ŏf-thăl-MŎM-ĕ-tĕr], device for measuring cornea curvature
-metry	measurement	*optometry* [ŏp-TŎM-ĕ-trē], specialty concerned with measurement of eye function
-oid	like, resembling	*cardioid* [KĂR-dē-ŏyd], resembling a heart
-oma (pl. -omata)	tumor, neoplasm	*myoma* (pl. *myomata*) [mī-Ō-mă (pl. mī-ō-MĂ-tă)], neoplasm of muscle tissue
-opia	vision	*diplopia* [dĭ-PLŌ-pē-ă], double vision
-opsia	vision	*chloropsia* [klō-RŎP-sē-ă], condition of seeing objects as green
-opsy	view of	*biopsy* [BĪ-ŏp-sē], cutting from living tissue to be viewed
-osis (pl. -oses)	condition, state, process	*halitosis* [hăl-ĭ-TŌ-sĭs], chronic bad breath

Suffixes	Meaning	Example
-ostomy	opening	*colostomy* [kō-LŎS-tō-mē], surgical opening in the colon
-oxia	oxygen	*anoxia* [ăn-ŎK-se-ă], lack of oxygen
-para	bearing	*primipara* [prī-MĬP-ăr-ă], woman who has given birth once
-parous	producing; bearing	*viviparous* [vī-VĬP-ă-rŭs], bearing living young
-paresis	slight paralysis	*monoparesis* [mŏn-ō-pă-RĒ-sĭs], paralysis of only one extremity
-pathy	disease	*osteopathy* [ŏs-tē-ŎP-ă-thē], bone disease
-penia	deficiency	*leukopenia* [lū-kō-PĒ-nē-ă], condition with fewer than normal white blood cells
-pepsia	digestion	*dyspepsia* [dĭs-PĔP-sē-ă], impaired digestion
-pexy	fixation, usually done surgically	*nephropexy* [NĔF-rō-pĕk-sē], surgical fixation of a floating kidney
-phage, -phagia, -phagy	eating, devouring	*polyphagia* [pŏl-ē-FĀ-jē-ă], excessive eating
-phasia	speaking	*aphasia* [ā-FĀ-zē-ă], loss of or reduction in speaking ability
-pheresis	removal	*leukapheresis* [lū-kă-fĕ-RĒ-sĭs], removal of leukocytes from drawn blood
-phil	attraction; affinity for	*cyanophil* [SĪ-ăn-nō-fĭl], element that turns blue after staining
-philia	attraction; affinity for	*hemophilia* [hē-mō-FĬL-ē-ă], blood disorder with tendency to hemorrhage
-phobia	fear	*acrophobia* [ăk-rō-FŌ-bē-ă], fear of heights
-phonia	sound	*neuraphonia* [nūr-ă-FŌ-nē-ă], loss of sounds
-phoresis	carrying	*electrophoresis* [ē-lĕk-trō-FŌR-ē-sĭs], movement of particles in an electric field
-phoria	feeling; carrying	*euphoria* [yū-FŌR-ēă], feeling of well-being
-phrenia	of the mind	*schizophrenia* [skĭz-ō-FRĔ-nē-ă], term for a common psychosis
-phthisis	wasting away	*hemophthisis* [hē-MŎF-thĭ-sĭs], anemia

Suffixes	Meaning	Example
-phylaxis	protection	*prophylaxis* [prō-fĭ-LĂK-sĭs], prevention of disease
-physis	growing	*epiphysis* [ĕ-PĬF-ĭ-sĭs], part of a long bone distinct from and growing out of the shaft
-plakia	plaque	*leukoplakia* [lū-kō-PLĀ-kē-ă], white patch on the mucous membrane
-plasia	formation	*dysplasia* [dĭs-PLĀ-zē-ă], abnormal tissue formation
-plasm	formation	*protoplasm* [PRŌ-tō-plăzm], living matter
-plastic	forming	*hemoplastic* [hē-mō-PLĂS-tĭk], forming new blood cells
-plasty	surgical repair	*rhinoplasty* [RĪ-nō-plăs-tē], plastic surgery of the nose
-plegia	paralysis	*quadriplegia* [KWĂH-drĭ-PLĒ-jē-ă], paralysis of all four limbs
-plegic	one who is paralyzed	*quadriplegic* [kwăh-drĭ-PLĒ-jĭk], person who has quadriplegia
-pnea	breath	*eupnea* [yūp-NĒ-ă], easy, normal respiration
-poiesis	formation	*erythropoiesis* [ĕ-RĬTH-rō-pŏy-Ē-sĭs], formation of red blood cells
-poietin	one that forms	*erythropoietin* [ĕ-RĬTH-rō-pŏy-ĕ-tĭn], an acid that aids in the formation of red blood cells
-poietic	forming	*erythropoietic* [ĕ-RĬTH-rō-pŏy-ĕt-ĭk], of the formation of red blood cells
-porosis	lessening in density	*osteoporosis* [ŎS-tē-ō-pō-RŌ-sĭs], lessening of bone density
-ptosis	falling down; drooping	*blepharoptosis* [blĕf-ă-RŎP-tō-sĭs], drooping eyelid
-rrhage	discharging heavily	*hemorrhage* [HĔM-ō-rĭj], to bleed profusely
-rrhagia	heavy discharge	*tracheorrhagia* [trā-kē-ō-RĀ-jē-ă], hemorrhage from the trachea
-rrhaphy	surgical suturing	*herniorrhaphy* [HĔR-nē-ŌR-ă-fē], surgical repair of a hernia
-rrhea	a flowing, a flux	*dysmenorrhea* [dĭs-mĕn-ŌR-ē-ă], difficult menstrual flow

Suffixes	Meaning	Example
-rrhexis	rupture	*cardiorrhexis* [kăr-dē-ō-RĔK-sĭs], rupture of the heart wall
-schisis	splitting	*spondyloschisis* [spŏn-dĭ-LŎS-kĭ-sĭs], failure of fusion of the vertebral arch in an embryo
-scope	instrument for observing	*microscope* [MĪ-krō-skōp], instrument for viewing small objects
-scopy	use of an instrument for observing	*microscopy* [mī-KRŎS-kō-pĕ], use of microscopes
-somnia	sleep	*insomnia* [ĭn-SŎM-nē-ă], inability to sleep
-spasm	contraction	*esophagospasm* [ĕ-SŎF-ă-gō-spăzm], spasm of the walls of the esophagus
-stalsis	contraction	*peristalsis* [pĕr-ĭ-STĂL-sĭs], movement of the intestines by contraction and relaxation of its tube
-stasis	stopping; constant	*homeostasis* [HŌ-mē-ō-STĀ-sĭs], state of equilibrium in the body
-stat	agent to maintain a state	*bacteriostat* [băk-TĒR-ē-ō-stăt], agent that inhibits bacterial growth
-static	maintaining a state	*hemostatic* [hē-mō-STĂT-ĭk], stopping blood flow within a vessel
-stenosis	narrowing	*stenostenosis* [STĔN-ō-stĕ-NŌ-sĭs], narrowing of the parotid duct
-stomy	opening	*colostomy* [kō-LŎS-tō-mē], surgical opening in the colon
-tome	cutting instrument, segment	*osteotome* [ŎS-tē-ō-tōm], instrument for cutting bone
-tomy	cutting operation	*laparotomy* [LĂP-ă-RŎT-ō-mē], incision in the abdomen
-trophic	nutritional	*atrophic* [ā-TRŌF-ĭk], of a wasting state, often due to malnutrition
-trophy	nutrition	*dystrophy* [DĬS-trō-fē], changes that result from inadequate nutrition
-tropia	turning	*esotropia* [ĕs-ō-TRŌ-pē-ă], crossed eyes
-tropic	turning toward	*neurotropic* [nūr-ō-TRŎP-ĭk], localizing in nerve tissue
-tropy	condition of turning toward	*neurotropy* [nū-RŎT-rō-pē], affinity of certain contrast mediums for nervous tissue

Suffixes	Meaning	Example
-uria	urine	*pyuria* [pī-YŪ-rē-ă], pus in the urine
-version	turning	*retroversion* [rĕ-trō-VĔR-zhŭn], a turning backward; said of the uterus

Word Roots and Combining Forms Exercises

Build Your Medical Vocabulary

Using the lists in this chapter, write the appropriate prefix, suffix, or combining form in the blank for each word part. The definition of each word part needed is given immediately under the blank. Exercise 1 is completed as an example.

1. *Osteo*(bone)myel*itis*(inflammation)

2. _____cardio_____
     (within)   (visual examining)

3. _____dactyly
     (together)

4. _____violet
     (beyond)

5. _____sensitive
     (overly)

6. entero_____ _____
     (disease)   (causing)

7. _____dermic
     (beneath)

8. _____therapy
     (sleep)

9. _____ost_____
     (together)   (condition)

10. _____tonsillar
     (above)

11. _____cranio_____
     (half)   (cutting)

12. _____ _____
     (old people)   (fear)

13. _____glandular
     (within)

14. _____blast
     (white)

15. _____ _____
     (structure)   (study of)

16. arterio_____
          (suture)

17. dermato_____
          (hemorrhage)

18. _____flexion
     (half)

19. _____algesia
     (heat)

20. fibr_____
        (resembling)

21. _____organsim
     (tiny)

22. _____plasm
     (new)

23. subcost_____
         (pain)

24. blepharo_____
          (paralysis)

25. _____myx_____
     (fiber)   (tumor)

Find a Match

Each of the words in the left-hand column contains a word part that matches one of the definitions in the right-hand column. Write the letter of the answer that best fits into the left-hand column. Exercise 26 is completed as an example.

26. _o_ antipsychotic		a. in the shape of
27. __ polycystic		b. without
28. __ acephaly		c. enlargement
29. __ tenosynovitis		d. abnormally low
30. __ myotrophy		e. nutrition
31. __ laryngoscope		f. self
32. __ dysgnosia		g. outside of
33. __ decontamination		h. inflammation
34. __ chyliform		i. instrument for viewing
35. __ autoinfection		j. abnormal
36. __ cardiomegaly		k. between
37. __ extrasensory		l. away from
38. __ intercerebral		m. condition
39. __ osteoporosis		n. many
40. __ hyposthenia		o. against

Find the Word Part

Complete the word for which the definition is given. Add a word part(s) learned in this chapter.

41. Any disease of the hair: tricho _____

42. Repair of a nose defect: rhino_____

43. Removal of the appendix: append_____

44. Having a jaw that protrudes abnormally forward: _____gnathic

45. Disease of the heart: cardio_____

46. Inflammation of the bronchi: bronch_____

47. Outer layer of a cell: _____blast

48. Rib-shaped: costi_____

49. Bone-forming cell: osteo_____

50. Above the nose: _____nasal

51. Study of the skin: dermato_____

52. Loss of the voice: _____phonia

53. Study of tissue: hist_____

54. Inflammation of the ovary: ovar _____

55. Inflammation of the ear: ot_____

56. Specialist in foot disorders: pod_____

57. Incision into a vein: phlebo_____

58. Study of the mind: psycho_____

59. Enlargement of the spleen:spleno _____

60. Removal of the kidney: nephr_____

Separate the Word Parts

Break apart the following words and define each part in the space allowed.

61. exocrine _____

62. endocranium _____

63. antidepressant _____

64. somatotropic _____

65. pseudesthesia _____

66. dextrotropic _____

67. algesic _____

68. xiphoid _____

69. litholysis _____

70. cryolysis _____

Find Where Word Parts Come From

Match the word part on the left with its etymology on the right.

71. __ xipho-

72. __ ambi-

73. __ -graph

74. __ -kinesia

75. __ ichthyo-

76. __ eosino-

77. __ bio-

78. __ xantho-

79. __ -phylaxis

80. __ -trophy

81. __ chrono-

82. __ melano-

83. __ -clasis

84. __ -plasia

85. __ lacto-

a. Greek *xanthos*, yellow

b. Greek *ichthys*, fish

c. Latin *lac*, milk

d. Greek *melas*, black

e. Greek *grapho*, to write

f. Greek *trophe*, nutrition

g. Greek *klastos*, broken

h. Greek *eos*, dawn

i. Greek *plasso*, to form

j. Greek *chronos*, time

k. Greek *xiphos*, sword

l. Greek *phylaxis*, protection

m. Latin *ambi-*, around; about

n. Greek *kinesis*, movement

o. Greek *bios*, life

Check for Accuracy

Circle T for true or F for false.

86. Lactoferrin is a form of iron found in the blood. T F

87. Hypoproteinemia means abnormally low amounts of protein in the blood. T F

88. Paraurethral means alongside the urethra. T F

89. Arteriotomy means a surgical incision into an artery. T F

90. Sphygmoid means like the pulse. T F

91. Pneumomalacia means black lung disease. T F

92. Tracheostenosis means narrowing of the trachea. T F

93. Pyrogenic means the lowering of fever. T F

94. Encephalogram is a machine for measuring the brain. T F

95. Angiokinesis and vasomotion are synonyms. T F

Root Out the Meaning

Match the word on the left with its synonym on the right.

96. __angiospasm   a. yellow skin

97. __arthrodynia   b. bradyrhythmia

98. __arthrometer   c. vaginofixation

99. __hemoconia   d. sleepwalking

100. __bradycardia   e. goniometer

101. __cancroid   f. phlebotomy

102. __cartilage cell   g. triplet

103. __cephalalgia   h. arthralgia

104. __xanthoderma   i. cancriform

105. __diplopia   j. headache

106. __venesection   k. blood dust

107. __vaginapexy   l. chondrocyte

108. __unicameral   m. double vision

109. __tridymus   n. monolocular

110. __somnambulism   o. vasospasm

USING THE http://www. INTERNET

Go to the FDA's News site (http://www.fda.gov/opacom/hpnews.html). Click the latest FDA news bulletin and find on the site at least ten combining forms, suffixes, and prefixes that you learned in this chapter.

Answers to Chapter Exercises

1. osteomyelitis
2. endocardiography
3. syndactyly
4. ultraviolet
5. hypersensitive
6. enteropathogenic
7. hypodermic
8. hypnotherapy
9. synostosis
10. supratonsillar
11. hemicraniotomy
12. gerontophobia
13. intraglandular
14. leukoblast
15. morphology
16. arteriorrhaphy
17. dermatorrhagia
18. semiflexion
19. thermalgesia
20. fibroid
21. microorganism
22. neoplasm
23. subcostalgia
24. blepharoplegia
25. fibromyxoma
26. o
27. n
28. b
29. h
30. e
31. I
32. j
33. l
34. a
35. f
36. c
37. g
38. k
39. m

40. d
41. trichopathy
42. rhinoplasty
43. appendectomy
44. prognathic
45. cardiopathy
46. bronchitis
47. ectoblast
48. costiform
49. osteoblast
50. supranasal
51. dermatology
52. aphonia
53. histology
54. ovaritis
55. otitis
56. podiatrist
57. phlebotomy
58. psychology
59. splenomegaly
60. nephrectomy
61. exo-, outside of; crin-, secreting
62. endo-, within; cranium
63. anti-, against; depressant
64. somato-, body; -tropic, turning toward
65. pseud-, false; -esthesia, sensation
66. dextro-, right; -tropic, turning toward
67. alges-, pain; -ic, pertaining to
68. xiph-, sword; -oid, resembling
69. litho, stone; -lysis, destruction of
70. cryo-, cold; -lysis, destruction of
71. k

72. m
73. e
74. n
75. b
76. h
77. o
78. a
79. l
80. f
81. j
82. d
83. g
84. I
85. c
86. F
87. T
88. T
89. T
90. T
91. F
92. T
93. F
94. F
95. T
96. o
97. h
98. e
99. k
100. b
101. I
102. l
103. j
104. a
105. m
106. f
107. c
108. n
109. g
110. d

3

Body Structure

After studying this chapter, you will be able to:

- ◆ Define the elements of human body structure

- ◆ Describe the planes of the body

- ◆ Locate the body cavities and list organs that are contained within each cavity

- ◆ Recognize combining forms that relate to elements and systems of the body

Body Structure and Organization

The body is organized from its smallest element, the **cell,** to the collection of systems, with all its interrelated parts. The entire body is made of cells that vary in size, shape, and function, but all cells have one thing in common: they need food, water, and oxygen to live and function.

Cells

The basic structures of the cell are the *cell membrane, nucleus,* and *cytoplasm* (Figure 3-1). The cell membrane is the outer covering of the cell, which holds substances inside the cell while helping the cell maintain its shape. The nucleus is the central portion of each cell. It directs the cell's activities and contains the *chromosomes,* the bearers of *genes*—those elements that control inherited traits such as eye color, height, inherited diseases, gender, and so on. The chromosomes are made of *deoxyribonucleic acid* or *DNA,* which contains all the genetic information for the cell. Surrounding the nucleus is the cytoplasm, the substance that performs the work of the cell, such as reproduction and movement.

Cephalo-
Encephalo-
Kerato-
Oculo-
Stomato-
Laryngo-
Tracheo-
Broncho-
Masto-
Cardio-
Arterio-
Thoraco-
Pleuro-
Phreno-
Hepato-
Entero-
Nephro-
Cysto-
Arthro-
Laparo-
Hemato-
Dermato
Osteo-
Phlebo-
Pod-

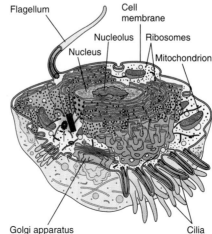

Flagellum
Cell membrane
Nucleolus   Ribosomes
Nucleus
Mitochondrion
Golgi apparatus
Cilia

Figure 3-1 A cell.

Cell Types

Cells all have specialized functions. Their shape influences their function. Nerve cells usually have long, thin extensions that can transmit nerve impulses over a distance. Epithelial cells that line the mouth are thin, flat, and tightly packed so that they form a protective layer over underlying cells. Muscle cells are slender rods that attach at the ends of the structures they move. As these types of cells specialize further, their shape and function change to fit a specific need.

Parts of a cell are also important to its function. For example, a cell membrane either allows or prevents passage of material through it, providing control over what materials move in and out of a cell.

Cell is from Latin cella, a store-room, chamber.

Tissues

Groups of cells that work together to perform the same task are called **tissue.** The body has four types of tissue:

- **Connective tissue** holds and connects body parts together. Examples are bones, ligaments, and tendons.

- **Epithelial tissue** covers the internal and external body surfaces. Skin and linings of internal organs (such as the intestines) are epithelial tissue.

- **Muscle tissue** expands and contracts, allowing the body to move.

- **Nervous tissue** carries messages to and from the brain and spinal cord from all parts of the body.

Organs

Groups of tissue that work together to perform a specific function are called **organs.** Examples are the *kidneys*, which maintain water and salt balance in the blood, and the *stomach*, which breaks down food into substances that the circulatory system can transport throughout the body as nourishment for its cells.

Systems

Groups of organs that work together to perform one of the body's major functions form a **system.** The terminology for each body system is provided in a separate chapter.

- The **integumentary system** consists of the skin and the accessory structures derived from it—hair, nails, sweat glands, and oil glands. (See Chapter 4.)

- The **musculoskeletal system** supports the body, protects organs, and provides body movement. It includes muscles, bones, and cartilage. (See Chapter 5.)

- The **cardiovascular system** includes the heart and blood vessels, which pump and transport blood throughout the body. Blood carries nutrients to and removes waste from the tissues. (See Chapter 6.)

- The **respiratory system** includes the lungs and the airways. This system performs respiration. (See Chapter 7.)

- The **nervous system** consists of the brain, spinal cord, and peripheral nerves. The nervous system regulates most body activities and sends and receives messages from the sensory organs. (See Chapter 8.) The two major sensory organs are covered in the sensory system. (See Chapter 16.)

- The **urinary system** includes the kidneys, ureters, bladder, and urethra. It eliminates metabolic waste, helps to maintain acid-base and water-salt balance, and helps regulate blood pressure. (See Chapter 9.)

- The **reproductive system** controls reproduction and heredity. The female reproductive system includes the ovaries, vagina, uterine (fallopian) tubes, uterus, and mammary glands. (See Chapter 10.) The male reproductive system includes the testes, penis, prostate gland, vas deferens, and the seminal vesicles. (See Chapter 11.)

- The **blood system** includes the blood and all its components. (See Chapter 12.)

- The **lymphatic and immune system** includes the lymph, the glands of the lymphatic system, lymphatic vessels, and the nonspecific and specific defenses of the immune system. (See Chapter 13.)

- The **digestive system** includes all the organs of digestion and excretion of waste. (See Chapter 14.)

- The **endocrine system** includes the glands that secrete hormones for regulation of many of the body's activities. (See Chapter 15.)

- The **sensory system** covers the eyes and ears and those parts of other systems that are involved in the reactions of the five senses. (See Chapter 16.)

Body Cavities

The body has two main cavities (spaces)—the dorsal and the ventral. The **dorsal cavity,** on the back side of the body, is divided into the **cranial cavity,** which holds the brain, and the **spinal cavity,** which holds the spinal cord. The **ventral cavity,** on the front side of the body, is divided (and separated by a muscle called the **diaphragm**) into the **thoracic cavity,** which holds the heart, lungs, and major blood vessels, and the **abdominal cavity,** which holds the organs of the digestive and urinary systems. The bottom portion of the abdominal cavity is called the **pelvic cavity.** It contains the reproductive system. Figure 3-2 shows the body cavities.

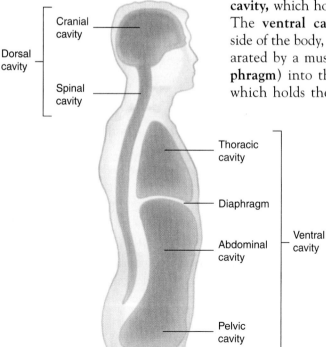

Figure 3-2 Body Cavities.

Body Structure and Organization Vocabulary Review

In the previous section, you learned terms relating to body structure and organization. Before going on to the exercises, review the terms below and refer to the previous section if you have any questions.

Term	Word Analysis	Definition
abdominal cavity	[ăb-DŎM-ĭ-năl]	Body space between the abdominal walls, above the pelvis, and below the diaphragm.
blood system	[blŭd] Old English *blud*.	Body system that includes blood and all its component parts.
cardiovascular system	[KĂR-dē-ō-VĂS-] kyū-lăr	Body system that includes the heart and blood vessels; circulatory system.
cell	[sĕl] Latin *cella*, storeroom	Smallest unit of a living structure.
connective tissue	[kŏn-NĔK-tĭv]	Fibrous substance that forms the body's supportive framework.
cranial cavity	[KRĀ-nē-ăl]	Space in the head that contains the brain.
diaphragm	[DĪ-ă-frăm]	Muscle that divides the abdominal and thoracic cavities.
digestive system	[dĭ-JĔS-tĭv]	Body system that includes all organs of digestion and waste excretion, from the mouth to the anus.
dorsal cavity	[DŌR-săl]	Main cavity on the back side of the body containing the cranial and spinal cavities.
endocrine system	[ĔN-dō-krĭn]	Body system that includes glands that secrete hormones to regulate certain body functions.
epithelial tissue	[ĕp-ĭ-THĒ-lē-ăl]	Tissue that covers or lines the body or its parts.
integumentary system	[ĭn-tĕg-yū-MĔN-tă-rē]	Body system that includes skin, hair, and nails.
lymphatic and immune system	[lĭm-FĂT-ĭk], [ĭ-MYŪN]	Body system that includes the lymph, glands of the lymphatic system, lymphatic vessels, and the specific and nonspecific defenses of the immune system.
muscle tissue	[MŬS-ĕl] Latin *musculus*, muscle, mouse	Tissue that is able to contract and relax.

Term	Word Analysis	Definition
musculoskeletal system	[MŬS-kyū-lō-SKĔL-ĕ-tăl]	Body system that includes muscles, bones, and cartilage.
nervous system	[NĔR-vŭs]	Body system that includes the brain, spinal cord, and nerves and controls most body functions by sending and receiving messages.
nervous tissue		Specialized tissue that forms nerve cells and is capable of transmitting messages.
organ	[ŌR-găn]	Group of specialized tissue that performs a specific function.
pelvic cavity	[PĔL-vĭk]	Body space below the abdominal cavity that includes the reproductive organs
reproductive system	[RĒ-prō-DŬK-tĭv]	Either the male or female body system that controls reproduction.
respiratory system	[RĔS-pĭ-ră-tōr-ē, rĕ-SPĪR-ă-tōr-ē]	Body system that includes the lungs and airways and performs breathing.
sensory system		Body system that includes the eyes and ears and those parts of other systems involved in the reactions of the five senses.
spinal cavity	[SPĪ-năl]	Body space that contains the spinal cord.
system	[SĬS-tĕm]	Any group of organs and ancillary parts that work together to perform a major body function.
thoracic cavity	[thō-RĂS-ĭk]	Body space above the abdominal cavity that contains the heart, lungs, and major blood vessels.
tissue	[TĬSH-ū]	Any group of cells that work together to perform a single function.
urinary system	[YŪR-ĭ-nār-ē]	Body system that includes the kidneys, ureters, bladder, and urethra and helps maintain homeostasis by removing fluid and dissolved waste.
ventral cavity	[VĔN-trăl]	Major cavity in the front of the body containing the thoracic, abdominal, and pelvic cavities.

Body Structure and Organization Exercises

Find the Match

Match the system to its function.

1. cardiovascular system   a. performs breathing

2. digestive system   b. removes fluid and dissolved waste

3. endocrine system   c. sends and receives messages

4. blood system   d. pumps and circulates blood to tissues

5. integumentary system   e. consists of blood and its elements

6. lymphatic and immune system   f. covers the body and its internal structures

7. musculoskeletal system   g. provides defenses for the body

8. nervous system   h. breaks down food

9. reproductive system   i. regulates through production of hormones

10. respiratory system   j. controls reproduction

11. urinary system   k. supports organs and provides movement

Complete the Sentence

12. The basic element of the human body is a(n) _____.

13. Groups of these basic elements form _____.

14. Tissue that covers the body or its parts is called _____ tissue.

15. The brain is contained within the _____ cavity.

16. The muscle separating the two main parts of the ventral cavity is called the _____.

17. The spinal and cranial cavities make up the _____ cavity.

18. The space below the abdominal cavity is called the _____ cavity.

19. The system that helps eliminate fluids is the _____ system.

20. The system that breaks down food is called the _____ system.

Directional Terms, Planes, and Regions

In making diagnoses or prescribing treatments, health care providers use standard terms to refer to different areas of the body. These terms describe each anatomical position as a point of reference. The anatomical position always means the body is standing erect, facing forward, with upper limbs at the sides and with the palms facing forward. For example, if a pain is described as *in the right lower quadrant* (RLQ), medical personnel immediately understand that to mean the lower right portion of the patient's body. Certain terms refer to a direction going to or from the body or in which the body is placed. Others divide the body into imaginary planes as a way of mapping the body when the person is in the anatomical position. Still others refer to specific regions of the body.

Anterior and ventral are both from Latin. The original meaning of anterior was near the surface or in front, while the meaning of ventral was belly, an organ near the surface (particularly the undersurface of animals). Posterior and dorsal also come from Latin. Posterior originally meant behind or following, and dorsal originally meant back.

Directional Terms

Directional terms locate a portion of the body or describe a position of the body. The front side (**anterior** or **ventral**) and the back side (**posterior** or **dorsal**) are the largest divisions of the body. Figure 3-3 on page 44 shows the body regions of the anterior and posterior sections. Some terms indicate a position relative to something else. **Inferior** means below another structure; for example, the vagina is inferior to (or below) the uterus. **Superior** means above another structure; for example, the stomach is superior to the large intestine. **Lateral** means to the side; for example, the eyes are lateral to the nose. **Medial** means middle or near the medial plane of the body; for example, the nose is medial to the eyes. **Deep** means through the surface (as in a deep cut), while **superficial** means on or near the surface (as a scratch on the skin). **Proximal** means near the point of attachment to the trunk; for example, the proximal end of the thighbone joins the hip bone. **Distal** means away from the point of attachment to the trunk; for example, the distal end of the thighbone joins the kneebone. For examination purposes, patients are either **supine** (lying on their spine face upward) or **prone** (lying on the stomach with their face down). Figure 3-4 on page 45 shows the directional terms.

Planes of the Body

For anatomical and diagnostic discussions, some standard terms are used for the planes and positions of the body. The imaginary planes of the body when it is vertical and facing front are: **frontal (coronal) plane,** which divides the body into anterior and posterior positions; **sagittal (lateral) plane,** which is the plane perpendicular to the medial; **medial or midsagittal plane,** which divides the body into equal left and right halves; and **transverse (cross-sectional) plane,** which intersects the body horizontally. Figure 3-5 on page 46 shows the planes of the body.

MORE ABOUT...
Areas of the Body

Pain is sometimes felt in only one region of the body (as a muscle pull in the RUQ or right upper quadrant). Other times, internal pain is felt in an area that is not the actual source of the pain. This is known as *"referred pain"* or *synalgia*. Such pain usually emanates from nerves or other deep structures within the body.

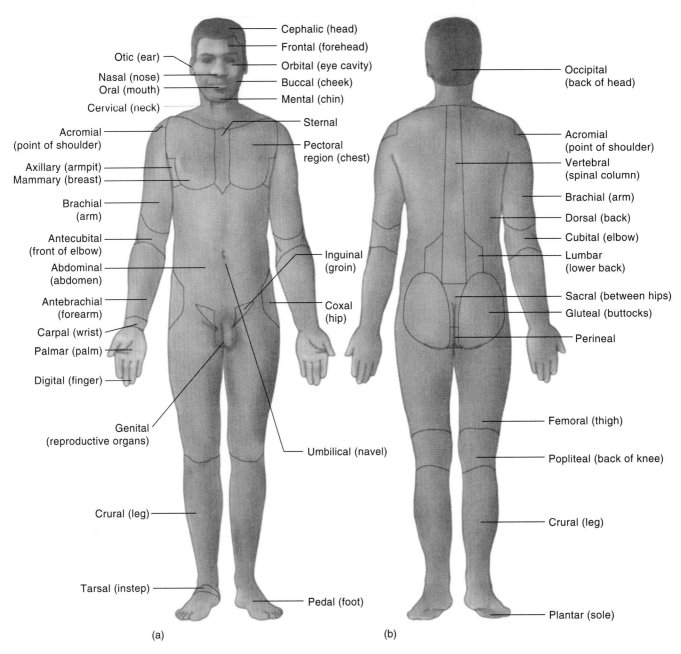

Figure 3-3 Anterior (a) and Posterior (b) regions.

Regions of the Body

Health care practitioners usually refer to a specific organ, area, or bone when speaking of the upper body. In the back, the spinal column is divided into specific regions (cervical, thoracic, lumbar, sacral, and coccygeal). Chapter 5 describes the spinal column in detail. The middle portion of the body (abdominal and pelvic cavities) is often the site of pain. Doctors use two standard sections to describe this area of the body. The larger section is divided into four quarters (Figure 3-6).

- **Right upper quadrant (RUQ):** On the right anterior side; contains part of the liver, the gallbladder, and parts of the pancreas and intestinal tract.

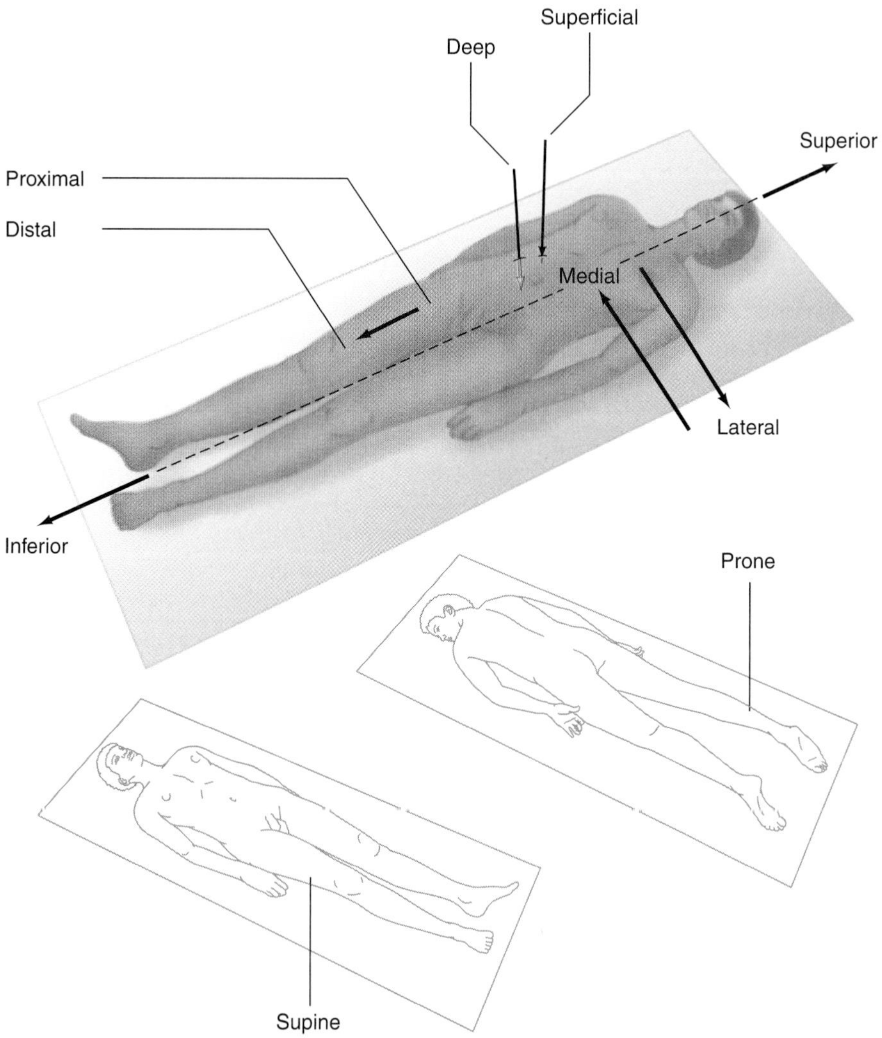

Figure 3-4 Directional terms used when referring to locations on the body.

Superficial

Deep

Proximal

Distal

Superior

Medial

Lateral

Inferior

Prone

Supine

+ **Right lower quadrant (RLQ):** On the right anterior side; contains the appendix, parts of the intestines, reproductive organs in the female, and urinary tract.

+ **Left upper quadrant (LUQ):** On the left anterior side; contains the stomach, spleen, and parts of the liver, pancreas, and intestines.

+ **Left lower quadrant (LLQ):** On the left anterior side; contains parts of the intestines, reproductive organs in the female, and urinary tract.

The smaller divisions of the abdominal and pelvic areas are the six regions, each of which correspond to a region near a specific point in the body (Figure 3-7).

+ **Epigastric region:** the area above the stomach.

+ **Hypochondriac regions** (left and right): the two regions just below the cartilage of the ribs, immediately over the abdomen.

+ **Umbilical region:** The region surrounding the umbilicus (navel).

The hypochondriac regions are immediately over the abdomen. The term hypochondriac also means someone who shows exaggerated concern for bodily functioning.

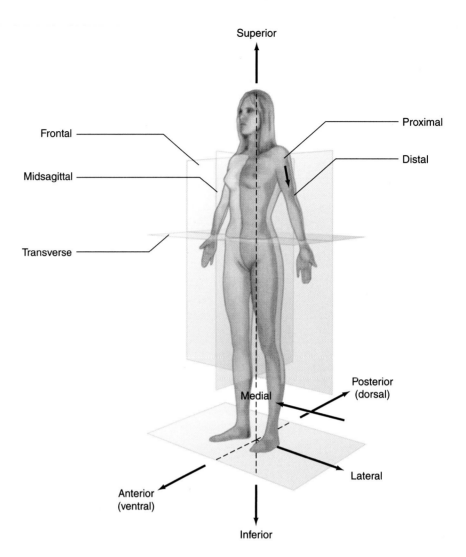

Figure 3-5 **Planes of and directions from the body.**

- ◆ **Lumbar regions** (left and right): the two regions near the waist.
- ◆ **Hypogastric region:** the area just below the umbilical region.
- ◆ **Iliac (inguinal) regions** (left and right): the two regions near the upper portion of the hip bone.

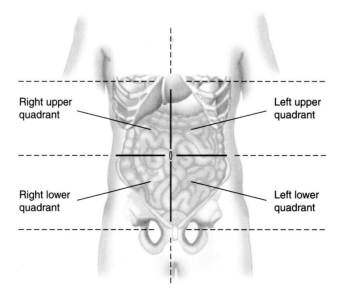

Figure 3-6 **Quadrants of the abdominopelvic area.**

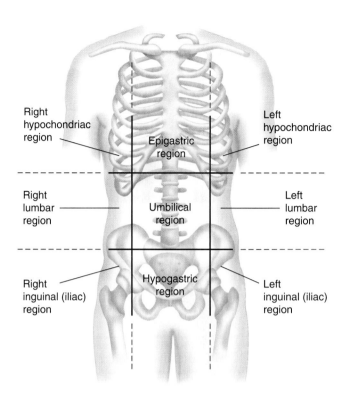

Right hypochondriac region

Epigastric region

Left hypochondriac region

Right lumbar region

Umbilical region

Left lumbar region

Right inguinal (iliac) region

Hypogastric region

Left inguinal (iliac) region

Figure 3-7 Regions of the abdominopelvic area.

Directional Terms, Planes, and Regions Vocabulary Review

In the previous section, you learned terms relating to directional terms, planes, and regions of the body. Before going on to the exercises, review the terms below and refer to the previous section if you have any questions.

Term	Word Analysis	Definition
anterior	[ăn-TĒR-ē-ŏr]	At or toward the front (of the body).
coronal plane	[KŌR-ŏ-năl]	Imaginary line that divides the body into anterior and posterior positions.
cross-sectional plane		Imaginary line that intersects the body horizontally.
deep		Away from the surface (of the body).
distal	[DĬS-tăl]	Away from the point of attachment to the trunk.
dorsal	[DŌR-săl]	At or toward the back of the body.
epigastric region	[ĕp-ĭ-GĂS-trĭk]	Area of the body immediately above the stomach.
frontal plane	[FRŬN-tăl]	Imaginary line that divides the body into anterior and posterior positions.
hypochondriac regions	[hĭ-pō-KŎN-drē-ăk]	Left and right regions of the body just below the cartilage of the ribs and immediately above the abdomen.

Term	Word Analysis	Definition
hypogastric region	[hī-pō-GĂS-trĭk]	Area of the body just below the umbilical region.
iliac regions	[ĬL-ē-ăk]	Left and right regions of the body near the upper portion of the hip bone.
inferior	[ĭn-FĒR-ē-ōr]	Below another body structure.
inguinal regions	[ĬN-gwĭ-năl]	Left and right regions of the body near the upper portion of the hip bone.
lateral	[LĂT-ĕr-ăl]	To the side.
lateral plane		Imaginary line that divides the body perpendicularly to the medial plane.
left lower quadrant (LLQ)		Quadrant on the lower left anterior side of the patient's body.
left upper quadrant (LUQ)		Quadrant on the upper left anterior side of the patient's body.
lumbar regions	[LŬM-băr]	Left and right regions of the body near the waist on the dorsal (or posterior) side.
medial	[MĒ-dē-ăl]	At or near the middle (of the body).
medial plane		Imaginary line that divides the body into equal left and right halves.
midsagittal plane	[mĭd-SĂJ-ĭ-tăl]	*See* medial plane.
posterior		At or toward the back side (of the body).
prone		Lying on the stomach with the face down.
proximal	[PRŎK-sĭ-măl]	At or near the point of attachment to the trunk.
right lower quadrant (RLQ)		Quadrant on the lower right anterior side of the patient's body.
right upper quadrant (RUQ)		Quadrant on the upper right anterior side of the patient's body.
sagittal plane	[SĂJ-ĭ-tăl]	Imaginary line that divides the body into right and left portions.
superficial	[sū-pĕr-FĬSH-ăl]	At or near the surface (of the body).
superior	[sū-PĒR-ē-ōr]	Above another body structure.

Term	Word Analysis	Definition
supine	[sū-PĪN]	Lying on the spine facing upward.
transverse plane		Imaginary line that intersects the body horizontally.
umbilical region	[ŭm-BĬL-ĭ-kăl]	Area of the body surrounding the umbilicus.
ventral	[VĔN-trăl]	At or toward the front (of the body).

C A S E S T U D Y

Locating a Problem

Dr. Lena Woodrow checked the chart of the next patient, Darlene Gordon. Darlene had called yesterday with a vague pain in her LUQ. She also experienced some nausea and general discomfort.

Dr. Woodrow suggested she make a morning appointment.

💡 Critical Thinking

21. What organs might be causing pain in the LUQ?

22. Is it possible for the source of the pain to be located elsewhere in the body?

Directional Terms, Planes, and Regions Exercises

Check For Accuracy

Circle T for true or F for false.

23. The epigastric region is below the hypogastric region. T F

24. The heart is deeper than the ribs. T F

25. The leg is inferior to the foot. T F

26. The nose is superior to the eyes. T F

27. The right lower quadrant contains the appendix. T F

28. The coronal plane divides the body horizontally. T F

29. The lateral plane is another name for the sagittal plane. T F

30. The wrist is proximal to the shoulder. T F

31. The spleen is in the left upper quadrant. T F

Complete the Diagram

32. Using any of the terms below, fill in the blanks on the following diagram.

distal

supine

inferior

deep

superficial

anterior

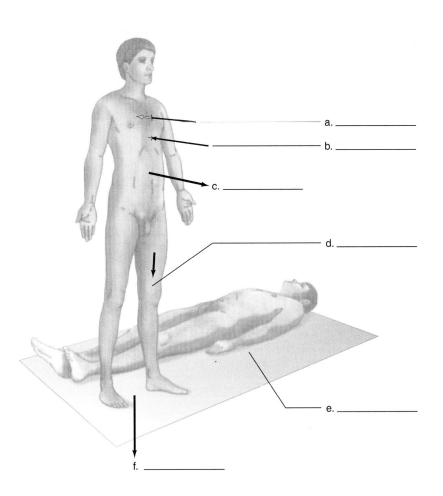

a. _____

b. _____

c. _____

d. _____

e. _____

f. _____

Combining Forms

Chapter 2 introduced many word roots, combining forms, prefixes, and suffixes used in medical terminology. The combining forms in this chapter relate to elements and systems of the body described here. Once you familiarize yourself with the word parts in Chapters 2 and 3, you will understand many medical terms.

Combining Form	Meaning	Example
abdomin(o)	abdomen	*abdominoplasty* [ăb-DŎM-ĭ-nō-plăs-tē], surgical repair of the abdomen
acetabul(o)	cup-shaped hip socket	*acetabulectomy* [ĂS-ĕ-tăb-yū-LĔK-tō-mē], excision of the acetabulum
aden(o)	gland	*adenitis* [ăd-ĕ-NĪ-tĭs], inflammation of a gland
adip(o)	fat	*adiposis,* [ĂD-ĭ-pōs], condition of excessive accumulation of fat
adren(o)	adrenal glands	*adrenotoxin* [ă-drē-nō-TŎK-sĭn], a substance toxic to the adrenal glands
alveol(o)	air sac, alveolus	*alveolitis* [ĂL-vē-ō-LĪ-tĭs], inflammation of alveoli
angi(o)	vessel	*angiomegaly* [ĂN-jē-ō-MĔG-ă-lē], enlargement of blood vessels
aort(o)	aorta	*aortitis* [ā-ōr-TĪ-tĭs], inflammation of the aorta

Combining Form	Meaning	Example
appendic(o)	appendix	*appendicitis* [ă-pĕn-dĭ-SĪ-tĭs], inflammation of the appendix
arteri(o)	artery	*arteriosclerosis* [ăr-TĒR-ē-ō-sklĕr-Ō-sĭs], hardening of the arteries
arteriol(o)	arteriole	*arteriolosclerosis* [ăr-tēr-ē-Ō-lō-sklĕr-Ō-sĭs], hardening of the arterioles, often seen in conjunction with chronic high blood pressure
arthr(o)	joint; articulation	*arthralgia* [ăr-THRĂL-jē-ă], severe joint pain
aur(i), auricul(o)	ear	*auriform* [ĂW-rĭ-fŏrm], ear-shaped; *auriculocranial* [ăw-RĬK-yū-lō-KRĀ-nē-ăl], of the ear and cranium
blephar(o)	eyelid	*blepharitis* [BLĔF-ă-RĪ-tĭs], inflammation of the eyelid
brachi(o)	arm	*brachialgia* [brā-kē-ĂL-jē-ă], pain in the arm
bronch(o), bronchi	bronchus	*bronchomycosis* [BRŎNG-kō-mĭ-KŌ-sĭs], fungal disease of the bronchi
bucc(o)	cheek	*buccolabial* [bŭk-ō-LĀ-bē-ăl], relating to both the cheeks and lips
burs(o)	bursa	*bursitis* [bĕr-SĪ-tĭs], inflammation of a bursa
calcane(o)	heel bone	*calcaneodynia* [kăl-KĀ-nē-ō-DĬN-ē-ă], heel pain
cardi(o)	heart; esophageal opening of the stomach	*cardiomegaly* [kăr-dē-ō-MĔG-ă-lē], enlargement of the heart
carp(o)	wrist bones	*carpopedal* [KĂR-pō-PĔD-ăl], relating to the wrist and the foot
celi(o)	abdomen	*celiorrhaphy* [sē-lē-ŌR-ă-fē], suture of an abdominal wound
cephal(o)	head	*cephalomegaly* [SĔF-ă-lō-MĔG-ă-lē], enlargement of the head
cerebell(o)	cerebellum	*cerebellitis* [sĕr-ĕ-bĕl-Ī-tĭs], inflammation of the cerebellum
cerebr(o)	cerebrum	*cerebrotomy* [sĕr-ĕ-BRŎT-ō-mē], incision into the brain
cervic(o)	neck; cervix	*cervicodynia* [SĔR-vĭ-kō-DĬN-ē-ă], neck pain
cheil(o), chil(o)	lip	*cheiloplasty*, *chiloplasty* [KĪ-lō-plăs-tē], plastic surgery of the lips

Combining Form	Meaning	Example
chir(o)	hand	*chiropractic* [kī-rō-PRĂK-tĭk], theory that uses manipulation of the spine to restore and maintain health
chol(e), cholo	bile	*cholelith* [KŌ-lē-lĭth], gallstone
chondri(o), chondr(o)	cartilage	*chondromalacia* [KŎN-drō-mă-LĀ-shē-ă], softening of cartilage
col(o), colon(o)	colon	*colonoscopy* [kō-lŏn-ŎS-kō-pē], visual examination of the colon
colp(o)	vagina	*colporrhagia* [kōl-pō-RĀ-jē-ă], vaginal hemorrhage
core(o)	pupil	*coreoplasty* [KŌR-ē-ō-plăs-tē], surgical correction of a pupil
cortic(o)	cortex	*corticectomy* [kōr-tĭ-SĔK-tō-mē], removal of a part of the cortex
costi, costo	rib	*costogenic* [kŏs-tō-JĔN-ĭk], arising from a rib
crani(o)	cranium	*craniotomy* [krā-nē-ŎT-ō-mē], opening into the skull
cyst(i), cysto	bladder; cyst	*cystoscopy* [sĭs-TŎS-kō-pē], examination of the interior of the bladder
cyt(o)	cell	*cytology* [sī-TŎL-ō-jē], study of cells
dactyl(o)	fingers, toes	*dactylitis* [dăk-tĭ-LĪ-tĭs], finger inflammation
dent(i), dento	tooth	*dentiform* [DĔN-tĭ-fŏrm], tooth-shaped
derm(o), derma, dermat(o)	skin	*dermatitis* [dĕr-mă-TĪ-tĭs], inflammation of the skin
duoden(o)	duodenum	*duodenoscopy* [dū-ō-dĕ-NŎS-kō-pē], examination of the interior of the duodenum
encephal(o)	brain	*encephalomyeloneuropathy* [ĕn-SĔF-ă-lō-MĪ-ĕ-lō-nū-RŎP-ă-thē], disease involving the brain, spinal cord, and nerves
enter(o)	intestines	*enteritis* [ĕn-tĕr-Ī-tĭs], inflammation of the intestine
episi(o)	vulva	*episiotomy* [ĕ-pĭz-ē-ŎT-ō-mē], surgical incision into the vulva at the time of birth to avoid tearing of the perineum
gastr(o)	stomach	*gastritis* [găs-TRĪ-tĭs], inflammation of the stomach

Combining Form	Meaning	Example
gingiv(o)	gum	*gingivitis* [jĭn-jĭ-VĪ-tĭs], inflammation of the gums
gloss(o)	tongue	*glossodynia* [GLŎS-ō-DĬN-ē-ă], pain in the tongue
gnath(o)	jaw	*gnathoplasty* [NĂTH-ō-plăs-tē], plastic surgery on the jaw
gonad(o)	sex glands	*gonadopathy* [gŏn-ă-DŎP-ă-thē], disease of the gonads
hem(a), hemat(o), hemo	blood	*hematoma* [hē-mă-TŌ-mă], mass of clotted blood
hepat(o), hepatic(o)	liver	*hepatoma* [hĕp-ă-TŌ-mă], malignant cancer of liver cells
hidr(o)	sweat	*hidropoeisis* [hī-DRŌ-pŏy-Ē-sĭs], production of sweat
histi(o), histo	tissue	*histolysis* [hĭs-TŎL-ĭ-sĭs], breakdown of tissue
hyster(o)	uterus, hysteria	*hysterectomy* [hĭs-tĕr-ĔK-tō-mē], removal of the uterus
ile(o)	ileum	*ileocolitis* [ĬL-ē-ō-kō-LĪ-tĭs], inflammation of the colon and the ileum
ili(o)	ilium	*iliospinal* [ĬL-ē-ō-SPĪ-năl], relating to the ilium and the spine
inguin(o)	groin	*inguinoperitoneal* [ĬNG-gwĭ-nō-PĔR-ĭ-tō-NĒ-ăl], relating to the groin and peritoneum
irid(o)	iris	*iridodilator* [ĬR-ĭ-dō-dī-LĀ-tĕr], agent that causes dilation of the pupil
ischi(o)	ischium	*ischialgia* [ĭs-kē-ĂL-jē-ă], hip pain
kary(o)	nucleus	*karyotype* [KĂR-ē-ō-tĭp], chromosomal characteristics of a cell
kerat(o)	cornea	*keratitis* [kĕr-ă-TĪ-tĭs], inflammation of the cornea
labi(o)	lip	*labioplasty* [LĀ-bē-ō-plăs-tē], plastic surgery of a lip
lamin(o)	lamina	*laminectomy* [LĂM-ĭ-NĔK-tō-mē], removal of a bony portion that forms the arch that surrounds the vertebra
lapar(o)	abdominal wall	*laparomyositis* [LĂP-ă-rō-mī-ō-SĪ-tĭs], inflammation of the abdominal muscles

Combining Form	Meaning	Example
laryng(o)	larynx	*laryngitis* [lăr-ĭn-JĪ-tĭs], inflammation of the larynx
linguo	tongue	*linguocclusion* [lĭng-gwō-KLŪ-zhŭn], displacement of a tooth toward the tongue
lip(o)	fat	*liposuctioning* [LĬP-ō-SŬK-shŭn-ĭng], removal of body fat by vacuum pressure
lymph(o)	lymph	*lymphuria* [lĭm-FŪ-rē-ă], discharge of lymph into the urine
mast(o)	breast	[măs-TĪ-tĭs], inflammation of the breast
maxill(o)	maxilla	*maxillitis* [MĂK-sĭ-LĪ-tĭs], inflammation of the jawbone
medull(o)	medulla	*medulloblastoma* [MĚD-ŭ-lō-blăs-TŌ-mă], tumor having cells similar to those in medullary substances
mening(o)	meninges	*meningitis* [měn-ĭn-JĪ-tĭs], inflammation of the membranes of the brain or spinal cord
muco	mucus	*mucolytic* [myū-kō-LĬT-ĭk], agent capable of dissolving mucus
my(o)	muscle	*myocarditis* [MĪ-ō-kăr-DĪ-tĭs], inflammation of the muscle tissue of the heart
myel(o)	spinal cord; bone marrow	*myelopathy* [mī-ĕ-LŎP-ă-thē], disease of the spinal cord
nephr(o)	kidney	*nephritis* [ně-FRĪ-tĭs], inflammation of the kidneys
neur, neuro	nerve	*neuritis* [nū-RĪ-tĭs], inflammation of a nerve
oculo	eye	*oculodynia* [ŎK-yū-lō-DĬN-ē-ă], eye pain
odont(o)	tooth	*odontalgia* [ō-dŏn-TĂL-jē-ă], toothache
onych(o)	nail	*onychoid* [ŎN-ĭ-kŏyd], resembling a fingernail
oo	egg	*oocyte* [Ō-ō-sīt], immature ovum
oophor(o)	ovary	*oophorectomy* [ō-ŏf-ōr-ĔK-tō-mē], removal of an ovary
ophthalm(o)	eye	*ophthalmoscope* [ŏf-THĂL-mō-skōp], device for examining interior of the eyeball

Combining Form	Meaning	Example
opto, optico	eye; sight	*optometer* [ŏp-TŎM-ĕ-tĕr], instrument for measuring eye refraction
or(o)	mouth	*orofacial* [ōr-ō-FĀ-shăl], relating to the mouth and face
orchi(o), orchido	testis	*orchialgia* [ōr-kē-ĂL-jē-ă], pain in the testis
osseo, ossi	bone	*ossiferous* [ō-SĬF-ĕr-ŭs], containing or generating bone
ost(e), osteo	bone	*osteochondritis* [ŎS-tē-ō-kŏn-DRĪ-tĭs], inflammation of a bone and its cartilage
ot(o)	ear	*otitis* [ō-TĪ-tĭs], earache
ovari(o)	ovary	*ovariopathy* [ō-vār-ē-ŎP-ă-thē], disease of the ovary
ovi, ovo	egg; ova	*oviduct* [Ō-vĭ-dŭkt], uterine (fallopian) tube through which ova pass
ped(o), pedi	foot; child	*pedicure* [PĔD-ĭ-kyūr], treatment of the feet; *pedophilia* [pĕ-dō-FĬL-ē-ă], abnormal sexual attraction to children
pelvi(o), pelvo	pelvic bone; hip	*pelviscope* [PĔL-vĭ-skōp], instrument for examining the interior of the pelvis
pharyng(o)	pharynx	*pharyngitis* [făr-ĭn-JĪ-tĭs], inflammation of the pharynx
phleb(o)	vein	*phlebitis* [flĕ-BĪ-tĭs], inflammation of a vein
phren(o), phreni, phrenico	mind; diaphragm	*phrenicocolic* [FRĔN-ĭ-kō-KŎL-ĭk], relating to the diaphragm and colon
pil(o)	hair	*pilonidal* [pī-lō-NĪ-dăl], having hair, as in a cyst
plasma, plasmo, plasmat(o)	plasma	*plasmacyte* [PLĂZ-mă-sīt], plasma cell
pleur(o), pleura	rib; side; pleura	*pleurography* [plūr-ŎG-ră-fē], imaging of the pleural cavity
pneum(a), pneumat(o), pneumo, pneumon(o)	lungs; air; breathing	*pneumonia* [nū-MŌ-nē-ă], disease of the lungs
pod(o)	foot	*podiatrist* [pō-DĪ-ă-trĭst], specialist in diseases of the foot
proct(o)	anus	*proctalgia* [prŏk-TĂL-jē-ă], pain in the anus or rectum

Combining Form	Meaning	Example
psych(o), psyche	mind	*psychomotor* [sī-kō-MŌ-tĕr], relating to psychological influence on body movement
pulmon(o)	lung	*pulmonitis* [pŭl-mō-NĪ-tĭs], inflammation of the lungs
pyel(o)	renal pelvis	*pyelitis* [pī-ĕ-LĪ-tĭs], inflammation of the cavity below the kidneys
rachi(o)	spine	*rachiometer* [rā-kē-ŎM-ĕ-tĕr], instrument for measuring curvature of the spine
rect(o)	rectum	*rectitis* [rĕk-TĪ-tĭs], inflammation of the rectum
reni, reno	kidney	*reniform* [RĚN-ĭ-fŏrm], kidney-shaped
rhin(o)	nose	*rhinitis* [rī-NĪ-tĭs], inflammation of the nasal membranes
sacr(o)	sacrum	*sacralgia* [sā-KRĂL-jē-ă], pain in the sacral area
sarco	fleshy tissue; muscle	*sarcopoietic* [SĂR-kō-pŏy-ĔT-ĭk], forming muscle
scler(o)	sclera	*sclerodermatitis* [SKLĒR-ō-dĕr-mă-TĪ-tĭs], inflammation and thickening of the skin
sial(o)	salivary glands; saliva	*sialism* [SĪ-ă-lĭzm], excessive production of saliva
sigmoid(o)	sigmoid colon	*sigmoidectomy* [sĭg-mŏy-DĔK-tō-mē], excision of the sigmoid colon
somat(o)	body	*somatophrenia* [SŌ-mă-tō-FRĒ-nē-ă], tendency to imagine bodily illnesses
sperma, spermato, spermo	semen; spermatozoa	*spermatocide* [SPĔR-mă-tō-sīd], agent that destroys sperm
splanchn(o), splanchni	viscera	*splanchnolith* [SPLĂNGK-nō-lĭth], stone in the intestinal tract
splen(o)	spleen	*splenectomy* [splē-NĔK-tō-mē], removal of the spleen
spondyl(o)	vertebra	*spondylitis* [spŏn-dĭ-LĪ-tĭs], inflammation of a vertebra
stern(o)	sternum	*sternalgia* [stĕr-NĂL-jē-ă], sternum pain
steth(o)	chest	*stethoscope* [STĔTH-ŏ-skōp], device for listening to chest sounds

Combining Form	Meaning	Example
stom(a), stomat(o)	mouth	*stomatopathy* [stō-mă-TŎP-ă-thē], disease of the mouth
ten(o), tendin(o), tendo, tenon(o)	tendon	*tenectomy* [tĕ-NĔK-tō-mē], *tenonectomy* [tĕn-ō-NĔK-tō-mē], removal of part of a tendon
test(o)	testis	*testitis* [tĕs-TĪ-tĭs], inflammation of the testis
thorac(o), thoracico	thorax, chest	*thoracalgia* [thōr-ă-KĂL-jē-ă], chest pain
thym(o)	thymus gland	*thymokinetic* [THĬ-mō-kĭ-NĔT-ĭk], agent that activates the thymus gland
thyr(o)	thyroid gland	*thyrotomy* [thĭ-RŎT-ō-mē], operation that cuts the thyroid gland
trache(o)	trachea	*tracheotomy* [trā-kē-ŎT-ō-mē], operation to create an opening into the trachea
trachel(o)	neck	*trachelophyma* [TRĀK-ĕ-lō-FĪ-mă], swelling of the neck
trich(o), trichi	hair	*trichoid* [TRĬK-ŏyd], hairlike
varico	varicosity	*varicophlebitis* [VĀR-ĭ-kō-flĕ-BĪ-tĭs], inflammation of varicose veins
vas(o)	blood vessel, duct	*vasoconstrictor* [VĀ-sō-kŏn-STRĬK-tĕr], agent that narrows blood vessels
vasculo	blood vessel	*vasculopathy* [văs-kyū-LŎP-ă-thĕ], disease of the blood vessels
veni, veno	vein	*venipuncture* [VĔN-ĭ-pŭnk-shŭr, VĒ-nĭ-pŭnk-shŭr], puncture of a vein, as with a needle
ventricul(o)	ventricle	*ventriculitis* [vĕn-trĭk-yū-LĪ-tĭs], inflammation of the ventricles in the brain
vertebro	vertebra	*vertebrosacral* [vĕr-tĕ-brō-SĀ-krăl], relating to the vertebra and the sacrum
vesic(o)	bladder	*vesicoprostatic* [VĔS-ĭ-kō-prŏs-TĂT-ĭk], relating to the bladder and the prostate

Combining Forms and Abbreviations Exercises

Build Your Medical Vocabulary.

Match each compound term with its meaning.

33. adrenomegaly   a. agent that stops the flow of blood

34. splanchnopathy   b. spasm of an artery

35. angiography   c. study of the hair and its diseases

36. osteosclerosis   d. inflammation of the liver

37. arteriospasm   e. destruction of sperm

38. trichology   f. relating to the abdomen and thorax

39. hepatitis   g. abnormal hardening of bone

40. spermatolysis   h. radiography of blood vessels

41. abdominothoracic   i. enlargement of the adrenal glands

42. hemostat   j. disease of the viscera

Add a Suffix

Add the suffix needed to complete the statement.

43. An inflammation of an artery is called arter_____.

44. Suturing of a tendon is called teno_____.

45. Death of muscle is called myo_____.

46. A name for any disorder of the spinal cord is myelo_____.

47. Cephal_____ means head pain.

48. Angio_____ means repair of a blood vessel.

49. Softening of the walls of the heart is called cardio_____.

50. Incision into the ileum is called an ileo_____.

51. Enlargement of the kidney is called nephro_____.

52. Any disease of the hair is called tricho_____.

Go to the National Institutes of Health's web site (http://www.nih.gov/health/) and click the NIH Clinical Center Research Studies. In the search box, enter the name of one of the body systems you have learned about in this chapter. Find the name of at least one disease being studied in a clinical trial (the process of testing a new medication by a pharmaceutical research company before it is approved as safe and effective by the Food and Drug Administration).

CHAPTER REVIEW

Definitions

Define the following terms and combining forms. Review the chapter before starting. Make sure you know how to pronounce each term as you define it. Check your answers in this chapter or in the glossary/index at the end of the book.

Term	Definition
abdominal [ăb-DŎM-ĭ-năl] cavity	
abdomin(o)	
acetabul(o)	
aden(o)	
adip(o)	
adren(o)	
alveol(o)	
angi(o)	
anterior [ăn-TĒR-ē-ōr]	
aort(o)	
appendic(o)	
arteri(o)	
arteriol(o)	
arthr(o)	
aur(i), auricul(o)	
blephar(o)	
brachi(o)	
blood [blŭd] system	
bronch(o), bronchi	
bucc(o)	
burs(o)	
calcane(o)	
cardi(o)	
cardiovascular system	
carp(o)	

Term	Definition
celi(o)	
cell [sĕl]	
cephal(o)	
cerebell(o)	
cerebr(o)	
cervic(o)	
cheil(o), chil(o)	
chir(o)	
chol(e), cholo	
chondri(o), chondro	
col(o), colon(o)	
colp(o)	
connective [kŏn-NĔK-tĭv] tissue	
core(o)	
coronal [KŌR-ō-năl] plane	
cranial [KRĀ-nē-ăl] cavity	
cortic(o)	
costi, costo	
crani(o)	
cross-sectional plane	
cyst(i), cysto	
cyt(o)	
dactyl(o)	
deep	
dent(i), dento	
derm(o), derma, dermat(o)	
diaphragm [DĪ-ă-frăm]	
digestive [dī-JĔS-tĭv] system	
distal [DĬS-tăl]	
dorsal [DŌR-săl]	
dorsal cavity	
duoden(o)	
encephal(o)	
endocrine [ĔN-dō-krĭn] system	

Term	Definition
enter(o)	
epigastric [ĕp-ĭ-GĂS-trĭk] region	
episi(o)	
epithelial [ĕp-ĭ-THĒ-lē-ăl] tissue	
frontal plane	
gastr(o)	
gingiv(o)	
gloss(o)	
gnath(o)	
gonad(o)	
hem(a), hemat(o), hemo	
hemic system	
hepat(o), hepatic(o)	
hidr(o)	
histi(o), histo	
hypochondriac [hī-pō-KŎN-drē-ăk] regions	
hypogastric [hī-pō-GĂS-trĭk] regions	
hyster(o)	
ile(o)	
ili(o)	
iliac [ĬL-ē-ăk] regions	
inferior [ĭn-FĒR-ē-ōr]	
inguin(o)	
inguinal [ĬNG-gwĭ-năl] regions	
integumentary [ĭn-tĕg-yū-MĔN-tă-rē] system	
irid(o)	
ischi(o)	
kary(o)	
kerat(o)	
labi(o)	
lamin(o)	
lapar(o)	

Term	Definition
laryng(o)	
lateral	
lateral plane	
left lower quadrant	
left upper quadrant	
linguo	
lip(o)	
lumbar regions	
lymph(o)	
lymphatic and immune system	
mast(o)	
maxill(o)	
medial	
medial plane	
medull(o)	
mening(o)	
midsagittal [mĭd-SĂJ-ĭ-tăl] plane	
muco	
muscle [MŬS-ĕl] tissue	
musculoskeletal [mŭs-kyū-lō-SKĔL-ĕ-tăl] system	
my(o)	
myel(o)	
nephr(o)	
nervous [NĔR-vŭs] system	
nervous tissue	
neur, neuro	
oculo	
odont(o)	
onych(o)	
oo	
oophor(o)	
ophthalm(o)	

Term	Definition
opto, optico	
or(o)	
orchi(o), orchid(o)	
organ [ŌR-găn]	
osseo, ossi	
ost(e), osteo	
ot(o)	
ovari(o)	
ovi, ovo	
ped(o), pedi	
pelvi(o), pelvo	
pelvic [PĔL-vĭk] cavity	
pharyng(o)	
phleb(o)	
phren(o), phreni, phrenico	
pil(o)	
plasma, plasmo, plasmat(o)	
pleur(o), pleura	
pneum(a), pneumat(o)	
pod(o)	
posterior	
proct(o)	
prone	
proximal [PRŎK-sĭ-măl]	
psych(o), psyche	
pulmon(o)	
pyel(o)	
rachi(o)	
rect(o)	
reni, reno	
reproductive [rē-prō-DŬK-tĭv] system	
respiratory [RĔS-pĭ-ră-tōr-ē, rĕ-SPĬR-ă-tōr-ē] system	
rhin(o)	

Term	Definition
right lower quadrant (RLQ)	
right upper quadrant (RUQ)	
sacr(o)	
sagittal [SĂJ-ĭ-tăl] plane	
sarco	
scler(o)	
sensory system	
sial(o)	
sigmoid(o)	
somat(o)	
sperma, spermato, spermo	
spinal [SPĪ-năl] cavity	
splanchn(o), splanchni	
splen(o)	
spondyl(o)	
stern(o)	
steth(o)	
stom(a), stomat(o)	
superficial	
superior	
supine [sū-PĪN]	
system [SĬS-těm]	
ten(o), tendin(o), tendo, tenon(o)	
test(o)	
thorac(o), thoracico	
thoracic [thō-RĂS-ĭk] cavity	
thym(o)	
thyr(o)	
tissue [TĬSH-ū]	
trache(o)	
trachel(o)	
transverse plane	
trich(o), trichi	

Term	Definition
umbilical [ŭm-BĬL-ĭ-kăl] region	
urinary [YŪR-ĭ-nār-ē] system	
varico	
vas(o)	
vasculo	
veni, veno	
ventral [VĔN-trăl]	
ventral cavity	
ventricul(o)	
vertebro	
vesic(o)	

Word Building

Build the Right Term

Using the vocabulary reviews in Chapters 1, 2, and 3, construct a medical term that fits each of the following definitions. The number following each definition tells you the number of word parts—combining forms, suffixes, or prefixes—you will need to use.

53. Disease of the heart muscle (3)

54. Reconstruction of an artery wall (2)

55. Muscle pain (2)

56. Incision into the intestines (2)

57. Study of poisons (2)

58. Relating to the bladder, uterus, and vagina (3)

59. Inflammation of the tissue surrounding a blood vessel (3)

60. Producing saliva (2)

61. Morbid fear of blood (2)

62. Paralysis of the heart (2)

63. Plastic surgery of the skin (2)

64. Causing death of an ovum (2)

Define the Terms

Using the information you have learned in Chapters 1, 2, and 3, and without consulting a dictionary, give the closest definition you can for each of the following terms.

65. otorhinolaryngology   _____

66. tracheomegaly   _____

67. cystopyelitis   _____

68. onychorrhexis   _____

69. fibroma   _____

70. oophorrhagia   _____

71. antiparasitic   _____

72. neopathy   _____

73. retropharynx   _____

74. lipocardiac   _____

Find a Match

Match the combining form with its definition.

75. adip(o)	a. rib	_____
76. blephar(o)	b. mouth	_____
77. carp(o)	c. eyelid	_____
78. celi(o)	d. fat	_____
79. core(o)	e. bone	_____
80. costo	f. wrist	_____
81. mening(o)	g. abdomen	_____
82. or(o)	h. meninges	_____
83. osseo	i. pupil	_____

Find What's Wrong

In each of the following terms, one or more word parts are misspelled. Replace the misspelled word part(s) and write the correct term in the space provided.

84. meningiitus   _____

85. polmonary   _____

86. abdomenal   _____

87. cardiomagaley   _____

88. ensephaloscope   _____

89. mielopathy   _____

90. larynjectomy   _____

91. ooocyte   _____

92. optimetrist   _____

93. hemoglobine   _____

94. athrodesis _____

95. yatrogenic _____

96. carcinsoma _____

97. paraplejic _____

98. mezomorph _____

99. simbiosis _____

100. schizofrenia _____

Find the Specialty

For each of the following diagnoses, name the appropriate specialist who would generally treat the condition. If you do not know the meaning of any of these conditions, look them up in the glossary/index at the back of the book.

101. myocarditis _____

102. dermatitis _____

103. bronchitis _____

104. ovarian cysts _____

105. prostatitis _____

106. cancer _____

107. glaucoma _____

108. colitis _____

109. neuritis _____

110. allergy to bee sting _____

1. d
2. h
3. i
4. e
5. f
6. g
7. k
8. c
9. j
10. a
11. b
12. cell
13. tissue
14. epithelial
15. cranial
16. diaphragm
17. dorsal
18. pelvic
19. urinary
20. digestive
21. stomach, spleen, intestines, liver, pancreas
22. Yes, pain may be "referred," felt in one part of the body but actually coming from another part.
23. F
24. T
25. F
26. F
27. T
28. F
29. T
30. F
31. T
32.

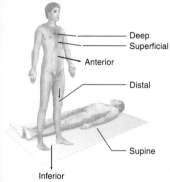

Deep
Superficial
Anterior
Distal
Supine
Inferior

33. i
34. j
35. h
36. g
37. b
38. c
39. d
40. e
41. f
42. a
43. itis
44. rrhaphy
45. necrosis
46. pathy
47. algia
48. plasty
49. malacia
50. tomy
51. megaly
52. pathy
53. cardiomyopathy
54. arterioplasty
55. myalgia or myodynia
56. enterotomy
57. toxicology
58. vesicouterovaginal
59. periangitis
60. sialogenous
61. hemophobia
62. cardioplegia
63. dermatoplasty
64. ovicidal
65. study of the ear, nose, and throat
66. abnormally enlarged trachea
67. inflammation of the bladder and the renal pelvis
68. abnormal breaking of the nails
69. benign neoplasm in fibrous tissues

70. ovarian hemorrhage
71. destructive to parasites
72. a new disease process
73. back part of the pharynx
74. relating to a fatty heart
75. d
76. c
77. f
78. g
79. i
80. a
81. h
82. b
83. e
84. meningitis
85. pulmonary
86. abdominal
87. cardiomegaly
88. encephaloscope
89. myelopathy
90. laryngectomy
91. oocyte
92. optometrist
93. hemoglobin
94. arthrodesis
95. iatrogenic
96. carcinoma
97. paraplegic
98. mesomorph
99. symbiosis
100. schizophrenia
101. cardiologist
102. dermatologist
103. pulmonologist
104. gynecologist
105. urologist
106. oncologist
107. opthalmologist
108. gastroenterologist
109. neurologist
110. allergist

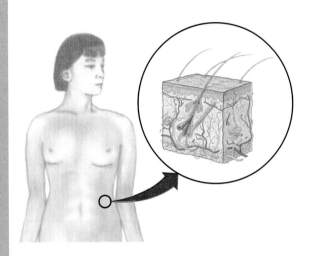

CHAPTER 4

The Integumentary System

After studying this chapter, you will be able to:

◆ Name the parts of the integumentary system and discuss the function of each part

◆ Define the combining forms used in building words that relate to the integumentary system

◆ Identify the meaning of related abbreviations

◆ Name the common diagnoses, laboratory tests, and clinical procedures used in testing and treating the integumentary system

◆ Define the major pathological conditions of the integumentary system

◆ Define surgical terms related to the integumentary system

◆ List common pharmacological agents used in treating the integumentary system

Structure and Function

The integumentary system includes the skin or **integument,** the *hair,* the **nails,** the **sweat glands** (also called the *sudoriferous glands*), and the oil-producing glands (also called the **sebaceous glands**). This system covers and protects the body, helps regulate the body's temperature, excretes some of the body's waste materials, and includes the body's sensors for pain and sensation. Figure 4-1a shows a cross-section of skin with the parts of the integumentary system labeled. Figure 4-1b is a diagram showing the three layers of skin and what they contain.

Skin

The skin is the largest body organ. The average adult has about 21.5 square feet of skin. The skin protects the body from injury and from the intrusion of harmful microorganisms and ultraviolet (UV) rays of the sun. It also helps to maintain the proper internal temperature of the body, serves as a site for excretion of waste materials through perspiration, and is an important sensory organ. The skin varies in thickness, depending on what part of the body it covers and what its function is in covering that part. For example, the skin on the upper back is about ten times thicker than the skin on the eyelid. The eyelid skin must be light, flexible, and movable, so it is thin. The skin on the upper back must cover and move with large muscle groups and bones, so it is thick to provide the necessary strength and protection.

The skin has three main parts or layers—the **epidermis,** the **dermis** or **corium,** and the **subcutaneous** or **hypodermis.**

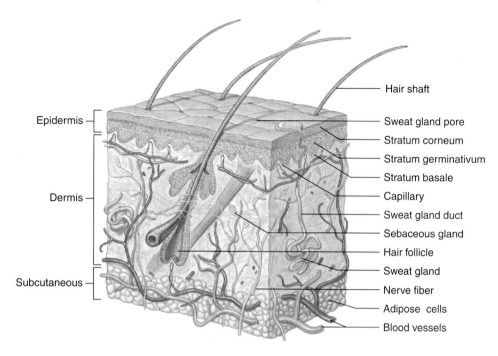

Figure 4-1 (a) The integumentary system consists of the skin with all its layers, hair, nails, and glands.

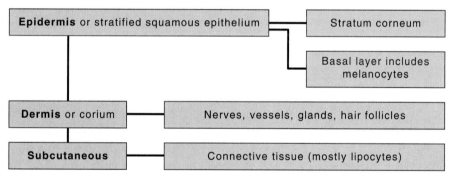

Figure 4-1 (b) A diagram showing the three layers of skin and what they contain.

Epidermis

The epidermis, the outer layer of skin, ranges from 1/200 to 1/20 of an inch thick, and consists of several **strata** (sublayers). The epidermis is made up of cells called **squamous epithelium,** a flat, scaly layer of cells. These layers are called **stratified squamous epithelium.** Not all parts of the body's skin contain all the sublayers of epidermis. The top sublayer is called the **stratum corneum.** It consists of a flat layer of dead cells arranged in parallel rows. As new cells are produced, the dead cells are sloughed off. As they die, the cells in the stratum corneum fill with **keratin**—a waterproof barrier to keep microorganisms out and moisture in. The keratin of the epidermis is softer than the hard keratin in nails. The bottom sublayer of the epidermis is called the **stratum germinativum.** Here new cells are produced and pushed up to the stratum corneum. The epidermis is a nonvascular layer of skin, meaning that it does not contain blood vessels.

Specialized cells called **melanocytes** produce a pigment called **melanin,** which helps to determine skin and hair color. Melanin is essential in screening out ultraviolet rays of the sun that can harm the body's cells.

Dermis

The dermis (also called the corium) contains two sublayers, a thin top one called the **papillary layer,** and a thicker one called the **reticular layer.** The dermis contains connective tissue that holds many capillaries, lymph cells, nerve endings, sebaceous and sweat glands, and hair follicles. These nourish the epidermis and serve as sensitive touch receptors. The connective tissue is composed primarily of **collagen** fibers that form a strong, elastic network. Collagen is a protein substance that is very tough, yet flexible. When the collagen fibers stretch, they form **striae** or stretch marks.

Subcutaneous Layer or Hypodermis

The subcutaneous layer is the layer between the dermis and the body's inner organs. It consists of **adipose** (or fatty) tissue and some layers of fibrous tissue. Within the subcutaneous layers lie blood vessels and nerves. The layer of fatty tissue serves to protect the inner organs and to maintain the body's temperature.

Hair

Hair grows out of the epidermis to cover various parts of the body. Hair serves to cushion and protect the areas it covers. Figure 4-2 shows a hair growing out of the epidermis. Hair has two parts. The *shaft* protrudes from the skin, and the *root* lies beneath the surface of the skin. The hair shaft is composed of outer layers of scaly cells filled with inner layers of soft and hard keratin. Hair grows upward from the root through the **hair follicles** (tubular sacs that hold the hair fibers). The shape of the follicle determines the shape of the hair (straight, curly, or wavy). Hair color is determined by the presence of melanin, which is produced by the melanocytes, cells in the epidermis. Gray hair occurs when melanocytes stop producing melanin. Hair growth, thickness, and curliness are generally determined by heredity. In addition to heredity, baldness or **alopecia** may result from disease, injury, or medical treatment (such as chemotherapy).

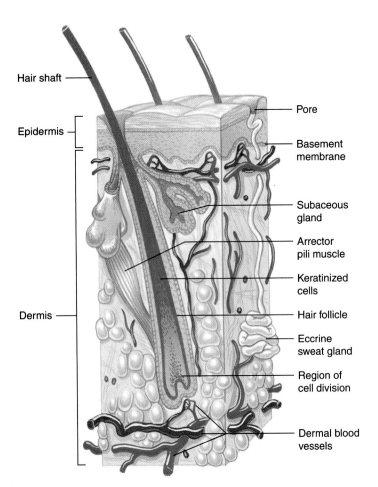

Hair shaft

Epidermis

Dermis

Pore

Basement membrane

Subaceous gland

Arrector pili muscle

Keratinized cells

Hair follicle

Eccrine sweat gland

Region of cell division

Dermal blood vessels

Figure 4-2 Hair growing out of the epidermis.

Hair Growth and Baldness

Scalp hair grows about 1 millimeter in length every 3 days for anywhere from two to four years at a time. Then, the hair stops growing for 3 to 4 months during a dormant phase. Normally, 10 to 100 hairs fall out every day. The fastest growth stage is from adolescence until the early 40s. Eyelash and eyebrow hair grow for only 3 to 4 months. As these hairs shed, they are replaced by new hairs that grow for only a few months, so they remain short as compared to scalp hair.

Hair loss occurs for a variety of reasons, such as emotional trauma, poor nutrition, disease, reaction to medication, radiation, or chemotherapy, or as part of a genetic code. *Pattern baldness* is a condition in which some parts of the scalp become devoid of hair while others retain hair. This patterning results from heredity and hormones. A man inherits the tendency for pattern baldness from his mother.

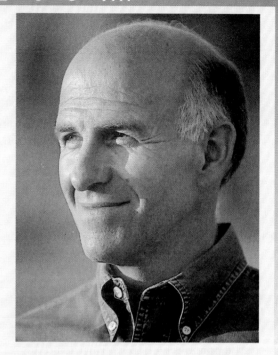

Male pattern baldness

Nails

Nails are plates made of hard keratin that cover the dorsal surface of the distal bone of the fingers and toes. Nails serve as a protective covering, help in the grasping of objects, and allow us to scratch. Healthy nails appear pinkish because the translucent nail covers vascular tissue. At the base of most nails, a **lunula,** or whitish half-moon, is an area where keratin and other cells have mixed with air. Nails are surrounded by a narrow band of epidermis called a **cuticle,** except at the top. The top portion of the nail grows above the level of the finger.

Glands

Sweat glands (also called sudoriferous glands) are found almost everywhere on the body surface. Glands that secrete outward toward the surface of the body through ducts are called **exocrine** glands. The excretion of sweat is called **diaphoresis.** Secretions exit the body through **pores** or tiny openings in the skin surface. There are also other kinds of

Nail Health

The nails sometimes offer a picture of inner health. In the photo at the top, the normal nails are healthy and pinkish, with no discolorations or white spots. The nails in the photo on the bottom have been altered by a fungal infection of the foot.

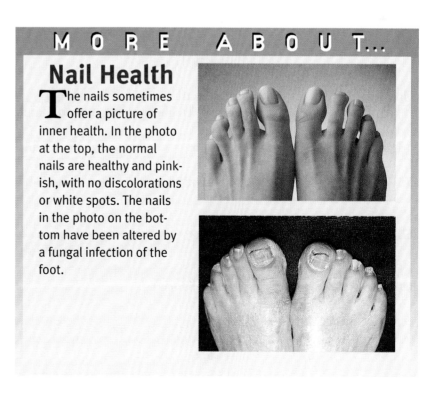

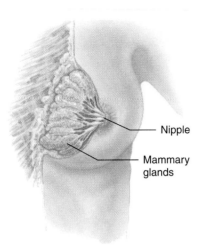

— Nipple

— Mammary
glands

Figure 4-3 The female breast is an apocrine gland.

sweat glands—eccrine and apocrine glands. **Eccrine** (or small sweat) **glands** are found on many places of the body. They excrete a colorless fluid that keeps the body at a constant temperature. The **apocrine glands** appear during and after puberty and secrete sweat from the armpits, near the reproductive organs, and around the nipples. The female breast is an apocrine gland that is adapted to secreting milk after childbirth (Figure 4-3).

Sebaceous glands, located in the dermis, secrete an oily substance called **sebum,** which is found at the base of the hair follicles. This substance serves to lubricate and protect the skin. Sebum forms a skin barrier against bacteria and fungi and also softens the surface of the skin.

Vocabulary Review

In the previous section, you learned terms relating to the integumentary system. Before going on to the exercise section, review the terms below and refer back to the previous section if you have any questions. Pronunciations are provided for certain terms.

Term	Word Analysis	Definition
adipose	[ĂD-ĭ-pōs]	Fatty; relating to fat.
alopecia	[ăl-ō-PĒ-shē-ă] Greek *alopekia*, mange	Lack of hair in spots; baldness.
apocrine glands	[ĂP-ō-krĭn] Greek *apo-krino*, to separate	Glands that appear during and after puberty and secrete sweat, as from the armpits.
collagen	KŎL-lă-jĕn] Greek *Koila*, glue + -gen	Major protein substance that is tough and flexible and that forms connective tissue in the body.
corium	KŌ-rē-ŭm	*See* dermis
cuticle	[KYŪ-tĭ-kl]	Thin band of epidermis that surrounds the edge of nails, except at the top.
dermis	[DĔR-mĭs]	Layer of skin beneath the epidermis containing blood vessels, nerves, and some glands.
diaphoresis	[DĪ-ă-fō-RĒ-sĭs]	Excretion of fluid by the sweat glands; sweating.
eccrine glands	[ĔK-rĭn] Greek *ek-krino*, to separate	Sweat glands that occur all over the body, except where the apocrine glands occur.

Term	Word Analysis	Definition
epidermis	[ĕp-ĭ-DĔRM-ĭs] epi-, upon + dermis, layer of skin	Outer portion of the skin containing several strata.
exocrine glands	[ĔK-sō-krĭn] exo-, outside + Greek *krino*, to separate	Glands that secrete through ducts toward the outside of the body.
hair follicle	[FŎL-ĭ-kl]	Tubelike sac in the epidermis out of which the hair shaft develops.
hair root		Portion of the hair beneath the skin surface.
hair shaft		Portion of the hair visible above the skin surface.
hypodermis	[hī-pō-DĔR-mĭs] hypo-, under + dermis, layer of skin	Subcutaneous skin layer; layer below the dermis.
integument	[ĭn-TĔG-yū-mĕnt] Latin *integumentum*, covering	Skin and all the elements that are contained within and arise from it.
keratin	[KĔR-ă-tĭn]	Hard, horny protein that forms nails and hair.
lunula (pl. lunulae)	[LŪ-nū-lă (LŪ-nū-lē)] Latin, little moon	Half-moon shaped area at the base of the nail plate.
melanin	[MĔL-ă-nĭn]	Pigment produced by melanocytes that determines skin, hair, and eye color.
melanocyte	[MĔL-ă-nō-sĭt] melano-, black + -cyte, cell	Cell in the epidermis that produces melanin.
nail		Thin layer of keratin that covers the distal portion of fingers and toes.
papillary layer	[PĂP-ĭ-lār-ē]	Thin sublayer of the dermis containing small papillae (nipple-like masses).
pore		Opening or hole, particularly in the skin.
reticular layer	[rĕ-TĬK-yū-lăr]	Bottom sublayer of the dermis containing reticula (network of structures with connective tissue between).
sebaceous glands	[sĕ-BĀ-shŭs]	Glands in the dermis that open to hair follicles and secrete sebum.

Term	Word Analysis	Definition
sebum	[SĒ-bŭm] Latin *sebum*, tallow	Oily substance, usually secreted into the hair follicle.
squamous epithelium	[SKWĂ-mŭs ĕp-ĭ-THĒ-lē-ŭm]	Flat, scaly layer of cells that makes up the epidermis.
stratified squamous epithelium		Layers of epithelial cells that make up the strata of the epidermis.
stratum (pl. strata)	[STRĂT-ŭm (STRĂ-tă)] Latin *stratum*, layer, bed cover	Layer of tissue, especially a layer of the skin.
stratum corneum	[KŌR-nē-ŭm]	Top sublayer of the epidermis.
stratum germinativum	[jĕr-mĭ-NĀT-ĭ-vŭm]	Bottom sublayer of the epidermis.
striae	[STRĪ-ē] Latin, plural of *stria*, furrow	Stretch marks made in the collagen fibers of the dermis layer.
subcutaneous layer	[sŭb-kyū-TĀ-nē-ŭs] sub-, beneath + Latin *cutis*, skin	Bottom layer of the skin containing fatty tissue.
sweat glands		Coiled glands of the skin that secrete perspiration to regulate body temperature and excrete waste products.

CASE STUDY

The Dermatologist's Office

Madeline Charles arrived at the office a few minutes early. She knew that Dr. Lin had a busy morning scheduled, and she wanted to set up before the doctor arrived. As secretary to Dr. Lin, Madeline handles incoming calls, scheduling, billing, new patient informa-tion forms, and insurance matters. She reports to James Carlson, the CMA and office manager for this small office. James assists the doctor with patients, oversees the work Madeline does, and helps when Madeline's load is too great. This morning, the first three patients are scheduled at 8:30, 9:00, and 9:30. Madeline looks at the schedule, realizes that one of the patients is new, and gets the folders for the other two. She sets up the clipboard with the forms the new patient will have to complete. She had previously asked the new patient to arrive 15 minutes early in order to have time to fill out the necessary forms.

Bob Luis, the first patient, is 48 years old and has a long history of diabetes. He sees Dr. Lin several times a year for treatment of skin irritations that do not seem to heal. Yesterday, Mr. Luis called with a specific problem. He has an extensive rash on his left ankle. It sounded serious

enough to warrant an appointment for the next morning. When Mr. Luis arrives, James escorts him to an examination room and helps him prepare for his visit.

Critical Thinking

1. What do we know about Mr. Luis's condition that

would warrant an immediate appointment with Dr. Lin?

2. Does a dermatologist treat a disease such as diabetes, or only symptoms related to the integumentary system?

Structure and Function Exercises

Build Your Medical Vocabulary

3. The dermis is a layer of skin. Using your knowledge of prefixes learned in Chapter 2, put the following words in order according to how close they are to the outside of the body.

    a. hypodermis _____

    b. epidermis_____

    c. dermis_____

4. Name the three types of glands, two of which were compound terms even in Ancient Greece.

Complete the Diagram

5. Fill in the missing labels on the figure shown here.

    a. _____

    b. _____

    c. _____

    d. _____

    e. _____

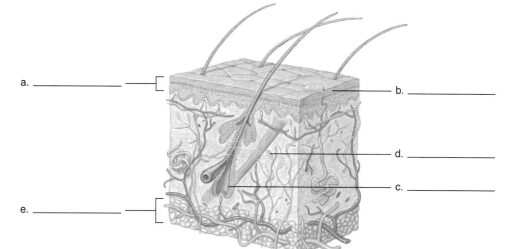

a. _____

b. _____

d. _____

c. _____

e. _____

Complete the Sentence

6. The thin layer of skin around the edge of a nail is called a(n) _____.

7. A hair follicle is in the _____ (layer of the skin).

8. The outer layer of skin is the _____.

9. The top sublayer of the dermis is called _____ _____.

10. Small sweat glands found all over the body are called _____.

11. The subcutaneous layer consists of _____ tissue.

12. A pinkish nail is a sign of a(n) _____ nail.

13. The area where keratin and other cells mix with air under the nail is called the _____.

14. Sebaceous glands secrete _____.

15. The female breast is a/an _____ gland.

Combining Forms and Abbreviations

The tables below include combining forms and abbreviations that relate specifically to the integumentary system. Pronunciations are included for the examples.

Combining Form	Meaning	Example
adip(o)	fatty	*adiposis* [ăd-ĭ-PŌ-sĭs], excessive accumulation of body fat
dermat(o)	skin	*dermatitis* [dĕr-mă-TĪ-tĭs], inflammation of the skin
derm(o)	skin	*dermabrasion* [dĕr-mă-BRĀ-zhŭn], surgical procedure to remove acne scars and marks, using an abrasive product to remove part of the skin
hidr(o)	sweat, sweat glands	*hidrosis* [hī-DRŌ-sĭs], production and excretion of sweat
ichthy(o)	fish, scaly	*ichthyosis* [ĭk-thē-Ō-sĭs], congenital skin disorder characterized by dryness and peeling
kerat(o)	horny tissue	*keratosis* [kĕr-ă-TŌ-sĭs], skin lesion covered by a horny layer of tissue
lip(o)	fatty	*liposuction* [lĭp-ō-SŬK-shŭn], removal of unwanted fat by suctioning through tubes placed under the skin

Combining Form	Meaning	Example
melan(o)	black, very dark	*melanoma* [mĕl-ă-NŌ-mă], malignancy arising from cells that form melanin
myc(o)	fungus	*mycosis* [mī-KŌ-sĭs], any condition caused by fungus
onych(o)	nail	*onychotomy* [ŏn-ĭ-KŎT-ō-mē] incision into a nail
pil(o)	hair	*pilocystic* [pī-lō-SĬS-tĭk], relating to a skin cyst with hair
seb(o)	sebum, sebaceous glands	*seborrhea* [sĕb-ō-RĒ-ă], excessive sebum caused by overactivity of the sebaceous glands
steat(o)	fat	*steatitis* [stē-ă-TĪ-tĭs], inflammation of fatty tissue
trich(o)	hair	*trichopathy* [trī-KŎP-ă-thē], disease of the hair
xanth(o)	yellow	*xanthoma* [zăn-THŌ-mă], yellow growth or discoloration of the skin
xer(o)	dry	*xeroderma* [zēr-ō-DĔR-mă], excessive dryness of the skin

Abbreviation	Meaning		Abbreviation	Meaning
bx	biopsy		PUVA	psoralen—ultraviolet A light therapy
DLE	discoid lupus erythematosus		SLE	systemic lupus erythematosus
PPD	purified protein derivative (of tuberculin)			

C A S E   S T U D Y

Understanding Information

While Dr. Lin is examining his first patient, the new patient arrives for the 9:00 appointment. Madeline explains which parts of the forms have to be filled out, asks for the patient's insurance card so she can copy it, and completes the file for Dr. Lin before 9:00. Meanwhile, Dr. Lin hands her his notes with a diagnosis for Bob Luis, including a new prescription for treatment of xeroderma. In addition, Dr. Lin gives Mr. Luis samples of a cream to relieve itching.

Critical Thinking

16. Why does the new patient have to fill out forms with questions about family history?

17. Mr. Luis is given samples of a prescription cream to try. Can the medical assistant decide which samples to give him?

Combining Forms and Abbreviations Exercises

Build Your Medical Vocabulary

Build a word for each of the following definitions. Use the combining form vocabulary review in this chapter and the combining forms for the body in Chapter 3.

18. Plastic surgery of the skin: _____

19. Inflammation of the skin and veins: _____

20. Horny growth on the epidermis: _____

21. Fungal eruption on the skin: _____

22. Excess pigment in the skin: _____

23. Fungal infection of the nail: _____

24. Repair of the nail: _____

25. Of the hair follicles and sebaceous glands: _____

26. Pigment-producing cell: _____

27. Examination of the hair: _____

28. Removal of fat by cutting: _____

29. Relating to both fatty and cellular tissue: _____.

30. Study of hair: _____

31. Disease of the nail: _____

32. Poison produced by certain fungi: _____

33. Virus that infects fungi: _____

34. Yellow coloration of the skin: _____

35. Condition of extreme dryness: _____

36. Removal or shedding of the horny layer of the epidermis: _____

37. Abnormally darkened skin: _____

38. Lessening of the rate of sweating: _____

Root Out the Meaning

Separate the following terms into word parts; define each word part.

39. trichoma _____

40. xerosis _____

41. mycocide _____

42. xanthoderma _____

43. onychoid _____

Diagnostic, Procedural, and Laboratory Terms

The field of **dermatology** studies, diagnoses, and treats ailments of the skin. The first diagnostic test is usually visual observation of the surface of the skin. Clinical procedures and laboratory tests can result in diagnosis and treatment of specific skin conditions.

Diagnostic Procedures and Tests

Once a visual assessment has been made, the dermatologist determines which procedures and tests will help find the underlying cause of a skin problem. Samples of **exudate** (material that passes out of tissues) or pus may be sent to a laboratory for examination. The laboratory can determine what types of bacteria are present. A scraping may also be taken and placed on a growth medium to be examined for the presence of fungi.

Skin is a reliable place to test for various diseases and allergies. A suspected *allergen*, something that provokes an allergic reaction, is mixed with a substance that can be used in tests. That substance containing the allergen is called an *antigen*. The **patch test** calls for placing a suspected antigen on a piece of gauze and applying it to the skin. If a reaction results, the test is considered positive. Other skin tests for allergies include the **scratch test** (in which a suspected antigen is scratched onto the skin, and redness or swelling within ten minutes indicates a positive reaction) and the **intradermal** test (in which a suspected antigen is injected between layers of skin). Infectious diseases may also be detected by an intradermal test. **PPD,** a purified protein derivative of tuberculin, is used in the **Mantoux test** for detecting tuberculosis. In the Mantoux test, the PPD is injected intradermally. A similar test, the **tine** test injects the tuberculin using a tine (an instrument with a number of pointed ends). The **Schick test** is a test for diphtheria in which a small amount of toxin is injected into the skin of one arm and a small amount of deactivated toxin is injected into the skin of the other arm for comparison. Figure 4-4 on page 82 shows the test for tuberculosis and a positive result.

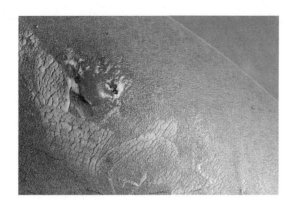

Figure 4-4 A positive test result for tuberculosis.

Vocabulary Review

In the previous section, you learned terms relating to diagnosis, clinical procedures, and laboratory tests. Before going on to the exercise section, review the terms below and refer to the previous section if you have questions.

Term	Word Analysis	Definition
dermatology	[dĕr-mă-TŎL-ō-jē] dermato-, skin + -logy, study	Medical specialty that deals with diseases of the skin.
exudate	[ĔKS-ū-dāt] ex-, out + Latin *sudo*, sweat	Any fluid excreted out of tissue, especially fluid excreted out of an injury to the skin.
intradermal	[ĬN-tră-DĔR-măl] intra-, within + derm(o)-, skin	From within the skin, particularly from the dermis.
Mantoux test	[măn-TŪ]	Test for tuberculosis in which a small dose of tuberculin is injected into the skin with a syringe.
patch test		Test for allergic sensitivity in which a small dose of antigen is applied to the skin on a small piece of gauze.
PPD		Purified protein derivative of tuberculin.
Schick test		Test for diphtheria.
scratch test		Test for allergic sensitivity in which a small amount of antigen is scratched onto the surface of the skin.
tine test	[tīn]	Test for tuberculosis in which a small dose of tuberculin is injected into a series of sites within a small space with a tine (instrument that punctures the surface of the skin).

Testing for Allergic Reactions

Several days ago, Dr. Lin had given a series of scratch tests to a teenager who had allergic skin rashes. The doctor had noted all the places where redness or swelling appeared within ten minutes. He had also noted the negative reactions, where no changes appeared within thirty minutes. There were also some mild, inconclusive reactions. Dr. Lin reviewed the results of the tests. He asked Madeline to send a report to the patient and to set up a phone appointment to discuss the results. Madeline thought the results looked interesting. She didn't know that people could be allergic to so many things at once.

Critical Thinking

44. What does a negative reaction to a scratch test indicate?

45. If the patient avoids the allergens that gave the most positive reactions, what is likely to happen to the rashes?

Diagnostic, Procedural, and Laboratory Terms Exercises

Check Your Knowledge

Circle T for true and F for false.

46. The Mantoux test detects allergies. T F

47. An intradermal test may detect an infectious disease. T F

48. PPD is used in the Mantoux test. T F

49. An intradermal injection usually reaches into the hypodermis. T F

50. Visual observation of the skin is a diagnostic tool. T F

Fill in the blanks

51. A scraping from the skin is placed on a growth medium to detect the presence of _____.

52. Samples of _____ may be sent to a laboratory for examination.

53. Scratch tests are often used to detect _____.

54. Suspected antigens are injected between layers of skin in a(n) _____ test.

Pathological Terms

The skin is a place where both abnormalities occur and some internal diseases show dermatological symptoms. **Lesions** are areas of tissues that are altered because of a pathological condition. Primary lesions appear on previously normal skin. Secondary lesions are abnormalities that result from changes in primary lesions. **Vascular lesions** are blood vessel lesions that show through the skin. Figure 4-5 shows various types of skin lesions.

Some common primary lesions are areas of discoloration, such as a **macule** (freckle or flat mole) or **patch.** Elevated, solid masses include: **papule,** a small elevated mass, also called a *pimple;* **plaque,** a small patch on the skin; **nodule,**

Figure 4-5 Types of skin lesions.

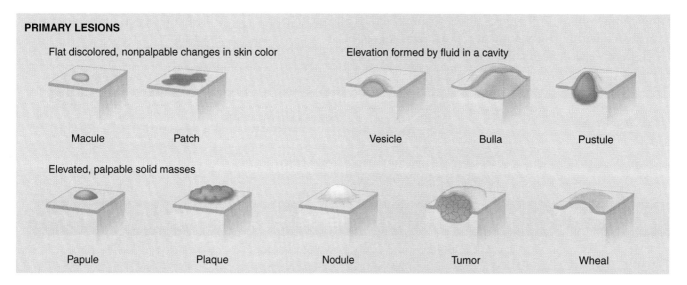

PRIMARY LESIONS

Flat discolored, nonpalpable changes in skin color

Macule   Patch

Elevation formed by fluid in a cavity

Vesicle   Bulla   Pustule

Elevated, palpable solid masses

Papule   Plaque   Nodule   Tumor   Wheal

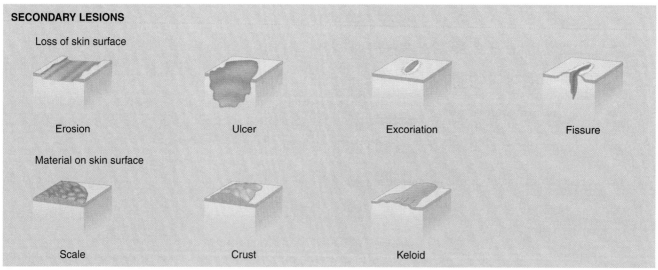

SECONDARY LESIONS

Loss of skin surface

Erosion   Ulcer   Excoriation   Fissure

Material on skin surface

Scale   Crust   Keloid

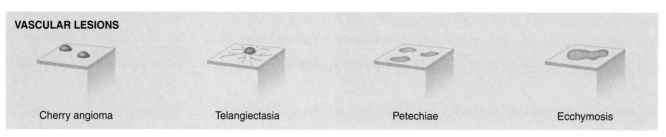

VASCULAR LESIONS

Cherry angioma   Telangiectasia   Petechiae   Ecchymosis

a large pimple or a small node; **polyp,** any mass that projects upward, either on a slender stalk (**pediculated polyp**) or from a broad base (**sessile polyp**); **tumor,** any swelling or, specifically, any abnormal tissue growth; and **wheal,** a smooth, slightly elevated area, usually associated with allergic itching. A **bulla,** a large blister; a **pustule,** a small elevated mass containing pus; and a **vesicle,** a small mass containing fluid are elevated skin pockets filled with fluid. A **cyst** may be solid or filled with fluid or gas. A **pilonidal cyst** contains hairs, and a **sebaceous cyst** contains yellow sebum.

Secondary lesions usually involve either loss of skin surface or material that forms on the skin surface. Lesions that involve loss of skin surface are: **erosion,** a shallow area of the skin worn away by friction or pressure; **excoriation,** a scratched area of the skin, usually covered with dried blood; **fissure,** a deep furrow or crack in the skin surface; and **ulcer,** a wound with loss of tissue and often with inflammation, especially **decubitus ulcers** or **pressure sores,** chronic ulcers on skin over bony parts that are under constant pressure. Lesions that form surface material are: **scale,** thin plates of epithelium formed on the skin's surface; **crust,** dried blood or pus that forms on the skin's surface; and **keloid,** a firm, raised mass of scar tissue. A **cicatrix,** a general word for scar, usually refers to internal scarring (as a lesion on the brain) or growth inside a wound.

> Any abnormal growth should be observed for changes and for certain characteristics that may indicate the presence of skin cancer.

Symptoms, Abnormalities, and Conditions

Symptoms of disease can appear on the skin. For example, **exanthematous viral diseases** are rashes that develop during a viral infection. Other common viral rashes are: **rubeola,** measles with an accompanying rash; **rubella,** disease with a rash caused by the rubella virus (also known as *German measles*); **roseola,** disease with small, rosy patches on the skin, usually caused by a virus; and **varicella,** disease with a rash known as *chicken pox,* caused by the varicella virus. Chicken pox does not usually cause harm (other than possible scarring) in young children. However, young adult males who become infected may become sterile. Infectious agents, such as staphylococci, may cause **impetigo,** a **pyoderma,** or pus-containing, contagious skin disease. At times, staphylococci infections can become deadly as is the case with flesh-eating bacteria, a fatal type of staph infection. Fungi may cause **tinea** or **ringworm,** a skin condition that causes intense **pruritus** or itching. **Candidiasis** is a yeast fungus that causes common rashes such as diaper rash. Other common fungi are *tinea pedis* or athlete's foot; *tinea capitis,* scalp ringworm; and *tinea barbae,* ringworm of the beard. Some autoimmune diseases, such as **pemphigus,** cause skin blistering.

Skin conditions, particularly skin irritations or **dermatitis,** can reflect systemic allergies or diseases. **Urticaria** or **hives** may arise from a food allergy; itching or pruritus can also be the result of allergies. **Eczema** is an acute form of dermatitis often caused by allergies.

Ecchymosis (plural, **ecchymoses**) is a bluish-purple skin mark that may result from a skin injury that can cause blood to leak out of blood vessels. **Petechiae** are tiny, pinpoint ecchymoses. **Purpura** is a condition with extensive hemorrhages into the skin covering a wide area. Purpura starts out with red areas, which turn purplish, and then brown, in a couple of weeks. **Rosacea** is a vascular disorder that appears as red blotches on the skin, particularly around the nose and cheeks.

Some diseases, infections, or inflammations cause skin conditions, such as a **furuncle,** a localized, pus-producing infection originating in a hair follicle; a **carbuncle,** a pus-producing infection that starts in subcutaneous tissue and

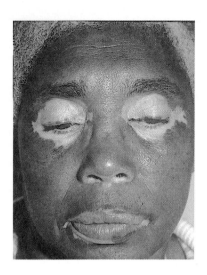

Figure 4-6 Vitiligo is a skin disorder with areas of extensive pigment surrounding areas that have lost pigment.

is usually accompanied by fever and an ill feeling; **abscess,** a localized infection usually accompanied by pus and inflammation; and **gangrene,** necrosis (death) of tissue due to loss of blood supply.

Some skin areas lack color, which may be the result of **depigmentation,** partial or complete loss of pigment; **leukoderma,** white patches on the skin; or **vitiligo** (Figure 4-6), patches with loss of pigment surrounded by patches with extensive pigment. These conditions often indicate a systemic autoimmune disease. A rare congenital condition called **albinism** causes either extensive or total lack of pigmentation. People with albinism often have very white, almost translucent, skin and white hair. A pigmented skin lesion found at birth is a **nevus** (plural, **nevi**) or **birthmark. Chloasma** is a group of fairly large, pigmented facial patches, often associated with pregnancy.

Herpes simplex virus Type 1, herpes simplex virus Type 2, and **herpes zoster** are all viral diseases caused by **herpes** viruses. Herpes 1, also called **cold sores** or **fever blisters,** usually appears around the mouth. Herpes 2, also known as **genital herpes,** affects the genital area. Herpes zoster or **shingles** is an inflammation that affects the nerves on one side of the body and results in skin blisters. It can be extremely painful.

A virus may also cause a **wart** or **verruca.** A **plantar wart** appears on the soles of the feet. *Lupus,* a chronic disease with erosion of the skin, may appear in different forms. Two common forms are **DLE** or **discoid lupus erythematosus,** a mild form of lupus that usually causes only superficial eruption of the skin, and **SLE** or **systemic lupus erythematosus,** a chronic inflammation of the collagen in the skin and joints that usually causes inflammation of connective tissue throughout the body and is often accompanied by fever, weakness, arthritis, and other serious symptoms. Inflammation of the dermis and subcutaneous skin layers is called **cellulitis,** which can spread infection via the blood to the brain.

Other skin conditions include **acne** (also called **acne vulgaris**), a skin condition with eruptions on the face and upper back. Acne usually starts around puberty and is often caused by overproduction of sebum. It usually includes several types of skin eruptions, such as **comedones** or **blackheads, whiteheads,** pustules, and nodules. Figure 4-7 shows a person with acne. **Scleroderma**

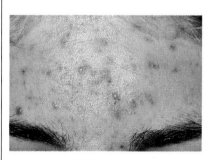

Figure 4-7 Acne usually affects adolescents.

is a chronic disease with abnormal thickening of the skin caused by the formation of new collagen. **Psoriasis,** a recurrent skin condition with scaly lesions on the trunk, arms, hands, legs, and scalp, is often associated with stress. **Seborrhea,** a condition with excessive production of sebum, is a result of overactivity of the sebaceous glands. *Seborrheic dermatitis* (also called *dandruff*), scaly eruptions on the face or scalp, is due to the overproduction of seborrhea.

Exposure of the skin to heat, chemicals, electricity, radiation, or other irritants may cause a **burn.** Different categories of burns indicate the amount or level of skin involvement. **First-, second-,** and **third-degree burns** are the standard categories. First-degree burns are superficial burns of the epidermis without blistering, but with redness and swelling; second-degree burns involve the epidermis and dermis and involve blistering; and third-degree burns involve complete destruction of the skin, sometimes reaching into the muscle and bone and causing extensive scarring. Figure 4-8 shows how the extent of a burn is estimated.

Some skin conditions are caused by insects. **Pediculosis** is an inflammation with lice, often on the head (*pediculosis capitis*) or the genital area (*pediculosis pubis*). **Scabies,** a contagious skin eruption that often occurs between fingers, on other areas of the trunk, or on the male genitalia, is caused by mites.

Inflammations of the nail can be caused by infection, irritation, or fungi. **Onychia** or **onychitis** is a nail inflammation. **Paronychia** is an inflammation in the *nail fold*, the flap of skin overlapping the edges of the nail. Both of these inflammations often occur spontaneously in debilitated people. They may also result from a slight trauma. A general term for disease of the nails is **onychopathy.**

Some abnormal growths or **neoplasms** are benign. The most common benign neoplasms are a **callus,** a hard, thickened area of skin; a **corn,** hardening or thickening of skin on a toe; **keratosis,** overgrowth of horny tissue on skin (especially **actinic keratosis**), such as overgrowth due to excessive sun exposure; and **leukoplakia,** thickened white patches of epithelium. A growth may be of fibrous tissue; for example, a cicatrix, which is a growth of fibrous tissue inside a wound that forms a scar.

Some neoplasms are malignant. **Basal cell carcinoma** is cancer of the basal layer of the epidermis; **squamous cell carcinoma** affects the squamous epithelium. **Kaposi's sarcoma** is often associated with AIDS. The incidence of **malignant melanoma** is rapidly increasing. Figure 4-9 shows examples of Kaposi's sarcoma and a malignant melanoma. This increase is thought to be due to the depletion of the Earth's ozone layer, which protects the skin from harmful UV rays. Many protective products, such as sunblock or sunscreen, are widely available. One of the odd results of widespread sunscreen use is that skin cancers have increased in people who use them. This is because people who use the screens actually feel that they can stay in the sun for much

Figure 4-8 Burns are classified as first-degree (minor), second-degree (serious), or third-degree (severe). One method of estimating the extent of burns is to use the "rule of nines." As shown in the illustration, the body is divided into sections with percentages. Depending on the percentage of the body burned and the depth of the burn in each area, a determination of degree is made. Slightly different percentages are used for young children. For example, a 10-percent burn area in a child is considered as serious as a 15-percent burn area in an adult.

New materials are manufactured for skin grafts. In severe burn cases, these new materials provide a protective covering and promote regrowth of damaged skin. Recently, material extracted from eggs is being tested for use as skin coverings for severe injuries.

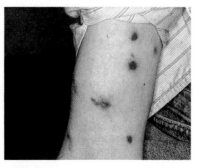
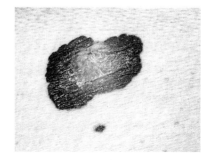

Figure 4-9 Two types of skin cancer—Kaposi's sarcoma (left) and malignant melanoma (right).

People at high risk for melanoma are those who have blond or red hair, a family history of melanoma, precancerous actinic keratoses, extensive freckling of the back, three or more blistering sunburns before age 20, and three or more summers spent in an outdoor summer job as a teen.

longer periods. The only effective skin cancer prevention is to avoid exposure to the sun as much as possible.

In most instances, hair loss is hereditary or due to a side effect of medication. However, hair loss can be a pathological condition, as in **alopecia areata,** a condition in which hair falls out in patches.

Vocabulary Review

In the previous section, you learned terms relating to pathology. Before going on to the exercises, review the terms below and refer to the previous section if you have questions.

Term	Word Analysis	Definition
abscess	[ĂB-sĕs] Latin *abscessus*, a going away	Localized collection of pus and other exudate, usually accompanied by swelling and redness.
acne	[ĂK-nē]	Inflammatory eruption of the skin, occurring in or near sebaceous glands on the face, neck, shoulder, or upper back.
acne vulgaris	[ĂK-nē vŭl-GĀR-ĕs]	*See* acne.
actinic keratosis	[ăk-TĬN-ĭk KĔR-ă-tō-sĭs]	Overgrowth of horny skin that forms from over-exposure to sunlight; sunburn.
albinism	[ĂL-bĭ-nĭzm] albin(o) + -ism, state	Rare, congenital condition causing either partial or total lack of pigmentation.
alopecia areata	[ăl-ō-PĒ-shē-ă ā-rē-Ā-tă]	Loss of hair in patches.
basal cell carcinoma		Slow-growing cancer of the basal cells of the epidermis, usually a result of sun damage.
birthmark		Lesion (especially a hemangioma) visible at or soon after birth; nevus.
blackhead		*See* comedo.
bulla (pl. bullae)	[BŬL-ă (BŬL-ī)]	Bubble-like blister on the surface of the skin.
burn		Damage to the skin caused by exposure to heat, chemicals, electricity, radiation, or other skin irritants.

Term	Word Analysis	Definition
callus	[KĂL-ŭs] Latin	Mass of hard skin that forms as a cover over broken skin on certain areas of the body, especially the feet and hands.
candidiasis	[kăn-dǐ-DĪ-ă-sǐs] Candid(a) + -iasis, condition	Yeastlike fungus on the skin, caused by Candida; characterized by pruritus, white exudate, peeling, and easy bleeding; examples are thrush and diaper rash.
carbuncle	[KĂR-bŭng-kl]	Infected area of the skin producing pus and usually accompanied by fever.
cellulitis	[sĕl-yū-LĪ-tǐs] cellul(ar) + -itis, inflammation	Severe inflammation of the dermis and subcutaneous portions of the skin, usually caused by an infection that enters the skin through an opening, as a wound; characterized by local heat, redness, pain, and swelling.
chloasma	[klō-ĂZ-mă] Greek chloazo, to become green	Group of fairly large, pigmented facial patches, often associated with pregnancy.
cicatrix	[SĬK-ă-trĭks] Latin	Growth of fibrous tissue inside a wound that forms a scar; also, general term for scar.
cold sore		Eruption around the mouth or lips; herpes simplex virus Type 1.
comedo (pl. comedos, comedones)	[KŌM-ē-dō, kō-MĒ-dō (KŌM-ē-dōz, kō-mē-DŌ-nĕz)] Latin, a glutton	Open hair follicle filled with bacteria and sebum; common in acne; blackhead.
corn		Growth of hard skin, usually on the toes.
crust		Hard layer, especially one formed by dried pus, as in a scab.
cyst	[sĭst] Greek kystis, bladder	Abnormal sac containing fluid.
decubitus (pl. decubiti) ulcer	[dĕ-KYŪ-bĭ-tŭs (dĕ-KYŪ-bĭ-tī)]	Chronic ulcer on skin over bony parts that are under constant pressure.
depigmentation	[dē-pĭg-mĕn-TĀ-shŭn] de-, removal + pigmentation	Loss of color of the skin.
dermatitis	[dĕr-mă-TĪ-tǐs] dermat-, skin + -itis	Inflammation of the skin.

Term	Word Analysis	Definition
discoid lupus erythematosus (DLE)	[DĬS-kŏyd LŪ-pŭs ĕr-ĭ-THĔM-ă-tō-sŭs]	Mild form of lupus.
ecchymosis (pl. ecchymoses)	[ĕk-ĭ-MŌ-sĭs (ĕk-ĭ-MŌ-sēz)] Greek	Purplish skin patch (bruise) caused by broken blood vessels beneath the surface.
eczema	[ĔK-zē-mă, ĔG-zē-mă] Greek	Severe inflammatory condition of the skin, usually of unknown cause.
erosion		Wearing away of the surface of the skin, especially that caused by friction.
exanthematous viral disease	[ĕg-zăn-THĔM-ă-tŭs]	Viral disease that causes a rash on the skin.
excoriation	[ĕks-KŌ-rē-Ā-shŭn] Latin excoriatio, to skin	Injury to the surface of the skin caused by a scratch, abrasion, or burn, usually accompanied by some oozing.
fever blister		Eruption around the mouth or lips; herpes simplex virus Type 1.
first-degree burn		Least severe burn, causes injury to the surface of the skin without blistering.
fissure	[FĬSH-ŭr] Latin fissura	Deep slit in the skin.
furuncle	[FYŪ-rŭng-kl]	Localized skin infection, usually in a hair follicle and containing pus; boil.
gangrene	[GĂNG-grēn] Greek gangraina, eating sore	Death of an area of skin, usually caused by loss of blood supply to the area.
genital herpes		See herpes simplex virus Type 2.
herpes	[HĔR-pēz] Greek, shingles	An inflammatory skin disease caused by viruses of the family Herpesviridae.
herpes simplex virus Type 1		Herpes that recurs on the lips and around the area of the mouth, usually during viral illnesses or states of stress.
herpes simplex virus Type 2		Herpes that recurs on the genitalia; can be easily transmitted from one person to another through sexual contact.
herpes zoster	[ZŎS-tĕr]	Painful herpes that affects nerve roots; shingles.

Term	Word Analysis	Definition
hives		*See* urticaria.
impetigo	[ĭm-pĕ-TĪ-gō] Latin	A type of pyoderma.
Kaposi's sarcoma	[KĂ-pō-sēz] After Moritz Kaposi (1837–1902), Hungarian dermatologist	Skin cancer associated with AIDS.
keloid	[KĒ-lŏyd] Greek *kele*, tumor + -oid, like	Thick scarring of the skin that forms after an injury or surgery.
keratosis	[kĕr-ă-TŌ-sĭs] kerat(o)-, horny layer + -osis, condition	Lesion on the epidermis containing keratin.
lesion	[LĒ-shŭn]	Wound, damage, or injury to the skin.
leukoderma	[lū-kō-DĔR-mă] euko-, white + -derma, skin	Absence of pigment in the skin or in an area of the skin.
leukoplakia	[lū-kō-PLĀ-kē-ă] leuko- + -plakia, plaque	White patch of mucous membrane on the tongue or cheek.
macule	[MĂK-yūl]	Small, flat, noticeably colored spot on the skin.
malignant melanoma		Virulent skin cancer originating in the melano-cytes, usually caused by overexposure to the sun.
neoplasm	[NĒ-ō-plăzm] neo-, recent, new + -plasm, formation	Abnormal tissue growth.
nevus (pl. nevi)	[NĒ-vŭs (NĒ-vĭ)]	Birthmark.
nodule	[NŎD-yūl]	Small knob of tissue.
onychia, onychitis	[ō-NĬK-ē-ă, ŏn-ĭ-KĪ-tĭs] onycho-, nail + -ia, condition; onych(o)- + -itis	Inflammation of the nail.
onychopathy	[ōn-ĭ-KŎP-ă-thē] onycho- + -pathy, disease	Disease of the nail.
papule	[PĂP-yūl]	Small, solid elevation on the skin.

Term	Word Analysis	Definition
paronychia	[păr-ŏ-NĬK-ē-ă] par(a)-, abnormal + Greek *onyx*, nail	Inflammation, with pus, of the fold surrounding the nail plate.
patch		Small area of skin differing in color from the surrounding area.
pediculated polyp	[pĕ-DĬK-yū-lā-tĕd]	Polyp that projects upward from a slender stalk.
pediculosis	[pĕ-DĬK-yū-LŌ-sĭs] Latin *pediculus*, louse + -osis	Lice infestation.
pemphigus	[PĔM-fĭ-gŭs] Greek *pemphix*, blister	Autoimmune disease that causes skin blistering.
petechia (pl. petechiae)	[pē-TĒ-kē-ă, pē-TĔK- ē-ă (pē-TĒ-kē-ē)]	Tiny hemorrhages beneath the surface of the skin.
pilonidal cyst	[pĭ-lō-NĪ-dăl] pilo-, hair + Latin *nidus*, nest	Cyst containing hair, usually found at the lower end of the spinal column.
plantar wart	[PLĂN-tăr]	Wart on the sole of the foot.
plaque	[plăk]	*See* patch.
polyp	[PŎL-ĭp]	Bulging mass of tissue that projects outward from the skin surface.
pressure sore		*See* decubitus ulcer.
pruritus	[prū-RĪ-tŭs]	Itching.
psoriasis	[sō-RĪ-ă-sĭs]	Chronic skin condition accompanied by scaly lesions with extreme pruritus.
purpura	[PŬR-pū-ră]	Skin condition with extensive hemorrhages underneath the skin covering a wide area.
pustule	[PŬS-tūl]	Small elevation on the skin containing pus.
pyoderma	[pĭ-ō-DĔR-mă] pyo-, pus + -derma, skin	Any inflammation of the skin that produces pus.
ringworm		Fungal infection; tinea.
rosacea	[rō-ZĀ-shē-ă]	Vascular disease that causes blotchy, red patches on the skin, particularly on the nose and cheeks.

Term	Word Analysis	Definition
roseola	[rō-ZĒ-ō-lǎ]	Skin eruption of small, rosy patches, usually caused by a virus.
rubella	[rū-BĔL-ǎ]	Disease that causes a viral skin rash; German measles.
rubeola	[rū-BĒ-ō-lǎ]	Disease that causes a viral skin rash; measles.
scabies	[SKĀ-bēz]	Skin eruption caused by a mite burrowing into the skin.
scale		Small plate of hard skin that falls off.
scleroderma	[sklēr-ō-DĔR-mǎ] sclero-, hardness + -derma, skin	Thickening of the skin caused by an increase in collagen formation.
sebaceous cyst	[sě-BĀ-shǔs]	Cyst containing yellow sebum.
seborrhea	[sěb-ō-RĒ-ǎ] sebo-, sebum + -rrhea, flowing	Overproduction of sebum by the sebaceous glands.
second-degree burn		Moderately severe burn that affects the epidermis and dermis; usually involves blistering.
sessile polyp	[SĔS-ĭl]	Polyp that projects upward from a broad base.
shingles	[SHĬN-glz]	Viral disease affecting peripheral nerves and caused by herpes zoster.
squamous cell carcinoma	[SKWĂ-mǔs]	Cancer of the squamous epithelium.
systemic lupus erythematosus (SLE)		Most severe form of lupus, involving internal organs.
third-degree burn		Most severe type of burn; involves complete destruction of an area of skin.
tinea	[TĬN-ē-ǎ]	Fungal infection; ringworm.
tumor	[TŪ-mǒr]	Any mass of tissue; swelling.
ulcer	[ŬL-sěr]	Open lesion, usually with superficial loss of tissue.
urticaria	[ĔR-tǐ-KĀR-ē-ǎ]	Group of reddish wheals, usually accompanied by pruritus and often caused by an allergy.

Term	Word Analysis	Definition
varicella	[vār-ĭ-SĔL-ă]	Contagious skin disease, usually occurring during childhood, and often accompanied by the formation of pustules; chicken pox.
vascular lesion		Lesion in a blood vessel that shows through the skin.
verruca (pl. verrucae)	[vĕ-RŪ-kă (vĕ-RŪ-kē)]	Flesh-colored growth, sometimes caused by a virus; wart.
vesicle	[VĔS-ĭ-kl]	Small, raised sac on the skin containing fluid.
vitiligo	[vĭt-ĭ-LĪ-gō]	Condition in which white patches appear on otherwise normally pigmented skin.
wart	[wōrt]	*See* verruca.
wheal	[hwēl]	Itchy patch of raised skin.
whitehead	[HWĪT-hĕd]	Closed comedo that does not contain the dark bacteria present in blackheads.

C A S E S T U D Y

Treating Adolescent Acne

Dr. Lin's new patient's name is Maria Cardoza. She is 17 years old and has a persistent case of acne. She had been treating it with soap and Oxy-10 with limited success in the past couple of years, but recently her condition has worsened and her pediatrician recommended that she see Dr. Lin. After careful examination and cleaning up of some comedones, Dr. Lin prescribed a course of antibiotics and asked Maria to return in three weeks. Dr. Lin put the following notes on Maria's chart:

Mild-to-moderate acne on the face, neck, and upper back. Lesions consist of macules, papules, mild oily comedones, and an occasional nodule, but no cysts or boils. erythromycin, 400 mg., t.i.d. for 3 months. Recheck in 3 months.

Critical Thinking

55. Dr. Lin recommended that Maria wash her face with soap three times a day. Acne occurs in the sebaceous glands. How will frequent washing help?

56. As Maria gets older, why might her acne improve even without treatment?

Pathological Terms Exercises

Build Your Medical Vocabulary

Put C for correct in the blank next to each word that is spelled correctly. Put the correct spelling next to words that are spelled incorrectly.

57. pemfigus _____

58. varicella _____

59. purpora _____

60. urticaria _____

61. rosola _____

Add the missing suffix to the following terms.

62. Nail inflammation: onych_____

63. Skin condition: dermat_____

64. Black tumor: melan_____

65. Hair disease: tricho_____

66. White skin: leuko_____

Check Your Knowledge

Circle T for true or F for false.

67. Basal cell carcinoma is characterized by blackened areas on the skin. T F

68. All neoplasms are malignant. T F

69. A nevus is a third-degree burn. T F

70. Pruritus can be present in many skin conditions. T F

71. Rubella is a viral skin rash. T F

72. Tinea barbae is ringworm of the feet. T F

73. Warts may be caused by a virus. T F

74. Seborrhea is abnormal pigmentation. T F

75. The herpes virus is not curable and recurs at various times. T F

76. Food allergies can cause skin eruptions. T F

Fill in the blanks.

77. Most adult hair loss is caused by _____ or _____.

78. Scabies is caused by _____.

79. Herpes simplex virus Type 1 usually occurs around the area of the _____.

80. Herpes simplex virus Type 2 usually occurs on the _____.

Surgical Terms

Skin surgery includes the repair of various conditions. Sutures, stitches, or staples hold skin together while healing takes place. Various types of plastic surgery may involve reconstructing areas of the skin, as after severe burns or radiation. Other types of skin surgery result in the removal of a part of a growth to test for the presence of cancer. Growths are also removed to keep a cancer from spreading.

Plastic surgery may involve the use of **skin grafts.** An **autograft** uses skin from one's own body. An **allograft** or **homograft** uses donor skin from another person. A **heterograft** or **xenograft** uses donor skin from one species to another (such as animal, for example a pig, to human). A *dermatome* is an implement used to remove layers of skin for grafts.

Plastic surgery may also use various methods to remove unwanted growths or scrape tissue or discolorations. **Cryosurgery** involves the removal of tissue by applying cold liquid nitrogen. **Dermabrasion** is the use of brushes and emery papers to remove wrinkles, scars, and tattoos. **Debridement** and **curettage** are the removal of dead tissue from a wound by scraping.

Some surgical procedures of the skin involve the use of electricity or lasers to stop bleeding, remove tissue, or excise tissues for examination. Wounds may be **cauterized** or burned to coagulate an area that is bleeding. They may be dried with electrical current (**electrodesiccation**). **Fulguration** is the use of electric sparks to destroy tissue.

A **biopsy** is a cutting of tissue for microscopic examination. A *needle biopsy* is the removal of tissue by aspirating it through a needle. A *punch biopsy* is the use of a cylindrical instrument to remove a small piece of tissue. A *shave biopsy* is the removal of a layer of skin using a surgical blade. **Moh's surgery** is the removal of thin layers of malignant growth until a nonmalignant area is reached. Figure 4-10 shows biopsied tissue observed through a microscope.

Figure 4-10 A biopsied piece of skin as it appears under a microscope. The darkened cells on the left are cancerous.

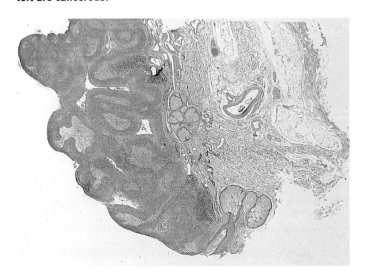

Vocabulary Review

In the previous section, you learned terms relating to surgery. Before going on to the exercises, review the terms below and refer to the previous section if you have any questions.

Term	Word Analysis	Definition
allograft	[ĂL-ō-grăft] allo-, other + graft	*See* homograft.
autograft	[ĂW-tō-grăft] auto-, self + graft	Skin graft using skin from one's own body.
biopsy	[BĪ-ŏp-sē] bi(o)-, life + -opsy, view of	Excision of tissue for microscopic examination.
cauterize	[KĂW-tĕr-īz]	To apply heat to an area to cause coagulation and stop bleeding.
cryosurgery	[krī-ō-SĔR-jĕr-ē] cryo-, cold + surgery	Surgery that removes tissue by freezing it with liquid nitrogen.
curettage	[kyū-rĕ-TĂHZH]	Removal of tissue from an area, such as a wound, by scraping.
debridement	[dā-brēd-MŎN]	Removal of dead tissue from a wound.
dermabrasion	[dĕr-mă-BRĀ-zhŭn] derm-, skin + abrasion	Removal of wrinkles, scars, tattoos, and other marks by scraping with brushes or emery papers.
electrodesiccation	[ē-LĔK-trō-dĕs-ĭ-KĀ-shŭn]	Drying with electrical current.
fulguration	[fŭl-gŭ-RĀ-shŭn]	Destruction of tissue using electric sparks.
heterograft	[HĔT-ĕr-ō-grăft] hetero-, other + graft	Skin graft using donor skin from one species to another.
homograft	[HŌ-mō-grăft] homo-, alike + graft	Skin graft using donor skin from one person to another.
Moh's surgery	[mōz]	Removal of thin layers of malignant tissue until nonmalignant tissue is found.
plastic surgery		Repair or reconstruction (as of the skin) by means of surgery.
skin graft		Placement of fresh skin over a damaged area.
xenograft	[ZĔN-ō-grăft] xeno-, foreign + graft	*See* heterograft.

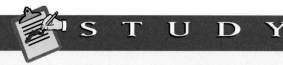

Skin Biopsy

Dr. Lin has hospital hours scheduled for tomorrow morning. He will see two patients in the one-day surgery unit for minor operations. The first patient is to have cryo-surgery for removal of several moles. Later, Dr. Lin will take a biopsy from a suspicious-looking skin patch of a patient who was treated earlier for a basal cell carcinoma. The pathology report follows:

```
The specimen consists of
two ellipses of skin, each
stated to be from the left
upper arm. The larger mea-
sures 1.7 x 0.7 cm. and
has a slightly raised and
roughened outer surface.
Sections of skin exhibit
a dermal nodular lesion
consisting of interlacing
bundles of elongated cells
surrounded by fibrous
stroma.
```

🔆 Critical Thinking

81. If the patch turns out to be a malignant melanoma, will that be more serious than the patient's earlier diagnosis?

82. What steps can you take to avoid permanent skin damage?

Surgical Terms Exercises

Build Your Medical Vocabulary

83. Tattoos can be removed through _____.

84. The repair of various conditions or the changing of one's appearance surgically is called _____ surgery.

85. Cauterizing a wound helps to stop _____.

86. The use of one's own skin to cover a wound is called a/an _____.

87. The use of someone else's skin to cover a wound is called a/an_____ or _____.

Pharmacological Terms

Treatment of skin disorders involves the use of various medications. A wide variety of topical preparations can relieve symptoms and even kill agents that cause disease. Other treatments involve heat, light, and radiation. Cancer of the skin is sometimes successfully treated by **chemotherapy.** In some cases, chemotherapy is combined with **radiation therapy.** Chemotherapy uses chemicals that destroy the malignant cells. Radiation destroys malignant cells by bombarding them with ionizing radiation.

The sun is beneficial in healing certain skin problems. Some lesions are treated with **ultraviolet light,** which imitates some of the sun's rays. On the other hand, sunlight may also be the cause of many skin problems, such as certain carcinomas.

Antihistamines are medications used to control allergic skin reactions. They do so by blocking the effects of *histamines*, chemicals present in tissues that heighten allergic reactions. Other skin conditions are controlled by different medications. For example, **antibiotics** kill or slow the growth of microorganisms on the skin. **Antiseptics** perform the same function. **Antifungals** and **antibacterials** kill or slow the growth of fungal infections. **Parasiticides** destroy insect parasites, such as lice and mites, that cause some skin conditions. **Anti-inflammatory** agents, particularly **corticosteroids,** reduce inflammation, and **antipruritics** control itching. Some skin conditions are painful because of nerve conduction near the skin surface. An **anesthetic** (especially, in the case of surface pain, a **topical anesthetic**) can relieve some of the pain associated with such conditions.

Some skin conditions result in either oversecretion of oils or extreme dryness. **Emollients** are agents that soothe or soften skin by moistening it or adding oils to it. **Astringents** temporarily lessen the formation of oily material on the surface of the skin. These types of agents are often present in over-the-counter products. Other vitamin-based products to control skin aging (often containing Vitamins A and C) are also often available over the counter. **Keratolytics** remove warts and corns from the skin surface. **Alpha-hydroxy acids** are fruit acids added to cosmetics to improve the skin's appearance. Table 4-1 lists drugs commonly used in treating skin conditions.

Table 4-1 Medications used to treat skin disorders

Drug Class	Purpose	Generic Name	Trade Name
anesthetic	to relieve pain	benzocaine	Anbesol, Orajel, Spec-T Anesthetic
		dibucaine	Nupercainal
antifungal	to slow or stop fungi growth	tolnaftate	Absorbine, Desenex, Tinactin
		clotrimazole	Lotrimin
antihistamine	to slow, stop, or prevent an allergic	diphenhydramine	Allerdryl, AllerMax, Benadryl, Benylin
		loratidine	Claritin
anti-infective	to relieve symptoms of infection	neomycin	Myciguent
		bacitracin	Neosporin
antipruritic	to relieve itching	hydrocortisone	Bactine Hydrocortisone, Caldecort, Cortaid, Hydrocortone
anti-inflammatory (corticosteroid)	to reduce inflammation	triamcinolone	Aristocort, Triamolone, Tri-Kort

Vocabulary Review

In the previous section, you learned terms relating to pharmacology. Before going on to the exercises, review the terms below and refer to the previous section if you have questions.

Term	Word Analysis	Definition
alpha-hydroxy acid	[ĂL-fă-hī-DRŎK-sē]	Agent added to cosmetics to improve the skin's appearance.
anesthetic	[ăn-ĕs-THĔT-ĭk] Greek *anaisthesia*, without sensation	Agent that relieves pain by blocking nerve sensations.
antibacterial	[ĂN-tē-băk-TĒR-ē-ăl] anti-, against + bacteria	Agent that kills or slows the growth of bacteria.
antibiotic	[ĂN-tē-bī-ŎT-ĭk] anti-, against + Greek *biosis*, life	Agent that kills or slows the growth of microorganisms.
antifungal	[ĂN-tē-FŬNG-găl] anti-, against + fungal	Agent that kills or slows the growth of fungi.
antihistamine	[ĂN-tē-HĬS-tă-mēn] anti-, against + histamine	Agent that controls allergic reactions by blocking the effectiveness of histamines in the body.
anti-inflammatory		Agent that relieves the symptoms of inflammations.
antipruritic	[ĂN-tē-prū-RĬT-ĭk] anti-, against + pruritic, relating to pruritus	Agent that controls itching.
antiseptic		Agent that kills or slows the growth of microorganisms.
astringent	[ăs-TRĬN-jĕnt]	Agent that removes excess oils and impurities from the surface of skin.
chemotherapy	[KĒ-mō-thār-ă-pē] chemo-, chemistry + therapy	Treatment of cancer that uses chemicals to destroy malignant cells.
corticosteroid	[KŌR-tĭ-kō-STĒR-ŏyd] cortico-, adrenal cortex + steroid	Agent with anti-inflammatory properties.
emollient	[ē-MŎL-ē-ĕnt]	Agent that smooths or softens skin.
keratolytic	[KĔR-ă-tō-LĬT-ĭk] kerato- + -lytic	Agent that aids in the removal of warts and corns.

Term	Word Analysis	Definition
parasiticide	[păr-ă-SĬT-ĭ-sīd] parasit(e) + -cide, killing	Agent that kills or slows the growth of parasites.
radiation therapy		Treatment of cancer that uses ionizing radiation to destroy malignant cells.
topical anesthetic		Anesthetic applied to the surface of the skin.
ultraviolet light	[ŭl-tră-VĪ-ō-lĕt]	Artificial sunlight used to treat some skin lesions.

CASE STUDY

Providing Relief

Dr. Lin has several patients in their mid-fifties who are concerned about dry skin, age spots, and wrinkling. One patient has dry skin with severe pruritus. Her skin is extremely rough in spots. Dr. Lin suggests that there may be a hormonal cause, since the patient is in menopause and since the production of hormones decreases during and after menopause. He refers her to her gynecologist. Meanwhile, he prescribes something to control the pruritus. Another patient is a young child with an allergic rash. The doctor writes the following prescriptions.

Critical Thinking

88. Prescription A is for which patient?

89. Prescription B is for what condition?

Dr. A. Lin
145 West 20th Street • Chicago, IL 55555 • (999)111–2222
PATIENT'S NAME _Michele Cortez_ AGE _53_
ADDRESS _____
CITY _____ DATE _9/1/XX_
℞
  Hydrocortisone ointment 0.5%, apply to affected area, q.i.d. for 2 wks.

LICENSE NO. 555   SIGNATURE _A. Lin, M.D._
(a)

Dr. A. Lin
145 West 20th Street • Chicago, IL 55555 • (999)111–2222
PATIENT'S NAME _Chester Banks_ AGE _6_
ADDRESS _____
CITY _____ DATE _9/1/XX_
℞
  Diphenhydramine lotion 1%, apply to affected area, b.i.d. for 1 wk.

LICENSE NO. 555   SIGNATURE _A. Lin, M.D._
(b)

Pharmacological Terms Exercises

Build Your Medical Vocabulary

Find and define at least one word part in each of the following words.

90. antiseptic

91. antipruritic

92. chemotherapy

93. fungicide

94. mycocide

95. keratolysis

Check Your Knowledge

Circle T for true or F for false.

96. Chemotherapy is the use of radiation to treat cancer. T F

97. Antibiotics are used to treat acne. T F

98. Histamines are always present in the body. T F

99. Astringents control pruritus. T F

100. Emollients can contain oils. T F

CHALLENGE SECTION

Dr. Lin has a patient with diabetes. Notes on the patient's chart are as follows:

Patient is a 48-year-old female with a history of diabetes. Patient noticed localized edema on lower aspect of leg. Area is very red and feels hot to the touch. The skin has the dimpled appearance *(peau d'orange)* of the outside of an orange, and appears "stretched." Patient has fever, chills, and headache. Also, patient feels fatigued.

Dr. Lin orders a CBC that shows an elevated WBC, indicating a bacterial infection. No pus has formed in the area. There is an indication of swollen lymph nodes. Treatment includes antibiotic (penicillin V 250 mg q.i.d. for 10–14 days), bed rest, and elevation of infected area with warm, moist compresses 6x daily.

Challenge Section Exercises

101. The patient has a diagnosis of cellulitis. What does that mean? Is it potentially dangerous if untreated?

102. What could happen if the patient feels better and stops the antibiotic early?

CHAPTER REVIEW

Definitions

Define the following terms and combining forms. Review the chapter before starting, and check your answers by looking in the vocabulary reviews in this chapter. Make sure you know how to pronounce each term.

Term	Definition
abscess [ĂB-sĕs]	
acne [ĂK-nē]	
acne vulgaris [ĂK-nē vŭl-GĀR-ĕs]	
actinic keratosis [ăk-TĬN-ĭk KĔR-ă-tō-sĭs]	
adip(o)	
adipose [ĂD-ĭ-pōs]	
allograft [ĂL-ō-grăft]	
albinism [ĂL-bĭ-nĭzm]	
alopecia [ăl-ō-PĒ-shē-ă]	
alopecia areata [ăl-ō-PĒ-shē-ă ā-rē-Ā-tă]	
alpha-hydroxy [ĂL-fă-hī-DRŎK-sē] acid	
anesthetic [ăn-ĕs-THĔT-ĭk]	
antibacterial [ĂN-tē-băk-TĒR-ē-ăl]	
antibiotic [ĂN-tē-bī-ŎT-ĭk]	
antifungal [ĂN-tē-FŬNG-ăl]	
antihistamine [ĂN-tē-HĬS-tă-mēn]	
anti-inflammatory	
antipruritic [ĂN-tē-prū-RĬT-ĭk]	
antiseptic	
apocrine [ĂP-ō-krĭn] gland	
astringent [ăs-TRĬN-jĕnt]	
autograft [ĂW-tō-grăft]	
basal cell carcinoma	

Term	Definition
biopsy [BĪ-ŏp-sē]	
birthmark	
blackhead	
bulla (pl. bullae) [BŬL-ă (BŬL-ī)]	
burn	
callus [KĂL-ŭs]	
candidiasis [kăn-dĭ-DĪ-ă-sĭs]	
carbuncle [KĂR-bŭng-kl]	
cauterize [KĂW-tĕr-īz]	
cellulitis [sĕl-yū-LĪ-tĭs]	
chemotherapy [KĒ-mō-thār-ă-pē]	
chloasma [klō-ĂZ-mă]	
cicatrix [SĬK-ă-trĭks]	
cold sore	
collagen [KŎL-lă-jĕn]	
comedo (pl. comedos, comedones) [KŎM-ē-dō, kō-MĒ-dō (KŎM-ē-dōz, kō-mē-DŌ-nĕz)]	
corium [KŌ-rē-ŭm]	
corn	
corticosteroid [KŌR-tĭ-kō-STĒR-ŏyd]	
crust	
cryosurgery [KRĪ-ō-SĔR-jĕr-ē]	
curettage [kyū-rĕ-TĂHZH]	
cuticle [KYŪ-tĭ-kl]	
cyst [sĭst]	
debridement [dā-brēd-MŎN]	
decubitus (pl. decubiti) [dĕ-KYŪ-bĭ-tŭs (dĕ-KYŪ-bĭ-tī)] ulcer	
depigmentation [dē-pĭg-mĕn-TĀ-shŭn]	
dermabrasion [dĕr-mă-BRĀ-zhŭn]	
dermatitis [dĕr-mă-TĪ-tĭs]	
dermat(o)	
dermatology [dĕr-mă-TŎL-ō-jē]	
dermis [DĔR-mĭs]	

Term	Definition
derm(o)	
diaphoresis [DĪ-ă-fō-RĒ-sĭs]	
discoid lupus erythematosus (DLE) [DĬS-kŏyd LŪ-pŭs ĕr-ĭ-THĔM-ă-tō-sŭs]	
ecchymosis (pl. ecchymoses) [ĕk-ĭ-MŌ-sĭs (ĕk-ĭ-MŌ-sēz)]	
eccrine [ĔK-rĭn] glands	
eczema [ĔK-zē-mă]	
electrodesiccation [ē-LĔK-trō-dĕs-ĭ-KĀ-shŭn]	
emollient [ē-MŎL-ē-ĕnt]	
epidermis [ĕp-ĭ-DĔRM-ĭs]	
erosion	
exanthematous [ĕks-zăn-THĔM-ă-tŭs] viral disease	
excoriation [ĕks-KŌ-rē-Ā-shŭn]	
exocrine [ĔK-sō-krĭn] glands	
exudate [ĔKS-yū-dāt]	
fever blister	
first-degree burn	
fissure [FĬSH-ŭr]	
fulguration [fŭl-gŭ-RĀ-shŭn]	
furuncle [FYŪ-rŭng-kl]	
gangrene [GĂNG-grēn]	
genital herpes	
hair follicle [FŎL-ĭ-kl]	
hair root	
hair shaft	
herpes [HĔR-pēz]	
herpes simplex virus Type 1	
herpes simplex virus Type 2	
herpes zoster [ZŎS-tĕr]	
heterograft [HĔT-ĕr-ō-grăft]	
hidr(o)	
hives	

Term	Definition
homograft [HŌ-mō-grăft]	
hypodermis [hĭ-pō-DĚR-mĭs]	
ichthy(o)	
impetigo [ĭm-pĕ-TĪ-gō]	
integument [ĭn-TĚG-yū-mĕnt]	
intradermal [ĭn-tră-DĚR-măl]	
Kaposi's [KĂ-pō-sēz] sarcoma	
keloid [KĒ-lŏyd]	
keratin [KĚR-ă-tĭn]	
kerat(o)	
keratolytic [KĚR-ā-tō-LĪT-ĭk]	
kcratosis [kcr-ă-TŌ-sĭs]	
lesion [LĒ-shŭn]	
leukoderma [lū-kō-DĚR-mă]	
leukoplakia [lū-kō-PLĀ-kē-ă]	
lip(o)	
lunula (pl. lunulae) [LŪ-nū-lă (LŪ-nū-lē)]	
macule [MĂK-yūl]	
malignant melanoma	
Mantoux [măn-TŪ] test	
melan(o)	
melanin [MĚL-ă-nĭn]	
melanocyte [MĚL-ă-nō-sīt]	
Moh's [mōz] surgery	
myc(o)	
nail	
neoplasm [NĒ-ō-plăzm]	
nevus (pl. nevi) [NĒ-vŭs (NĒ-vī)]	
nodule [NŎD-yūl]	
onych(o)	
onychia, onychitis [ō-NĬK-ē-ă, ŏn-ĭ-KĪ-tĭs]	
onychopathy [ŏn-ĭ-KŎP-ă-thē]	
papillary [PĂP-ĭ-lār-ē] layer	

Term	Definition
papule [PĂP-yūl]	
parasiticide [păr-ă-SĬT-ĭ-sīd]	
paronychia [păr-ŏ-NĬK-ē-ă]	
patch	
patch test	
pediculated [pĕ-DĬK-yū-lā-tĕd] polyp	
pediculosis [pĕ-DĬK-yū-lō-sĭs]	
pemphigus [PĔM-fĭ-gŭs]	
petechia (pl. petechiae) [pē-TĒ-kē-ă, pē-TĔK-ē-ă (pē-TĒ-kē-ē)]	
pil(o)	
pilonidal [pī-lō-NĪ-dăl] cyst	
plantar [PLĂN-tăr] wart	
plaque [plăk]	
plastic surgery	
polyp [PŎL-ĭp]	
pore	
pressure sore	
pruritus [prū-RĪ-tŭs]	
psoriasis [sō-RĪ-ă-sĭs]	
purpura [PŬR-pū-ră]	
pustule [PŬS-tūl]	
pyoderma [pī-ō-DĔR-mă]	
radiation therapy	
reticular [rĕ-TĬK-ū-lăr] layer	
ringworm	
rosacea [rō-ZĀ-shē-ă]	
roseola [rō-ZĒ-ō-lă]	
rubella [rū-BĔL-ă]	
rubeola [rū-BĒ-ō-lă]	
scabies [SKĀ-bēz]	
scale	
Schick test	
scleroderma [sklēr-ō-DĔR-mă]	

Term	Definition
scratch test	
sebaceous [sĕ-BĀ-shŭs] cyst	
sebaceous glands	
seb(o)	
seborrhea [sĕb-ō-RĒ-ă]	
sebum [SĒ-bŭm]	
second-degree burn	
sessile [SĔS-ĭl] polyp	
shingles [SHĬN-glz]	
skin graft	
squamous cell carcinoma	
squamous epithelium [SKWĂ-mŭs ĕp-ĭ-THĒ-lē-ŭm]	
steat(o)	
stratified squamous epithelium	
stratum (pl. strata)[STRĂT-ŭm (STRĂ-tă)]	
stratum corneum [KŌR-nē-ŭm]	
stratum germinativum [jĕr-mĭ-NĀT-ĭ-vŭm]	
striae [STRĪ-ē]	
subcutaneous [sŭb-kyū-TĀ-nē-ŭs] layer	
sweat glands	
systemic lupus erythematosus (SLE)	
third-degree burn	
tine [tīn] test	
tinea [TĬN-ē-ă]	
topical anesthetic	
trich(o)	
tumor [TŪ-mŏr]	
ulcer [ŬL-sĕr]	
ultraviolet [ŭl-tră-VĪ-ō-lĕt] light	
urticaria [ĔR-tĭ-KĀR-ē-ă]	
varicella [vār-ĭ-SĔL-ă]	
vascular lesion	

Term	Definition
verruca (pl. verrucae) [vĕ-RŪ-kă (vĕ-RŪ-kē)]	
vesicle [VĔS-ĭ-kl]	
vitiligo [vĭt-ĭ-LĪ-gō]	
wart [wōrt]	
wheal [hwēl]	
whitehead [HWĪT-hĕd]	
xanth(o)	
xenograft [ZĔN-ō-grăft]	
xer(o)	

Abbreviations

Write the full meaning of each abbreviation.

Abbreviation	Meaning
bx	
DLE	
PPD	
PUVA	
SLE	

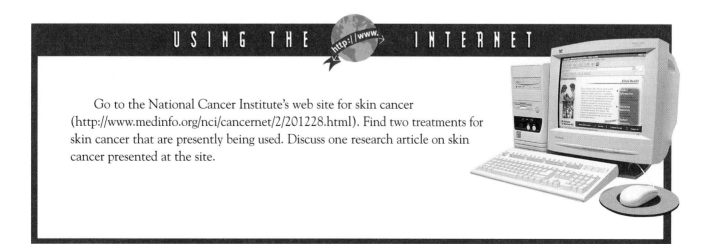

USING THE http://www. INTERNET

Go to the National Cancer Institute's web site for skin cancer (http://www.medinfo.org/nci/cancernet/2/201228.html). Find two treatments for skin cancer that are presently being used. Discuss one research article on skin cancer presented at the site.

Answers to Chapter Exercises

1. He is a diabetic and has a stubborn skin rash, which may become infected.
2. symptoms
3. a. 3; b. 1; c. 2
4. apocrine, eccrine, and exocrine
5. a. epidermis
   b. stratum corneum
   c. hair follicle
   d. sebaceous gland
   e. subcutaneous layer
6. cuticle
7. epidermis
8. epidermis
9. papillary layer
10. eccrine
11. adipose
12. healthy
13. lunula
14. sebum
15. apocrine
16. Family history can give clues to hereditary disorders.
17. No, only a medical doctor may order prescription medication whether in sample form or not.
18. dermatoplasty
19. dermophlebitis
20. keratoderma
21. mycodermatitis
22. melanoderma
23. onychomycosis
24. onychoplasty
25. pilosebaceous
26. melanocyte
27. trichoscopy
28. lipotomy
29. adipocellular
30. trichology
31. onychopathy
32. mycotoxin
33. mycovirus

34. xanthoderma
35. xerosis
36. keratolysis
37. melanoderma
38. hidromeiosis
39. tricho-, hair + -oma tumor
40. xer(o)-, dry + -osis, condition
41. myco-, fungus + - cide, killing
42. xantho-, yellow + - derma, skin
43. onych(o)-, nail + - oid, resembling
44. Patient does not have allergies to the allergens being tested.
45. The rashes would subside or even disappear.
46. F
47. T
48. T
49. F
50. T
51. fungi
52. exudate
53. allergies
54. intradermal
55. Washing helps to remove excess sebum from the skin.
56. Hormonal changes that occur as one ages affect the occurrence of acne.
57. pemphigus
58. C
59. purpura
60. C
61. roseola
62. -itis
63. -osis
64. -oma
65. -pathy
66. -derma
67. F

68. F
69. F
70. T
71. T
72. F
73. T
74. F
75. T
76. T
77. heredity or medication
78. mites
79. mouth
80. genitalia
81. yes
82. Avoid baking in the sun; use protectant lotions; wear a hat outside.
83. dermabrasion
84. plastic
85. bleeding
86. autograft
87. allograft/homograft
88. for the woman
89. allergic rash
90. anti-, against
91. anti-, against
92. chemo-, chemistry
93. fungi-, fungus/-cide, killing
94. myco-, fungus/-cide, killing
95. kerato-, horny tissue/-lysis, destruction of
96. F
97. T
98. T
99. F
100. T
101. Inflammation of the dermis and subcutaneous skin layers. Yes, infection can spread via bloodstream
102. The infection will not be destroyed and may recur.

CHAPTER 5

The Musculoskeletal System

After studying this chapter you will be able to:

- ◆ Name the parts of the musculoskeletal system and discuss the function of each part

- ◆ Define combining forms used in building words that relate to the musculoskeletal system

- ◆ Identify the meaning of related abbreviations

- ◆ Name the common diagnoses, laboratory tests, and clinical procedures used in treating the musculoskeletal system

- ◆ Define the major pathological conditions of the musculoskeletal system

- ◆ Define surgical terms related to the musculoskeletal system

- ◆ List common pharmacological agents used in treating the musculoskeletal system

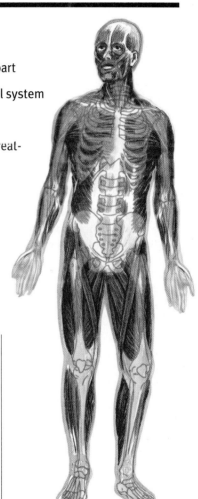

Structure And Function

The **musculoskeletal system** forms the framework that holds the body together, enables it to move, and protects and supports all the internal organs. This system includes **bones, joints,** and **muscles.** Figure 5-1 shows the musculoskeletal system.

Bones are made of **osseous tissue** and include a rich network of blood vessels and nerves. The cells of bone, called **osteocytes,** are part of a dense network of connective tissue. The cells themselves are surrounded by calcium salts. During fetal development, bones are softer and flexible and are composed of **cartilage** until the hardening process begins. Bone-forming cells are called **osteoblasts.** As bone tissue develops, some of it dies and is reabsorbed by **osteoclasts** (also called **bone phagocytes**). The reabsorption of dead bone cells prevents the bone from becoming overly thick and heavy. Later, if a bone breaks, osteoblasts will add new mineral matter to repair the break and the osteoclasts will remove any bone debris, thereby smoothing over the break. The hardening process and development of the osteocytes is called **ossification.** This process is largely dependent on **calcium, phosphorus,** and **vitamin D.**

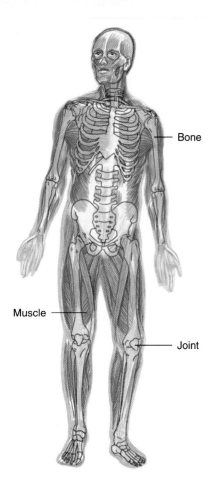

Figure 5-1 **Muscles and bones hold the body together, enable it to move and protect the internal organs.**

In Latin, the word *foramen* means an opening.

The **skeleton** of the body is made up of bones and joints. A mature adult has 206 bones that work together with joints and muscles to move the various parts of the body. The *axial* portion of the skeleton includes the trunk and head. The *appendicular* portion of the skeleton includes the limbs.

Bones

There are many types of bones. The five most common categories include **long bones, short bones, flat bones, irregular bones,** and **sesamoid bones.** Long bones form the extremities of the body. The legs and arms include this type of bone. The longest portion of a long bone is called the shaft. The outer portion is **compact bone,** solid bone that does not bend easily. Compact bone is where oxygen and nutrients are brought from the bloodstream to the bone. This shaft is also called the **diaphysis** or place where bone growth occurs first. Each end of the shaft has an area shaped to connect to other bones by means of ligaments and muscle. These ends are called the *proximal epiphysis* and the *distal epiphysis*. As long bones grow, the **metaphysis,** the space between the diaphysis and the two epiphyses, develops. The **epiphyseal plate** is cartilaginous tissue that is replaced during growth years, but eventually calcifies and disappears when growth has stopped. The epiphysis is covered by **articular cartilage,** a thin, flexible substance that provides protection at movable points. Inside the compact bone is **cancellous bone** (which has a latticelike structure and is also called **spongy bone**) that covers the **medullary cavity** or empty space in which **marrow** is stored. Spongy bone is also in the epiphyses. The medullary cavity has a lining called the **endosteum.** The outside of the bone is covered by a fibrous membrane called the **periosteum.** Figure 5-2 shows the parts of long bones.

Short bones are the small, cube-shaped bones of the wrists, ankles, and toes. Short bones consist of an outer layer of compact bone with an inner layer of cancellous bone.

Flat bones generally have large, somewhat flat surfaces that cover organs or that provide a surface for large areas of muscle. The shoulder blades, pelvis, and skull include flat bones.

Irregular bones are specialized bones with specific shapes. The bones of the ears, vertebrae, and face are irregular bones.

Sesamoid bones are bones formed in a tendon near joints. The patella (kneecap) is a sesamoid bone. Sesamoid bones are also found in the hands and feet.

Commonly, bones have various extensions and depressions that serve as sites for attaching muscles and tendons. Bone extensions are the **bone head,** the end of a bone, often rounded, that attaches to other bones or connective material; the **crest,** a bony ridge; the **process,** any bony projection; the **tubercle,** a slight elevation on a bone's surface where muscles or ligaments are attached; the **trochanter,** a bony extension near the upper end of the femur; a **tuberosity,** a large elevation on the surface of a bone; and a **condyle,** a rounded surface protrusion at the end of a bone, usually where it articulates with another bone. Depressions in bone are a **fossa,** a pit in bone; a **foramen,** an opening through bone; a **fissure,** a deep cleft in bone; a **sulcus,** a groove or furrow on the surface of a bone; and a **sinus,** a hollow space or cavity in a bone. Figure 5-3 shows the types of bone extensions.

Marrow is soft connective tissue and serves important functions in the production of blood cells. *Red bone marrow* is generally found in infant bones and in the flat bones of adults. It is the site where red blood cells start to develop.

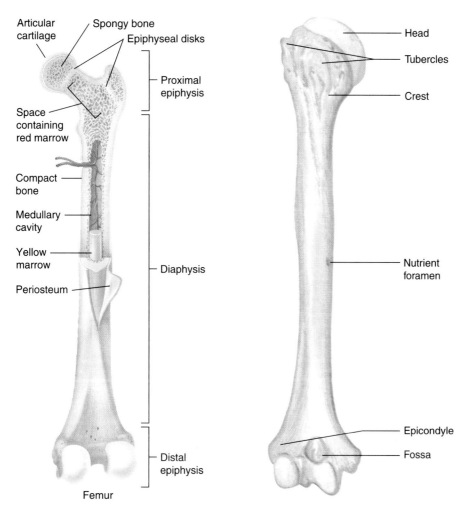

Figure 5-2 Parts of a long bone. The legs and arms are made up of long bones.

Labels for Figure 5-2:
Articular cartilage · Spongy bone · Epiphyseal disks · Proximal epiphysis · Space containing red marrow · Compact bone · Medullary cavity · Yellow marrow · Periosteum · Diaphysis · Distal epiphysis · Femur

Figure 5-3 Bone extensions allow each bone to connect to other bones.

Labels for Figure 5-3:
Head · Tubercles · Crest · Nutrient foramen · Epicondyle · Fossa

Yellow bone marrow is found in most other adult bones and is made up of connective tissue filled with fat.

Bones of the Head

Cranial bones form the skull, which protects the brain and the structures inside the skull. The skull or cranial bones join at points called **sutures.** The skull of a newborn is not completely joined and has soft spots, called **fontanelles.** The skull contains the **frontal bone** (the forehead and roof of the eye sockets), the **ethmoid bone** (the nasal cavity and the orbits of the eyes), the **parietal bone** (top and upper parts of the sides of the skull), and the **temporal bone** (lower part of the skull and the lower sides, including the openings for the ears). The **temporomandibular joint (TMJ)** is the connection point for the temporal bone and the mandible (lower jawbone). A round extension behind the temporal bone is the **mastoid process.** It sits behind the ear. The **styloid process** is a peg-shaped protrusion from a bone, as the one that extends down from the temporal bone. The back and base of the skull are covered by the **occipital bone.** An opening in the occipital bone, the **foramen magnum,** is the structure through which the spinal cord passes. The skull bones are held together by the **sphenoid bone,** which joins the frontal, occipital, and ethmoid bones and forms the base of the cranium. The pituitary gland sits in the **sella turcica,** a depression in the sphenoid bone.

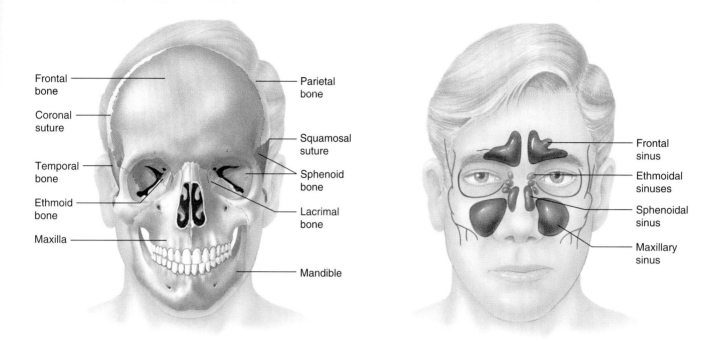

Figure 5-4 Cavities in the skull make the skull lighter.

The skull has sinuses, specific cavities that reduce its weight. The **frontal sinuses** are above the eyes. The **sphenoid sinus** is above and behind the nose. The **ethmoid sinuses** are a group of small sinuses on both sides of the nasal cavities, between each eye and the sphenoid sinus. The **maxillary sinuses** are on either side of the **nasal cavity** below the eyes. Figure 5-4 shows the bones of the skull and the location of the sinuses.

The head also has facial bones, each with a specific function. **Nasal bones** form the bridge of the nose; **lacrimal bones** hold the lacrimal gland and the canals for the tear ducts; the **mandibular bone** or **mandible** is the lower jaw-bone and contains the sockets for the lower teeth. The mandible is the only movable bone in the face. **Maxillary bones** form the upper jawbone and contain the sockets for the upper teeth. The **vomer** is a flat bone that joins with the ethmoid bone to form the nasal septum, and **zygomatic bones** form the prominent shape of the cheek. The **palatine bone** sits behind the maxillary bones and helps to form the nasal cavity and the hard palate. Figure 5-5 shows the bones of the face.

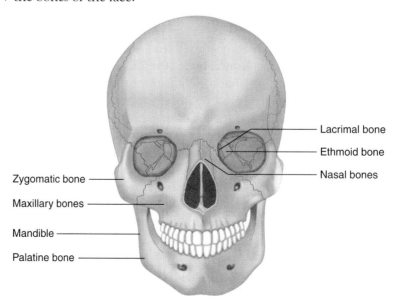

Figure 5-5 Facial bones form cavities and supports that allow facial movement and functioning.

Spinal Column

The **spinal column** (also called the **vertebral column**) consists of five sets of **vertebrae.** Each vertebra is a bone segment with a thick, **cartilaginous disk** (also called *intervertebral disk* or **disk,** sometimes spelled **disc**) that separates the vertebrae. In the middle of the disk is a fibrous mass called the **nucleus pulposus.** The disks cushion the vertebrae and help in movement and flexibility of the spinal column. The space between the **vertebral body** and the back of the vertebra is called the **neural canal.** This is the space through which the spinal cord passes. At the back of the vertebra, the **spinous process, transverse process,** and **lamina** form the posterior side of the spinal column.

The five divisions of vertebrae are: (1) the **cervical vertebrae,** the seven vertebrae of the neck bone, which include the first vertebra, called the **atlas,** and the second vertebra, called the **axis;** (2) the **thoracic vertebrae** (also called the **dorsal vertebrae**), the twelve vertebrae that connect to the ribs; (3) the **lumbar vertebrae,** the five bones of the middle back; (4) the **sacrum,** the curved bone of the lower back, consisting of five separate bones at birth that fuse together in early childhood; and (5) the **coccyx,** the tailbone, formed from four bones fused together. Figure 5-6 shows the divisions of the spinal column.

Bones of the Chest

At the top of the **thorax** (chest cavity) are the **clavicle** (anterior collar bone) and **scapula** (posterior shoulder bone). The scapula joins with the clavicle at a point called the **acromion.** Next is the **sternum** (breastbone), which extends down the middle of the chest. Extending out from the sternum are the twelve pairs of **ribs.** The first seven pairs of ribs, the **true ribs,** are joined both to the vertebral column and to the sternum by costal cartilage. The next three pairs of ribs, called *false ribs*, attach to the vertebral column but not to the sternum. Instead, they join the seventh rib. The last two ribs, which are also called false ribs, are known as *floating ribs* because they do not attach to the sternum anteriorly.

Bones of the Pelvis

Below the thoracic cavity is the pelvic area. The **pelvic girdle** is a large bone that forms the hips and supports the trunk of the body. It is composed of

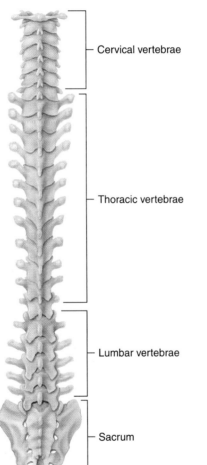

Figure 5-6 The spinal column is divided into five groups of vertebrae.

- Cervical vertebrae
- Thoracic vertebrae
- Lumbar vertebrae
- Sacrum
- Coccyx

three fused bones, including the **ilium, ischium,** and **pubes** (the anteroinferior portion of the hip bone). It is also the point of attachment for the legs. Inside the pelvic girdle is the **pelvic cavity.** In the pelvic cavity are located the female reproductive organs, the sigmoid colon, the bladder, and the rectum. The area where the two pubic bones join is called the **pubic symphysis.**

Bones of the Extremities

The upper arm bone, the **humerus,** attaches to the scapula and clavicle. The two lower arm bones are the **ulna,** which has a bony protrusion called the **olecranon (elbow),** and the **radius,** which attaches to the eight **carpals,** the wrist bones. The **metacarpals** are the five bones of the palm that radiate out to the finger bones, the **phalanges.** Each **phalanx** (except for the thumbs and great toes) has a *distal* (furthest from the body), *middle,* and *proximal* (nearest to the body) segment.

The hip bone has a cup-shaped depression or socket called the **acetabulum** into which the **femur** (thigh bone) fits. The femur is the longest bone in the body. It meets the two bones of the lower leg, the **tibia** (also called the **shin**) and **fibula,** at the kneecap or **patella.** The tibia and fibula have bony protrusions near the foot called the **malleoli.** The protrusion of the tibia is called the *medial malleolus.* The protrusion of the fibula is called the *lateral malleolus.* The malleoli and the **tarsals** form the **ankle.** The largest tarsal is the **calcaneus (heel).** The **metatarsals** connect to the phalanges of the toes.

Joints

Joints are also called **articulations,** points where bones connect. The movement at a particular joint varies depending on the body's needs. **Diarthroses** are joints that move freely, such as the knee joint. **Amphiarthroses** are cartilaginous joints that move slightly, such as the joints between vertebrae. **Synarthroses** do not move; examples are the fibrous joints between the skull bones. **Symphyses** are cartilaginous joints that unite two bones firmly; an example is the pubic symphysis. Bones are connected to other bones with **ligaments,** bands of fibrous tissue. **Tendons** are bands of fibrous tissue that connect muscles to bone. Movement takes place at the joints using the muscles, ligaments, and tendons. **Synovial joints** are covered with a **synovial membrane,** which secretes **synovial fluid,** a joint lubricant, and which helps the joint move easily. The hip joint is an example of a synovial joint. Some spaces between tendons and joints have a **bursa,** a sac lined with a synovial membrane. Bursae help the movement of hands and feet. Figure 5-7 shows the parts of a joint.

Muscles

Muscles contract and extend to provide body movement. The **voluntary (striated) muscles** can be contracted at will. These muscles are called skeletal muscles, as they are responsible for the movement of all skeletal bones, including facial bones, such as the mandible. The **involuntary (smooth or visceral) muscles** control movement that is not controlled by

Figure 5-7 The range of joint movement depends on the purpose of the joint.

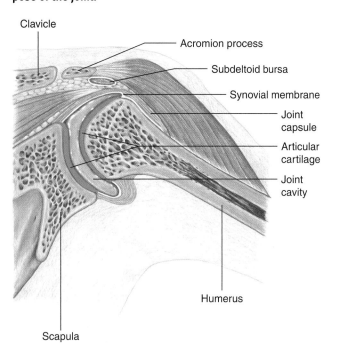

Clavicle

Acromion process

Subdeltoid bursa

Synovial membrane

Joint capsule

Articular cartilage

Joint cavity

Humerus

Scapula

will, such as respiration, urination, and digestion. Involuntary muscles move the internal organs and systems, such as the digestive system and the blood. **Cardiac muscle,** which controls the contractions of the heart, is the only involuntary muscle that is also striated. Most muscles are covered by **fascia,** a band of connective tissue that supports and covers the muscle. Muscles attach to a stationary bone at a point called the **origin.** They attach to a movable bone at a point called the **insertion.** Figure 5-8 shows the various types of muscle.

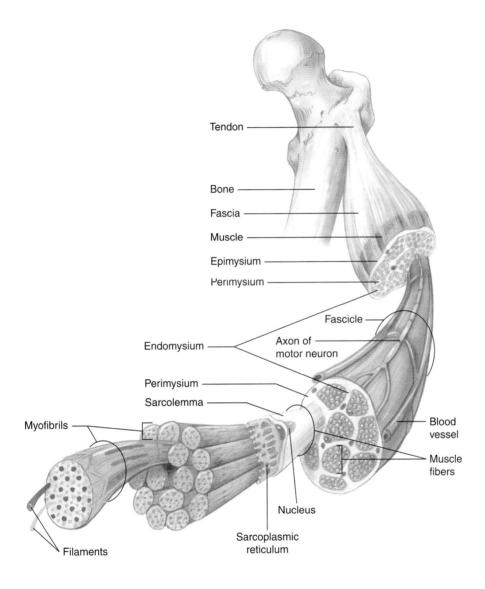

Figure 5-8 Muscles are the primary elements in body movement.

Vocabulary Review

In the previous section, you learned terms relating to the musculoskeletal system. Before going on to the exercises, review the terms below and refer to the previous section if you have any questions.

Term	Word Analysis	Definition
acetabulum	[ăs-ĕ-TĂB-yū-lŭm]	Cup-shaped depression in the hip bone into which the top of the femur fits.

Term	Word Analysis	Definition
acromion	[ă-KRŌ-mē-ōn]	Part of the scapula that connects to the clavicle.
amphiarthrosis (pl. amphiarthroses)	[ĂM-fĭ-ăr-THRŌ-sĭs (pl. -sēs)] Greek *amphi-*, both + *arthrosis*, joint	Cartilaginous joint having some movement at the union of two bones.
ankle	[ĂNG-kl]	Hinged area between the lower leg bones and the bones of the foot.
articular cartilage	[ăr-TĬK-yū-lăr]	Cartilage at a joint.
articulation	[ăr-tĭk-yū-LĀ-shŭn]	Point at which two bones join together to allow movement.
atlas	[ĂT-lăs]	First cervical vertebra.
axis	[ĂK-sĭs]	Second cervical vertebra.
bone		Hard connective tissue that forms the skeleton of the body.
bone head		Upper, rounded end of a bone.
bone phagocyte	[FĂG-ō-sīt]	Bone cell that ingests dead bone and bone debris.
bursa	[BĔR-să]	Sac lined with a synovial membrane that fills the spaces between tendons and joints.
calcaneus	[kăl-KĀ-nē-ŭs]	Heel bone.
calcium	[KĂL-sē-ŭm]	Mineral important in the formation of bone.
cancellous bone	[KĂN-sĕ-lŭs]	Spongy bone with a latticelike structure.
cardiac muscle	[KĂR-dē-ăk]	Striated involuntary muscle of the heart.
carpus, carpal bone	[KĂR-pŭs, KĂR-păl]	Wrist bone.
cartilage	[KĂR-tĭ-lĭj]	Flexible connective tissue found in joints, fetal skeleton, and the lining of various parts of the body.
cartilaginous disk	[kăr-tĭ-LĂJ-ĭ-nŭs]	Thin, circular mass of cartilage between the vertebrae of the spinal column.
cervical vertebrae	[SĔR-vĭ-kăl]	Seven vertebrae of the spinal column located in the neck.
clavicle	[KLĂV-ĭ-kl]	Curved bone of the shoulder that joins to the scapula; collar bone.

Term	Word Analysis	Definition
coccyx	[KŎK-sĭks]	Small bone consisting of four fused vertebrae at the end of the spinal column; tailbone.
compact bone		Hard bone with a tightly woven structure.
condyle	[KŎN-dīl]	Rounded surface at the end of a bone.
crest		Bony ridge.
diaphysis	[dī-ĂF-ĭ-sĭs] Greek, a growing between	Long middle section of a long bone; shaft.
diarthroses	[dī-ăr-THRŌ-sēz] Greek, articulations	Freely movable joints.
disk, disc	[dĭsk] Latin *discus*	*See* cartilaginous disk.
dorsal vertebrae		Thoracic vertebrae.
elbow	[ĔL-bō]	Joint between the upper arm and the forearm.
endosteum	[ĕn-DŎS-tē-ŭm] end(o)-, within + Greek *osteon*, bone	Lining of the medullary cavity.
epiphyseal plate	[ĕp-ĭ-FĬZ-ē-ăl]	Cartilaginous tissue that is replaced during growth years, but eventually calcifies and disappears when growth stops.
ethmoid bone	[ĔTH-mŏyd]	Irregular bone of the face attached to the sphenoid bone.
ethmoid sinuses		Sinuses on both sides of the nasal cavities between each eye and the sphenoid sinus.
fascia	[FĂSH-ē-ă]	Sheet of fibrous tissue that encloses muscles.
femur	[FĒ-mŭr]	Long bone of the thigh.
fibula	[FĬB-yū-lă]	Smallest long bone of the lower leg.
fissure	[FĬSH-ŭr]	Deep furrow or slit.
flat bones		Thin, flattened bones that cover certain areas, as of the skull.
fontanelle	[FŎN-tă-nĕl]	Soft, membranous section on top of an infant's skull.

Term	Word Analysis	Definition
foramen	[fō-RĀ-mĕn]	Opening or perforation through a bone.
foramen magnum	[MĂG-nŭm]	Opening in the occipital bone through which the spinal cord passes.
fossa	[FŎS-ă]	Depression, as in a bone.
frontal bone	[FRŬN-tăl]	Large bone of the skull that forms the top of the head and forehead.
frontal sinuses		Sinuses above the eyes.
heel	[hēl]	Back, rounded portion of the foot.
humerus	[HYŪ-mĕr-ŭs]	Long bone of the arm connecting to the scapula on top and the radius and ulna at the bottom.
ilium	[ĬL-ē-ŭm]	Wide portion of the hip bone.
insertion		Point at which muscles attach to a movable bone.
involuntary muscle		Muscle not movable at will.
irregular bones		Any of a group of bones with a special shape to fit into certain areas of the skeleton, such as the skull.
ischium	[ĬS-kē-ŭm]	One of three fused bones that form the pelvic girdle.
joint	[jŏynt]	Place of joining between two or more bones.
lacrimal bone	[LĂK-rĭ-măl]	Thin, flat bone of the face.
lamina (pl. laminae)	[LĂM-ĭ-nă (LĂM-ĭ-nē)]	Thin, flat part of either side of the arch of a vertebra.
ligament	[LĬG-ă-mĕnt]	Sheet of fibrous tissue connecting and supporting bones; attaches bone to bone.
long bone		Any bone of the extremities with a shaft.
lumbar vertebrae	[LŬM-băr]	Five vertebrae of the lower back.
malleolus (pl. malleoli)	[mă-LĒ-ō-lŭs (mă-lē-Ō-lī)]	Rounded protrusion of the tibia or fibula on either side of the ankle.
mandible	[MĂN-dĭ-bl]	U-shaped bone of the lower jaw.
mandibular bone	[măn-DĬB-yū-lăr]	Mandible.
marrow	[MĂR-ō]	Connective tissue filling the medullary cavity, often rich in nutrients.

Term	Word Analysis	Definition
mastoid process	[MĂS-tŏyd]	Protrusion of the temporal bone that sits behind the ear.
maxillary bone	[MĂK-sĭ-lār-ē]	Bone of the upper jaw.
maxillary sinus		Sinus on either side of the nasal cavity below the eyes.
medullary cavity	[MĔD-ū-lār-ē]	Soft center cavity in bone that often holds marrow.
metacarpal	[MĔT-ă-KĂR-păl] meta-, behind + carpal, of the wrist	One of five bones of the hand between the wrist and the fingers.
metaphysis	[mĕ-TĂF-i-sĭs] meta-, behind + Greek *physis*, growth	Section of a long bone between the epiphysis and diaphysis.
metatarsal bones	[MĔT-ă-TĂR-săl] meta-, behind + tarsus	Bones of the foot between the instep (arch) and the toes.
muscle	[MŬS-ĕl]	Contractile tissue that plays a major role in body movement.
musculoskeletal system	[MŬS-kyū-lō-SKĔL-ĕ-tăl] musculo-, muscle + skeletal	System of the body including the muscles and skeleton.
nasal bones		Bones that form the bridge of the nose.
nasal cavity		Cavity on either side of the nasal septum.
neural canal	[NŪR-ăl]	Space through which the spinal cord passes.
nucleus pulposus	[NŪ-klē-ŭs pŭl-PŌ-sŭs]	Fibrous mass in the center portion of the intervertebral disk.
occipital bone	[ŏk-SĬP-ĭ-tăl]	Bone that forms the lower back portion of the skull.
olecranon	[ō-LĔK-ră-nŏn]	Curved end of the ulna to which tendons of the arm muscles attach; bony prominence of the elbow.
origin		Point at which muscles attach to stationary bone.
osseous tissue	[ŎS-ē-ŭs]	Connective tissue into which calcium salts are deposited.
ossification	[ŎS-ĭ-fĭ-KĀ-shŭn]	Hardening into bone.

Term	Word Analysis	Definition
osteoblast	[ŎS-tē-ō-blăst] osteo-, bone + -blast, forming	Cell that forms bone.
osteoclast	[ŎS-tē-ō-klăst] osteo-, bone + -clast, breaking	Large cell that reabsorbs and removes osseous tissue.
osteocyte	[ŎS-tē-ō-sīt] osteo-, bone + -cyte, cell	Bone cell.
palatine bone	[PĂL-ĭ-tĭn]	Bone that helps form the hard palate and nasal cavity; located behind the maxillary bones.
parietal bone	[pă-RĪ-ĕ-tăl]	Flat, curved bone on either side of the upper part of the skull.
patella	[pă-TĚL-ă]	Large, sesamoid bone that forms the kneecap.
pelvic cavity	[PĚL-vĭk]	Cup-shaped cavity formed by the large bones of the pelvic girdle; contains female reproductive organs, sigmoid colon, bladder, and rectum.
pelvic girdle		Hip bones.
pelvis	[PĚL-vĭs]	Cup-shaped ring of bone and ligaments at the base of the trunk.
periosteum	[pĕr-ē-ŎS-tē-ŭm]	Fibrous membrane covering the surface of bone.
phalanges (sing. phalanx)	[fă-LĂN-jēz (FĂ-lăngks)]	Long bones of the fingers and toes.
phosphorus	[FŎS-fōr-ŭs]	Mineral important to the formation of bone.
process	[PRŌ-sĕs, PRŎS-ĕs]	Bony outgrowth or projection.
pubes	[PYŪ-bĭs]	Anteroinferior portion of the hip bone.
pubic symphysis	[PYŪ-bĭk SĬM-fĭ-sĭs]	Joint between the two pubic bones.
radius	[RĀ-dē-ŭs]	Shorter bone of the forearm.
rib		One of twenty-four bones that form the chest wall.
sacrum	[SĀ-krŭm]	Next-to-last spinal vertebra made up of five fused bones; vertebra that forms part of the pelvis.
scapula	[SKĂP-yū-lă]	Large flat bone that forms the shoulder blade.

Term	Word Analysis	Definition
sella turcica	[SĔL-ă TŬR-sĭ-kă]	Bony depression in the sphenoid bone where the pituitary gland is located.
sesamoid bone	[SĔS-ă-mŏyd]	Bone formed in a tendon over a joint.
shin	[shĭn]	Anterior ridge of the tibia.
short bones		Square-shaped bones with approximately equal dimensions on all sides.
sinus	[SĪ-nŭs]	Hollow cavity, especially either of two cavities on the sides of the nose.
skeleton	[SKĔL-ĕ-tŏn]	Bony framework of the body.
smooth muscle		Fibrous muscle of internal organs that acts involuntarily.
sphenoid bone	[SFĒ-nŏyd]	Bone that forms the base of the skull.
sphenoid sinus		Sinus above and behind the nose.
spinal column		Column of vertebrae at the posterior of the body, from the neck to the coccyx.
spinous process	[SPĪ-nŭs]	Protrusion from the center of the vertebral arch.
spongy bone		Bone with an open latticework filled with connective tissue or marrow.
sternum	[STĔR-nŭm]	Long, flat bone that forms the midline of the anterior of the thorax.
striated muscle	[strĭ-ĀT-ĕd]	Muscle with a ribbed appearance that is controlled at will.
styloid process	[STĪ-lŏyd]	Peg-shaped protrusion from a bone.
sulcus	[SŬL-kŭs]	Groove or furrow in the surface of bone.
suture	[SŪ-chūr]	Joining of two bone parts with a fibrous membrane.
symphysis	[SĬM-fĭ-sĭs] Greek, from *sym-*, together + *physis*, joint	Type of cartilaginous joint uniting two bones.
synarthrosis	[SĬN-ăr-THRŌ-sĭs] Greek, from *syn-*, together + *arthrosis*, articulation	Fibrous joint with no movement.

Term	Word Analysis	Definition
synovial fluid	[sǐ-NŌ-vē-ăl]	Fluid that serves to lubricate joints.
synovial joint		A joint that moves.
synovial membrane		Connective tissue lining the cavity of joints and producing the synovial fluid.
tarsus, tarsal bones	[TĂR-sŭs, TĂR-săl]	Seven bones of the instep (arch of the foot).
temporal bone	[TĔM-pō-răl]	Large bone forming the base and sides of the skull.
temporomandibular joint	[TĔM-pō-rō-măn-DĬB-yū-lăr]	Joint of the lower jaw between the temporal bone and the mandible.
tendon	[TĔN-dŏn]	Fibrous band that connects muscle to bone or other structures.
thoracic vertebrae	[thō-RĂS-ĭk]	Twelve vertebrae of the chest area.
thorax	[THŌ-răks]	Part of the trunk between the neck and the abdomen; chest.
tibia	[TĬB-ē-ă]	Larger of the two lower leg bones.
transverse process		Protrusion on either side of the vertebral arch.
trochanter	[trō-KĂN-tĕr]	Bony protrusion at the upper end of the femur.
true ribs		Seven upper ribs of the chest that attach to the sternum.
tubercle	[TŪ-bĕr-kl]	Slight bony elevation to which a ligament or muscle may be attached.
tuberosity	[TŪ-bĕr-ŎS-ĭ-tē]	Large elevation in the surface of a bone.
ulna	[ŬL-nă]	Larger bone of the forearm.
vertebra (pl. vertebrae)	[VĔR-tĕ-bră (VĔR-tĕ-brē)]	One of the bony segments of the spinal column.
vertebral body		Main portion of the vertebra, separate from the arches of the vertebra.
vertebral column		Spinal column.
visceral muscle	[VĬS-ĕr-ăl]	Smooth muscle.
vitamin D		Vitamin important to the formation of bone.

Term	Word Analysis	Definition
voluntary muscle		Striated muscle.
vomer	[VŌ-mĕr]	Flat bone forming the nasal septum.
zygomatic bone	[ZĪ-gō-MĂT-ĭk]	Bone that forms the cheek.

C A S E   S T U D Y

Seeing a Specialist

Mary Edgarton was referred to Dr. Alana Wolf, a rheumatologist, by her internist. Mary's five-month history of joint pain, swelling, and stiffness had not shown improvement. Dr. Wolf gave her a full musculoskeletal examination to check for swelling, abnormalities, and her ability to move her joints. Even though Mary remains a fairly active person, her movement in certain joints is now limited. She shows a moderate loss of grip strength.

In checking earlier for a number of systemic diseases, Mary's internist felt that Mary's problems were the result of some disease of her musculoskeletal system. Many of the laboratory tests that were forwarded to Dr. Wolf showed normal levels.

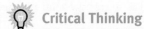 **Critical Thinking**

1. What lubricates the joints allowing movement?

2. Exercise is usually a recommended activity for most people to alleviate musculoskeletal problems. Is it possible to exercise both involuntary and voluntary muscles?

Structure and Function Exercises

Check Your Knowledge

Fill in the blanks.

3. The extremities of the body include mostly _____ bones.

4. A mature adult has a total of _____ bones.

5. Soft connective tissue with high nutrient content in the center of some bones is called _____.

6. An infant's skull generally has soft spots known as _____.

7. Disks in the spinal column have a soft, fibrous mass in the middle called the _____

   _____.

8. The scapula and the clavicle join at a point called the _____.

9. Ribs that attach to both the vertebral column and the sternum are called _____ _____.

10. Another name for kneecap is _____.

11. The largest tarsal is called the _____ or heel.

12. The only muscle that is both striated and involuntary is the _____ muscle.

Circle T for true or F for false

13. Compact bone is another name for cancellous bone. T F

14. Yellow bone marrow is found in adults. T F

15. The mandible is the upper jawbone. T F

16. The twelve vertebrae that connect to the ribs are the dorsal vertebrae. T F

17. Joints are lubricated with synovial fluid. T F

COMBINING FORMS AND ABBREVIATIONS

The lists below include combining forms and abbreviations that relate specifically to the musculoskeletal system. Pronunciations are provided for the examples.

Combining Form	Meaning	Example
acetabul(o)	acetabulum	*acetabulectomy* [ĂS-ĕ-tăb-yū-LĔK-tō-mē], excision of the acetabulum
acromi(o)	end point of the scapula	*acromioscapular* [ă-KRŌ-mē-ō-SKĂP-yū-lăr], relating to the acromion and the body of the scapula
ankyl(o)	bent, crooked	*ankylosis* [ĂNG-kĭ-LŌ-sĭs], fixation of a joint in a bent position, usually resulting from a disease
arthr(o)	joint	*arthrogram* [ĂR-thrō-grăm], x-ray of a joint
brachi(o)	arm	*brachiocephalic* [BRĀ-kē-ō-sĕ-FĂL-ĭk], relating to both the arm and head
burs(o)	bursa	*bursitis* [bĕr-SĪ-tĭs], inflammation of a bursa
calcane(o)	heel	*calcaneodynia* [kăl-KĀ-nē-ō-DĬN-ē-ă], heel pain
calci(o)	calcium	*calciokinesis* [KĂL-sē-ō-kĭ-NĒ-sĭs], mobilization of stored calcium in the body

Combining Form	Meaning	Example
carp(o)	wrist	*carpopedal* [KĂR-pō-PĔD-ăl], relating to the wrist and foot
cephal(o)	head	*cephalomegaly* [SĔF-ă-lō-MĔG-ă-lē], abnormally large head
cervic(o)	neck	*cervicodynia* [SĔR-vĭ-kō-DĬN-ē-ă], neck pain
chondr(o)	cartilage	*chondroplasty* [KŎN-drō-plăs-tē], surgical repair of cartilage
condyl(o)	knob, knuckle	*condylectomy* [kŏn-dĭ-LĔK-tō-mē], excision of a condyle
cost(o)	rib	*costiform* [KŎS-tĭ-fŏrm], rib-shaped
crani(o)	skull	*craniotomy* [krā-nē-ŎT-ō-mē], incision into the skull
dactyl(o)	fingers, toes	*dactylitis* [dăk-tĭ-LĪ-tĭs], inflammation of the finger(s) or toe(s)
fasci(o)	fascia	*fasciotomy* [făsh-ē-ŎT-ō-mē], incision through a fascia
femor(o)	femur	*femorocele* [FĔM-ō-rō-sēl], hernia in the femur
fibr(o)	fiber	*fibroma* [fī-BRŌ-mă], benign tumor in fibrous tissue
humer(o)	humerus	*humeroscapular* [HYŪ-mĕr-ō-SKĂP-yū-lăr], relating to both the humerus and the scapula
ili(o)	ilium	*iliofemoral* [ĬL-ē-ō-FĔM-ō-răl], relating to the ilium and the femur
ischi(o)	ischium	*ischiodynia* [ĬS-kē-ō-DĬN-ē-ă], pain in the ischium
kyph(o)	hump; bent	*kyphoscoliosis* [KĪ-fō-skō-lē-Ō-sĭs], kyphosis and scoliosis combined
lamin(o)	lamina	*laminectomy* [LĂM-ĭ-NĔK-tō-mē], removal of part of one or more of the thick cartilaginous disks between the vertebrae
leiomy(o)	smooth muscle	*leiomyosarcoma* [LĪ-ō-MĪ-ō-săr-KŌ-mă], malignant tumor of smooth muscle
lumb(o)	lumbar	*lumboabdominal* [LŬM-bō-ăb-DŎM-ĭ-năl], relating to the lumbar and abdominal regions
maxill(o)	upper jaw	*maxillofacial* [măk-SĬL-ō-FĀ-shăl], pertaining to the jaws and face

Combining Form	Meaning	Example
metacarp(o)	metacarpal	*metacarpectomy* [MĔT-ă-kăr-PĔK-tō-mē], excision of a metacarpal
my(o)	muscle	*myocardium* [mī-ō-KĂR-dē-ŭm], cardiac muscle in the middle layer of the heart
myel(o)	spinal cord; bone marrow	*myelocyst* [MĪ-ĕ-lō-sĭst], cyst that develops in bone marrow
oste(o)	bone	*osteoarthritis* [ŎS-tē-ō-ăr-THRĪ-tĭs], arthritis characterized by erosion of cartilage and bone and joint pain
patell(o)	knee	*patellectomy* [PĂT-ĕ-LĔK-tō-mē], excision of the patella
ped(i), pedo-	foot	*pedometer* [pĕ-dŏm-ĕ-tĕr], instrument for measuring walking distance
pelv(i)	pelvis	*pelviscope* [PĔL-vĭ-skōp], instrument for viewing the pelvic cavity
phalang(o)	finger or toe bone	*phalangectomy* [făl-ăn-JĔK-tō-mē], removal of a finger or toe
pod(o)	foot	*podalgia* [pō-DĂL-jē-ă], foot pain
pub(o)	pubis	*puborectal* [PYŪ-bō-RĔK-tăl], relating to the pubis and the rectum
rachi(o)	spine	*rachiometer* [rā-kē-ŎM-ĕ-tĕr], instrument for measuring spine curvature
radi(o)	forearm bone	*radiomuscular* [RĀ-dē-ō-MŬS-kyū-lăr], relating to the radius and nearby muscles
rhabd(o)	rod-shaped	*rhabdosphincter* [RĂB-dō-SFĬNGK-tĕr], striated muscular sphincter
rhabdomy(o)	striated muscle	*rhabdomyolysis* [RĂB-dō-mī-ŎL-ĭ-sĭs], acute disease that includes destruction of skeletal muscle
scapul(o)	scapula	*scapulodynia* [SKĂP-yū-lō-DĬN-ē-ă], scapula pain
scoli(o)	curved	*scoliokyphosis* [SKŌ-lē-ō-kī-FŌ-sĭs], lateral and posterior curvature of the spine
spondyl(o)	vertebra	*spondylitis* [spŏn-dĭ-LĪ-tĭs], inflammation of a vertebra
stern(o)	sternum	*sternodynia* [stĕr-nō-DĬN-ē-ă], sternum pain
synov(o)	synovial membrane	*synovitis* [sĭn-ō-VĪ-tĭs], inflammation of a synovial joint

Combining Form	Meaning	Example
tars(o)	tarsus	*tarsomegaly* [tăr-sō-MĔG-ă-lē], congenital abnormality with overgrowth of a tarsal bone
ten(o), tend(o), tendin(o)	tendon	*tenodynia* [tĕn-ō-DĬN-ē-ă], tendon pain; *tendoplasty* [TĔN-dō-plăs-tē], surgical repair of a tendon; *tendinitis* [tĕn-dĭ-NĪ-tĭs], tendon inflammation
thorac(o)	thorax	*thoracoabdominal* [THŌR-ă-kō-ăb-DŎM-ĭ-năl], relating to the thorax and the abdomen
tibi(o)	tibia	*tibiotarsal* [tĭb-ē-ō-TĂR-săl], relating to the tarsal and tibia bones
uln(o)	ulna	*ulnocarpal* [ŬL-nō-KĂR-păl], relating to the ulna and the wrist
vertebr(o)	vertebra	*vertebroarterial* [VĔR-tĕ-brō-ăr-TĒR-ē-ăl], relating to a vertebral artery or to a vertebra and an artery

Abbreviation	Meaning
A-K	above the knee (amputation)
B-K	below the knee (amputation)
C_1, C_2, etc.	first cervical vertebra, second cervical vertebra, etc.
ca	calcium
CTS	carpal tunnel syndrome
DJD	degenerative joint disease
DTR	deep tendon reflex
EMG	electromyogram
fx	fracture
IM	intramuscularly
L_1, L_2, etc.	first lumbar vertebra, second lumbar vertebra, etc.
MCP	metacarpophalangeal
NSAID	nonsteroidal anti-inflammatory drug
P	phosphorus
PIP	proximal interphalangeal joint
ROM	range of motion
T_1, T_2, etc.	first thoracic vertebra, second thoracic vertebra, etc.
TMJ	temporomandibular joint

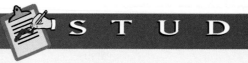

Checking Medication

Dr. Wolf's next patient, Laura Spinoza, is in for a follow-up visit for fibromyalgia, a disease that causes chronic muscle pain. In addition, Laura has tested positive for CTS. The patient suffers from depression, for which she is currently being treated. Laura has had earlier reactions to some of the medications meant to relieve the symptoms of fibromyalgia. She is receiving new prescriptions for the fibromyalgia as well as directions for an exercise program. Dr. Wolf sent a follow-up letter to Laura's primary care physician after her visit.

 Critical Thinking

18. Dr. Wolf gets referrals from general practitioners and internists. As a specialist in rheumatology, most of her cases involve diseases of the musculoskeletal system. Refer to the letter from Dr. Wolf and use the combining forms list to provide definitions of two diseases given as examples.

19. Laura has a physical condition in addition to fibromyalgia. What is it? Give both the abbreviation and the full spelling.

Alana Wolf, M.D.
285 Riverview Road
Belle Harbor, MI 09999

March 12, 20XX

Dr. Robert Johnson
16 Tyler Court
Newtown, MI 09990

Dear Dr. Johnson

I saw Laura Spinoza on March the 7th for evaluation of her fibromyalgia. I reviewed her history with her and discussed her treatment for depression. The history suggests that there has not been any new development of an inflammatory rheumatic disease process within the last two years. She does have right thumb-carpal pain, which represents some osteoarthritis. Headaches are frequent but she is receiving no specific therapy. Her sleep pattern remains disturbed at times.

Her height was 62 inches, her weight was 170 lbs, while her BP was 162/100 in the right arm in the reclining position. Pelvic and rectal examinations were not done. The abdominal examination revealed some mild tenderness in the right lower quadrant without other abnormalities. The musculoskeletal examination revealed rotation and flexion to the left with no other cervical abnormalities. The remainder of the musculoskeletal examination revealed hypermobility in the elbow and knees and slight bony osteoarthritic enlargement of the thumb-carpal joint. Slight deformity was noted in the right knee with mild patellar-femoral crepitus. Severe bilateral pas planus was present, with the right foot more involved than the left, and ankle vagus deformity with mild bony osteoarthritic enlargement of both 1st MTP joints.

Hope these thoughts are helpful. I want to thank you for the consultation. If I can be of future service with her or other rheumatic-problem patients, please do not hesitate to contact me.

Alana Wolf, MD

Alana Wolf, M.D.

Combining Forms and Abbreviations Exercises

Build Your Medical Vocabulary

Complete the words using combining forms listed in this chapter.

20. Joint pain: _____dynia

21. Plastic surgery of the skull: _____plasty

22. Of the upper jaw and its teeth: _____dental

23. Relating to the large area of the hip bone and the tibia: _____tibial

24. Operation on the instep of the foot: _____tomy

25. Relating to the head and chest: cephalo_____

26. Production of fibrous tissue: _____plasia

27. Inflammation of the foot: _____itis

28. Instrument for measuring spine curvature: _____meter

29. Incision through the sternum: _____tomy

Find the Word Parts

Give the term that fits the definition given below. Each term must contain at least one of the combining forms given in the previous section. You may refer to the Appendix of combining forms at the back of the book.

30. Joint pain _____.

31. Removal of a bursa_____.

32. Inflammation of cartilage_____.

33. Removal of a vertebra_____.

34. Bone-forming cell _____.

35. Abnormal bone hardening _____.

36. Plastic surgery on the neck _____.

37. Inflammation of the spinal cord _____.

38. Foot spasm _____.

39. Of the ulna and the carpus _____.

Find the misspelled word part. Write the corrected word part in the space with its definition

40. sinovotomy_____

41. myellogram_____

42. arthrodunia_____

43. ostiomyelitis_____

44. rakiometer_____

Diagnostic, Procedural, and Laboratory Terms

The musculoskeletal system is often the site of pain caused by conditions in the system itself or by symptoms of other systemic conditions. Specialists in the musculoskeletal system include **orthopedists,** physicians who treat disorders of the musculoskeletal system; **osteopaths,** physicians who combine manipulative procedures with conventional treatment; **rheumatologists,** physicians who treat disorders of the joints, specifically, and the musculoskeletal system, generally; **podiatrists,** medical specialists who treat disorders of the foot; and **chiropractors,** health care professionals who manipulate the spine to treat certain ailments.

Diagnosing bone and muscle ailments often involves taking x-rays, scans, or radiographs or performing internal examinations to determine if an abnormality is present. **Arthrography** is the examination of joints using radiography; **arthroscopy** is the examination of a joint internally using an instrument; and **diskography** is the examination of disks by injecting a contrast medium and using radiography. Computed tomography (CT) scans can reveal joint, bone, or connective tissue disease. **Myelography** is the use of radiography of the spinal cord to identify spinal cord conditions. An **electromyogram** is a graphic image of the electrical activity of muscles. Magnetic resonance imaging (MRI) may be used to detect disorders of the musculoskeletal system, especially of soft tissue. A **bone scan** is used to detect tumors. Figure 5-9 is a bone scan showing a malignant tumor.

Physicians examine bones and joints externally, often using small rubber mallets to provoke responses. **Tinel's sign** is a "pins and needles" sensation felt when an injured nerve site is tapped. The sign indicates a partial lesion in a nerve and is a common test for carpel tunnel syndrome.

Laboratory tests measure the levels of substances found in some musculo-

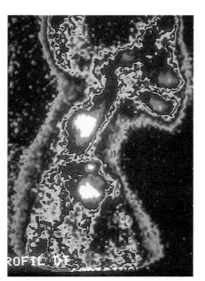

Figure 5-9 The spot in the image is a tumor that appears to be malignant.

skeletal disorders. Rheumatoid arthritis may be confirmed by a **rheumatoid factor test.** High **serum creatine phosphokinase (CPK)** levels appear in some disorders such as a skeletal injury. The measurement of **serum calcium**

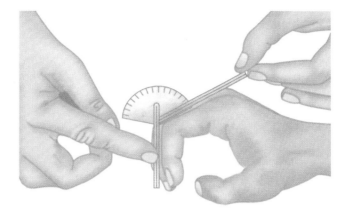

Figure 5-10 A goniometer is used to measure the range of motion of a joint.

and **serum phosphorus** in the blood indicates the body's incorporation of those substances in the bones. **Uric acid tests** can detect gout. Tests for range of motion (ROM) in certain joints can indicate movement or joint disorders. A **goniometer** is used to measure motion in the joints (Figure 5-10). A **densitometer** uses light and x-ray images to measure bone density for osteoporosis, a disease with bone fractures that is most common in post-menopausal women.

Vocabulary Review

In the previous section, you learned terms relating to diagnosis, clinical procedures, and laboratory tests. Before going on to the exercises, review the terms below and refer to the previous section if you have any questions.

Term	Word Analysis	Definition
arthrography	[ăr-THRŎG-ră-fĕ] arthro-, joint + -graphy, process of recording	Radiography of a joint.
arthroscopy	[ăr-THRŎS-kō-pē] arthro-, joint + -scopy, a viewing with an instrument	Examination with an instrument that explores the interior of a joint.
bone scan		Radiographic or ultrasound image of a bone.
chiropractor	[kī-rō-PRĂK-tōr] chiro-, hand + Greek *praktikos*, efficient	Health care professional who works to align the spinal column so as to treat certain ailments.
densitometer	[dĕn-sĭ-TŎM-ĕ-tĕr]	Device that measures bone density using light and x-rays.

Term	Word Analysis	Definition
diskography	[dĭs-KŎG-ră-fē]	Radiographic image of an intervertebral disk by injection of a contrast medium into the center of the disk.
electromyogram	[ĕ-lĕk-trō-MĪ-ō-grăm] electro-, electrical + myo-, muscle + -gram, recording	A graphic image of muscular action using electrical currents.
goniometer	[gō-nē-ŎM-ĕ-tĕr] Greek *gonia*, angle + -meter, measuring device	Instrument that measures angles or range of motion in a joint.
myelography	[MĪ-ĕ-LŎG-ră-fē] myelo-, spinal cord + -graphy, process of recording	Radiographic imaging of the spinal cord.
orthopedist	[ōr-thō-PĒ-dĭst] ortho-, straight + Greek *pais (paid-)*, child	Physician who examines, diagnoses, and treats disorders of the musculoskeletal system.
osteopath	[ŎS-tē-ō-păth] osteo-, bone + -path(y), disease	Physician who combines manipulative treatment with conventional therapeutic measures.
podiatrist	[pō-DĪ-ă-trĭst]	Medical specialist who examines, diagnoses, and treats disorders of the foot.
rheumatoid factor test		Test used to detect rheumatoid arthritis.
rheumatologist	[rū-mă-TŎL-ō-jĭst]	Physician who examines, diagnoses, and treats disorders of the joints and musculoskeletal system.
serum calcium		Test for calcium in the blood.
serum creatine phosphokinase	[SĒR-ŭm KRĒ-ă-tēn fŏs-fō-KĪ-nās]	Enzyme active in muscle contraction, usually elevated after a myocardial infarction and in the presence of other degenerative muscle diseases.
serum phosphorus		Test for phosphorus in the blood.
Tinel's sign		"Pins and needles" sensation felt when an injured nerve site is tapped.
uric acid test		Test for acid content in urine; elevated levels may indicate gout.

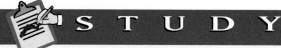

CASE STUDY

Preventing Disease

Louella Jones (age 48) visited her gynecologist, Dr. Phillips, for her annual examination. During the past year, Louella had stopped menstruating. She had some symptoms of menopause, but they did not bother her tremendously. Louella is tall and very thin. Dr. Phillips sent her for a bone density test. The densitometer measured the density of Louella's bones and found that there was a slight increase in her bones' porosity from three years ago. Dr. Phillips suggested hormone replacement therapy and a program of weight-bearing exercises. However, Louella wanted more information about the treatments' potential impact on her condition before beginning therapy.

Critical Thinking

45. Why are bone density measurements important in the diagnosis?

46. Louella wanted more information before taking medication and starting an exercise program. What kind of information might she be given?

Diagnostic, Procedural, and Laboratory Terms Exercises

Test Your Knowledge

Answer the following questions.

47. Tests for calcium and phosphorus are given to determine blood levels of these minerals. What significance do these minerals have for the musculoskeletal system?

_____

_____

_____

48. Is it likely that a chiropractor would order a uric acid test? Why or why not?

_____

_____

_____

49. Would a bone scan be likely to show bone cancer? _____

50. How is an osteopath like a chiropractor? _____

_____

51. What might a goniometer show about a muscle's action? _____

_____

Pathological Terms

Musculoskeletal disorders arise from congenital conditions, injury, degenerative disease, or other systemic disorders. Birth defects, such as **spina bifida,** affect the development of the spinal cord. Injuries to the spinal cord may produce paralysis. In some situations, surgery on the fetus while it is in utero can alleviate some of the effects of spina bifida. In such surgery, the abnormal spinal cord opening is repaired. A **herniated disk,** in which the center of the disk is compressed and presses on nerves in the neural canal, can lead to **sciatica,** pain radiating down the leg from the lower back. Some diseases, such as **rickets,** which causes deformities in the legs, may result from a vitamin D deficiency.

Foot deformities may occur in or involve the ankle joint. **Talipes calcaneus** is a deformity of the heel due to weakened calf muscles; **talipes valgus** is *eversion* (a turning outward) of the foot; and **talipes varus** is *inversion* (a turning inward) of the foot. A **calcar** or **spur** is a bony projection growing out of a bone.

Fractures are breaks or cracks in bones. A **closed fracture** is a break with no open wound. An **open (compound) fracture** is a break with an open wound. A **simple (hairline** or **closed) fracture** does not move any part of the bone out of place. A **complex fracture** is a separation of part of the bone and usually requires surgery for repair. A **greenstick fracture** is an incomplete break of a soft (usually, a child's) bone. An **incomplete fracture** is a break that does not go entirely through any type of bone. A **comminuted fracture** is a break in which the bone is fragmented or shattered. A **Colles' fracture** is a break of the lower end of the radius. A **complicated fracture** involves extensive soft tissue injury. An **impacted fracture** occurs when a fragment from one part of a fracture is driven into the tissue of another part. A **pathological fracture** occurs at the site of bone already damaged by disease. A **compression fracture** is a break in one or more vertebrae caused by a *compressing* or squeezing of the space between the vertebrae. Compression fractures often result from loss of bone density as in osteoporosis. Figure 5-11 shows types of fractures.

Injury or trauma to the joints or muscle may cause a **sprain.** Overuse of a muscle may cause a **strain.** Overworking a joint may cause **tendinitis (tendonitis),** an inflammation of a tendon. **Dislocation** may result from an injury or from a strenuous, sudden movement. A **subluxation** is a partial dislocation. Bones may lose their density (**osteoporosis**).

Pain in the musculoskeletal system may appear in the bones (**osteoalgia, osteodynia**), muscles (**myalgia, myodynia**), or joints (**arthralgia**). Stiffness of the joints (**ankylosis**) may be an indicator of several diseases. **Spastic** muscles have abnormal contractions (**spasms**) in diseases such as multiple sclerosis. An abnormal increase in muscle size is **hypertrophy. Flaccid** muscles are flabby in tone. **Hypotonia** is abnormally reduced muscle tension, and **rigor** (also called **rigidity**) is abnormal muscle stiffness as seen in lockjaw. **Dystonia** is abnormal tone (tension) in a muscle. A painfully long muscle contraction is **tetany.** Shaking (**tremors**) appears in a number of diseases such as Parkinson's Disease.

Talipes is a combination of Latin *talus,* ankle, and *pes,* foot.

MORE ABOUT...

Fractures

Fractures can be caused by many types of injuries or diseases. Osteoporosis in older people may result in hip fractures which, in many cases, are thought to precede the actual fall. A twisting fracture may result from a twisting injury in a sports game. A comminuted fracture may result from the impact of a car crash. The type of fracture often gives clues as to how the initial injury occurred.

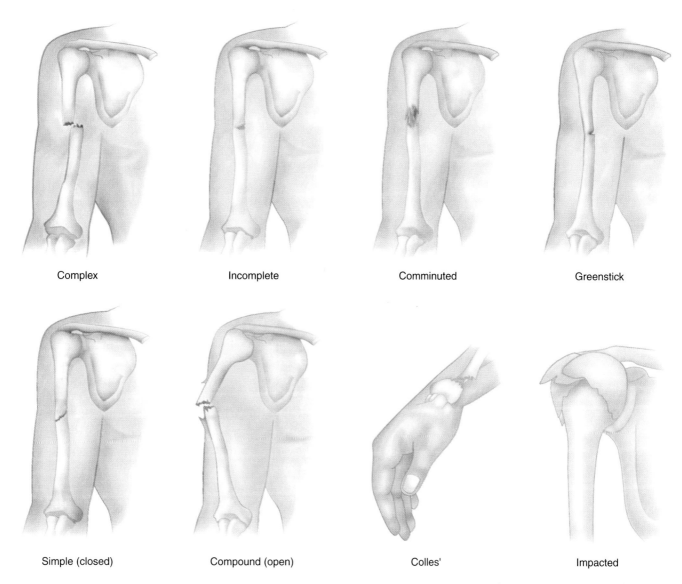

Complex   Incomplete   Comminuted   Greenstick

Simple (closed)   Compound (open)   Colles'   Impacted

Figure 5-11 Intervention in the case of fractures varies from virtually no treatment (as in fractured toes) to extensive surgery (as in complex fractures).

Some muscles **atrophy** (shrink) as a result of disuse or specific diseases such as **muscular dystrophy,** a progressive, degenerative disorder affecting skeletal muscles. A muscle inflammation is **myositis.**

Some bone tissue dies (**bony necrosis, sequestrum**), often as a result of loss of blood supply. Abnormal bone growths may be capped with cartilage, as in **exostosis.** The bursa may become inflamed, causing **bursitis.** Inflammation of the bursa in the big toe causes a **bunion.** The epiphyses may also become inflamed, causing **epiphysitis.** A common inflammation of the joints is **arthritis.** Arthritis is a name for many different joint diseases, such as osteoarthritis or **degenerative arthritis** (arthritis characterized by erosion of joint cartilage), **rheumatoid arthritis** (a systemic disease affecting connective tissue), and **gouty arthritis** (disease characterized by joint pain, as in **podagra,** pain in the big toe). Figure 5-12 shows symptoms of arthritis. Certain types of arthritis

Bunion is from an Old French term meaning a bump on the head. The exact path to how it became a bump on the foot is unknown.

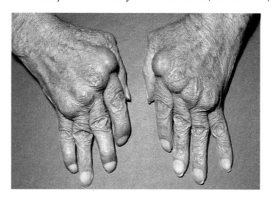

Figure 5-12 Arthritis is a general name for many joint diseases including osteoarthritis shown here.

Cartilage

The replacement of damaged or lost cartilage is now possible. The procedure is to remove some of a patient's cartilage through a small incision, grow more cartilage in the laboratory using the patient's own cells, and inject them back into the small incision.

may cause *crepitation* (also called *crepitus*) noise made when affected surfaces rub together. Infections in the bone may cause **osteomyelitis.**

Cartilage may soften (**chondromalacia**) or become fragmented, as in a herniated disk. Disks may also slip or become misaligned with other vertebrae (**spondylolisthesis**) or become stiff (**spondylosis**). Various tumors may develop in the muscle, bone, bone marrow, and joints. **Myeloma, myoma, leiomyoma, leiomyosarcoma, rhabdomyoma, rhabdomyosarcoma, osteoma,** and **osteosarcoma** are types of musculoskeletal tumors.

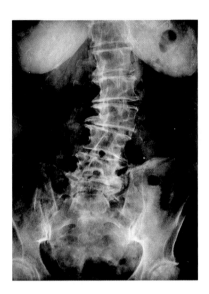

Figure 5-13 **Many abnormalities of the spinal column are congenital. The image of the spine shown here is of someone who was born with several vertebrae curving out of alignment.**

Some abnormal posture conditions (spinal curvature, **kyphosis, lordosis,** and scoliosis) may cause pain (Figure 5-13). Pain may even be felt in limbs that have been paralyzed or amputated. **Phantom limb** or **phantom pain** afflicts many who are paralyzed or are missing a limb. Repetitive motion of the hand may cause carpal tunnel syndrome, pain and paresthesia (numbness or tingling) of the hand. Chiropractors treat some spinal conditions by manipulation. Physical therapy is movement therapy to restore use of damaged areas of the body.

Vocabulary Review

In the previous section, you learned terms relating to the pathology. Before going on to the exercises, review the terms below and refer to the previous section if you have any questions.

Term	Word Analysis	Definition
ankylosis	[ĂNG-kĭ-LŌ-sĭs]	Stiffening of a joint, especially as a result of disease.
arthralgia	[ăr-THRĂL-jē-ă] arthro-, joint + -algia, pain	Severe joint pain.
arthritis	[ăr-THRĪ-tĭs] Greek, from arthro-, joint + -itis, inflammation	Any of various conditions involving joint inflammation.

Term	Word Analysis	Definition
atrophy	[ĂT-rō-fē] Greek *atrophia*, without nourishment	Wasting away of tissue, organs, and cells, usually as a result of disease or loss of blood supply.
bony necrosis	[BŌN-ē nĕ-KRŌ-sĭs]	Death of portions of bone.
bunion	[BŬN-yŭn]	An inflamed bursa at the foot joint, between the big toe and the first metatarsal bone.
bursitis	[bĕr-SĪ-tĭs] burs(a) + -itis, inflammation	Inflammation of a bursa.
calcar	[KĂL-kăr]	Another name for spur.
carpal tunnel syndrome	[KĂR-păl]	Pain and paresthesia in the hand due to repetitive motion injury of the median nerve.
chondromalacia	[KŎN-drō-mă-LĀ-shē-ă] chondro-, cartilage + -malacia, softening	Softening of cartilage.
closed fracture		Fracture with no open skin wound.
Colles' fracture	[kōlz]	Fracture of the lower end of the radius.
comminuted fracture	[KŎM-ĭ-nū-tĕd]	Fracture with shattered bones.
complex fracture		Fracture with part of the bone displaced.
complicated fracture		Fracture involving extensive soft tissue injury.
compound fracture		Fracture with an open skin wound; open fracture.
compression fracture		Fracture of one or more vertebrae caused by compressing of the space between the vertebrae.
degenerative arthritis		Arthritis with erosion of the cartilage.
dislocation		Movement of a joint out of its normal position as a result of an injury or sudden, strenuous movement.
dystonia	[dĭs-TŌ-nē-ă]	Abnormal tone in tissues.
epiphysitis	[ĕ-pĭf-ĭ-SĪ-tĭs]	Inflammation of the epiphysis.
exostosis	[ĕks-ŏs-TŌ-sĭs] ex-, out of + ost(eo)-, bone + -osis, condition	Abnormal bone growth capped with cartilage.

Term	Word Analysis	Definition
flaccid	[FLĂK-sĭd]	Without tone; relaxed.
fracture	[FRĂK-chūr]	A break, especially in a bone.
gouty arthritis, gout	[gŏwt]	Inflammation of the joints, present in gout; usually caused by uric acid crystals.
greenstick fracture		Fracture with twisting or bending of the bone but no breaking; usually occurs in children.
hairline fracture		Fracture with no bone separation or fragmentation.
herniated disk	[HĔR-nē-ā-tĕd]	Protrusion of an intervertebral disk into the neural canal.
hypertrophy	[hī-PĔR-trō-fē] hyper-, excessive + -trophy, nutrition	Abnormal increase as in muscle size.
hypotonia	[HĪ-pō-TŌ-nē-ă] hypo-, subnormal + Greek *tonos*, tone	Abnormally reduced muscle tension.
impacted fracture		Fracture in which a fragment from one part of the fracture is driven into the tissue of another part.
incomplete fracture		Fracture that does not go entirely through a bone.
kyphosis	[kī-FŌ-sĭs]	Abnormal posterior spine curvature.
leiomyoma	[LĪ-ō-mī-Ō-mă] leio-, smooth + my(o)-, muscle + -oma, tumor	Benign tumor of smooth muscle.
leiomyosarcoma	[LĪ-ō-MĪ-ō-săr-KŌ-mă] leio-, smooth + myo-, muscle + sarcoma	Malignant tumor of smooth muscle.
lordosis	[lōr-DŌ-sĭs]	Abnormal anterior spine curvature resulting in a sway back.
muscular dystrophy	[MŬS-kyū-lăr DĬS-trō-fē]	Progressive degenerative disorder affecting the musculoskeletal system and, later, other organs.
myalgia	[mī-ĂL-jē-ă] my(o)-, muscle + -algia, pain	Muscle pain.

Term	Word Analysis	Definition
myeloma	[mī-ĕ-LŌ-mă] myel(o)-, bone marrow + -oma, tumor	Bone marrow tumor.
myodynia	[MĪ-ō-DĬN-ē-ă] myo-, muscle + -dynia, pain	Muscle pain.
myoma	[mī-Ō-mă] my(o)-, muscle +-oma, tumor	Benign muscle tumor.
myositis	[mī-ō-SĪ-tĭs] myo-, muscle + -itis, inflammation	Inflammation of a muscle.
open fracture		Fracture with an open skin wound; compound fracture.
ostealgia	[ŏs-tē-ĂL-jē-ă] oste(o)-, bone + algia, pain	Bone pain.
osteoarthritis	[ŎS-tē-ō-ăr-THRĪ-tĭs] osteo-, bone + arthritis	Arthritis with loss of cartilage.
osteodynia	[ŏs-tē-ō-DĬN-ē-ă] osteo-, bone + -dynia, pain	Bone pain.
osteoma	[ŏs-tē-Ō-mă] osteo-, bone + -oma, tumor	Benign tumor, usually on the skull or mandible.
osteomyelitis	[ŎS-tē-ō-mī-ĕ-LĪ-tĭs] osteo-, bone + myel(o)-, bone marrow + -itis, inflammation	Inflammation of the bone marrow and surrounding bone.
osteoporosis	[ŎS-tē-ō-pō-RŌ-sĭs] osteo-, bone + por(e) + -osis, condition	Degenerative thinning of bone.
osteosarcoma	[ŎS-tē-ō-săr-KŌ-mă] osteo-, bone + sarcoma	Malignant tumor of bone.
pathological fracture		Fracture occurring at the site of already damaged bone.

Term	Word Analysis	Definition
phantom limb; phantom pain		Pain felt in a paralyzed or amputated limb.
physical therapy		Movement therapy to restore use of damaged areas of the body.
podagra	[pō-DĂG-ră]	Pain in the big toe, often associated with gout.
rhabdomyoma	[RĂB-dō-mī-Ō-mă] rhadbdo-, rod-shaped + my(o)-, muscle + -oma, tumor	Benign tumor in striated muscle.
rhabdomyosarcoma	[RĂB-dō-mī-ō-săr-KŌ-mă] rhabdo-, rod-shaped + myo-, muscle + sarcoma	Malignant tumor in striated muscle.
rheumatoid arthritis		Autoimmune disorder affecting connective tissue.
rickets	[RĬK-ĕts]	Disease of the skeletal system, usually caused by vitamin D deficiency.
rigidity		Stiffness.
rigor	[RĬG-ĕr]	Stiffening.
sciatica	[sī-ĂT-ĭ-kă]	Pain in the lower back, usually radiating down the leg, from a herniated disk or other injury or condition.
scoliosis	[skō-lē-Ō-sĭs]	Abnormal lateral curvature of the spinal column.
sequestrum	[sē-KWĔS-trŭm]	Piece of dead tissue or bone separated from the surrounding area.
simple fracture		Fracture with no open skin wound.
spasm	[spăzm]	Sudden, involuntary muscle contraction.
spastic	[SPĂS-tĭc]	Tending to have spasms.
spina bifida	[SPĪ-nă BĬF-ĭ-dă]	Congenital defect with deformity of the spinal column.
spinal curvature		Abnormal curvature of the spine.
spondylolisthesis	[SPŎN-dĭ-lō-lĭs-THĒ-sĭs] spondyl(o)-, vertebrae + Greek olisthesis, slipping	Degenerative condition in which one vertebra misaligns with the one below it.

Term	Word Analysis	Definition
spondylolysis	[spŏn-dĭ-LŎL-ĭ-sĭs] spondylo-, vertebrae + -lysis, destruction of	Degenerative condition of the moving part of a vertebra.
sprain	[sprān]	Injury to a joint without dislocation or fracture.
spur	[spĕr]	Bony projection growing out of a bone.
strain	[strān]	Injury to a muscle as a result of overuse.
subluxation	[sŭb-lŭk-SĀ-shŭn]	Partial dislocation, as between joint surfaces.
talipes calcaneus	[TĂL-ĭ-pēz kăl-KĀ-nē-ŭs]	Deformity of the heel resulting from weakened calf muscles.
talipes valgus	[TĂL-ĭ-pēz VĂL-gŭs]	Foot deformity characterized by eversion of the foot.
talipes varus	[TĂL-ĭ-pēz VĀ-rŭs]	Foot deformity characterized by inversion of the foot.
tendinitis, tendonitis		Inflammation of a tendon.
tetany	[TĔT-ă-nē]	Painfully long muscle contraction.
tremor	[TRĔM-ĕr]	Abnormal, repetitive muscle contractions.

C A S E   S T U D Y

Making a Referral

Dr. Millet, a chiropractor, sees many patients for back pain. His treatments consist primarily of spinal manipulation, heat, and nutritional and exercise counseling. He currently sees a group of patients, mainly middle-aged men, who complain of sciatica. He has been able to relieve the pain for about 50 percent of them. The others seem to have more persistent pain. Dr. Millet is not allowed to prescribe medications because he is not a licensed medical doctor. He refers some of his patients to Dr. Wolf, a specialist, who believes that Dr. Millet provides a valuable service.

Critical Thinking

52. Chiropractic is one way for some people to manage pain. Why might spinal manipulation help?

53. If spinal manipulation does not work, why should the patient see a medical specialist?

Pathological Terms Exercises

Build Your Medical Vocabulary

Match the word roots on the left with the proper definition on the right.

54. myo-   a. bone

55. myelo-   b. hand

56. rhabdo-   c. rod

57. osteo-   d. joint

58. arthro-   e. bone marrow

59. chiro-   f. muscle

Know The Word Parts

Match the following terms with the letter that gives the best definition.

60. myeloma   a. malignant tumor of smooth muscle

61. myoma   b. benign tumor in striated muscle

62. leiomyoma   c. benign tumor of smooth muscle

63. leiomyosarcoma   d. benign muscle tumor

64. rhabdomyoma   e. malignant bone tumor

65. rhabdomyosarcoma   f. bone marrow tumor

66. osteoma   g. malignant tumor in striated muscle

67. osteosarcoma   h. benign tumor, usually on the skull or mandible

Check Your Knowledge

Fill in the blanks.

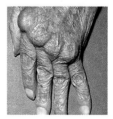

68. The photograph at the right shows a patient with _____.

69. Fractures that are most likely to occur in young children are called _____.

70. Osteoporosis is usually a disease found in _____ women.

71. Playing tennis too vigorously may cause _____ of the elbow.

72. Underworked muscles may become _____.

73. A muscle tumor is a/an _____.

74. A slipped disk is called _____.

75. A compound fracture is a break accompanied by a/an _____ wound.

76. Arthritis is a general term for a number of _____ diseases.

77. Paralysis may be caused by an injury to the _____ _____.

Surgical Terms

Orthopedic surgery may involve repair, grafting, replacement, excision, or reconstruction of parts of the musculoskeletal system. Surgeons also make incisions to take biopsies. Almost any major part of the musculoskeletal system can now be surgically replaced. In some situations (as with loss of circulation in diabetes, cancer of a limb, or severe infection), **amputation** may be necessary. **Prosthetic devices** now routinely replace knees and hips, as when injury or degenerative disease has worn down joints (Figure 5-14). **Bone grafting** can be used to repair a defect. An **orthosis** or **orthotic** may be used to provide support and prevent movement during treatment. Fractures are treated by **casting, splinting,** surgical manipulation, or placement in **traction.** Casts and splints are considered **external fixation devices**—devices that surround a fractured body part to hold the bones in place while healing. They may be used in combination with an **internal fixation device,** such as a pin placed internally to hold bones together. Pins for internal fixation are usually metal or hard plastic. A pin may be placed permanently or it may be removed after the bone has healed. **Reduction** is the return of a part to its normal position. An *open reduction* is done surgically; a *closed* reduction is external manipulation used for dislocated bones, such as a shoulder bone.

Osteoplasty is repair of a bone. **Osteoclasis** is the breaking of bone for the purpose of repairing it (as when a fracture has not healed properly). **Osteotomy** is an incision into a bone. **Tenotomy** is the cutting into a tendon to repair a muscle. **Myoplasty** is muscle repair. **Arthroplasty** is joint repair. **Arthrocentesis** is a puncture into a joint. A **synovectomy** is the removal of part or all of the synovial membrane of a joint. **Arthrodesis** and **spondylosyndesis** are two types of fusion. A **bursectomy** is the removal of an affected bursa. A **bunionectomy** is the removal of a bunion. This operation it usually performed on the *great toe*. Other types of toe repair may correct such things as *hammer toe*, one or more toes permanently flexed to one side. Some musculoskeletal surgery is done by arthroscopy. **Laminectomy** or removal of part of a spinal disk may alleviate the pain of a herniated disk.

Historically, before the advent of antibiotics, limb amputations were often necessary due to infections or wounds that would have no way to heal. Now, amputations are much rarer. New techniques of bone repair and infection control make it more likely that they can be avoided.

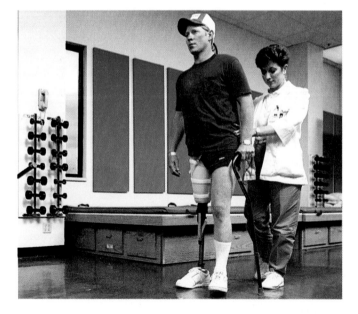

Figure 5-14 **Prosthetic devices provide a way for people who have lost limbs to walk, maintain balance, and use their arms and/or hands.**

Vocabulary Review

In the previous section, you learned terms relating to surgery. Before going on to the exercises, review the terms below and refer to the previous section if you have questions.

Term	Word Analysis	Definition
amputation	[ĂM-pyū-TĀ-shŭn]	Cutting off of a limb or part of a limb.
arthrocentesis	[ĂR-thrō-sĕn-TĒ-sĭs] arthro-, joint + Greek *kentesis*, puncture	Removal of fluid from a joint with use of a puncture needle.
arthrodesis	[ăr-thrō-DĒ-sĭs] arthro- + Greek *desis*, a binding	Surgical fusion of a joint to stiffen it.
arthroplasty	[ĂR-thrō-plăs-tē] arthro- + -plasty, repair	Surgical replacement or repair of a joint.
bone grafting		Transplantation of bone from one site to another.
bunionectomy	[bŭn-yŭn-ĔK-tō-mē] bunion +-ectomy, removal	Removal of a bunion.
bursectomy	[bĕr-SĔK-tō-mĕ] burs(a) + -ectomy, removal	Removal of a bursa.
casting		Forming of a cast in a mold; placing of fiberglass or plaster over a body part to prevent its movement.
external fixation device		Device applied externally to hold a limb in place.
internal fixation device		Device, such as a pin, inserted in bone to hold it in place.
laminectomy	[LĂM-ĭ-NĔK-tō-mē] lamin(a) + -ectomy, removal	Removal of part of an invertebral disk.
myoplasty	[MĪ-ō-plăs-tē] myo-, muscle + -plasty, repair	Surgical repair of muscle tissue.
orthosis, orthotic	[ōr-THŌ-sĭs, ōr-THŎT-ĭk]	External appliance used to immobilize or assist the movement of the spine or limbs.
osteoclasis	[ŎS-tē-ŎK-lā-sĭs] osteo-, bone + -clasis, breaking	Breaking of a bone in order to repair or reposition it.

Term	Word Analysis	Definition
osteoplasty	[ŎS-tē-ō-plăs-tē] osteo-, bone + -plasty, repair	Surgical replacement or repair of bone.
osteotomy	[ŏs-tē-ŎT-ō-mē] osteo-, bone + -tomy, cutting	Cutting of bone.
prosthetic device	[prŏs-THĔT-ĭk]	Artificial device used as a substitute for a missing or diseased body part.
reduction		Return of a part to its normal position.
splinting		Applying a splint to immobilize a body part.
spondylosyndesis	[SPŎN-dĭ-lō-sĭn-DĒ-sĭs] spondylo-, vertebrae + Greek *syndesis*, a binding together	Fusion of two or more spinal vertebrae.
synovectomy	[sĭn-ō-VĔK-tō-mē] synovi(o)-, synovial fluid + -ectomy, removal	Removal of part or all of a joint's synovial membrane.
tenotomy	[tĕ-NŎT-ō-mē] teno-, tendon + -tomy, cutting	Surgical cutting of a tendon.
traction	[TRĂK-shŭn]	Dragging or pulling or straightening of something, as a limb, by attachment of elastic or other devices.

C A S E S T U D Y

Musculoskeletal Injury

John Positano, a track star at a large university, suffered a knee injury during a meet. The team physician prescribed rest and medication first, then, a gradual program of physical therapy. John missed about six weeks of meets and seemed fine until the end of the season, when a particularly strenuous run in which he twisted his knee left him writhing in pain. It was the same knee on which fluid had accumulated during the previous week. X-rays showed no fractures. Later, after examination by a specialist, arthroscopic surgery was recommended. John had to go through another rehabilitative program (rest, medication, and physical therapy) after the surgery.

 Critical Thinking

78. A program of physical therapy was prescribed for John. Which one of his tests was most important in determining whether or not he could exercise?

79. Is physical therapy always appropriate for a musculoskeletal injury?

Surgical Terms Exercises

Build Your Medical Vocabulary

Form two surgical words for each of the following word roots by adding suffixes learned in Chapter 2.

80. osteo-_____

81. arthro-_____

82. myo-_____

83. spondylo-_____

Find a Match

Match the terms in the second column to the terms in the first.

84. amputation   a. replacement device

85. prosthesis   b. molding

86. orthosis, orthotic   c. muscle repair

87. traction   d. bone cutting

88. casting   e. removal

89. splinting   f. bone repair

90. myoplasty   g. external immobilizing device

91. osteoplasty   h. wrapping to immobilize

92. osteotomy   i. pulling to straighten

93. arthroplasty   j. joint repair

Pharmacological Terms

Most medications for treatment of the musculoskeletal system treat symptoms, not causes. Pain medications, such as **analgesics, narcotics, anti-inflammatories, muscle relaxants,** and **nonsteroidal anti-inflammatory drugs (NSAIDs),** all relieve or relax the area of pain either by numbing the area or by reducing the inflammation. Table 5-1 shows some common medications.

Table 5-1 Some Medication for the Musculoskeletal System

Drug Class	Purpose	Generic	Trade Name
analgesic	to relieve pain	aspirin acetaminophen (NSAIDS are also analgesics.)	Bayer, Excedrin, and various Tylenol and various
anti-inflammatory (steroids)	to reduce inflammation	desoximetasone prednisone fluocinonide (Aspirin and NSAIDS also reduce inflammation.)	Topicort Apo-Prednisone, Deltasone, Orasone Lidex
muscle relaxant	to relieve stiffness	baclofen carisoprodol cyclobenzaprine methocarbamol	Lioresal Rela, Sodol, Soridal Cycloflex, Flexeril Delaxin, Robaxin
NSAIDS	to reduce inflammation	ibuprofen ketoprofen naproxen ketorolac tromethamine nabutemone	Advil, Excedrin, Motrin, Nuprin Orudis, Oruvail Naprosyn Toradol (IV) Relafen

Vocabulary Review

In the previous section, you learned terms relating to pharmacology. Before going on to the exercises, review the terms below and refer to the previous section if you have questions.

Term	Word Analysis	Definition
analgesic	[ăn-ăl-JĒ-zĭk]	Agent that relieves pain.
anti-inflammatory		Agent that reduces inflammation.
muscle relaxant		Agent that relieves muscle stiffness.
narcotic		Agent that relieves pain by affecting the body in ways that are similar to opium.
nonsteroidal anti-inflammatory drug (NSAIDs)	[nŏn-STĔR-ŏy-dăl]	Agent that reduces inflammation without the use of steroids.

CASE STUDY

Treating the Symptoms

In her follow-up letter on Laura Spinoza's visit, Dr. Wolf listed a number of medications to treat the symptoms of fibromyalgia. Part of the difficulty in treating musculoskeletal disorders is that many of the diseases are degenerative, and damage cannot be reversed. Some of these diseases, such as muscular dystrophy, currently have no cure. Many forms of arthritis are degenerative and, short of replac-ing joints, cannot be improved significantly. Alleviating the pain is the only available course of treatment in many instances.

 Critical Thinking

94. Narcotics can be addictive. The long-term use of steroids can cause other health prob-lems. What does Dr. Wolf prescribe to avoid these two problems?

95. Many athletes use anabolic steroids illegally for strength and endurance building. (Corticosteroids are not used for this purpose.) Anabolic-steroid use can cause heart damage and many other seri-ous health problems. What are some ways to increase strength and endurance without the use of dangerous drugs?

Pharmacological Terms Exercises

Choose one of the following terms to fill in each blank. Each term may be used more than once.

analgesic

anti-inflammatory

antibiotic

96. Treatment for bursitis _____.

97. Treatment for myalgia _____.

98. Treatment for bone infection _____.

99. Treatment for arthritis _____.

100. Treatment for arthralgia _____.

CHALLENGE SECTION

The notes of Janet Azrah's examination give the results of all observations and tests. The treatment protocol is described.

Janet Azrah was in on March 7th for what I think is recent onset of rheumatoid arthritis. We discussed her five-month history of joint pain, swelling, and stiffness which is quite familiar to you, and I will not review it in great detail. I detected nothing else that suggested any other type of rheumatic disease process. The remainder of the review of systems covered a history of irritable bowel syndrome and otherwise reveals that she has been a reasonably healthy and active person throughout her years.

The examination revealed a blood pressure of 150/94 in the right arm in a sitting position. The general examination did not include a rectal or pelvic examination. Many molars were absent and the remainder of the examination of the ears, nose, and throat were normal. The musculoskeletal examination revealed a one-third reduction of all range of motion of the neck. Slight inflammatory swelling was noted in wrists, MCP and PIP joints with mild tenderness and a moderate loss in grip strength. Tinel's sign was positive on the right and negative on the left with bilateral positive Phalen's signs. Bony osteo-arthritic enlargement was noted in the thumb DIP joints. Moderate edema was present in the ankles. Tenderness of mild to moderate severity was noted in the tarsal joints and metatarsal joints.

The Westergren sedimentation rate was elevated to 78 mm per hour when checked in my office. Copies of my lab results are enclosed. I want to thank you for your sending copies of your record, as these were a great help. I had originally started 5 mg of Prednisone in a dose of 30 mg b.i.d. and tapered to a dose of 10 mg b.i.d. by the time of her return. Her symptomology was vastly improved as one would expect. I outlined a program to reduce Prednisone further to 7.5 mg per day. I added 200 mg of Plaquenil b.i.d. and provided information sheets on those drugs as well as an information booklet on rheumatoid arthritis.

Challenge Section Exercises

101. The notes in this section indicate a probable diagnosis of rheumatoid arthritis. Was the musculoskeletal examination normal?

102. Why might a physician perform a general examination on a patient who only shows symptoms related to the musculoskeletal system?

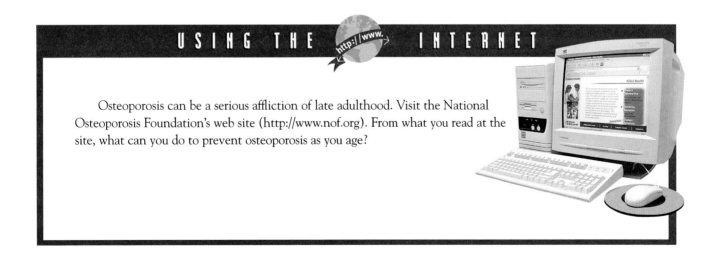

USING THE INTERNET

Osteoporosis can be a serious affliction of late adulthood. Visit the National Osteoporosis Foundation's web site (http://www.nof.org). From what you read at the site, what can you do to prevent osteoporosis as you age?

CHAPTER REVIEW

Define the following terms and combining forms. Review the chapter before starting. Make sure you know how to pronounce each term as you define it.

Word	Definitions
acetabul(o)	
acetabulum [ăs-ĕ-TĂB-yū-lŭm]	
acromi(o)	
acromion [ă-KRŌ-mē-ōn]	
amphiarthroses [ĂM-fĭ-ăr-THRŌ-sĕs]	
amputation [ĂM-pyū-TĀ-shŭn]	
analgesic [ăn-ăl-JĒ-zĭk]	
ankle [ĂNG-kl]	
ankyl(o)	
ankylosis [ĂNG-kĭ-LŌ-sĭs]	
anti-inflammatory	
arthr(o)	
arthralgia [ăr-THRĂL-jē-ă]	
arthritis [ăr-THRĪ-tĭs]	
arthrocentesis [ĂR-thrō-sĕn-TĒ-sĭs]	
arthrodesis [ăr-thrō-DĒ-sĭs]	
arthrography [ăr-THRŎG-ră-fĕ]	
arthroplasty [ĂR-thrō-plăs-tē]	
arthroscopy [ăr-THRŎS-kŏ-pē]	
articular [ăr-TĬK-yū-lăr] cartilage	
articulation [ār-tĭk-yū-LĀ-shūn]	
atlas [ĂT-lăs]	
atrophy [ĂT-rō-fē]	
axis [ĂK-sĭs]	
bone	

Word	Definitions
bone grafting	
bone head	
bone phagocyte [FĂG-ō-sīt]	
bone scan	
bony necrosis [BŌN-ē nĕ-KRŌ-sĭs]	
brachi(o)	
bunion [BŬN-yŭn]	
bunionectomy [bŭn-yŭn-ĔK-tō-mē]	
burs(o)	
bursa [BĔR-să]	
bursectomy [bĕr-SĔK-tō-mē]	
bursitis [bĕr-SĪ-tĭs]	
calcane(o)	
calcaneus [kăl-KĀ-nē-ŭs]	
calcar [KĂL-kăr]	
calci(o)	
calcium [KĂL-sē-ŭm]	
cancellous [KĂN-sĕ-lŭs] bone	
cardiac [KĂR-dē-ăk] muscle	
carp(o)	
carpal [KĂR-păl] tunnel syndrome	
carpus, carpal [KĂR-pŭs, KĂR-păl] bone	
cartilage [KĂR-tĭ-lĭj]	
cartilaginous [kăr-tĭ-LĂJ-ĭ-nŭs] disk	
casting	
cephal(o)	
cervic(o)	
cervical [SĔR-vĭ-kăl] vertebrae	
chiropractor [kī-rō-PRĂK-tōr]	
chondr(o)	
chondromalacia [KŎN-drō-mă-LĀ-shē-ă]	
clavicle [KLĂV-ĭ-kl]	

Word	Definitions
closed fracture	
coccyx [KŎK-sĭks]	
Colles' [kōlz] fracture	
comminuted [KŎM-ĭ-nū-tĕd] fracture	
compact bone	
complex fracture	
complicated fracture	
compound fracture	
compression fracture	
condyl(o)	
condyle [KŎN-dĭl]	
cost(o)	
crani(o)	
crest	
dactyl(o)	
degenerative arthritis	
densitometer [dĕn-sĭ-TŎM-ĕ-tĕr]	
diaphysis [di-AF-i-sis]	
diarthroses [di-ar-THRO-sez]	
disk, disc [dĭsk]	
diskography [dĭs-KŎG-ră-fē]	
dislocation	
dorsal vertebrae	
dystonia [dĭs-TŌ-nē-ă]	
elbow [ĔL-bō]	
electromyogram [ĕ-lĕk-trō-MĪ-ō-grăm]	
endosteum [ĕn-DŎS-tē-ŭm]	
epiphyseal [ĕp-ĭ-FĬZ-ē-ăl] plate	
epiphysitis [ĕ-pĭf-ĭ-SĪ-tĭs]	
ethmoid [ĔTH-mŏyd] bone	
ethmoid sinuses	
exostosis [ĕks-ŏs-TŌ-sĭs]	
external fixation device	

Word	Definitions
fasci(o)	
fascia [FĂSH-ē-ă]	
femor(o)	
femur [FĒ-mūr]	
fibr(o)	
fibula [FĬB-yū-lă]	
fissure [FĬSH-ŭr]	
flaccid [FLĂK-sĭd]	
flat bones	
fontanelle [FŎN-tă-nĕl]	
foramen [fō-RĀ-mĕn]	
foramen magnum [MĂG-nŭm]	
fossa [FŎS-ă]	
fracture [FRĂK-chūr]	
frontal [FRŬN-tăl] bone	
frontal sinuses	
goniometer [gō-nē-ŎM-ĕ-tĕr]	
gouty arthritis, gout [gowt]	
greenstick fracture	
hairline fracture	
heel [hēl]	
herniated [HĔR-nē-ā-tĕd] disk	
humer(o)	
humerus [HYŪ-mĕr-ŭs]	
hypertrophy [hī-PĔR-trō-fē]	
hypotonia [HĪ-pō-TŌ-nē-ă]	
ili(o)	
ilium [ĬL-ē-ŭm]	
impacted fracture	
incomplete fracture	
insertion	
internal fixation device	

Word	Definitions
involuntary muscle	
irregular bones	
ischi(o)	
ischium [ĬS-kē-ūŭm]	
joint [jŏynt]	
kyph(o)	
kyphosis [kī-FŌ-sĭs]	
lacrimal [LĂK-rĭ-măl] bone	
lamin(o)	
lamina (pl. laminae) [LĂM-ĭ-nă (LĂM-ĭ-nē)]	
laminectomy [LĂM-ĭ-NĔK-tō-mē]	
leiomy(o)	
leiomyoma [LĪ-ō-mĭ-Ō-mă]	
leiomyosarcoma [LĪ-ō-MĬ-ō-săr-KŌ-mă]	
ligament [LIG-a-ment]	
long bone	
lordosis [lōr-DŌ-sĭs]	
lumb(o)	
lumbar [LŬM-băr] vertebrae	
malleolus (pl. malleoli) [mă-LĒ-ō-lŭs (mă-lē-Ō-lī)]	
mandible [MĂN-dĭ-bl]	
mandibular [măn-DĬB-yū-lăr] bone	
marrow [MĂR-ō]	
mastoid [MĂS-tŏyd] process	
maxill(o)	
maxillary [MĂK-sĭ-lār-ē] bone	
maxillary sinus	
medullary [MĔD-ū-lār-ē] cavity	
metacarp(o)	
metacarpal [MĔT-ă-KĂR-păl]	
metaphysis [mĕ-TĂF-ĭ-sĭs]	

Word	Definitions
metatarsal [MĔT-ă-tăr-săl] bones	
muscle [MŬS-ĕl]	
muscle relaxant	
muscular dystrophy [MŬS-kyū-lăr DĬS-trō-fē]	
musculoskeletal [MŬS-kyū-lō-SKĔL-ĕ-tăl] system	
my(o)	
myalgia [mī-ĂL-jē-ă]	
myel(o)	
myelography [MĪ-ĕ-LŎG-ră-fē]	
myeloma [mī-ĕ-LŌ-mă]	
myodynia [MĪ-ō-dĭn-ē-ă]	
myoma [mī-Ō-mă]	
myoplasty [MĪ-ō-plăs-tē]	
myositis [mī-ō-SĪ-tĭs]	
narcotic	
nasal bones	
nasal cavity	
neural [NŪR-ăl] canal	
nonsteroidal [nŏn-STĔR-ŏy-dăl] anti-inflammatory drug	
nucleus pulposus [NŪ-klē-ŭs pŭl-PŌ-sŭs]	
occipital [ŏk-SĬP-ĭ-tăl] bone	
olecranon [ō-LĔK-ră-nŏn]	
open fracture	
origin	
orthopedist [ōr-thō-PĒ-dĭst]	
orthosis [ōr-THŌ-sĭs], orthotic [ōr-THŎT-ĭk]	
osseus [ŎS-ē-ŭs] tissue	
ossification [ŎS-ĭ-fĭ-KĀ-shŭn]	
oste(o)	
ostealgia [ŏs-tē-ĂL-jē-ă]	

Word	Definitions
osteoarthritis [ŎS-tē-ō-ăr-THRĪ-tĭs]	
osteoblast [ŎS-tē-ō-blăst]	
osteoclasis [ŎS-tē-ŎK-lā-sĭs]	
osteoclast [ŎS-tē-ō-klăst]	
osteocyte [ŎS-tē-ō-sīt]	
osteodynia [ŏs-tē-ō-DĬN-ē-ă]	
osteoma [ŏs-tē-Ō-mă]	
osteomyelitis [ŎS-tē-ō-mī-ĕ-LĪ-tĭs]	
osteopath [ŎS-tē-ō-păth]	
osteoplasty [ŎS-tē-ō-plăs-tē]	
osteoporosis [ŎS-tē-ō-pō-RŌ-sĭs]	
osteosarcoma [ŎS-tē-ō-săr-KŌ-mă]	
osteotomy [ŏs-tē-ŎT-ō-mē]	
palatine [PĂL-ĭ-tīn] bone	
parietal [pă-RĪ-ĕ-tăl] bone	
patell(o)	
patella [pă-TĔL-ă]	
pathological fracture	
ped(i), pedo	
pelv(i)	
pelvic [PĔL-vĭk] cavity	
pelvic girdle	
pelvis [PĔL-vĭs]	
periosteum [pĕr-ē-ŎS-tē-ŭm]	
phalang(o)	
phalanges (sing. phalanx) [fă-LĂN-jĕz (FĂ-lăngks)]	
phantom limb; phantom pain	
phosphorus [FŎS-fōr-ŭs]	
physical therapy	
pod(o)	
podagra [pō-DĂG-ră]	
podiatrist [pō-DĪ-ă-trĭst]	
process [PRŌS-sĕs, PRŎS-ĕs]	

Word	Definitions
prosthetic [prŏs-THĔT-ĭk] device	
pub(o)	
pubes [PYŪ-bĭs]	
pubic symphysis [PYŪ-bĭk SĬM-fĭ-sĭs]	
rachi(o)	
radi(o)	
radius [RĀ-dē-ŭs]	
reduction	
rhabd(o)	
rhabdomy(o)	
rhabdomyoma [RĂB-dō-mī-Ō-mă]	
rhabdomyosarcoma [RĂB-dō-mī-ō-săr-KŌ-mă]	
rheumatoid arthritis	
rheumatoid factor test	
rheumatologist [rū-mă-TŎL-ō-jĭst]	
rib	
rickets [RĬK-ĕts]	
rigidity	
rigor [RĬG-ĕr]	
sacrum [SĀ-krŭm]	
scapul(o)	
scapula [SKĂP-yū-lā]	
sciatica [sī-ĂT-ĭ-kă]	
scoli(o)	
scoliosis [skō-lē-Ō-sĭs]	
sella turcica [SĔL-ă-TŬR-sĭ-kă]	
sequestrum [sē-KWĔS-trŭm]	
serum calcium	
serum creatine phosphokinase [SĒR-ŭm KRĒ-ă-tēn fŏs-fō-KĪ-nās]	
serum phosphorus	
sesamoid [SĔS-ă-mŏyd] bone	
shin [shĭn]	

Word	Definitions
short bones	
simple fracture	
sinus [SĪ-nŭs]	
skeleton [SKĔL-ĕ-tŏn]	
smooth muscle	
spasm [spăzm]	
spastic [SPAS-tik]	
sphenoid [SFĒ-nŏyd] bone	
sphenoid sinus	
spina bifida [SPĪ-nă-BĬF-ĭ-dă]	
spinal column	
spinal curvature	
spinous [SPĪ-nŭs] process	
splinting	
spondyl(o)	
spondylolisthesis [SPŎN-dĭ-lō-lĭs-THĒ-sĭs]	
spondylolysis [spŏn-dĭ-LŎL-ĭ-sĭs]	
spondylosyndesis [SPŎN-dĭ-lō-sĭn-DĒ-sĭs]	
spongy bone	
sprain [sprān]	
spur [spĕr]	
stern(o)	
sternum [STĔR-nŭm]	
strain [strān]	
striated [strī-ĀT-ĕd] muscle	
styloid [STĪ-lŭyd] process	
subluxation [sŭb-lŭk-SĀ-shŭn]	
sulcus [SŬL-kŭs]	
suture [SŪ-chūr]	
symphysis [SĬM-fĭ-sĭs]	
synarthrosis [SĬN-ăr-THRŌ-sĭs]	
synov(o)	

Word	Definitions
synovectomy [sĭn-ō-VĔK-tō-mē]	
synovial [sĭ-NŌ-vē-ăl] fluid	
synovial joint	
synovial membrane	
talipes calcaneus [TĂL-ĭ-pēz kăl-KĀ-nē-ŭs]	
talipes valgus [TĂL-ĭ-pēz VĂL-gŭs]	
talipes varus [TĂL-ĭ-pēz VĀ-rŭs]	
tars(o)	
tarsus, tarsal [TĂR-sŭs, TĂR-săl] bones	
temporal [TĔM-pō-RĂL] bone	
temporomandibular [TĔM-pō-rō-măn-DĬB-yū-lăr] joint	
ten(o), tend(o), tendin(o)	
tendinitis, tendonitis	
tendon [TĔN-dŏn]	
tenotomy [tĕ-NŎT-ō-mē]	
tetany [TĔT-ă-nē]	
thorac(o)	
thoracic [thō-RĂS-ĭk] vertebrae	
thorax [THŌ-răks]	
tibi(o)	
tibia [TĬB-ē-ă]	
Tinel's sign	
traction [TRĂK-shŭn]	
transverse process	
tremor [TRĔM-ĕr]	
trochanter [trō-KĂN-tĕr]	
true ribs	
tubercle [TŪ-bĕr-kl]	
tuberosity [TŪ-bĕr-ŏs-ĭ-tē]	
uln(o)	
ulna [ŬL-nă]	
uric acid test	

Word	Definitions
vertebr(o)	
vertebra (pl. vertebrae) [VĔR-tĕ-bră (VĔR-tĕ-brē)]	
vertebral body	
vertebral column	
visceral [VĬS-ĕr-ăl] muscle	
vitamin D	
voluntary muscle	
vomer [VŌ-mĕr]	
zygomatic [ZĪ-gō-MĂT-ĭk] bone	

Abbreviations

Write out the full meaning of each abbreviation.

Abbreviation	Meaning
A-K	
B-K	
C_1, C_2, etc.	
ca	
CTS	
DJD	
DTR	
EMG	
fx	
IM	
L_1, L_2, etc.	
MCP	
NSAID	

P   _____

PIP   _____

ROM   _____

T₁, T₂, etc.   _____

TMJ   _____

Answers to Chapter Exercises

1. Synovial fluid lubricates joints.
2. Yes, exercise can increase breathing and heart rate which can exercise certain involuntary muscles. Voluntary muscles may be exercised at will.
3. long
4. 206
5. marrow
6. fontanelles
7. nucleus pulposus
8. acromion
9. true ribs
10. patella
11. calcaneus
12. cardiac
13. F
14. T
15. F
16. T
17. T
18. fibromyalgia, pain in the fibrous tissue of muscles; osteoarthritis, arthritis of the bone
19. CTS, carpel tunnel syndrome
20. arthro
21. cranio
22. maxillo
23. ilio
24. tarso
25. thoracic
26. fibro
27. pod
28. rachio
29. sterno
30. arthralgia, arthrodynia
31. bursectomy
32. chondritis
33. spondylectomy
34. osteoblast
35. osteosclerosis
36. cervicoplasty
37. myelitis
38. podospasm
39. ulnocarpal
40. synovo-, synovial fluid; synovial membrane
41. myelo-, spinal cord; bone marrow
42. -dynia, pain

43. osteo-, bone
44. rachio-, spine
45. Porous bone can result in breakage.
46. alternative treatment plans, side effects, potential benefits, potential risks, and the negative effect of not taking the medicine
47. These elements are crucial to bone formation.
48. No. Chiropractors are concerned with spinal manipulation.
49. Yes, the picture of the bone should show abnormalities.
50. Both believe in spinal manipulation.
51. A goniometer can measure range of motion of a muscle.
52. It may help ease pain by loosening and realigning.
53. Because the pain may be due to a condition other than back misalignment.
54. f.
55. e.
56. c.
57. a.
58. d.
59. b.
60. f
61. d
62. c
63. a
64. b
65. g
66. h
67. e
68. arthritis
69. greenstick
70. older
71. tendinitis
72. flaccid
73. myoma
74. spondylolisthesis
75. open
76. joint
77. spinal cord
78. The x-rays showed no fractures; therefore, no area needed to be held in place for a long period of time to allow the bone to heal.

79. No, not if there are certain kinds of fractures that must heal before movement is attempted.

Answers to 80-83 may vary. Sample answers are shown below.

80. osteotomy, osteoplasty, osteoclasis
81. arthroplasty, arthrotomy
82. myotomy, myoplasty
83. spondylotomy, spondylectomy
84. e
85. a
86. g
87. i
88. b
89. h
90. c
91. f
92. d
93. j
94. He suggests no narcotics, since the patient has fairly continuous pain episodes, and he suggests switching to nonsteroidal compounds.
95. diet, weight-bearing exercises, cardiovascular exercise, aerobics
96. anti-inflammatory
97. analgesic
98. anti-inflammatory, antibiotic
99. anti-inflammatory
100. analgesic
101. no
102. to eliminate possible diseases (such as multiple sclerosis) that might mimic symptoms of musculoskeletal diseases

CHAPTER 6

The Cardiovascular System

After studying this chapter, you will be able to:

- Name the parts of the cardiovascular system and discuss the function of each part

- Define combining forms used in building words that relate to the cardiovascular system

- Identify the meaning of related abbreviations

- Name the common diagnoses, clinical procedures, and laboratory tests used in treating the cardiovascular system

- List and define the major pathological conditions of the cardiovascular system

- Explain the meaning of surgical terms related to the cardiovascular system

- Recognize common pharmacological agents used in treating the cardiovascular system

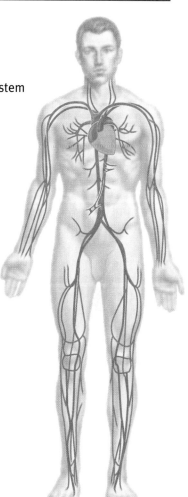

Structure and Function

The cardiovascular system is the body's delivery service. Figure 6-1 on page 166 shows the routes of blood circulation throughout the cardiovascular system. The **heart** pumps **blood** through the **blood vessels** to all the cells of the body. The average adult heart is about 5 inches long and 3.5 inches wide and weighs anywhere from 7 ounces to almost 14 ounces, depending on an individual's size and gender. The heart is covered by the **pericardium,** a protective sac. The pericardium has two layers: the *visceral pericardium* (the layer next to the heart) and the *parietal pericardium* (the outer portion of the pericardium). Inside the pericardium, the heart has three layers of tissue. The outermost layer is the **epicardium.** The second layer is the **myocardium,** a layer of muscular tissue. The inner layer, the **endocardium,** forms a membranous lining for the chambers and valves of the heart.

The heart is divided into right and left sides. Each side has two chambers. The **right atrium** and **right ventricle** on the right side are separated from the **left atrium** and **left ventricle** on the left side by a partition called a **septum** (plural, **septa**). The part of the septum between the two **atria** (plural of **atrium**) is called the *interatrial septum;* the part between the two **ventricles** is called the *interventricular septum.* Fibers in the ventricles called **Purkinje fibers** cause the

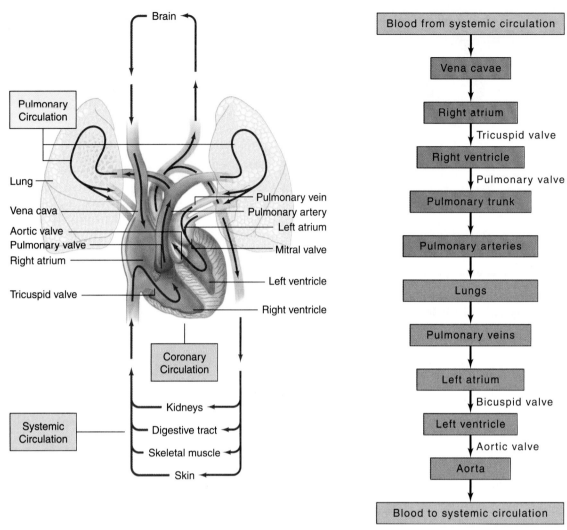

Brain

Pulmonary
Circulation

Lung

Vena cava

Aortic valve

Pulmonary valve

Right atrium

Tricuspid valve

Pulmonary vein
Pulmonary artery
Left atrium
Mitral valve

Left ventricle

Right ventricle

Coronary
Circulation

Kidneys

Systemic
Circulation

Digestive tract

Skeletal muscle

Skin

(a)

Blood from systemic circulation

Vena cavae

Right atrium

Tricuspid valve

Right ventricle

Pulmonary valve

Pulmonary trunk

Pulmonary arteries

Lungs

Pulmonary veins

Left atrium

Bicuspid valve

Left ventricle

Aortic valve

Aorta

Blood to systemic circulation

(b)

Figure 6-1 The heart pumps blood throughout the cardiovascular system via the blood vessels—arteries and veins. Arteries are shown in red, and veins are shown in blue (a). The cardiovascular system includes: coronary circulation, pulmonary circulation, and systemic circulation (b).

ventricles to contract. Blood flows through the chambers of the heart in only one direction, with the flow regulated by **valves.** The blood is pumped throughout the body through the system of **arteries** and **veins.** Arteries carry blood *away* from the heart. Veins carry blood *toward* the heart. The arteries carry oxygenated blood, except in pulmonary circulation. The veins carry deoxygenated blood, except in pulmonary circulation. Arteries have a lining called the **endothelium,** which secretes enzymes and other substances into the blood. The space within the arteries through which blood flows is called the **lumen.**

The valves of the heart also control the blood flow to and from the heart. The two **atrioventricular valves**—the **tricuspid valve** and the **bicuspid valve** (also called the **mitral valve**)—control the flow of blood within the heart between the atria and ventricles. The two **semilunar valves**—the **pulmonary valve** and the **aortic valve**—prevent the backflow of blood into the heart. The tricuspid valve has three cusps (flaps) that open and close to allow blood to flow from the right atrium into the right ventricle. The two cusps of the bicuspid valve are said to resemble a bishop's miter (hat), so this valve is commonly known as the *mitral valve.* The bicuspid valve controls blood flow on the left side of the heart, from the atrium to the ventricle. Figure 6-2 shows the heart and the structures leading to and from it.

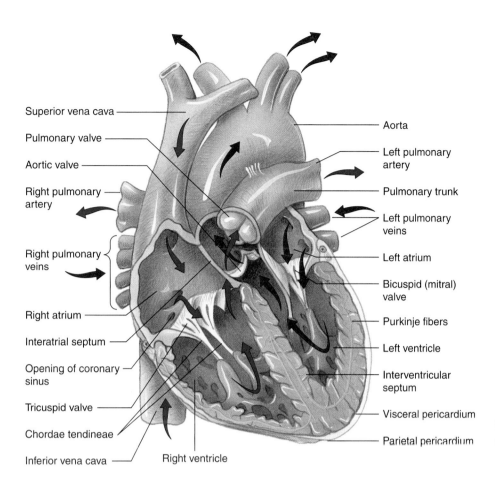

Superior vena cava

Pulmonary valve

Aortic valve

Right pulmonary artery

Right pulmonary veins

Right atrium

Interatrial septum

Opening of coronary sinus

Tricuspid valve

Chordae tendineae

Inferior vena cava

Right ventricle

Aorta

Left pulmonary artery

Pulmonary trunk

Left pulmonary veins

Left atrium

Bicuspid (mitral) valve

Purkinje fibers

Left ventricle

Interventricular septum

Visceral pericardium

Parietal pericardium

Oxygenated blood

Deoxygenated blood

Figure 6-2 Blood flow through a cross section of the heart.

The Vessels of the Cardiovascular System

Arteries and veins are the vessels that carry blood to and from the heart and lungs and to and from the heart and the rest of the body. This circulation of blood is the essential function of the cardiovascular system, which includes *coronary circulation,* the circulation of blood within the heart; *pulmonary circulation,* the flow of blood between the heart and lungs; and *systemic circulation,* the flow of blood between the heart and the cells of the body.

Coronary Circulation

The **coronary arteries,** which branch off the **aorta** (the body's largest artery and the artery through which blood exits the heart), supply blood to

MORE ABOUT...

The Heart

The heart is the body's main pump, sending blood to sustain all parts of the body. The heart is surprisingly small for such a large body function—only the size of an average adult fist. Although the heart has two sides, its shape is not symmetrical.

the heart muscle. The aortic semilunar valves control this flow of blood. The heart needs more oxygen than any other organ except the brain. The amount of blood pumped to the heart through the coronary arteries is about 100 gallons per day. The atrioventricular valves control the circulation of blood within the heart, between the atria and the ventricles. Figure 6-3 diagrams coronary circulation.

Pulmonary Circulation

The **pulmonary arteries** carry blood that is low in oxygen (*deoxygenated blood*) to the lungs from the right ventricle of the heart to get oxygen. Blood that is rich in oxygen (*oxygenated blood*) flows from the lungs to the left atrium of the heart through the **pulmonary veins.** Figure 6-4 traces the circulation of blood from the heart to the lungs and back.

Systemic Circulation

The heart pumps blood through the arteries to the cells of the body. The blood moves in a surge caused by the muscular contraction of the heart. This surge is called the **pulse.** The blood that goes from the heart to the cells of the body (except the lungs) is oxygenated. Specialized arteries carry the oxygen-rich blood to different areas of the body. For example, the **carotid artery** supplies the head and neck; the **femoral artery** supplies the thigh; and the **popliteal artery** supplies the back of the knee. The arteries divide into smaller vessels called **arterioles,** which then divide into very narrow vessels called **capillaries.** The capillaries are the transfer station of the delivery system. The capillaries provide the cells they serve with essential nutrients and, in turn, remove waste products (including **carbon dioxide, CO_2**) from the cells, sending it to the **venules,**

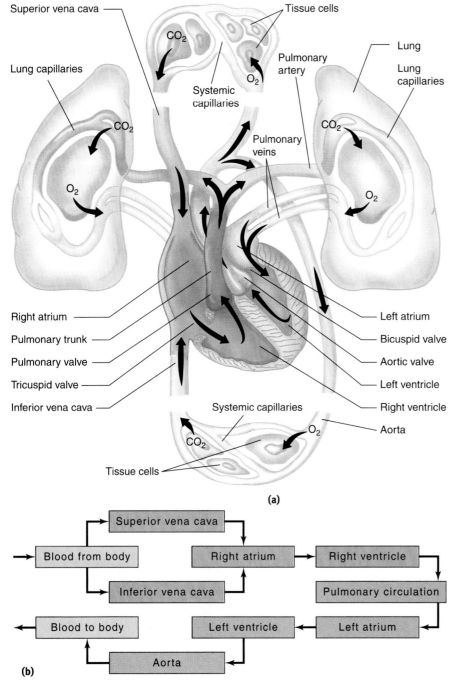

(a)

(b)

Figure 6-3 Coronary circulation is the circulation of blood within the heart (a). The flowchart (b) gives an overview of this type of circulation.

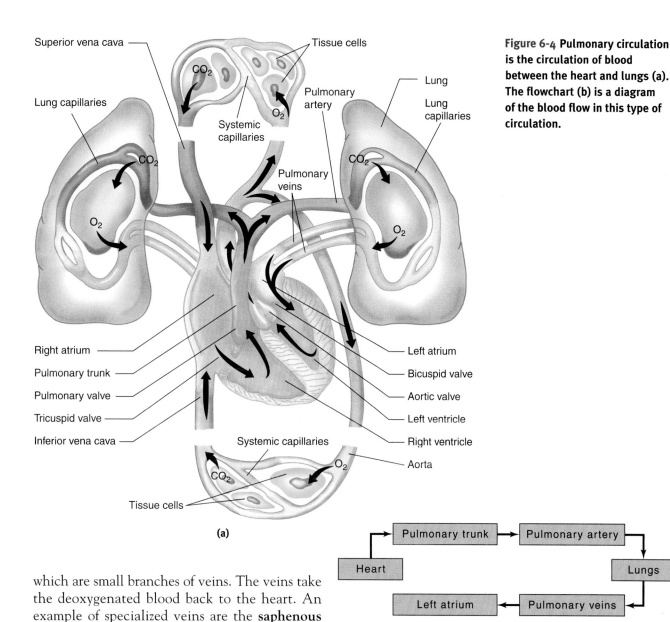

Superior vena cava

Tissue cells

Lung capillaries

CO_2

Systemic capillaries

Pulmonary artery

O_2

Lung

Lung capillaries

CO_2

Pulmonary veins

O_2

CO_2

O_2

Right atrium

Pulmonary trunk

Pulmonary valve

Tricuspid valve

Inferior vena cava

Systemic capillaries

Left atrium

Bicuspid valve

Aortic valve

Left ventricle

Right ventricle

Aorta

O_2

CO_2

Tissue cells

(a)

Figure 6-4 Pulmonary circulation is the circulation of blood between the heart and lungs (a). The flowchart (b) is a diagram of the blood flow in this type of circulation.

Heart → Pulmonary trunk → Pulmonary artery → Lungs → Pulmonary veins → Left atrium

(b)

which are small branches of veins. The veins take the deoxygenated blood back to the heart. An example of specialized veins are the **saphenous veins,** which remove oxygen-poor blood from the legs. Veins move the blood by gravity, skeletal muscle contractions, and respiratory activity. The veins contain small valves that prevent the blood from flowing backward. The blood from the upper part of the body is collected and carried to the heart through a large vein called the **superior vena cava**; the blood from the lower part of the body goes to the other large vein called the **inferior vena cava** and then to the heart. Both of these large veins, the **venae cavae** (plural of **vena cava**), bring the blood to the right atrium of the heart. Figure 6-5 on page 170 shows the major pathways in the systemic circulation.

Blood Pressure Blood pressure measures the force of the blood surging against the walls of the arteries. Each heartbeat consists of two parts. The first is the contraction, called **systole,** and the second is the relaxation, the **diastole. Blood pressure** is the measurement of the *systolic pressure* followed by the *diastolic pressure*. Normal blood pressure for an adult is 120/80. The number 120 represents the pressure within the walls of an artery during systole; the number 80 represents the pressure within the arterial wall during diastole. Figure 6-6 on page 171 shows a sphygmomanometer being used to measure blood pressure and a detail of the scale on it.

Controlling High Blood Pressure

High blood pressure is a dangerous condition with virtually no symptoms felt by the patient. At almost every doctor visit, blood pressure is measured, usually with a sphygmomanometer. Blood pressure measurements are characterized as normal, low, or high, but there is disagreement as to the ranges of normal. The ranges of measurements for an adult, taken from the Framingham Heart Study, are:

Normal: 120/80, or slightly above or below
High: Above 139/89

High blood pressure is sometimes the result of lifestyle factors. Overeating leading to overweight, smoking, lack of exercise, and stress are lifestyle factors that affect blood pressure. For systolic pressures above 160, most doctors recommend lifestyle changes along with medication. The American Heart Association regards any blood pressure over 139/89 as high blood pressure.

Conduction System The **conduction system** that controls the impulses that cause the heart to contract is contained in special heart tissue called *conductive tissue* in the right atrium. This region is called the **sinoatrial node (SA node)** and is known as the heart's **pacemaker** because its electrical impulse causes the regular contractions that result in a regular heartbeat or pulse. The contractions take place in the myocardium, which cycles through **polarization** (resting state) to **depolarization** (contracting state) to **repolarization** (recharging from contracting to resting) in the heartbeat. The electrical current from the SA node passes to a portion of the interatrial septum called the **atrioventricular node (AV node)**, which sends the charge to a group of specialized muscle fibers called the **atrioventricular bundle,** also called the **bundle of His.** The bundle of His divides into left and right bundle branches and causes the ventricles to contract, forcing blood away from the heart during systole.

Heart rate can vary depending on a person's health, physical activity, or emotions at any one time. The repeated beating of the heart takes place in the

Figure 6-5 Systemic circulation is the flow of blood between the heart and the cells of the entire body. In addition to arteries and veins, smaller blood vessels branch off to connect with cellular material. Specific arteries and veins are named for the area of the body that they serve. The brachiocephalic artery serves the arms and head, the subclavian arteries and veins serve the area beneath the shoulder or collar bone, the iliac arteries and veins serve the small intestines, the hepatic vessels serve the liver, and the jugular veins serve the throat and neck.

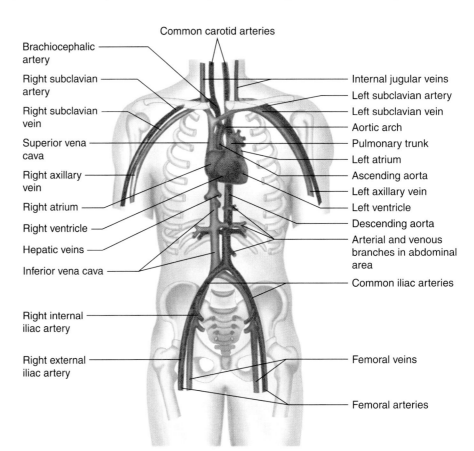

Common carotid arteries

Brachiocephalic artery

Right subclavian artery

Right subclavian vein

Superior vena cava

Right axillary vein

Right atrium

Right ventricle

Hepatic veins

Inferior vena cava

Right internal iliac artery

Right external iliac artery

Internal jugular veins

Left subclavian artery

Left subclavian vein

Aortic arch

Pulmonary trunk

Left atrium

Ascending aorta

Left axillary vein

Left ventricle

Descending aorta

Arterial and venous branches in abdominal area

Common iliac arteries

Femoral veins

Femoral arteries

cardiac cycle, during which the heart contracts and relaxes as it circulates blood. Normal heart rhythm is called **sinus rhythm.**

Fetal Circulation

The circulatory system of the fetus bypasses pulmonary circulation, because a fetus's lungs do not function until after birth. The umbilical cord contains arteries and a vein. Fetal blood is transported back and forth to the placenta, where deoxygenated blood is oxygenated and returned to the fetus. Three structures are important to fetal circulation (Figure 6-7). The **ductus venosus** is the connection from the umbilical vein to the fetus's inferior vena cava, through which oxygenated blood is delivered to the fetal heart, bypassing the fetal liver. Deoxygenated blood flows from the fetal heart through the **ductus arteriosus** and back through the umbilical cord to the placenta. The septum between the atria of the fetal heart has a small opening called the **foramen ovale,** which allows blood to flow from the right atrium intro the left atrium. After birth, this opening closes. Chapter 17 discusses fetal development.

Figure 6-6 A sphygmomanometer measures blood pressure.

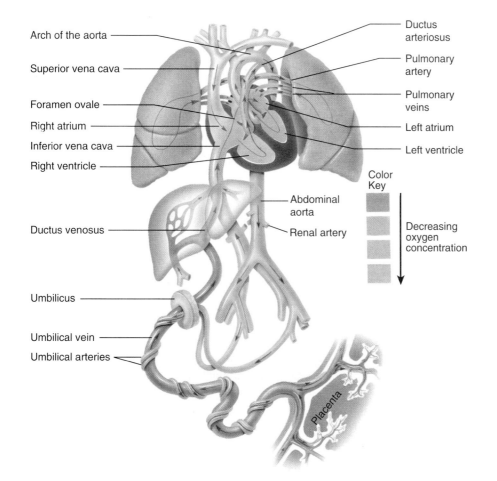

Arch of the aorta

Superior vena cava

Foramen ovale

Right atrium

Inferior vena cava

Right ventricle

Ductus venosus

Umbilicus

Umbilical vein

Umbilical arteries

Ductus arteriosus

Pulmonary artery

Pulmonary veins

Left atrium

Left ventricle

Abdominal aorta

Renal artery

Color Key

Decreasing oxygen concentration

Placenta

Figure 6-7 Fetal blood moves back and forth between the placenta and the growing fetus. The diagram shows the flow of oxygenated and deoxygenated blood from the fetus's heart through its nonfunctioning lungs to the umbilicus to the placenta. Structures unique to the fetus that change after birth are the foramen ovale and the ductus venosus.

Vocabulary Review

In the previous section, you learned terms relating to the cardiovascular system. Before going on to the exercises, review the terms below and refer to the previous section if you have any questions.

Term	Word Analysis	Definition
aorta	[ā-ŌR-tă] Greek *aorte*	Largest artery of the body; artery through which blood exits the heart.
aortic valve		Valve between the aorta and the left ventricle.
arteriole	[ăr-TĒ-rē-ōl] arteri-, artery + -ole, small	A tiny artery connecting to a capillary.
artery	[ĂR-tĕr-ē] Latin and Greek *arteria*	A thick-walled blood vessel that, in systemic circulation, carries oxygenated blood away from the heart.
atrioventricular bundle	[Ā-trē-ō-vĕn-TRĬK-yū-lăr] atrio-, atrium + ventricular	Bundle of fibers in the interventricular septum that transfer charges in the heart's conduction system; also called *bundle of His*.
atrioventricular node (AV node)		Specialized part of the interatrial septum that sends a charge to the bundle of His.
atrioventricular valve		One of two valves that control blood flow between the atria and ventricles.
atrium (pl. atria)	[Ā-trē-ŭm, (Ā-trē-ă)]	Either of the two upper chambers of the heart.
bicuspid valve	[bī-KŬS-pĭd] bi-, two + cuspid, having one cusp	Atrioventricular valve on the left side of the heart.
blood	[blŭd] Old English *blod*	Essential fluid containing plasma and other elements that circulates throughout the body; delivers nutrients to and removes waste from the body's cells.
blood pressure		Measure of the force of blood surging against the walls of the arteries.
blood vessel		Any of the tubular passageways in the cardiovascular system through which blood travels.
bundle of His	[hĭz, hĭs] After Wilhelm His (1863–1934), German Physician	*See* atrioventricular bundle.

Term	Word Analysis	Definition
capillary	[KĂP-ĭ-lār-ē]	A tiny blood vessel that forms the exchange point between the arterial and venous vessels.
carbon dioxide		Waste material transported in the venous blood.
cardiac cycle		Repeated contraction and relaxation of the heart as it circulates blood within itself and pumps it out to the rest of the body or the lungs.
carotid artery	[kă-RŎT-ĭd]	Artery that transports oxygenated blood to the head and neck.
conduction system		Part of the heart containing specialized tissue that sends charges through heart fibers, causing the heart to contract and relax at regular intervals.
coronary artery	[KŌR-ō-nār-ē] Latin *coronarius* from *corona*, crown	Blood vessel that supplies oxygen-rich blood to the heart.
depolarization	[dē-pō-lă-rĭ-ZĀ-shŭn] de-, away from + polarization	Contracting state of the myocardial tissue in the heart's conduction system.
diastole	[dī-ĂS-tō-lē] Greek, dilation	Relaxation phase of a heartbeat.
ductus arteriosus	[DŬK-tŭs ăr-tēr-ē-Ō-sŭs]	Structure in the fetal circulatory system through which blood flows to bypass the fetus's nonfunctioning lungs.
ductus venosus	[vĕn-Ō-sŭs]	Structure in the fetal circulatory system through which blood flows to bypass the fetal liver.
endocardium	[ĕn-dō-KĂR-dē-ŭm] endo-, within + Greek *kardia*, heart	Membranous lining of the chambers and valves of the heart; the innermost layer of heart tissue.
endothelium	[ĕn-dō-THĒ-lē-ŭm] endo- + Greek *thele*, nipple	Lining of the arteries that secretes substances into the blood.
epicardium	[ĕp-ĭ-KĂR-dē-ŭm] epi-, upon + Greek *kardia*, heart	Outermost layer of heart tissue.
femoral artery	[FĔM-ŏ-răl, FĒ-mŏ-răl]	An artery that supplies blood to the thigh.
foramen ovale	[fō-RĀ-mĕn ō-VĂ-lē]	Opening in the septum of the fetal heart that closes at birth.

Term	Word Analysis	Definition
heart	[hărt] Old English *heorte*	Muscular organ that receives blood from the veins and sends it into the arteries.
inferior vena cava	[VĒ-nă KĂ-vă, KĀ-vă]	Large vein that draws blood from the lower part of the body to the right atrium.
left atrium		Upper left heart chamber.
left ventricle		Lower left heart chamber.
lumen	[LŪ-mĕn]	Channel inside an artery through which blood flows.
mitral valve	[MĪ-trăl]	*See* bicuspid valve.
myocardium	[mī-ō-KĂR-dē-ŭm] myo-, muscle + Greek kardia, *heart*	Muscular layer of heart tissue between the epicardium and the endocardium.
pacemaker		Term for the sinoatrial node (SA node); also, an artificial device that regulates heart rhythm.
pericardium	[pĕr-ĭ-KĂR-dē-ŭm] peri-, around + Greek *kardia*, heart	Protective covering of the heart.
polarization	[pō-lăr-ĭ-ZĀ-shŭn]	Resting state of the myocardial tissue in the conduction system of the heart.
popliteal artery	[pŏp-LĬT-ē-ăl]	An artery that supplies blood to the cells of the area behind the knee.
pulmonary artery		One of two arteries that carry blood that is low in oxygen from the heart to the lungs.
pulmonary valve		Valve that controls the blood flow between the right ventricle and the pulmonary arteries.
pulmonary vein		One of four veins that bring oxygenated blood from the lungs to the left atrium.
pulse	[pŭls]	Rhythmic expansion and contraction of a blood vessel, usually an artery.
Purkinje fibers	[pŭr-KĬN-jē] After Johannes E. Purkinje (1787–1869), Bohemian physiologist	Fibers in the ventricle that cause it to contract.

Term	Word Analysis	Definition
repolarization	[rē-pō-lă-rĭ-ZĀ-shŭn] re, again + polarization	Recharging state; transition from contraction to resting that occurs in the conduction system of the heart.
right atrium		Upper right chamber of the heart.
right ventricle		Lower right chamber of the heart.
saphenous vein	[să-FĒ-nŭs]	Any of a group of veins that transport deoxygenated blood from the legs.
semilunar valve	[sĕm-ē-LŪ-năr] semi-, half + Latin *luna*, moon	One of the two valves that prevent the backflow of blood flowing out of the heart into the aorta and the pulmonary artery.
septum (pl. septa)	[SĔP-tŭm, (SĔP-tă)]	Partition between the left and right chambers of the heart.
sinoatrial node (SA node)	[sī-nō-Ā-trē-ăl]	Region of the right atrium containing specialized tissue that sends electrical impulses to the heart muscle, causing it to contract.
sinus rhythm		Normal heart rhythm.
superior vena cava		Large vein that transports blood collected from the upper part of the body to the heart.
systole	[SĬS-tō-lē]	Contraction phase of the heartbeat.
tricuspid valve	[trī-KŬS-pĭd] tri-, three + cuspid, having one cusp	Atrioventricular valve on the right side of the heart.
valve	[vălv]	Any of various structures that slow or prevent fluid from flowing backward or forward.
vein	[vān]	Any of various blood vessels carrying deoxygenated blood toward the heart, except the pulmonary vein.
vena cava	[VĒ-nă KĂ-vă, KĀ-vă]	*See* superior vena cava and inferior vena cava.
ventricle	[VĔN-trĭ-kl]	Either of the two lower chambers of the heart.
venule	[VĔN-yūl, VĒ-nūl]	A tiny vein connecting to a capillary.

CASE STUDY

A Cardiovascular Emergency

On a hot summer afternoon, Joseph Davino entered the emergency room at Stone General Hospital with severe shortness of breath (SOB). Dr. Mary Woodard was the cardiologist on call that day. She immediately started examining Mr. Davino and made a preliminary diagnosis based upon the physical assessment and the patient's history. She learned that Mr. Davino is 44 years old, is a smoker, is overweight, and has a sedentary lifestyle.

Mr. Davino's past medical history shows that he has a high cholesterol level, has a history of angina, and takes medication to control high blood pressure. The physical exam shows normal temperature and a blood pressure of 190/100. Dr. Woodard orders an ECG and cardiac enzymes.

 Critical Thinking

1. Shortness of breath may indicate cardiovascular disease. What lifestyle factors put Mr. Davino at risk?

2. Was Mr. Davino's blood pressure normal?

Structure and Function Exercises

Finish the Picture

Fill in the blanks.
Label the parts of the heart on the diagram. Describe the function of each part in the space below.

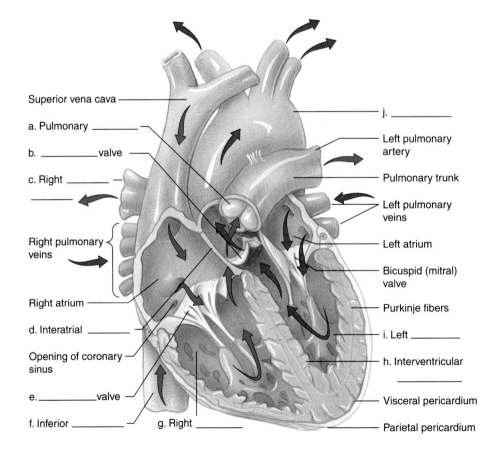

Superior vena cava

a. Pulmonary _____

b. _____ valve

c. Right _____
_____

Right pulmonary veins

Right atrium

d. Interatrial _____

Opening of coronary sinus

e. _____ valve

f. Inferior _____

g. Right _____

j. _____

Left pulmonary artery

Pulmonary trunk

Left pulmonary veins

Left atrium

Bicuspid (mitral) valve

Purkinje fibers

i. Left _____

h. Interventricular
_____

Visceral pericardium

Parietal pericardium

3. a. _____

   _____

   b. _____

   _____

   c. _____

   _____

   d. _____

   _____

   e. _____

   _____

   f. _____

   _____

   g. _____

   _____

   h. _____

   _____

   i. _____

   _____

   j. _____

Spell It Correctly

For each of the following words, write C if the spelling is correct. If it is not, write the correct spelling.

4. atriaventricular _____

5. capillairy _____

6. ductus arteriosus _____

7. Purkine fibers _____

8. myocardium _____

9. arteryole _____

10. bundle of His _____

11. popliteal _____

12. sistole _____

Test Your Knowledge

Fill in the blanks.

13. A vessel that carries oxygenated blood is a(n) _____.

14. Deoxygenated blood flows through the _____.

15. The innermost layer of heart tissue is called the _____.

16. The two atrioventricular valves control the flow of blood between the _____ and the _____.

17. Carbon dioxide is carried back to the heart via the _____.

18. Three lifestyle factors that may result in high blood pressure are _____,
    _____, and _____.

19. The fetal circulatory system does not include _____ circulation.

20. The lining of the arteries that secretes substances into the blood is called the_____.

21. Pulmonary circulation is the flow of blood between the _____ and _____.

22. The head and neck receive oxygen-rich blood via the _____ _____.

23. Fill in the missing part in the following sequence: pulmonary arteries ⟶ _____ ⟶
    pulmonary veins.

Combining Forms and Abbreviations

The lists below include combining forms and abbreviations that relate specifically to the cardiovascular system. Pronunciations are provided for the examples.

Combining Form	Meaning	Example
angi(o)	blood vessel	*angiogram* [ĂN-jē-ō-grăm], image of a blood vessel
aort(o)	aorta	*aortitis* [ā-ōr-TĪ-tĭs], inflammation of the aorta
arteri(o), arter(o)	artery	*arteriosclerosis* [ăr-TĒR-ē-ō-sklĕr-Ō-sĭs], hardening of the arteries
ather(o)	fatty matter	*atherosclerosis* [ĂTH-ĕr-ō-sklĕr-ō-sĭs], hardening of the arteries with irregular plaque deposits
atri(o)	atrium	*atrioventricular* [Ā-trē-ō-vĕn-TRĬK-yū-lăr], relating to the atria and ventricles of the heart
cardi(o)	heart	*cardiomyopathy* [KĂR-dē-ō-mī-ŎP-ă-thē], disease of the heart muscle
hemangi(o)	blood vessel	*hemangioma* [hĕ-MĂN-jē-ō-mă], abnormal mass of blood vessels
pericardi(o)	pericardium	*pericarditis* [PĔR-ĭ-kăr-DĪ-tĭs], inflammation of the pericardium
phleb(o)	vein	*phlebitis* [flĕ-BĪ-tĭs], inflammation of a vein

Combining Form	Meaning	Example
sphygm(o)	pulse	*sphygmomanometer* [SFĬG-mō-mă-NŎM-ĕ-tĕr], instrument for measuring blood pressure
thromb(o)	blood clot	*thrombocytosis* [THRŎM-bō-sī-TŌ-sŭs], abnormal increase in blood platelets in the blood
vas(o)	blood vessel	*vasodepressor* [VĀ-sō-dē-PRĔS-ĕr], agent that lowers blood pressure by relaxing blood vessels
ven(o)	vein	*venography* [vē-NŎG-ră-fē], radiographic imaging of a vein

Abbreviation	Meaning	Abbreviation	Meaning
AcG	accelerator globulin	ECHO	echocardiogram
AF	atrial fibrillation	ETT	exercise tolerance test
AS	aortic stenosis	GOT	glutamic oxaloacetic transaminase
ASCVD	arteriosclerotic cardiovascular disease	HDL	high-density lipoprotein
ASD	atrial septal defect	LDH	lactate dehydrogenase
ASHD	arteriosclerotic heart disease	LDL	low-density lipoprotein
AV	atrioventricular	LV	left ventricle
BP	blood pressure	LVH	left ventricular hypertrophy
CABG	coronary artery bypass graft	MI	mitral insufficiency; myocardial infarction
CAD	coronary artery disease	MR	mitral regurgitation
cath	catheter	MS	mitral stenosis
CCU	coronary care unit	MUGA	multiple-gated acquisition scan
CHD	coronary heart disease	MVP	mitral valve prolapse
CHF	congestive heart failure	PTCA	percutaneous transluminal coronary angioplasty
CO	cardiac output	PVC	premature ventricular contraction
CPK	creatine phosphokinase	SA	sinoatrial
CPR	cardiopulmonary resuscitation	SV	stroke volume
CVA	cerebrovascular accident	tPA, TPA	tissue plasminogen activator
CVD	cardiovascular disease	VLDL	very low-density lipoprotein
DSA	digital subtraction angiography	VSD	ventricular septal defect
DVT	deep venous thrombosis	VT	ventricular tachycardia
ECG, EKG	electrocardiogram		

CASE STUDY

Marking the Chart

The nurse on duty the night of Mr. Davino's admittance observed that his blood pressure dropped gradually from 190/100 to 160/90. The nurse, Joan Aquino, marked each change of blood pressure on his chart. In addition to blood pressure, she also took Mr. Davino's temperature and pulse every two hours. All his measurements seemed to show improvement, except that Mr. Davino was running a slight fever. However, Joan did not like Mr. Davino's appearance. His skin had a gray pallor and he seemed very disoriented. Dr. Mirkhan, the cardiologist on call that night, spoke with Nurse Aquino and looked over the results of the tests ordered earlier. The doctor also made the notes shown on the chart.

Critical Thinking

24. Nurse Aquino made very specific comments to Dr. Mirkhan about her observations of Mr. Davino's appearance. What are the two items that Nurse Aquino noticed?

25. Referring to Mr. Davino's chart and the doctor's notes on page 188, how long did Mr. Davino's temperature remain slightly elevated?

MEDICAL RECORD	PROGRESS NOTES
DATE 8/15/XX	3:30 pm Chest clear to auscultation bilaterally with mild crackles; Heart rate and rhythm regular; no audible murmur; no rubs; ECG, blood gases, and SED rate were ordered. Recommended transfer to CCU.—A. Mirkhan, M.D.
8/15/XX	4 pm BP 190/100; temp 100.4°; no urine in catheter bag.—J. Aquino, R.N.
8/15/XX	5 pm BP 182/95; temp 100.5°; still no urine in catheter bag; if no urine by 8 pm, notify Dr. Mirkhan.—J. Aquino, R.N.
8/15/XX	6 pm BP 176/97; temp 100.6°; catheter bag empty.—J. Aquino, R.N.
8/15/XX	7 pm Catheter bag empty.—J. Aquino, R.N.
8/15/XX	8 pm BP 168/94; temp 100.7°; catheter bag empty; paged Dr. Mirkhan.—J. Aquino, R.N.
8/15/XX	9 pm BP 162/96; temp 100.8°; start IV; ECG, blood gases.—A. Mirkhan, M.D.
8/15/XX	10 pm Catheter bag contains 50 ml of urine; patient resting comfortably.—J. Aquino, R.N.
8/15/XX	11 pm Catheter bag contains about 200 ml of urine; patient still sleeping.—J. Aquino, R.N.
8/15/XX	12 pm Woke patient; BP 160/90; temp 100.2°; 300 ml of urine.—J. Aquino, R.N.

PATIENT'S IDENTIFICATION (For typed or written entries give: Name—last, first, middle; grade; rank; hospital or medical facility)

REGISTER NO.

WARD NO.
4B

Combining Forms and Abbreviations Exercises

Build Your Medical Vocabulary

Build a word for each of the following definitions. Use the combining forms in this chapter as well as in Chapters 2 and 3.

26. Disease of the heart muscle _____

27. Inflammation of the membrane surrounding the heart _____

28. X-ray of a vein _____

29. Inflammation of a vein _____

30. Operation for reconstruction of an artery _____

31. A disease involving both nerves and blood vessels _____

32. Tending to act on the blood vessels _____

33. Of cardiac origin _____

34. Enlargement of the heart _____

35. Inflammation of the artery with a thrombus _____

Use the following combining forms and the suffixes and prefixes you learned in Chapters 2 and 3 to fill in the missing word parts: atrio-, arterio-, phlebo-, thrombo-, veno-.

36. _____ itis, inflammation of a vein

37. _____ ectomy, surgical removal of a thrombus

38. _____ plasty, vein repair

39. _____ megaly, enlargement of the atrium

40. _____ graph, radiograph of veins

Give the term that fits each definition. Each term must contain at least one of the combining forms shown in the previous section. You may also refer to Chapters 2 and 3.

41. Enlargement of the heart _____

42. Relating to the heart and lungs _____

43. Establishing an opening into the pericardium _____

44. Inflammation of the endocardium _____

45. Repair of a vein _____

46. Paralysis of a blood vessel _____

47. Suturing of a blood vessel _____

Check Your Knowledge

Fill in the blanks.

48. An inflammation of a vein is _____.

49. Atherosclerosis is hardening of the _____.

50. A venogram is an x-ray of a(n) _____.

51. An abbreviation for a term meaning heart attack is _____.

52. CABG is a surgical procedure that bypasses a blocked _____.

Define these abbreviations used on Mr. Davino's chart.

53. ECG _____

54. CCU _____

55. MI _____

56. BP _____

57. ECHO _____

Diagnostic, Procedural, and Laboratory Terms

Treatment of cardiovascular disease requires a precise understanding of the condition of the heart and of the parts of the body that affect the heart's functioning. Doctors order many types of diagnostic tests based on their observations of a patient. They may order clinical procedures whose results will indicate certain specific conditions or they may order laboratory tests to find disease-causing factors or evidence of a specific disease.

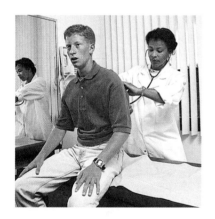

Figure 6-8 Auscultation sounds are usually heard with a stethoscope.

Diagnostic Procedures and Tests

Doctors who specialize in the diagnosis and treatment of cardiovascular disease (*cardiology*) are called *cardiologists*. Cardiologists usually see patients who already have some type of cardiovascular problem or indication of disease. The cardiologist often starts an examination with **auscultation** (listening to sounds within the body through a stethoscope). Some abnormal sounds a physician may hear are a *murmur*, a *bruit*, or a *gallop*. Each sound is a clue to the patient's condition. Figure 6-8 illustrates auscultation as part of a normal checkup.

One common diagnostic test is a **stress test** or *exercise tolerance test (ETT)*. Patients are asked to exercise on a treadmill while technicians take certain measurements, such as heart rate and respiration. Another common test is **electrocardiography,** which produces an *electrocardiogram* (**ECG, EKG**), which measures the amount of electricity flowing through the heart by means of electrodes placed on the patient's skin at specific points surrounding the heart. Figure 6-9 shows a patient having an electrocardiogram and Figure 6-10 illustrates the printout that results. Figure 6-11 on page 184 illustrates some abnormalities that show up on ECGs. A **Holter monitor** is a portable type of *electrocardiograph* or instrument that performs an electrocardiogram over a 24-hour period.

Various diagnostic procedures can be performed by producing some type of image. Taking x-rays after a dye has been injected is called **angiocardiography** (x-ray of the heart and its large blood vessels), **angiography** (x-ray of the heart's large blood vessels), **arteriography** (x-ray of a specific artery), **aortography** (x-ray of the aorta), or **venography** or **phlebography** (x-ray of a specific vein). The tests are called an *angiocardiogram, angiogram, arteriogram, aortogram, or veno-gram or phlebogram.* A **ventriculogram** is an x-ray showing the ventricles. Ventriculograms measure *stroke volume* (SV), the amount of blood going out of a ventricle in one contraction; *cardiac output* (CO), the amount of blood ejected from a ventricle every minute; and the **ejection fraction,** the percentage of volume of the contents of the left ventricle ejected with each contraction. Another x-ray test, **digital subtraction angiography (DSA)**, requires two angiograms with different contrast material to compare the results of the two tests in a computer.

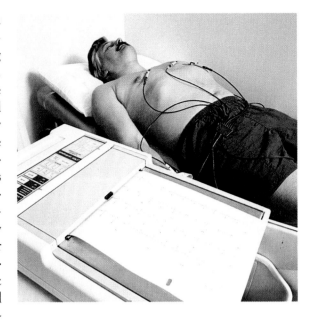

Ultrasound tests, or *ultrasonography* or **sonography,** produce images by measuring the echoes of sound waves against various structures. **Doppler ultrasound** measures blood flow in certain blood vessels. **Echocardiography** records sound waves to show the structure and movement of the heart. The test itself is called an *echocardiogram.* Figure 6-12 on page 184 shows an echocardiogram.

Radioactive substances that are injected into to the patient can provide information in a **cardiac scan,** a test that measures movement of areas of the heart, or in *nuclear medicine imaging.* **Positron emission tomography (PET) scans** are one form of nuclear imaging. A PET scan of the heart reveals images of the heart's blood flow and its cellular metabolism. Another form of nuclear

Figure 6-9 An ECG produces a picture of the heartbeat in the form of a graph. Six leads are used in most ECGs, as shown. Some ECGs are performed using more leads, such as twelve, to map electrical changes in other areas of the heart.

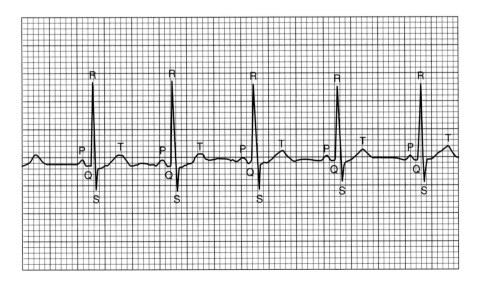

Figure 6-10 A normal ECG. The waves of electrical changes in the heart are mapped as P, QRS, and T waves. The P wave is electrical change occurring in the atria, the QRS wave represents change in the ventricles, and the T wave represents relaxation of the ventricles.

Figure 6-11 An abnormal ECG taken in the emergency room. Note the irregularities compared to Figure 6-10. These irregularities show atrial fibrillation and a blockage. In atrial fibrillation, the heart's rhythm is irregular, with as many as 350 beats per minute. It results from the atria discharging blood simultaneously. If not treated with medication, it can result in heart failure. Heart blockage represents a delay in the heart's conduction system.

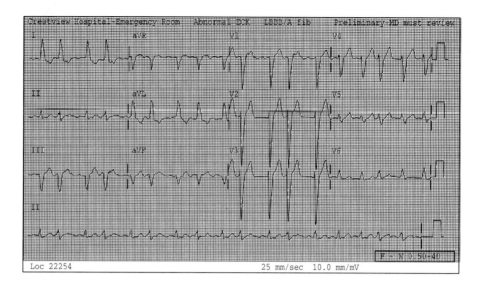

imaging is **multiple-gated acquisition (MUGA) angiography.** A MUGA scan is a noninvasive method of assessing cardiac muscle function. Figure 6-13 shows a nuclear image of the heart.

Magnetic resonance imaging (MRI) uses magnetic waves to produce images. A **cardiac MRI** provides a detailed image of the heart and shows any lesions in the large blood vessels of the heart.

Other procedures require actual insertion of a device, such as a catheter, into a vein or artery, and the device is guided to the heart. **Cardiac catheterization** allows withdrawal of blood samples from the heart and measures certain pressures and blood flow patterns within the heart. The catheter can be directed to the left side of the heart for measurements and images involving the coronary arteries or to the right side of the heart for measurement of oxygenated blood.

Figure 6-12 An echocardiogram is an ultrasound test that produces an image of the heart. The device that transmits the image in an echocardiogram allows the heart to be viewed from all angles. In this illustration, the device has been placed near the ventricles so the heart appears upside down.

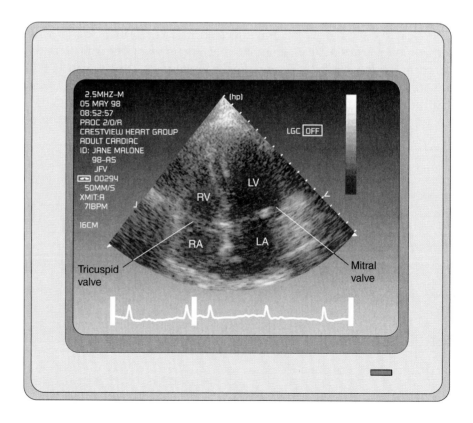

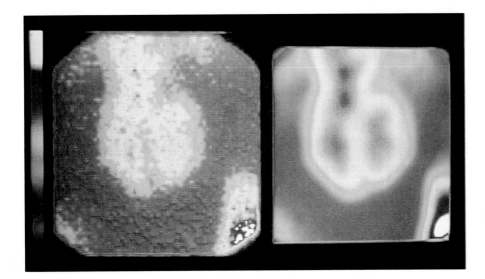

Figure 6-13 The nuclear imaging test shown here is a set of two images of the heart. The image on the right is an enhanced version of the image on the left. The red areas show the flow of blood as it moves through the heart's chambers.

Laboratory Tests

Laboratory tests are crucial for determining what may be happening to a patient or for evaluating risk factors for heart disease. Drug therapy, clinical procedures, and lifestyle changes may all be recommended largely on the basis of laboratory test results.

The flow of blood in the arteries is affected by the amount of **cholesterol** and **triglycerides** (fatty substances or *lipids*) contained in the blood. Lipids are carried through the blood by *lipoproteins*. *Low-density lipoproteins (LDL)* and *very low-density lipoproteins (VLDL)* cause cholesterol to form blockages in the arteries. *High-density lipoproteins (HDL)* actually remove lipids from the arteries and help protect people from the formation of blockages. One factor that increases LDL and VLDL is a diet high in *saturated fats* (animal fats and some vegetable fats that tend to be solid). *Polyunsaturated fats* (certain vegetable oils such as safflower or olive) do not raise LDL or VLDL. Laboratory tests performed on blood samples determine the levels of lipoproteins in the blood. Adult cholesterol readings below 200 are considered to pose little risk for coronary artery disease. The importance of cholesterol testing is evidenced by the fact that the chance of heart disease is reduced by 2 to 3 percent for each 1 percent reduction in the cholesterol level. A **lipid profile** (a series of laboratory tests performed on a blood sample) gives the lipid, triglyceride, glucose, and other values that help in evaluating a patient's risk factors. Figure 6-14 is an example of a patient's lipid profile.

A laboratory test that can be used to diagnose a myocardial infarction earlier than most other laboratory tests measures the levels of *troponin T* and *troponin I*, proteins found in the heart. As levels of the two rise, it usually indicates the early states of an acute myocardial infarction. If only one level rises, it can indicate a number of conditions not related to the heart, such as kidney failure or muscle trauma.

Another important laboratory test of blood is the **cardiac enzyme test** or

Physicians use many tests to determine the type and extent of cardiovascular disease. Diagnostic imaging is used to track circulation, heart function, and the presence of abnormalities. Laboratory tests for cardiovascular disease mainly involve testing blood for high levels of enzymes, an indicator of heart damage. A common heart enzyme test is CPK. Normal laboratory values may vary according to gender, and sometimes, race.

Other blood and urine tests provide information about lifestyle and illness-related factors that affect the cardiovascular system. A cholesterol reading below 200 mg/dL (milligrams per deciliter) is considered normal. Readings above 200 mg/dL may be indicative of coronary artery disease.

Laboratory Report
Embar Diagnostics
Three Riverview Drive
Wesley, OH 66666
(800) 999-0000

PATIENT NAME _Mary Helfer_
PATIENT ID _777-888-6666_
DATE RECEIVED _06/14/XXXX_
DATE REPORTED _06/15/XXXX_

TEST	RESULTS OUT OF RANGE	WITHIN RANGE	REFERENCE RANGE/UNITS
HDL	36 mg/dL		>40 mg/dL
LDL	192 mg/dL		<130mg/dL
Triglycerides	204 mg/dL		40–199 mg/dL
Cholesterol	208 mg/dL		120–199mg/dL

Figure 6-14 The lipid profile reveals the need to cut cholesterol in the patient's diet.

study (also called a **serum enzyme test**), which measures the levels of enzymes released into the blood by damaged heart muscle during a myocardial infarction. The three enzymes that help evaluate the condition of the patient are GOT *(glutamic oxaloacetic transaminase)*, CPK *(creatine phosphokinase)*, and LDH *(lactate dehydrogenase)*. The enzymes may indicate the degree of injury to the heart or the seriousness of an attack.

Vocabulary Review

In the previous section, you learned terms relating to diagnosis, clinical procedures, and laboratory tests. Before going on to the exercises, review the terms below and refer to the previous section if you have questions.

Term	Word Analysis	Definition
angiocardiography	[ăn-jē-ō-kăr-dē-ŎG-ră-fē] angio-, vessel + cardio-, heart + -graphy, a recording	Viewing of the heart and its major blood vessels by x-ray after injection of a contrast medium.
angiography	[ăn-jē-ŎG-ră-fē] angio- + -graphy	Viewing of the heart's major blood vessels by x-ray after injection of a contrast medium.
aortography	[ā-ōr-TŎG-ră-fē] aorto-, aorta + -graphy	Viewing of the aorta by x-ray after injection of a contrast medium.
arteriography	[ăr-tēr-ē-ŎG-ră-fē] arterio-, artery + -graphy	Viewing of a specific artery by x-ray after injection of a contrast medium.
auscultation	[ăws-kŭl-TĀ-shŭn]	Process of listening to body sounds via a stethoscope.
cardiac catheterization	[kăth-ĕ-tĕr-ĭ-ZĀ-shŭn]	Process of passing a thin catheter through an artery or vein to the heart to take blood samples, inject a contrast medium, or measure various pressures.
cardiac enzyme studies		Blood tests for determining levels of enzymes during a myocardial infarction; serum enzyme tests.
cardiac MRI		Viewing of the heart by magnetic resonance imaging.
cardiac scan		Process of viewing the heart muscle at work by scanning the heart of a patient into whom a radioactive substance has been injected.
cholesterol	[kō-LĔS-tĕr-ōl]	Fatty substance present in animal fats; cholesterol circulates in the bloodstream, sometimes causing arterial plaque to form.
digital subtraction angiography		Use of two angiograms done with different dyes to provide a comparison between the results.

Term	Word Analysis	Definition
Doppler ultrasound	[DŎP-lĕr] After Christian Doppler (1803–1853), Austrian physicist	Ultrasound test of blood flow in certain blood vessels.
echocardiography	[ĕk-ō-kăr-dē-ŎG-ră-fē] echo-, sound + cardio- + -graphy	Use of sound waves to produce images showing the structure and motion of the heart.
ejection fraction		Percentage of the volume of the contents of the left ventricle ejected with each contraction.
electrocardiography	[ē-lĕk-trō-kăr-dē-ŎG-ră-fē] electro-, electrical + cardio- + -graphy	Use of the electrocardiograph in diagnosis.
Holter monitor	[HŌL-tĕr] After Norman Holter (1914–1983), U.S. biophysicist	Portable device that provides a 24-hour electrocardiogram.
lipid profile	Greek *lipos*, fat	Laboratory test that provides the levels of lipids, triglycerides, and other substances in the blood.
multiple-gated acquisition (MUGA) angiography		Radioactive scan showing heart function.
phlebography	[flĕ-BŎG-ră-fē] phlebo-, vein + -graphy	Viewing of a vein by x-ray after injection of a contrast medium.
positron emission tomography scans	[tō-MŎG-ră-fē]	Type of nuclear image that measures movement of areas of the heart.
serum enzyme tests		Laboratory tests performed to detect enzymes present during or after a myocardial infarction; cardiac enzyme studies.
sonography	[sō-NŎG-ră-fē] Latin *sonus*, sound + -graphy	Production of images based on the echoes of sound waves against structures.
sphygmomanometer	[SFĬG-mō-mă-NŎM-ĕ-tĕr] sphygmo-, pulse + Greek *manos*, thin + -meter	Device for measuring blood pressure.
stress test		Test that measures heart rate, blood pressure, and other body functions while the patient is exercising on a treadmill.

Term	Word Analysis	Definition
triglyceride	[trī-GLĬS-ĕr-īd] tri-, three + glyceride	Fatty substance; lipid.
venography	[vē-NŎG-ră-fē] veno-, vein + -graphy	Viewing of a vein by x-ray after injection of a contrast medium.
ventriculogram	[vĕn-TRĬK-yū-lō-grăm] ventricle + -gram, a recording	X-ray of a ventricle taken after injection of a contrast medium.

C A S E · S T U D Y

Diagnosing the Problem

Dr. Woodard, the admitting physician, made notations on the patient's chart. She had left in the early evening, before the results of the tests she had ordered were in. The doctor on call that night was Dr. Mirkhan, a cardiologist. He agreed with Nurse Aquino that the patient's pallor and disorientation warranted further tests. First, Dr. Mirkhan reviewed the ECG that Dr. Woodard had ordered. It showed a sinus rhythm with Q waves in 2 AVF and a mild ST elevation in V2 and V3. Dr. Mirkhan ordered some laboratory tests to help in his diagnosis of Mr. Davino's current condition. He made the additions to Mr. Davino's chart. He also made some notes for Mr. Davino's personal physician.

 Critical Thinking

58. From the notations added to the chart, is his cholesterol still high?

59. Which of his laboratory tests shows an abnormal level that can often be corrected by dietary changes?

MEDICAL RECORD	PROGRESS NOTES
DATE 8/15/XX	3:30 pm Have reviewed nursing notes. Chest clear to auscultation bilaterally with mild crackles; Heart rate and rhythm regular; no audible murmur; no rubs; ECG, blood gases, and SED rate were ordered. Recommend transfer to CCU.—A. Mirkhan, M.D.
8/15/XX	9 pm BP 162/96; temp 100.8°; start IV; ECG, blood gases.—A. Mirkhan, M.D.
8/16/XX	2 am ECG—sinus rhythm with Q waves in 2AVF; mild ST elevation in V2 and V3; cholesterol 296; SED rate 15 mm/1 hr.—A. Mirkhan, M.D.

PATIENT'S IDENTIFICATION *(For typed or written entries give: Name—last, first, middle; grade; rank; hospital or medical facility)*

Davino, Joseph A.
000-77-9999

REGISTER NO.

WARD NO.
4B

PROGRESS NOTES
STANDARD FORM 509

Dr. Mirkhan also works in private practice. Patients' notes from his practice give you an idea of the types of clinical problems he treats.

Patient name _Angela O'Toole_ **Age** _57_ **Current Diagnosis** _angina_

DATE/TIME	
9/7/XX 9:30	Exercise thallium test with no post-exercise changes; continue current medication.

Patient name _Marvin Hochstadter_ **Age** _64_ **Current Diagnosis** _arteriosclerosis_

DATE/TIME	
9/7/XX 10:15	Two-year post angioplasty; SOB; cardiac pain; schedule cardiac catheterization.

Patient name _Lou Lawisky_ **Age** _49_ **Current Diagnosis** _unstable angina_

DATE/TIME	
9/7/XX 1:20	Negative stress cardiolite scan to 12 MET; peak heart rate of 153/min with no ischemia or infarction; epigastric burning, no angina; recommend Tagamet to control reflux.

Patient name _Marlena Castelli_ **Age** _68_ **Current Diagnosis** _R/O MI_

DATE/TIME	
9/7/XX 2:30	Neck and jaw discomfort; two previous MIs (last 1/23/XX); PTCA 2/6/XX; BP 126/84, pulse 88, heart: Apical impulse discrete. S1 and S2 are regular in rate and intensity. There is an S4 gallop, no S3 gallop, no cardiac murmur. Laboratory: Sodium 142, potassium 3.7, CO_2 29, chloride 103, creatinine 1.1, BUN 13, cholesterol 293, triglycerides 28; HDL 35; LDL 156; CPK 133.

---

60. What is Marvin's diagnosis? _____

61. List five laboratory tests Dr. Mirkhan reviewed on 9/7/xx.

_____

_____

_____

_____

_____

Pathological Terms

Cardiovascular disease (CVD) can have many causes and can take many forms. Some diseases are caused by a congenital anomaly, whereas others may be caused by other pathology or by lifestyle factors (**risk factors**), such as poor diet, smoking, and lack of exercise.

Heart Rhythm

The rhythm of the heart maintains the blood flow through and in and out of the heart. Abnormal rhythms are called **arrhythmias.** Heart rates may be too slow (**bradycardia**), too fast (**tachycardia**), or irregular (also called **atrial fibrillation, fibrillation,** or **dysrhythmia**). A **flutter** is a rapid but regular heartbeat. The heart rate may be regular, but the sound of the heartbeat may be abnormal (**bruit,** heard on auscultation of the carotid artery or, **murmur** a soft humming sound), which may indicate valve leakage. A new murmur heard during a heart attack may indicate a rupture of the heart muscle, which is an instant surgical emergency. Other sounds indicate specific problems; for example, a **rub** (a frictional sound) usually indicates a pericardial murmur, and a **gallop** (a triple heart sound) usually indicates serious heart disease. Some pulsations of the heart (**palpitations**) can be felt by the patient as thumping in the chest. An **atrioventricular block** or **heart block** is caused by a blocking of impulses from the AV node. The electrical impulses of the heart control contractions. Irregularities in the heart's contractions, such as **premature atrial contractions (PACs)** or **premature ventricular contractions (PVCs),** can cause palpitations.

Blood Pressure

Abnormalities in blood pressure can damage the heart as well as other body systems (**hypertensive heart disease**). If the blood pressure is too high (**hypertension** or **high blood pressure**) or too low (**hypotension** or **low blood pressure**), the blood vessels do not have the proper pressure of blood flowing through them. **Essential hypertension** is high blood pressure that is *idiopathic* or without any known cause. **Secondary hypertension** has a known cause, such as a high-salt diet, renal disease, adrenal gland disease, and so on. Hypertension is the most common cardiovascular disease. Hypotension often results from another disease process or trauma (as in shock). Hypotension may lead to fainting or becoming unconscious. Extremely low hypotension may lead to death.

Diseases of the Blood Vessels

Blood vessels can become diseased, as when **plaque,** buildup of fatty material, is deposited on the wall of an artery. An **atheroma** is plaque specifically on the wall of an artery, which can build up to cause **atherosclerosis.** An **embolus** is a mass traveling through the bloodstream causing a blockage in the vessel. A **thrombus** is a stationary blood clot, usually formed from elements of the blood. Figure 6-15 shows the difference between an embolus and a thrombus. **Thrombophlebitis** is an inflammation of a vein with a thrombus. **Thrombosis** is the presence of a thrombus in a blood vessel. **Deep vein thrombosis** forms in a deep vein or vein within a structure rather than one on the surface of a structure. **Thrombotic occlusion** is the occlusion or closing of a vessel caused by a thrombus.

Blood vessels can have a **constriction,** or narrowing, due to contraction. An **occlusion** is the closing off of a blood vessel due to a blockage. A weakness in an artery wall can cause a ballooning or **aneurysm,** which can fatally rupture. Loss of elasticity or hardening of the arteries (**arteriosclerosis**) can lessen blood flow. Inadequate blood supply, particularly to the blood vessels in the legs, causes **claudication,** limping. **Intermittent claudication,** irregular attacks of claudication, is helped by resting. **Peripheral vascular disease** is a general term for vascular disease in the lower extremities. A sudden drop in the supply of blood to a vessel (an **infarction**) can cause an area of dead

Figure 6-15 A thrombus is a stationary blood clot, while an embolus is a traveling mass of material that blocks a blood vessel.

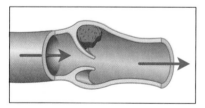

A thrombus.

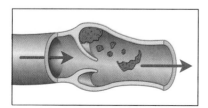

An embolus.

tissue, or **necrosis** (an **infarct**). The general term for lack of flow through a blood vessel is **perfusion deficit.** An area of blood insufficiency in the body is called **ischemia.** Insufficiently oxygenated areas of the body may develop **cyanosis,** a bluish or purplish discoloration of the skin caused by deficient oxygenation of the blood.

Veins sometimes become twisted or enlarged (**varicose veins**). **Hemorrhoids** are varicose veins in the anal region. An inflammation of a vein is called **phlebitis.** An inflammation of an artery is called **arteritis.** Minute hemorrhages in the blood vessels in the skin are called **petechiae.** Numbness or pain in the fingers caused by arterial spasms is called **Raynaud's phenomenon.** Raynaud's phenomenon may be an indicator of some serious connective tissue or autoimmune diseases. Most often, it is a reaction to cold or to emotional stress. Once a "trigger" starts the phenomenon, three color changes usually take place. First, the finger(s) turn absolutely white when the blood flow is blocked by the spasm; second, the finger becomes cyanotic from the slow return of blood to the site; and third, as blood fills the finger, a darker red color appears. Treatment of Raynaud's not linked to another disease is usually as simple as wearing gloves when removing items from the freezer and when going out in cold weather.

Coronary Artery Disease

Coronary artery disease (CAD) refers to any condition that reduces the nourishment the heart receives from the blood flowing through the arteries of the heart. Such diseases include **aortic stenosis** or narrowing of the aorta. **Coarctation of the aorta** is also an abnormal narrowing of the aorta. **Stenosis** is any narrowing of a blood vessel. **Pulmonary artery stenosis** slows the flow of blood to the lungs. **Angina** or **angina pectoris** (sometimes referred to as cardiac pain) can result from lack of oxygen to the heart muscle. Angina is usually categorized in degrees from class I to class IV. A person with class I angina (able to withstand prolonged exertion) will have no limits to normal activity. Severe angina (class IV) requires strict limitations on any activity except rest.

General Heart and Lung Diseases

When the heart suffers an attack that causes insufficient blood flow to the heart or ischemia, one is said to have a *coronary* or *heart attack*. These are informal terms for a **myocardial infarction,** a disruption in the heart's activity usually caused by blockage (a clot or plaque) of blood flow to a coronary artery. Myocardial infarctions are often classified by the location of the area to which blood flow is restricted; for example, an anterior myocardial infarction is one in which the anterior wall of the heart is affected, and a posterior one involves the heart's posterior wall.

Cardiac arrest or **asystole** is a sudden stopping of the heart. Such an attack can be fatal or, with treatment, can be a warning to make medical and lifestyle changes to ward off a further attack. Approximately 1.5 million people suffer heart attacks annually. One-third of these people do not survive. Before age 50, men are much

---

M O R E   A B O U T...

Familiar Terms

Cardiovascular disease is a common ailment of middle and old age. Many familiar terms are used by lay people to describe common cardiovascular diseases and procedures. A myocardial infarction may be called a *coronary* or a *heart attack*. Arteriosclerosis is often referred to as *hardening of the arteries*. Congestive heart failure may be called *heart failure. Vein stripping* is a common term for removal of veins for transplanting elsewhere or for treating varicosities.

more likely to suffer heart attacks than are women, who are thought to be protected by their production of estrogen before menopause. After menopause, the risk for women is approximately the same as for men.

Some diseases of the heart are specific inflammations, such as **endocarditis, myocarditis, pericarditis,** or **bacterial endocarditis.** Other conditions of the heart have to do with fluid accumulation. **Congestive heart failure** occurs when the heart is unable to pump the necessary amount of blood. People suffering from congestive heart failure usually experience shortness of breath, edema, enlarged organs and veins, and irregular breathing patterns. **Pulmonary edema** or accumulation of fluid in the lungs can result from this failure. Fluid accumulation in the pericardial sac causes **cardiac tamponade.**

An **intracardiac tumor** is a tumor in a heart chamber. **Cardiomyopathy** is disease of the heart muscle.

Valve Conditions

The heart valves control the flow of blood into, through, and out of the heart. Valve irregularities affecting the flow of blood can be serious. **Aortic regurgitation** or **reflux** is a backward flow of blood through the aortic valve. An abnormal narrowing of the opening of the mitral valve (**mitral stenosis**) affects the opening and closing of the valve. **Mitral insufficiency** or **reflux** is a backward flow of blood through the mitral valve. Similarly, **mitral valve prolapse** is a backward flow of blood, but it is due to the abnormal protrusion of one or both of the mitral cusps into the left atrium. **Tricuspid stenosis** is an abnormal narrowing of the opening of the tricuspid valve.

Sometimes, infections or inflammation may cause valve damage. **Valvulitis** is the general term for a heart valve inflammation. **Rheumatic heart disease** is damage to the heart, usually to the valves, caused by an untreated streptococcal infection. Some infections can cause a clot on a heart valve or opening (**vegetation**).

Congenital Heart Conditions

Congenital heart disease results from a condition present at birth. Some common conditions are **patent ductus arteriosus,** a disease in which a small duct remains open at birth; **septal defect,** an abnormal opening in the septum between the atria or ventricles; and **tetralogy of Fallot,** actually a combination of four congenital heart abnormalities (ventricular septal defect, pulmonary stenosis, incorrect position of the aorta, and right ventricular hypertrophy) that appear together.

Vocabulary Review

In the previous section, you learned terms relating to pathology. Before going on to the exercises, review the terms below and refer to the previous section if you have questions.

Term	Word Analysis	Definition
aneurysm	[ĂN-yū-rĭzm] Greek *aneurysma,* dilation	Ballooning of the artery wall caused by weakness in the wall.

Term	Word Analysis	Definition
angina	[ĂN-ji-nă, ăn-JĪ-nă] Latin, sore throat	Angina pectoris.
angina pectoris	[PĔK-tōr-ĭs, pĕk-TŌR-ĭs] Latin, sore throat of the chest	Chest pain, usually caused by a lowered oxygen or blood supply to the heart.
aortic regurgitation or reflux	[rē-GŬR-ji-TĀ-shŭn]	Backward flow or leakage of blood through a faulty aortic valve.
aortic stenosis	[stĕ-NŌ-sĭs]	Narrowing of the aorta.
arrhythmia	[ā-RĬTH-mē-ă] a-, without + Greek *rhythmos*, rhythm	Irregularity in the rhythm of the heartbeat.
arteriosclerosis	[ăr-TĒR-ē-ō-sklĕr-Ō-sĭs] arterio-, artery + sclerosis	Hardening of the arteries.
arteritis	[ăr-tĕr-Ī-tĭs] arter-, artery + -itis inflammation	Inflammation of an artery or arteries.
asystole	[ā-SĬS-tō-lē] a- + Greek *systole*, a contracting	Cardiac arrest.
atheroma	[ăth-ĕr-Ō-mă] ather-, fatty matter + -oma, tumor	A fatty deposit (plaque) in the wall of an artery.
atherosclerosis	[ĂTH-ĕr-ō-sklĕr-ō-sĭs] athero-, fatty matter + sclerosis	Hardening of the arteries caused by the buildup of atheromas.
atrial fibrillation	[fĭ-brĭ-LĀ-shŭn]	An irregular, usually rapid, heartbeat caused by overstimulation of the AV node.
atrioventricular block	atrio-, atrium + ventricle	Heart block; partial or complete blockage of the electrical impulses from the atrioventricular node to the ventricles.
bacterial endocarditis		Bacterial inflammation of the inner lining of the heart.
bradycardia	[brād-ē-KĂR-dē-ă] brady-, slow + Greek *kardia*, heart	Heart rate of fewer than 60 beats per minute.

Term	Word Analysis	Definition
bruit	[brū-Ē] French, noise	Sound or murmur, especially an abnormal heart sound heard on auscultation, especially of the carotid artery.
cardiac arrest		Sudden stopping of the heart; also called *asystole*.
cardiac tamponade	[tăm-pō-NĀD]	Compression of the heart caused by fluid accumulation in the pericardial sac.
cardiomyopathy	[KĂR-dē-ō-mī-ŎP-ă-thē] cardio-, heart + myo-, muscle + -pathy, disease	Disease of the heart muscle.
claudication	[klăw-dĭ-KĀ-shŭn] Latin *claudicatio*, limping	Limping caused by inadequate blood supply during activity; usually subsides during rest.
coarctation of the aorta	[kō-ărk-TĀ-shŭn] Latin *coarcto*, to press together	Abnormal narrowing of the aorta.
congenital heart disease		Heart disease (usually a type of malformation) that exists at birth.
congestive heart failure		Inability of the heart to pump enough blood out during the cardiac cycle; collection of fluid in the lungs results.
constriction	[kŏn-STRĬK-shŭn]	Compression or narrowing caused by contraction, as of a vessel.
coronary artery disease		Condition that reduces the flow of blood and nutrients through the arteries of the heart.
cyanosis	[sī-ă-NŌ-sĭs] Greek, dark blue color	Bluish or purplish coloration, as of the skin, caused by deficient oxygenation of the blood.
deep vein thrombosis	[thrŏm-BŌ-sĭs]	Formation of a thrombus (clot) in a deep vein, such as a femoral vein.
dysrhythmia	[dĭs-RĬTH-mē-ă] dys-, difficult + Greek *rhythmos*, rhythm	Abnormal heart rhythm.
embolus	[ĔM-bō-lŭs] Greek *embolos*, plug	Mass of foreign material blocking a vessel.
endocarditis	[ĔN-dō-kăr-DĪ-tĭs] endo-, within + card-, heart + -itis, inflammation	Inflammation of the endocardium, especially one caused by a bacterial (for example, staphylococci) or fungal agent.

Term	Word Analysis	Definition
essential hypertension		High blood pressure without any known cause.
fibrillation	[fĭ-brĭ-LĀ-shŭn] Latin *fibrilla*, little fiber	Random, chaotic, irregular heart rhythm.
flutter		Regular but very rapid heartbeat.
gallop		Triple sound of a heartbeat, usually indicative of serious heart disease.
heart block		*See* atrioventricular block.
hemorrhoids	[HĔM-ō-rŏydz] From Greek *haima*, blood + *rhoia*, flow	Varicose condition of veins in the anal region.
high blood pressure		*See* hypertension.
hypertension	[HĪ-pĕr-TĔN-shŭn] hyper-, excessive + tension	Chronic condition with blood pressure greater than 140/90.
hypertensive heart disease		Heart disease caused, or worsened, by high blood pressure.
hypotension	[HĪ-pō-TĔN-shŭn] hypo-, below normal + tension	Chronic condition with blood pressure below normal.
infarct	[ĬN-fărkt] Latin *infarcto*, to stuff into	Area of necrosis caused by a sudden drop in the supply of arterial or venous blood.
infarction	[ĭn-FĂRK-shŭn]	Sudden drop in the supply of arterial or venous blood, often due to an embolus or thrombus.
intermittent claudication		Attacks of limping, particularly in the legs, due to ischemia of the muscles.
intracardiac tumor	[ĭn-tră-KĂR-dē-ăk] intra-, within + cardiac	A tumor within one of the heart chambers.
ischemia	[ĭs-KĒ-mē-ă] From Greek *ischo*, to keep back + *haima*, blood	Localized blood insufficiency caused by an obstruction.
low blood pressure		*See* hypotension.
mitral insufficiency or reflux	[MĪ-trăl]	Backward flow of blood due to a damaged mitral valve.

Term	Word Analysis	Definition
mitral stenosis		Abnormal narrowing at the opening of the mitral valve.
mitral valve prolapse		Backward flow of blood into the left atrium due to protrusion of one or both mitral cusps into the left atrium during contractions.
murmur		Soft heart humming sound heard between normal beats.
myocardial infarction	myocardi(um) + -al, pertaining to	Sudden drop in the supply of blood to an area of the heart muscle, usually due to a blockage in a coronary artery.
myocarditis	[MĪ-ō-kăr-DĪ-tĭs] myocard(ium) + -itis	Inflammation of the myocardium.
necrosis	[nĕ-KRŌ-sĭs] Greek *nekrosis*, death	Death of tissue or an organ or part due to irreversible damage; usually a result of oxygen deprivation.
occlusion	[ŏ-KLŪ-zhŭn] From Latin *ob-*, against + *claudo*, to close	The closing of a blood vessel.
palpitations	[păl-pĭ-TĀ-shŭnz] Latin *palpito*, to throb	Uncomfortable pulsations of the heart felt as a thumping in the chest.
patent ductus arteriosus	[PĂ-tĕnt DŬK-tŭs ăr-tēr-ē-Ō-sŭs]	A condition at birth in which the ductus arteriosus, a small duct between the aorta and the pulmonary artery, remains abnormally open.
perfusion deficit		Lack of flow through a blood vessel, usually caused by an occlusion.
pericarditis	[PĔR-ĭ-kăr-DĪ-tĭs] pericard(ium) + -itis	Inflammation of the pericardium.
peripheral vascular disease		Vascular disease in the lower extremities, usually due to blockages in the arteries of the groin or legs.
petechiae	[pĕ-TĒ-kē-ē, pĕ-TĔK-ē-ē, pĕ-TĒ-kē-ă] Italian *petecchie*	Minute hemorrhages in the skin.
phlebitis	[flĕ-BĪ-tĭs] phleb-, vein + itis	Inflammation of a vein.

Term	Word Analysis	Definition
plaque	[plăk] French, plate	Buildup of solid material, such as a fatty deposit, on the lining of an artery.
premature atrial contractions (PACs)		Atrial contractions that occur before the normal impulse; can be the cause of palpitations.
premature ventricular contractions (PVCs)		Ventricular contractions that occur before the normal impulse; can be the cause of palpitations.
pulmonary artery stenosis		Narrowing of the pulmonary artery, preventing the lungs from receiving enough blood from the heart to oxygenate.
pulmonary edema		Abnormal accumulation of fluid in the lungs.
Raynaud's phenomenon	[rā-NŌZ] After Maurice Raynaud (1834–1881), French physician	Spasm in the arteries of the fingers causing numbness or pain.
rheumatic heart disease	Greek *rheumatikos*, subject to flux, the discharge of fluids	Heart valve and/or muscle damage caused by an untreated streptococcal infection.
risk factor		Any of various factors considered to increase the probability that a disease will occur; for example, high blood pressure and smoking are considered risk factors for heart disease.
rub		Frictional sound heard between heartbeats, usually indicating a pericardial murmur.
secondary hypertension		Hypertension having a known cause, such as kidney disease.
septal defect		Congenital abnormality consisting of an opening in the septum between the atria or ventricles.
stenosis	[stĕ-NŌ-sĭs]	Narrowing, particularly of blood vessels or of the cardiac valves.
tachycardia	[TĂK-ĭ-KĂR-dē-ă] tachy-, fast + Greek *kardia*, heart	Heart rate greater than 100 beats per minute.
tetralogy of Fallot	[fă-LŌ] After Étienne-Louis A. Fallot (1850–1911), French physician	Set of four congenital heart abnormalities appearing together that cause deoxygenated blood to enter the systemic circulation: ventricular septal defect, pulmonary stenosis, incorrect position of the aorta, and right ventricular hypertrophy.

Term	Word Analysis	Definition
thrombophlebitis	[THRŎM-bō-flĕ-BĪ-tĭs] thrombo-, thrombus + phleb- + -itis	Inflammation of a vein with a thrombus.
thrombosis	[thrŏm-BŌ-sĭs] Greek, a clotting	Presence of a thrombus in a blood vessel.
thrombotic occlusion		Narrowing caused by a thrombus.
thrombus	[THRŎM-bŭs] Latin, clot	Stationary blood clot in the cardiovascular system, usually formed from matter found in the blood.
tricuspid stenosis		Abnormal narrowing of the opening of the tricuspid valve.
valvulitis	[văl-vyū-LĪ-tĭs] New Latin valvula, value + -itis	Inflammation of a heart valve.
varicose vein	[VĂR-ĭ-kōs] Latin varix, dilated vein	Dilated, enlarged, or twisted vein, usually on the leg.
vegetation	[vĕj-ĕ-TĀ-shŭn]	Clot on a heart valve or opening, usually caused by infection.

C A S E S T U D Y

Applying Medical Technology to Reimbursement

The billing department of the hospital has just received the charts and notes for Mr. Davino. Mr. Davino's insurance company will pay the claim once the hospital fills out a HCFA [HĬK-fă] (Health Care Financing Admin-istration) form and submits it for payment. The filled-out form is shown on page 199.

Critical Thinking

62. On the HCFA form, what is the procedure code for the service provided to Mr. Davino?
63. On the HCFA form, what is the code for Mr. Davino's diagnosis?

APPROVED OMB-0938-0008

CARRIER

PLEASE
DO NOT
STAPLE
IN THIS
AREA

| | PICA | | | | **HEALTH INSURANCE CLAIM FORM** | PICA | | |

1. MEDICARE	MEDICAID	CHAMPUS	CHAMPVA	GROUP HEALTH PLAN (SSN or ID)	FECA BLK LUNG (SSN)	OTHER (ID)	1a. INSURED'S I.D. NUMBER (FOR PROGRAM IN ITEM 1)
☐ (Medicare #)	☐ (Medicaid #)	☐ (Sponsor's SSN)	☐ (VA File #)	☒	☐	☐	000-77-9999

2. PATIENT'S NAME (Last Name, First Name, Middle Initial)
Davino, Joseph

3. PATIENT'S BIRTH DATE   SEX
MM 07 | DD 12 | YY XXXX   M ☒   F ☐

4. INSURED'S NAME (Last Name, First Name, Middle Initial)
same

5. PATIENT'S ADDRESS (No., Street)
2025 Lapointe St.

6. PATIENT RELATIONSHIP TO INSURED
Self ☒   Spouse ☐   Child ☐   Other ☐

7. INSURED'S ADDRESS (No., Street)

CITY
Wesley   STATE *OH*

8. PATIENT STATUS
Single ☐   Married ☒   Other ☐

CITY   STATE

ZIP CODE *66666*
TELEPHONE (Include Area Code) (600) 555-1234

Employed ☒   Full-Time Student ☐   Part-Time Student ☐

ZIP CODE
TELEPHONE (INCLUDE AREA CODE) ( )

9. OTHER INSURED'S NAME (Last Name, First Name, Middle Initial)

10. IS PATIENT'S CONDITION RELATED TO:

11. INSURED'S POLICY GROUP OR FECA NUMBER

a. OTHER INSURED'S POLICY OR GROUP NUMBER

a. EMPLOYMENT? (CURRENT OR PREVIOUS)
☐ YES   ☒ NO

a. INSURED'S DATE OF BIRTH
MM 07 | DD 21 | YY XXXX   SEX   M ☐   F ☐

b. OTHER INSURED'S DATE OF BIRTH
MM | DD | YY   SEX   M ☐   F ☐

b. AUTO ACCIDENT?   PLACE (State)
☐ YES   ☒ NO

b. EMPLOYER'S NAME OR SCHOOL NAME
Steelworks

c. EMPLOYER'S NAME OR SCHOOL NAME

c. OTHER ACCIDENT?
☐ YES   ☒ NO

c. INSURANCE PLAN NAME OR PROGRAM NAME
MD Health Plan of Ohio

d. INSURANCE PLAN NAME OR PROGRAM NAME

10d. RESERVED FOR LOCAL USE

d. IS THERE ANOTHER HEALTH BENEFIT PLAN?
☐ YES   ☒ NO   *If yes,* return to and complete item 9 a-d.

READ BACK OF FORM BEFORE COMPLETING & SIGNING THIS FORM.
12. PATIENT'S OR AUTHORIZED PERSON'S SIGNATURE I authorize the release of any medical or other information necessary to process this claim. I also request payment of government benefits either to myself or to the party who accepts assignment below.
SIGNED *Joseph Davino*   DATE *08/15/XXXX*

13. INSURED'S OR AUTHORIZED PERSON'S SIGNATURE I authorize payment of medical benefits to the undersigned physician or supplier for services described below.
SIGNED

14. DATE OF CURRENT: ◄ ILLNESS (First symptom) OR INJURY (Accident) OR PREGNANCY (LMP)
MM 08 | DD 15 | YY XXXX

15. IF PATIENT HAS HAD SAME OR SIMILAR ILLNESS, GIVE FIRST DATE
MM 12 | DD 09 | YY XXXX

16. DATES PATIENT UNABLE TO WORK IN CURRENT OCCUPATION
FROM MM | DD | YY   TO MM | DD | YY

17. NAME OF REFERRING PHYSICIAN OR OTHER SOURCE
Dr. Mirkhan

17a. I.D. NUMBER OF REFERRING PHYSICIAN
BY0S987

18. HOSPITALIZATION DATES RELATED TO CURRENT SERVICES
FROM MM 08 | DD 15 | YY XXXX   TO MM | DD | YY

19. RESERVED FOR LOCAL USE

20. OUTSIDE LAB? $ CHARGES
☐ YES   ☒ NO

21. DIAGNOSIS OR NATURE OF ILLNESS OR INJURY. (RELATE ITEMS 1,2,3, OR 4 TO ITEM 24E BY LINE)
1. 414.0
2. |___.___
3. |___.___
4. |___.___

22. MEDICAID RESUBMISSION
CODE | ORIGINAL REF. NO.

23. PRIOR AUTHORIZATION NUMBER

24. A. DATE(S) OF SERVICE						B. Place of Service	C. Type of Service	D. PROCEDURES, SERVICES, OR SUPPLIES (Explain Unusual Circumstances) CPT/HCPCS MODIFIER	E. DIAGNOSIS CODE	F. $ CHARGES		G. DAYS OR UNITS	H. EPSDT Family Plan	I. EMG	J. COB	K. RESERVED FOR LOCAL USE
From MM 08	DD 15	YY XXXX	To MM	DD	YY			82803	1	74	00	1				

25. FEDERAL TAX I.D. NUMBER   SSN ☒ EIN ☐
12-34-56789

26. PATIENT'S ACCOUNT NO.
000-77-9999

27. ACCEPT ASSIGNMENT? (For govt. claims, see back)
☒ YES   ☐ NO

28. TOTAL CHARGE
$ 74 | 00

29. AMOUNT PAID
$

30. BALANCE DUE
$ 74 | 00

31. SIGNATURE OF PHYSICIAN OR SUPPLIER INCLUDING DEGREES OR CREDENTIALS (I certify that the statements on the reverse apply to this bill and are made a part thereof.)
SIGNED *Andar Mirkhan, M.D.*   DATE 08/22/XXXX

32. NAME AND ADDRESS OF FACILITY WHERE SERVICES WERE RENDERED (if other than home or office)
Glenview Clinic
14 Woodrow Blvd.
Andover, OH 66666

33. PHYSICIAN'S OR SUPPLIER'S NAME, ADDRESS, ZIP CODE & TELEPHONE NO.
Andar Mirkhan, M.D.
16 Courtyard Lane
Andover, Ohio 66666
PIN# *BY0S987*   GRP# *3218B*

(APPROVED BY AMA COUNCIL ON MEDICAL SERVICE 8/88)   ***PLEASE PRINT OR TYPE***

FORM HCFA-1500 (12-90)
FORM OWCP-1500   FORM RRB-1500

PATIENT AND INSURED INFORMATION

PHYSICIAN OR SUPPLIER INFORMATION

Pathological Terms Exercises

Make an Educated Guess

For each of the following four situations, insert the likely age of the patient from the following age ranges. Use each range only once.

A. 0–2   B. 11–18   C. 40–55   D. 67–90

64. A patient going into surgery for a septal defect _____

65. Arteriosclerosis with pulmonary edema _____

66. Cardiac arrest of an athlete during a stressful game _____

67. Hypertension due to stress _____

Check Your Knowledge

Fill in the blanks.

68. Heart rhythms may be dangerously fast (called _____) or dangerously slow (called _____).

69. Atrial fibrillation is another name for _____ or _____, irregular rhythm.

70. An embolus travels in the blood while a(n) _____ is stationary.

71. An abnormal sound heard on auscultation is called a(n) _____.

72. An abnormal heartbeat with a soft humming sound is called a(n) _____.

73. The most common cardiovascular disease is _____.

74. Smoking, poor diet, and lack of exercise are _____ _____ for heart disease.

75. A heart attack is also called a(n) _____ _____.

Surgical Terms

Cardiovascular surgery usually involves opening up or repairing blood vessels or valves; removal, repair, or replacement of diseased portions of blood vessels; or bypass of blocked areas. The goal of most cardiovascular surgery is to improve blood flow, thereby allowing proper oxygenation and nourishment of all the cells of the body. Many types of heart surgery are now *minimally invasive procedures*. Most heart operations require opening up the chest to access the heart. However, devices such as lasers and miniature surgical instruments now allow surgeons to perform certain procedures through a "keyhole," a small opening in the chest.

A balloon catheter is used in **balloon catheter dilation** (also called **percutaneous transluminal coronary angioplasty** or **PTCA**) to open the passageway inside a blood vessel so that blood can flow freely (see Figure 6-16). A **balloon valvuloplasty** involves the use of a balloon catheter to open narrowed cardiac valve openings. Similarly, **angioplasty** or **coronary angioplasty** is the opening of a blood vessel using a balloon catheter. *Cardiac catheterization* uses a catheter threaded through an artery or vein into the heart to observe blood flow. It is the most common type of operation performed in the United States; over 1 million operations are performed annually. **Angioscopy** uses a fiberoptic catheter to view the interior of a blood vessel. Surgery that involves the use of cardiac catheterization is called **endovascular surgery.** During surgery, a **stent** or an **intravascular stent** (Figure 6-17) may be inserted to hold a blood vessel passageway open. Such procedures also help to break up blockages.

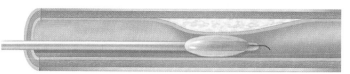

Narrowed artery with balloon catheter positioned.

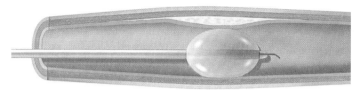

Inflated balloon presses against arterial wall.

Figure 6-16 Balloon catheter dilation is a surgical procedure to open a blocked blood vessel.

Sometimes it becomes necessary to create a detour or a **bypass** around blockages. **Coronary bypass surgery** or **CABG** (coronary artery bypass graft) is performed to attach the vessel to be used for the bypass. A **graft**, particularly of a blood vessel from another part of the body, can be used to bypass an arterial blockage. Saphenous (leg)

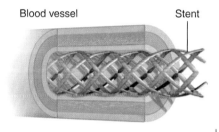

Blood vessel   Stent

Figure 6-17 An intravascular stent holds a blood vessel passageway open to allow the flow of blood.

veins or mammary (chest) arteries are two types of vessels used for this procedure. The number of arteries that are bypassed determines whether a CABG is a triple (three arteries bypassed) bypass, a quadruple (four) bypass, and so on. **Fontan's operation** creates a bypass from the right atrium to the main pulmonary artery. Sometimes it is necessary to divert blood flow from the heart during surgery. This procedure, **cardiopulmonary bypass** (also called *extracorporeal circulation*), circulates the blood through a heart-lung machine and back into systemic circulation.

Surgical removal and replacement of the entire heart is called a **heart transplant.** **Valve replacement** is the removal and replacement of a heart valve. Surgical removal of a thrombus is a **thrombectomy**; of an embolus, an **embolectomy**; of an atheroma, an **atherectomy**; and of hemorrhoids, a **hemorrhoidectomy.** An **endarterectomy** removes the diseased lining of an artery, while an **arteriotomy** is an incision into an artery, as to remove a clot. A **valvotomy** is the incision into a cardiac valve to remove an obstruction. **Venipuncture** is a small puncture for the purpose of drawing blood (**phlebotomy**). Figure 6-18 shows a phlebotomist drawing blood from a patient.

Some surgeries are for the purpose of reconstruction or repair—a **valvuloplasty** is done to reconstruct a cardiac valve (see Figure 6-19 on page 202). Other surgical procedures, such as **anastomosis,** are performed to connect blood vessels and to implant devices, such as *pacemakers*, that help regulate

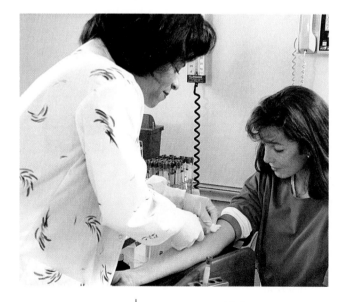

Figure 6-18 Phlebotomists must follow standard precautions when drawing blood.

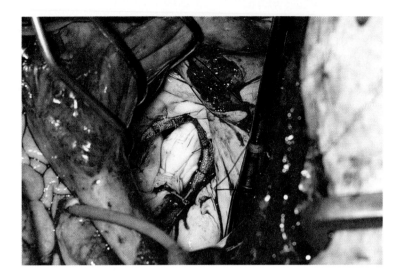

Figure 6-19 Valvuloplasty is a surgical reconstruction of a cardiac valve.

body functions. Pacemakers are small computers that provide electrical stimulation to regulate the heart rate. They can be attached temporarily (usually with a small box worn outside the body and a sensor attached to the outside of the chest) or permanently (the lead is surgically inserted into a blood vessel leading to the heart).

Vocabulary Review

In the previous section, you learned terms relating to surgery. Before going on to the exercises, review the terms below and refer to the previous section if you have questions.

Term	Word Analysis	Definition
anastomosis	[ă-năs-tō-MŌ-sĭs] Greek, to furnish with a mouth	Surgical connection of two blood vessels to allow blood flow between them.
angioplasty	[ĂN-jē-ō-plăs-tē] Angio-, vessel + -plasty, repair	Opening of a blocked blood vessel, as by balloon dilation.
angioscopy	[ăn-jē-ŎS-kō-pē] angio- + -scopy, viewing	Viewing of the interior of a blood vessel using a fiberoptic catheter inserted or threaded into the vessel.
arteriotomy	[ăr-tēr-ē-ŎT-ō-mē] arterio-, artery + -tomy, cutting	Surgical incision into an artery, especially to remove a clot.
atherectomy	[ăth-ĕ-RĔK-tō-mē] ather-, fatty matter + -ectomy, removal	Surgical removal of an atheroma.

Term	Word Analysis	Definition
balloon catheter dilation		Insertion of a balloon catheter into a blood vessel to open the passage so blood can flow freely.
balloon valvuloplasty	[VĂL-vyū-lō-PLĂS-tē]	Procedure that uses a balloon catheter to open narrowed orifices in cardiac valves.
bypass		A structure (usually a vein graft) that creates a new passage for blood to flow from one artery to another artery or part of an artery; used to create a detour around blockages in arteries.
cardiopulmonary bypass		Procedure used during surgery to divert blood flow to and from the heart through a heart-lung machine and back into circulation.
coronary angioplasty		*See* angioplasty.
coronary bypass surgery		*See* bypass.
embolectomy	[ĕm-bō-LĔK-tō-mē] embol(us) + -ectomy	Surgical removal of an embolus.
endarterectomy	[ĕnd-ăr-tēr-ĔK-tō-mē] end-, within + arter-, artery + -ectomy	Surgical removal of the diseased portion of the lining of an artery.
endovascular surgery	endo-, within + vascular	Any of various procedures performed during cardiac catheterization, such as angioscopy and atherectomy.
Fontan's operation	[FŎN-tănz] After François Fontan (1929–), French surgeon	Surgical procedure that creates a bypass from the right atrium to the main pulmonary artery; Fontan's procedure.
graft		Any tissue or organ implanted to replace or mend damaged areas.
heart transplant		Implantation of the heart of a person who has just died into a person whose diseased heart cannot sustain life.
hemorrhoidectomy	[HĔM-ō-rŏy-DĔK-tō-mē] hemorrhoid + -ectomy	Surgical removal of hemorrhoids.
intravascular stent	intra-, within + vascular	Stent placed within a blood vessel to allow blood to flow freely.

Term	Word Analysis	Definition
percutaneous transluminal coronary angioplasty	[pĕr-kyū-TĀ-nē-ŭs trăns-LŪ-mĭn-ăl]	*See* balloon catheter dilation.
phlebotomy	[flĕ-BŎT-ō-me] phlebo-, vein + -tomy	Drawing blood from a vein via a small incision.
stent	[stĕnt]	Surgically implanted device used to hold something (as a blood vessel) open.
thrombectomy	[thrŏm-BĔK-tō-mē] thromb-, thrombus + -ectomy	Surgical removal of a thrombus.
valve replacement		Surgical replacement of a coronary valve.
valvotomy	[văl-VŎT-ō-mē] valve + -tomy	Incision into a cardiac valve to remove an obstruction.
valvuloplasty	[VĂL-vyū-lō-PLĂS-tē] New Latin *valvula*, valve + -plasty	Surgical reconstruction of a cardiac valve.
venipuncture	[VĔN-ĭ-pŭnk-chŭr, VĒ-nĭ-PŬNK-chŭr] veni-, vein + punture	Small puncture into a vein, usually to draw blood or inject a solution.

C A S E   S T U D Y

Surgery Helps

Mr. Davino's progress is poor after three days in the hospital. After determining that his heart has extensive blockages, the doctors decide to perform a CABG on him. The surgeon implants two stents, and Mr. Davino has a smoother recovery. He is told that he must make some lifestyle changes and will have to attend a cardiac rehabilitation center as an outpatient.

 Critical Thinking

76. What are some of the lifestyle changes the staff at the cardiac rehabilitation center will probably recommend?

77. Evaluate your own general cardiovascular health based on your lifestyle. What changes should you make to prevent heart disease?

Surgical Terms Exercises

Check Your Knowledge

Define the following terms.

78. Anastomosis is _____

_____

79. Valvuloplasty is _____

_____

80. Valvotomy is _____

_____

81. Embolectomy is _____

_____

82. Angioplasty is _____

_____

_____

_____

Spell It Correctly

Check the spelling of the following terms. If the term is spelled correctly, put "C" in the blank. If not, put the correct spelling.

83. thromboctomy _____

84. atherectomy _____

85. arteritomy _____

86. angiascopy _____

87. hemorrrhoidectomy _____

88. valvitomy _____

89. veinipuncture _____

90. valvuloplasty _____

91. coronery _____

Pharmacological Terms

Drug therapy for the cardiovascular system generally treats the following conditions: angina, heart attack, high blood pressure, high cholesterol, congestive heart failure, rhythm disorders, and vascular problems. Many of the pharmacological agents treat several problems at once. Table 6-1 lists some of the medications commonly used to treat the cardiovascular system.

Antianginals relieve the pain and prevent attacks of angina. Three categories of drugs—**nitrates,** *beta blockers,* and **calcium channel blockers**—are used as antianginals. Figure 6-20 illustrates how antianginals can be administered. **Thrombolytics** are used to dissolve blood clots in heart-attack victims. **Tissue-type plasminogen activator (tPA)** is an agent used to prevent the formation of a thrombus. **Nitrates** and beta blockers are used to treat myocardial infarctions.

High blood pressure may require treatment with one drug or a combination of drugs. Beta blockers and calcium channel blockers are used along with a number of agents that affect the control centers in the brain that regulate blood pressure. **Vasodilators** relax the walls of the blood vessels. Other treatments for high blood pressure include **diuretics,** to relieve edema (swelling) and increase kidney function; **angiotensin converting enzyme (ACE) inhibitors,** which dilate arteries thus making it easier for blood to flow out of the heart; and agents that affect the nerves of the body. Congestive heart failure is treated with ACE inhibitors, diuretics, and **cardiotonics,** which increase myocardial contractions. In certain situations, **vasoconstrictors,** may be needed to narrow blood vessels.

Rhythm disorders are treated with a number of medications that normalize heart rate by affecting the nervous system that controls the heart rate. Beta blockers and calcium channel blockers may also be used for rhythm disorders.

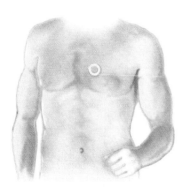

Figure 6-20 The most common antianginal is nitroglycerin, which can be administered sublingually under the tongue, or via a patch on the skin.

Table 6-1 Medications for the Cardiovascular System

Drug Class	Purpose	Generic Name	Trade Name
coronary vasodilators	dilate veins, arteries, and coronary arteries; used to treat angina, myocardial infarction, congestive heart failure	nitroglycerin	Nitrostat, Nitrostat IV, Nitrolingual, Nitrogard, Nitrol, Nitro-Bid, Nitro-disc, Nitro-Dur, Transderm-Nitro, Deponit (patches), Minitran
		isosorbide dinitrate	Isordil, Sorbitrate, Dilatrate
		pentaerythritol tetranitrate	Peritrate
		erythrityl tetranitrate	Cardilate
beta blockers	reduce contraction strength of heart muscle; lower blood pressure; slow heartbeat	propanolol	Inderal
		metroprolol	Lopressor
		nadolol	Corgard
		atenolol	Tenormin
		acebutolol	Sectral
		betaxolol	Kerlone
		labetalol	Normodyne, Trandate
		penbutolol	Levatol

Table 6-1 (continued)

Drug Class	Purpose	Generic Name	Trade Name
beta blockers *(continued)*		pindolol timolol carteolol esmolol	Visken Blocadren Cartrol Brevibloc
calcium channel blockers	inhibit ability of calcium ions to enter heart muscle and blood vessel muscle cells; reduce heart rate; lower squeezing strength of heart contraction; lower blood pressure; dilate coronary arteries to enhance blood flow; normalize some fast or irregular heartbeats	verapamil nifedipine nicardipine diltiazem isradipine felodipine bepridil	Calan, Isoptin, Verlan Procardia, Adalat Cardene Cardizem, Dilacor XR DynaCirc Plendil Vascor
thrombolytics	dissolve blood clots	urokinase Tissue plasminogen activator (tPA,TPA) streptokinase anistreplase	Abbokinase Activase Kabikinase, Streptase Eminase
bile acid sequestrants	lipid-lowering medications that bind to bile acids and require more body cholesterol to create other bile acids; more cholesterol used up and hence lowered	cholestyramine colestipol	Questran, Cholybar, Lipocol, Lismol, Quantalan, Colestrol, Vasosan Colestid
lipid-lowering medications	reduce triglycerides and cholesterol (but mechanisms not totally understood)	gemfibrozil lovastatin pravastatin simvastatin niacin clofibrate probucol dextrothyroxine	Lopid Mevacor Pravachol Zocor Nia-Bid, Niacels, Nicobid, Nicolar, Slo-Niacin, Nicotinex Atromid-S Lorelco Choloxin
centrally acting hypertensive agents, antihypertensive	decrease blood pressure by affecting brain control centers	methyldopa guanfacine guanabenz clonidine	Aldomet Tenex Wytensin Catapres
direct-acting vasodilators	lower blood pressure by relaxing walls of blood vessels	hydralazine minoxidil	Apresoline Loniten
peripherally acting hypertensive agents	lower blood pressure by affecting nerves involved in blood pressure regulation	guanadrel guanethidine mecamylamine prazosin rauwolfia alkaloids trazosin doxazosin	Hylorel Ismelin Inversine Minipress Harmonyl, Raudixin, Rauzide, Serpasil Hytrin Cardura

(continued on page 208)

Table 6-1 (continued)

Drug Class	Purpose	Generic Name	Trade Name
ACE inhibitors	ease heart pumping and lower blood pressure by dilating arteries	captopril enalapril lisinopril benazepril fosinopril ramipril	Capoten Vasotec Zestril, Prinivil Lotensin Monopril Altace
diuretics	promote removal of water by kidneys to lower blood pressure and relieve edema	chlorthalidone chlorothiazide hydrochlorothiazide methyclothiazide metolazone amiloride spironolactone triamterene bumetanide ethacrynic acid furosemide	Hygroton, Thalitone Diuril Esidrix, Hydrodiuril Aquatensen, Enduron Diulo, Zaroxolyn Midamor Aldactone Dyrenium Bumex Edecrin Lasix
combination diuretics		hydrochlorothiazide plus amiloride hydrochlorothiazide plus spironolactone hydrochlorothiazide plus triamterene	Moduretic Aldactazide Dyazide, Maxzide
inotropic agents	increase amount of blood heart is able to pump by increasing squeezing strength of heart muscle	digitalis milrinone digoxin digitoxin dopamine dobutamine amrinone	 Primacor Lanoxin, Lanoxicaps Crystodigin Intropin Dobutrex Inocor
antiarrhythmics	alter the electrical flow through the heart's conduction system thereby regulating fast or irregular heartbeats	quinidine procainamide disopyramide lidocaine phenytoin mexiletine tocainide sotalol flecainide moricizine propafenone bretylium amiodarone adenosine	Cardioquin, Cin-Quin Duraquin, Quinaglute, Quinalan, Quinidex, Quinora Procan SR, Pronestyl, Pronestyl-SR Norpace, Norpace CR Xylocaine Dilantin Mexitil Tonocard Betapace Tambocor Ethmozine Rhythmol Bretylol Cordarone Adenocard

Table 6-1 (continued)

Drug Class	Purpose	Generic Name	Trade Name
medications for slow heartbeats	affect control of heart rate in the nervous system	atropine isoproterenol	(numerous) Isuprel
anticoagulants, anticlotting	reduce proteins involved in blood clotting so clots cannot form as readily	warfarin enoxaparin dicumarol heparin	Coumadin, Panwarfin Lovenox
antiplatelet medications	reduce ability of blood platelets to clot	aspirin dipyridamole	(numerous) Persantine
hemorrheologic	decrease viscosity of blood making flow easier; used to treat claudication	pentoxifylline	Trental

Cholesterol is a substance the body needs in certain quantities. Excesses of certain kinds of cholesterol such as LDL can cause fatty deposits or plaque to form on blood vessels. Figure 6-21 compares a normal artery with a plaque-filled artery. **Lipid-lowering** drugs work in various ways (some of which are not understood) to help the body excrete unwanted cholesterol. Blood clotting in vessels can cause dangerous blockages. **Anticoagulants** and *antiplatelet* medications inhibit the ability of the blood to clot. Other medications used for vascular problems may include drugs that decrease the thickness of the blood, or drugs that increase the amount of blood the heart is able to pump.

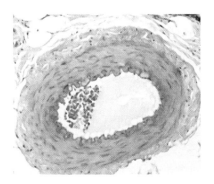
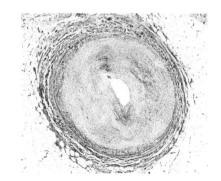

Vocabulary Review

In the previous section, you learned terms relating to pharmacology. Before going on to the exercises, review the terms below and refer to the previous section if you have questions.

Agent	Word Analysis	Purpose
angiotensin converting enzyme (ACE) inhibitor	[ăn-jē-ō-TĔN-sĭn] angio-, vessel + (hyper)tension	Medication used for heart failure and other cardiovascular problems; acts by dilating arteries to lower blood pressure and makes heart pump easier.

Agent	Word Analysis	Purpose
antianginal	[ăn-tē-ĂN-jĭ-năl] anti-, against + angina	Agent used to relieve or prevent attacks of angina.
antiarrhythmic	[ăn-tē-ā-RĬTH-mĭk] anti- + arrhythmic	Agent used to help normalize cardiac rhythm.
anticlotting	anti- + clotting	*See* anticoagulant.
anticoagulant	anti- + coagulant	Agent that prevents the formation of dangerous clots.
antihypertensive	anti- + hypertensive	Agent that helps control high blood pressure.
calcium channel blocker		Medication that lessens the ability of calcium ions to enter heart and blood vessel muscle cells; used to lower blood pressure and normalize some arrhythmias.
cardiotonic	[KĂR-dē-ō-TŎN-ĭk] cardio-, heart + Greek *tonos*, tension	Medication for congestive heart failure; increases the force of contractions of the myocardium.
diuretic	[dī-yū-RĔT-ĭk] di-, throughout + Greek *uresis*, urine	Medication that promotes the excretion of urine.
heparin	[HĔP-ă-rĭn] From Greek *hepar*, liver	Anticoagulant present in the body; also, synthetic version administered to prevent clotting.
lipid-lowering		Helpful in lowering cholesterol levels.
nitrate		Any of several medications that dilate the veins, arteries, or coronary arteries; used to control angina.
thrombolytic	[thrŏm-bō-LĬT-ĭk] thrombo-, thrombus + -lytic, destroying	Agent that dissolves a thrombus.
tissue-type plasminogen activator (tPA, TPA)	[plăz-MĬN-ō-jĕn]	Agent that prevents a thrombus from forming.
vasoconstrictor	[VĀ-sō-kŏn-STRĬK-tĕr] vaso-, vessel + constrictor	Agent that narrows the blood vessels.
vasodilator	[VĀ-sō-dī-LĀ-tĕr] vaso- + dilator	Agent that dilates or widens the blood vessels.

C A S E S T U D Y

The Long-Term Treatment

As part of Mr. Davino's long-term rehabilitation, medication has been prescribed, as shown on the prescription forms given to him upon his release.

Critical Thinking

92. For what condition is Mr. Davino's medication (a) most likely being prescribed?

93. Prescription form (b) prescribes a medication for what other condition?

Dr. Andar Mirkhan
16 Courtyard Lane • Andover, Ohio 66666
PATIENT'S NAME *Joseph Davino* AGE *44*
ADDRESS
CITY *Wesley* DATE *9/1/XX*
℞
Questran 4g ac TID
#90
DEA NO. 54321x *Andar Mirkhan, M.D.*
LICENSE NO. 12345y SIGNATURE

(a)

Dr. Andar Mirkhan
16 Courtyard Lane • Andover, Ohio 66666
PATIENT'S NAME *Joseph Davino* AGE *44*
ADDRESS
CITY *Wesley* DATE *9/1/XX*
℞
Lasix 80 mg q12h
#60
DEA NO. 54321x *Andar Mirkhan, M.D.*
LICENSE NO. 12345y SIGNATURE

(b)

Pharmacological Terms Exercises

Using Table 6-1, describe the condition for which each combination of medications is probably being prescribed.

94. metroprolol, Vasotec, and Diazide _____

_____

95. Coumadin, aspirin, and pentoxifylline _____

_____

96. nitroglycerin, lidocaine, and esmolol _____

_____

Check Your Knowledge

From Table 6-1, name at least one medication used to treat each of the following conditions.

97. hypertension _____

98. water retention _____

99. arrhythmia _____

100. bradycardia _____

101. clotting _____

102. arterial plaque _____

103. angina _____

104. congestive heart failure _____

The cardiologists on the hospital staff have a weekly meeting to review cases. Dr. Woodard and Dr. Mirkhan have discussed the admission of Mr. Davino to the CCU and have reported on his progress. Another interesting case is a 50-year-old woman who presented with no symptoms except chest pain when she was admitted for possible coronary disease. After she was stabilized in the emergency room, the cardiologist on call examined her closely. The patient was found to have very few risk factors (nonsmoker, normal weight, normal BP). However, upon discussions with her, they found she has a high-stress job and a moderate-to-poor diet. The notes on the woman's chart are shown here.

Referring physician: Margaret Lao, M.D.

Examination: Resting pulse was 78 beats per minute. The blood pressure was 126/80 mm/Hg. Lungs clear. Soft systolic ejection murmur along left sternal border.

ECG: Patient's resting, modified 12-lead ECG had no resting abnormalities.

Patient was given a stress electrocardiogram one month ago. Her doctor noted no exercise-associated arrythmias and found mild-to-moderate hypokinesis of inferior and posterior segments. Her improved contractility with exercise suggested adequate myocardial perfusion.

105. From the cardiologist's notes, describe the patient's condition.

_____

_____

_____

USING THE http://www. INTERNET

If you search the World Wide Web for the American Heart Association (http://www.amhrt.org), you will find many discussions of all aspects of heart disease. Use the Internet to find and list at least three inherited or genetic risk factors and at least three acquired risk factors for heart disease.

CHAPTER REVIEW

Definitions

Define the following terms and combining forms. Review the chapter before starting. Make sure you know how to pronounce each term as you define it.

Term	Definition
anastomosis [ă-năs-tō-MŌ-sĭs]	
aneurysm [ĂN-yū-rĭzm]	
angina [ĂN-jĭ-nă, ăn-JĪ-nă]	
angina pectoris [PĔK-tōr-ĭs, pĕk-TŌR-ĭs]	
angi(o)	
angiocardiography [ăn-jē-ō-kăr-dē-ŎG-ră-fē]	
angiography [ăn-jē-ŎG-ră-fē]	
angioplasty [ĂN-jē-ō-plăs-tē]	
angioscopy [ăn-jē-ŎS-kō-pē]	
angiotensin [ăn-jē-ō-TĔN-sĭn] converting enzyme (ACE) inhibitor	
antianginal [ăn-tē-ĂN-jĭ-năl]	
antiarrhythmic [ăn-tē-ā-RĬTH-mĭk]	
anticlotting	
anticoagulant	
antihypertensive	
aorta [ā-ŌR-tă]	
aort(o)	
aortic regurgitation [rē-GŬR-jĭ-TĀ-shŭn]	
aortic stenosis [stĕ-NŌ-sĭs]	
aortic valve	
aortography [ā-ōr-TŎG-ră-fe]	

Term	Definition
arrhythmia [ā-RĬTH-mē-ă]	
arteri(o), arter(o)	
arteriography [ăr-tēr-ē-ŎG-ră-fē]	
arteriole [ăr-TĒ-rē-ōl]	
arteriosclerosis [ăr-TĒR-ē-ō-sklĕr-Ō-sĭs]	
arteriotomy [ăr-tēr-ē-ŎT-ō-mē]	
arteritis [ăr-tēr-Ī-tĭs]	
artery [ĂR-tēr-ē]	
asystole [ā-SĬS-tō-lē]	
ather(o)	
atherectomy [ăth-ĕ-RĔK-tō-mē]	
atheroma [ăth-ĕr-Ō-mă]	
atherosclerosis [ĂTH-ĕr-ō-sklĕr-ō-sĭs]	
atri(o)	
atrial fibrillation [fĭ-brĭ-LĀ-shŭn]	
atrioventricular block	
atrioventricular [Ā-trē-ō-vĕn-TRĬK-yū-lăr] bundle	
atrioventricular node (AV node)	
atrioventricular valve	
atrium (pl. atria) [Ā-trē-ŭm (Ā-trē-ă)]	
auscultation [ăws-kŭl-TĀ-shŭn]	
bacterial endocarditis	
balloon catheter dilation	
balloon valvuloplasty [VĂL-vyū-lō-PLĂS-tē]	
bicuspid [bī-KŬS-pĭd] valve	
blood [blŭd]	
blood pressure	
blood vessel	
bradycardia [brād-ē-KĂR-dē-ă]	
bruit [brū-Ē]	

Term	Definition
bundle of His [hĭz, hĭs]	
bypass	
calcium channel blocker	
capillary [KĂP-ĭ-lār-ē]	
carbon dioxide	
cardi(o)	
cardiac arrest	
cardiac catheterization [kăth-ĕ-tĕr-ĭ-ZĀ-shŭn]	
cardiac cycle	
cardiac enzyme studies	
cardiac MRI	
cardiac scan	
cardiac tamponade [tăm-pō-NĀD]	
cardiomyopathy [KĂR-dē-ō-mī-ŎP-ă-thē]	
cardiopulmonary bypass	
cardiotonic [KĂR-dē-ō-TŎN-ĭk]	
carotid [kă-RŎT-ĭd] artery	
cholesterol [kō-LĔS-tĕr-ōl]	
claudication [klăw-dĭ-KĀ-shŭn]	
coarctation [kō-ărk-TĀ-shŭn] of the aorta	
conduction system	
congenital heart disease	
congestive heart failure	
constriction [kŏn-STRĬK-shŭn]	
coronary angioplasty	
coronary [KŌR-ō-nār-ē] artery	
coronary artery disease	
coronary bypass surgery	
cyanosis [sī-ă-NŌ-sĭs]	
deep vein thrombosis [thrŏm-BŌ-sĭs]	
depolarization [dē-pō-lă-rĭ-ZĀ-shŭn]	

Term	Definition
diastole [dī-ĂS-tō-lē]	
digital subtraction angiography	
diuretic [dī-yū-RĔT-ĭk]	
Doppler [DŎP-lĕr] ultrasound	
ductus arteriosus [DŬK-tŭs ăr-tēr-ē-Ō-sŭs]	
ductus venosus [vĕn-Ō-sĭs]	
dysrhythmia [dĭs-RĬTH-mē-ă]	
echocardiography [ĕk-ō-kăr-dē-ŎG-ră-fē]	
ejection fraction	
electrocardiography [ē-lĕk-trō-kăr-dē-ŎG-ră-fē]	
embolectomy [ĕm-bō-LĔK-tō-mē]	
embolus [ĔM-bō-lŭs]	
endarterectomy [ĕnd-ăr-tēr-ĔK-tō-mē]	
endocarditis [ĔN-dō-kăr-DĪ-tĭs]	
endocardium [ĕn-dō-KĂR-dē-ŭm]	
endothelium [ĕn-dō-THĒ-lē-ŭm]	
endovascular surgery	
epicardium [ĕp-ĭ-KĂR-dē-ŭm]	
essential hypertension	
femoral [FĔM-ŏ-răl, FĒ-mŏ-răl] artery	
fibrillation [fĭ-brĭ-LĀ-shŭn]	
flutter	
Fontan's [FŎN-tănz] operation	
foramen ovale [fō-RĀ-mĕn ō-VĂ-lē]	
gallop	
graft	
hardening of the arteries	
heart [hărt]	
heart block	

Term	Definition
heart transplant	
hemangi(o)	
hemorrhoidectomy [HĔM-ō-rŏy-DĔK-tō-mē]	
hemorrhoids [HĔM-ō-rŏydz]	
heparin [HĔP-ă-rĭn]	
high blood pressure	
Holter [HŌL-tĕr] monitor	
hypertension [HĪ-pĕr-TĔN-shŭn]	
hypertensive heart disease	
hypotension [HĪ-pō-TĔN-shŭn]	
infarct [ĬN-fărkt]	
infarction [ĭn-FĂRK-shŭn]	
inferior vena cava [VĒ-nă KĂ-vă, KĀ-vă]	
intermittent claudication	
intracardiac [ĭn-tră-KĂR-dē-ăk] tumor	
intravascular stent	
ischemia [ĭs-KĒ-mē-ă]	
left atrium	
left ventricle	
lipid-lowering	
lipid profile	
low blood pressure	
lumen [LŪ-mĕn]	
mitral [MĪ-trăl] insufficiency or reflux	
mitral stenosis	
mitral [MĪ-trăl] valve	
mitral valve prolapse	
multiple-gated acquisition angiography	
murmur	
myocardial infarction	

Term	Definition
myocarditis [MĪ-ō-kăr-DĪ-tĭs]	
myocardium [mī-ō-KĂR-dē-ŭm]	
necrosis [nĕ-KRŌ-sĭs]	
nitrate	
occlusion [ŏ-KLŪ-zhŭn]	
pacemaker	
palpitations [păl-pĭ-TĀ-shŭnz]	
patent ductus arteriosus [PĂ-tĕnt DŬK-tŭs ăr-tēr-ē-Ō-sŭs]	
percutaneous transluminal [pĕr-kyū-TĀ-nē-ŭs trăns-LŪ-mĭn-ăl] coronary angioplasty	
perfusion deficit	
pericardi(o)	
pericarditis [PĔR-ĭ-kăr-DĪ-tĭs]	
pericardium [pĕr-ĭ-KĂR-dē-ŭm]	
peripheral vascular disease	
petechiae [pĕ-TĒ-kē-ē, pĕ-TĔK-ē-ē, pĕ-TĒ-kē-ă]	
phleb(o)	
phlebitis [flĕ-BĪ-tĭs]	
phlebography [flĕ-BŎG-ră-fē]	
phlebotomy [flĕ-BŎT-ō-mē]	
plaque [plăk]	
polarization [pō-lăr-ĭ-ZĀ-shŭn]	
popliteal [pŏp-LĬT-ē-ăl] artery	
positron emission tomography [tō-MŎG-ră-fē]	
premature atrial contractions (PACs)	
premature ventricular contractions (PVCs)	
pulmonary artery	
pulmonary artery stenosis	
pulmonary edema	

Term	Definition
pulmonary valve	
pulmonary vein	
pulse [pŭls]	
Purkinje [pŭr-KĬN-jē] fibers	
Raynaud's [rā-NŌZ] phenomenon	
repolarization [rē-pō-lăr-ĭ-ZĀ-shŭn]	
rheumatic heart disease	
right atrium	
right ventricle	
risk factor	
rub	
saphenous [să-FĒ-nŭs] vein	
secondary hypertension	
semilunar [sĕm-ē-LŪ-năr] valve	
septal defect	
septum (pl. septa) [SĔP-tŭm (SĔP-tă)]	
serum enzyme tests	
sinoatrial [sī-nō-Ā-trē-ăl] node (SA node)	
sinus rhythm	
sonography [sō-NŎG-ră-fē]	
sphygm(o)	
sphygmomanometer [SFĬG-mō-mă-NŎM-ĕ-tĕr]	
stenosis [stĕ-NŌ-sĭs]	
stent [stĕnt]	
stress test	
superior vena cava	
systole [SĬS-tō-lē]	
tachycardia [TĂK-ĭ-KĂR-dē-ă]	
tetralogy of Fallot [fă-LŌ]	
thromb(o)	

Term	Definition
thrombectomy [thrŏm-BĔK-tō-mē]	
thrombolytic [thrŏm-bō-LĬT-ĭk]	
thrombophlebitis [THRŎM-bō-flĕ-BĪ-tĭs]	
thrombosis [thrŏm-BŌ-sĭs]	
thrombotic occlusion	
thrombus [THRŎM-bŭs]	
tissue-type plasminogen [plăz-MĬN-ō-jĕn] activator (tPA, TPA)	
tricuspid stenosis	
tricuspid [trī-KŬS-pĭd] valve	
triglyceride [trī-GLĬS-ĕr-īd]	
valve [vălv]	
valve replacement	
valvotomy [văl-VŎT-ō-mē]	
valvulitis [văl-vyū-LĪ-tĭs]	
valvuloplasty [VĂL-vyū-lō-PLĂS-tē]	
varicose [VĂR-ĭ-kōs] vein	
vas(o)	
vasoconstrictor [VĀ-sō-kŏn-STRĬK-tĕr]	
vasodilator [VĀ-sō-dī-LĀ-tĕr]	
vegetation [vĕj-ĕ-TĀ-shŭn]	
vein [vān]	
vena cava [VĒ-nă KĂ-vă, KĀ-vă]	
ven(o)	
venipuncture [VĔN-ĭ-pŭnk-chŭr, VĒ-nĭ-PŬNK-chŭr]	
venography [vē-NŎG-ră-fē]	
ventricle [VĔN-trĭ-kl]	
ventriculogram [vĕn-TRĬK-yū-lō-grăm]	
venule [VĔN-yūl, VĒ-nūl]	

Abbreviations

Write the full meaning of each abbreviation.

Abbreviation	Meaning
AcG	
AF	
AS	
ASCVD	
ASD	
ASHD	
AV	
BP	
CABG	
CAD	
cath	
CCU	
CHD	
CHF	
CO	
CPK	
CPR	
CVA	
CVD	
DSA	
DVT	
ECG, EKG	
ECHO	
ETT	
GOT	
HDL	
LDH	
LDL	
LV	
LVH	
MI	
MR	

MS _____

MUGA _____

MVP _____

PTCA _____

PVC _____

SA _____

SV _____

tPA, TPA _____

VLDL _____

VSD _____

VT _____

1. overweight, sedentary, smoker
2. no
3. a. pulmonary valve—controls blood flow between the right ventricle and the pulmonary arteries
   b. aortic valve—controls blood flow between the aorta and the left ventricle
   c. right pulmonary artery—one of two arteries that carry blood that is low in oxygen from the heart to the lungs
   d. interatrial septum—partition separating the two atria
   e. tricuspid valve—atrioventricular valve on the right side of the heart
   f. inferior vena cava—large vein that draws blood from the lower part of the body to the right atrium
   g. right ventricle—one of the heart's four chambers
   h. interventricular septum—part of the septum between two ventricles
   i. left ventricle—one of the heart's four chambers
   j. aorta—artery through which blood exits the heart
4. atrioventricular
5. capillary
6. C
7. Purkinje fibers
8. C
9. arteriole
10. C
11. C
12. systole
13. artery
14. veins
15. endocardium
16. atria and ventricles
17. blood
18. poor diet, smoking, lack of exercise
19. pulmonary
20. endothelium
21. heart and lungs
22. carotid artery
23. lungs
24. Skin color and disorientation
25. 8 hours
26. cardiomyopathy
27. pericarditis
28. venogram
29. phlebitis
30. arterioplasty
31. vasoneuropathy
32. vasotropic
33. cardiogenic
34. cardiomegaly
35. thromboarteritis
36. phlebitis
37. thrombectomy
38. phleboplasty
39. atriomegaly
40. phlebograph, venograph
41. cardiomegaly
42. cardiopulmonary
43. pericardiostomy
44. endocarditis
45. phleboplasty
46. vasoparalysis
47. angiorrhaphy
48. phlebitis
49. arteries
50. vein
51. MI
52. artery
53. ECG–electrocardiogram
54. CCU–coronary care unit
55. MI—myocardial infarction
56. BP—blood pressure
57. ECHO—echocardiogram
58. yes
59. Cholesterol
60. arteriosclerosis
61. sodium, potassium, chloride, creatinine, BUN, cholesterol, CPK, thallium HDL, LDL, CO_2
62. 99222
63. 414.0
64. A
65. D
66. B
67. C
68. tachycardia, bradycardia
69. arrhythmia, dysrhythmia
70. thrombus
71. bruit
72. murmur
73. hypertension
74. risk factors
75. myocardial infarction
76. dietary changes, quit smoking, exercise program, stress reduction
77. depends on individual, but maintaining a healthy lifestyle will help prevent heart disease
78. surgical connection of two blood vessels
79. repair of a cardiac valve
80. incision into a cardiac valve to remove an obstruction
81. surgical removal of an embolus
82. surgical repair of a blocked blood vessel
83. thrombectomy
84. C
85. arteriotomy
86. angioscopy
87. C
88. valvotomy
89. venipuncture
90. C
91. coronary
92. high blood cholesterol
93. excess urine and high blood pressure
94. high blood pressure
95. clotting in blood vessels; anticoagulants
96. myocardial infarction
97. Inderal
98. Diuril
99. Cardioquin
100. Duraquin
101. Coumadin
102. Abbokinase
103. Nitrostat
104. Cardilate
105. Patient's condition showed no evidence of cardiac disease. She has low risk factors; however, she has stress-related problems and a poor diet that may eventually cause more serious health problems if not corrected.

CHAPTER 7

The Respiratory System

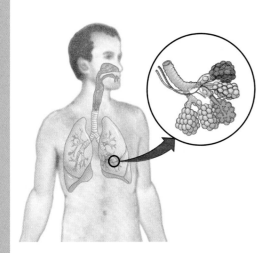

After studying this chapter, you will be able to:

- Name the parts of the respiratory system and discuss the function of each part
- Define combining forms used in building words that relate to the respiratory system and its parts
- Identify the meaning of related abbreviations
- Name the common diagnoses, clinical procedures, and laboratory tests used in treating disorders of the respiratory system
- List and define the major pathological conditions of the respiratory system
- Explain the meaning of surgical terms related to the respiratory system

Structure And Function

The respiratory system performs two major tasks—**external respiration,** breathing or exchanging air between the body and the outside environment, and **internal respiration,** bringing oxygen to the cells and removing carbon dioxide from them. The respiratory system includes the **lungs,** the **respiratory tract** (passageways through which air moves in and out of the lungs), and the muscles that move air into and out of the lungs (Figures 7-1a and 7-1b). In the upper part of the trachea is the larynx, where most of the sound used in speech and singing is produced.

External Respiration

Inspiration (breathing in or **inhalation**) brings air from the outside environment into the **nose** (or mouth). The **nostrils** (also called **external nares**) are the two external openings at the base of the external portion of the nose. The external nose is supported by the nasal bones and is divided into two halves by the **nasal septum,** a strip of cartilage. After air enters the nose, it passes into the **nasal cavity** and the **paranasal sinuses,** where it is warmed by blood in the mucous membranes that line these areas. **Cilia** (hairs) in the nasal cavity filter out foreign bodies.

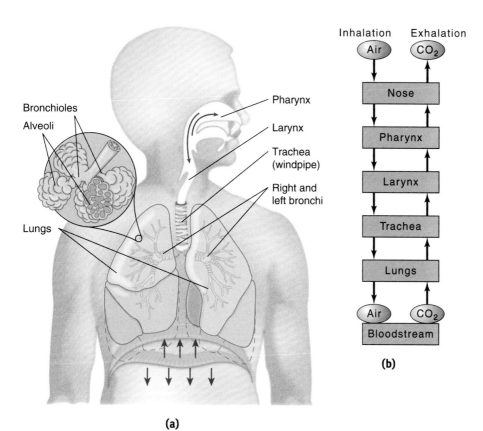

Inhalation — Air
Exhalation — CO2

Nose

Pharynx

Larynx

Trachea

Lungs

Air — CO2

Bloodstream

(b)

(a)

Bronchioles
Alveoli

Lungs

Pharynx

Larynx

Trachea (windpipe)

Right and left bronchi

Figure 7-1 (a). The respiratory system performs the process of inhaling air and exhaling carbon dioxide. (b). The diagram shows the pathways of inhaled air (containing oxygen) and exhaled air (containing carbon dioxide).

The air next reaches the **pharynx (throat)**, which is a passageway for both air and food. The pharynx is divided into three sections. The **nasopharynx** lies above the **soft palate**, which is a flexible muscular sheet that separates the nasopharynx from the rest of the pharynx. The nasopharynx contains the **pharyngeal tonsils**, more commonly known as the **adenoids**, which aid in the body's immune defense. Sometimes, particularly in children, these tonsils become repeatedly infected and may swell and obstruct air passageways. In some cases, they are surgically removed to alleviate this condition.

The next division of the pharynx is the **oropharynx**, the back portion of the mouth. It contains the *palatine tonsils*, lymphatic tissue that works as part of the immune system. The oropharynx is part of the mechanism of the mouth that triggers swallowing.

The bottom and third section of the pharynx is the **laryngopharynx** (also called the **hypopharynx**). It is at this point that the respiratory tract divides into the esophagus, the passageway for food, and the **larynx** or **voice box**, through which air passes to the **trachea** or **windpipe.**

Food is prevented from going into the larynx by the **epiglottis**, a movable flap of cartilage that covers the opening to the larynx (called the **glottis**) every time one swallows. Food then passes only into the esophagus. Occasionally, a person may swallow and inhale at the same time, allowing some food to be pulled (or *aspirated*) into the larynx. Usually, a strong cough forces out the food, but sometimes an individual may choke, and the food must be dislodged with help from another person in a technique called the **Heimlich maneuver** (Figure 7-2) on page 226. This technique has saved many people from choking to death.

Air goes into the larynx, which serves both as a passageway to the trachea and as the area where the sounds of speech and singing are produced. The

Larynx and pharynx are both directly from Greek. The meanings remain basically the same as in ancient times.

Figure 7-2 The Heimlich maneuver is used widely to aid victims of choking.

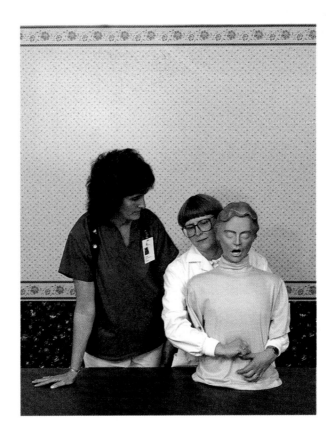

A thoracic surgeon, Harry J. Heimlich (born 1920), devised and helped to publicize the Heimlich maneuver.

larynx contains **vocal cords,** strips of epithelial tissue that vibrate when muscular tension is applied (Figure 7-3). The size and thickness of the cords determine the pitch of sound. The male's thicker and longer vocal cords produce a lower pitch than do the shorter and thinner vocal cords of most women. Children's voices tend to be higher in pitch because of the smaller size of their vocal cords. Sound volume is regulated by the amount of air that passes over the vocal cords. The larynx is supported by various cartilaginous structures, one of which consists of two disks joined at an angle to form the **thyroid cartilage** or **Adam's apple** (larger in males than in females).

The trachea is a tube that connects the larynx to the right and left **bronchi,** tubular branches into which the larynx divides. The point at which the trachea divides is called the **mediastinum,** a general term for a median area, especially one with a **septum** or cartilaginous division. The mediastinum contains the heart, lungs, esophagus, trachea, and thymus gland. The median portion of the thoracic cavity is also known as the *mediastinum*. Both bronchi

Figure 7-3 Vocal cords are the primary instruments of sound.

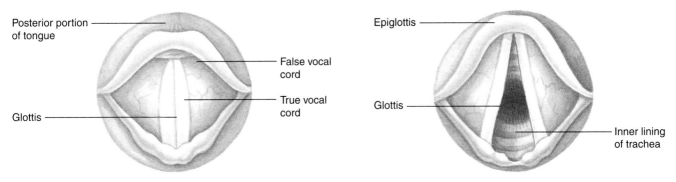

Posterior portion of tongue

False vocal cord

True vocal cord

Glottis

Epiglottis

Glottis

Inner lining of trachea

contain cartilage and mucous glands and are the passageways through which air enters the right and left lungs. Air that is pushed out of the lungs travels up through the respiratory tract during **expiration** (breathing out or **exhalation**), where air is expelled into the environment.

Internal Respiration

The bronchi further divide into many smaller branches called **bronchioles.** Inside the lungs, the structures resemble tree branches, with smaller parts branching off. At the end of each bronchiole is a cluster of air sacs. Each air sac is called an **alveolus** (plural, **alveoli**). There are about 300 million alveoli in the lungs. The one-celled, thin-walled alveoli connect to capillaries in the lungs. Oxygen is exchanged from the alveoli into the capillaries of the bloodstream and carbon dioxide is returned from the capillaries into the alveoli. Oxygen is then delivered to the body's other cells during this phase of respiration called internal respiration. This type of respiration is affected by how well the cardiovascular system supplies oxygenated blood. Carbon dioxide is expelled back up through the respiratory tract during expiration.

The lungs take up most of the thoracic cavity (or **thorax**), reaching from the collarbone to the diaphragm. The outside of the lungs is a moist, double layer of membrane called the **pleura** (plural, **pleurae**). The outer layer, the **parietal pleura,** and the inner layer, the **visceral pleura,** both make lung movement in the thoracic cavity easier by protecting the lungs and providing the moisture that allows movement. The space between the two pleurae is called the **pleural cavity.** Each lung has an **apex,** or topmost section; a middle area called the **hilum** or **hilus**; and a lower section called the **base.** The hilum is the area where the bronchi, blood vessels, and nerves enter the lungs. The right, larger lung is divided into three lobes—a **superior lobe,** a **middle lobe,** and an **inferior lobe.** The left lung is divided into two lobes— a superior lobe and an inferior lobe (Figure 7-4). Humans can function with one or more lobes removed or even an entire lung removed, as is necessary in some cases of lung cancer.

Muscles for Breathing

Muscular contractions enlarge the volume of the thoracic cavity during inspiration and decrease the volume when they relax during expiration. The major muscles that contract are the **diaphragm** and the **intercostal muscles** (the muscles

Figure 7-4 The lungs are divided into lobes—three on the right and two on the left.

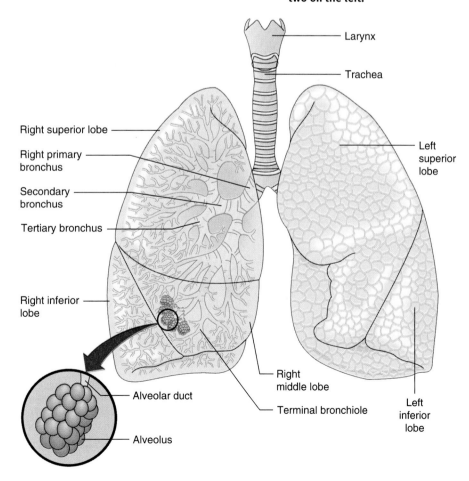

- Larynx
- Trachea
- Left superior lobe
- Right superior lobe
- Right primary bronchus
- Secondary bronchus
- Tertiary bronchus
- Right inferior lobe
- Alveolar duct
- Alveolus
- Right middle lobe
- Terminal bronchiole
- Left inferior lobe

Lung Capacity

Normal inspiration brings about 500 milliliters of air into the lungs. Normal expiration expels about the same amount from the lungs. Forced inspiration brings extra air (even up to six times the normal amount) into the lungs. Forced expiration can expel up to three times the normal amount of air from the lungs.

Some quantity of air always remains in the lungs so that newly inhaled air mixes with the remaining air. This helps to maintain the proper concentrations of oxygen and carbon dioxide in the lungs.

between the ribs). The diaphragm lowers itself when it contracts, allowing more space in the thoracic cavity, and the intercostal muscles pull the ribs upward and outward when they contract, also enlarging the thoracic cavity.

Vocabulary Review

In the previous section, you learned terms relating to the respiratory system. Before going on to the exercises, review the terms below and refer to the previous section if you have any questions.

Term	Word Analysis	Definition
Adam's apple		Thyroid cartilage, supportive structure of the larynx; larger in males than in females.
adenoids	[ĂD-ĕ-nŏydz] Greek *aden*, gland + *eidos*, resembling	Collection of lymphoid tissue in the nasopharynx; pharyngeal tonsils.
alveolus (pl. alveoli)	[ăl-VĒ-ō-lŭs (ăl-VĒ-ō-lī)] Latin, little sac	Air sac at the end of each bronchiole.
apex	[Ā-pĕks] Latin, summit	Topmost section of the lung.
base	[bās] Latin *basis*, bottom	Bottom section of the lung.
bronchiole	[BRŎNG-kē-ōl] bronchi-, bronchus + -ole, small	Fine subdivision of the bronchi made of smooth muscle and elastic fibers.
bronchus (pl. bronchi)	[BRŎNG-kŭs (BRŎNG-kī)] Latin *bronchus*, windpipe	One of the two airways from the trachea to the lungs.
cilia	[SĬL-ē-ă] Latin, plural of *cilium*, hair	Hairlike extensions of a cell's surface that usually provide some protection by sweeping foreign particles away.

Term	Word Analysis	Definition
diaphragm	[DĪ-ă-frăm] Greek *diaphragma*, from *dia-*, through + *phrassein*, to enclose	Membranous muscle between the abdominal and thoracic cavities that contracts and relaxes during the respiratory cycle.
epiglottis	[ĕp-ĭ-GLŎT-ĭs] Greek, from *epi-*, on + *glottis*, mouth of the windpipe	Cartilaginous flap that covers the larynx during swallowing to prevent food from entering the airway.
exhalation	[ĕks-hă-LĀ-shŭn] Latin *exhalo*, to breathe out	Breathing out.
expiration	[ĕks-pĭ-RĀ-shŭn] Latin *expiro*, to breathe out	Exhalation.
external nares	[ĕks-TĔR-năl NĀR-ēz]	*See* nostrils.
external respiration		Exchange of air between the body and the outside environment.
glottis	[GLŎT-ĭs]	Part of the larynx consisting of the vocal folds of mucous membrane and muscle.
Heimlich maneuver	[HĪM-lĭk]	Procedure to prevent choking to death. One person places his or her hands on the midsection of the choking person's abdomen and thrusts upward until the obstruction is dislodged.
hilum (also hilus)	[HĪ-lŭm (HĪ-lŭs)] Latin, small bit	Midsection of the lung where the nerves and vessels enter and exit.
hypopharynx	[HĪ-pō-FĂR-ĭnks] hypo-, below + pharynx	Laryngopharynx.
inferior lobe	[ĭn-FĒ-rē-ōr lŏb]	Bottom lobe of the lung.
inhalation	[ĭn-hă-LĀ-shŭn] Latin *inhalo*, to breathe in	Breathing in.
inspiration	[ĭn-spĭ-RĀ-shŭn] Latin *inspiro*, to breath in	Inhalation.
intercostal muscles	[ĭn-tĕr-KŎS-tăl MŬS-ĕlz] inter-, between + Latin *costa*, rib	Muscles between the ribs.

Term	Word Analysis	Definition
internal respiration		Exchange of oxygen and carbon dioxide between the cells.
laryngopharynx	[lă-RĬNG-gō-făr-ĭngks] laryngo-, larynx + pharynx	Part of the pharynx below and behind the larynx.
larynx	[LĂR-ĭngks] Greek, larynx	Organ of voice production in the respiratory tract, between the pharynx and the trachea; voice box.
lung	[lŭng] Old English lungen	One of two organs of respiration (left lung and right lung) in the thoracic cavity where oxygenation of blood takes place.
mediastinum	[MĒ-dē-ăs-TĪ-nŭm]	Median portion of the thoracic cavity; septum between two areas of an organ or cavity.
middle lobe		Middle section of the right lung.
nasal cavity		Opening in the external nose where air enters the body.
nasal septum	[NĀ-zăl SĔP-tŭm]	Cartilaginous division of the external nose.
nasopharynx	[NĀ-zō-FĂR-ĭngks] naso-, nose + pharynx	Portion of the throat above the soft palate.
nose	[nōz] Old English nosu	External structure supported by nasal bones and containing nasal cavity.
nostrils	[NŎS-trĭls]	External openings at the base of the nose; also called external nares.
oropharynx	[ŌR-ō-FĂR-ĭngks] oro-, mouth + pharynx	Back portion of the mouth, a division of the pharynx.
paranasal sinuses	[păr-ă-NĀ-săl SĪ-nŭs-ĕz] para-, beside + nasal	Area of the nasal cavity where external air is warmed by blood in the mucous membrane lining.
parietal pleura	[pă-RĪ-ĕ-tăl PLŪR-ă]	Outer layer of the pleura.
pharyngeal tonsils	[fă-RĬN-jē-ăl TŎN-sĭls]	Adenoids.
pharynx	[FĂR-ĭnks] Greek, pharynx	Passageway at back of mouth for air and food; throat.
pleura (pl. pleurae)	[PLŪR-ă (PLŪR-ē)] Greek, rib	Double layer of membrane making up the outside of the lungs.
pleural cavity	[PLŪR-ăl KĂV-ĭ-tē]	Space between the two pleura.

Term	Word Analysis	Definition
respiratory tract	[RĔS-pĭ-ră-tōr-ē, rĕ-SPĪR-ă-tōr-ē]	Passageways through which air moves into and out of the lungs.
septum	[SĔP-tŭm]	Cartilaginous division, as in the nose or mediastinum.
soft palate	[sŏft PĂL-ăt]	Flexible muscular sheet that separates the nasopharynx from the rest of the pharynx.
superior lobe		Topmost lobe of each lung.
thorax	[THŌ-răks] From Greek, breastplate	Chest cavity.
throat	[thrōt]	See pharynx.
thyroid cartilage		See Adam's apple.
trachea	[TRĀ-kē-ă]	Airway from the larynx into the bronchi; windpipe.
visceral pleura	[VĬS-ĕr-ăl PLŪR-ă]	Inner layer of the pleura.
vocal cords		Strips of epithelial tissue that vibrate and play a major role in the production of sound.
voice box		See larynx.
windpipe		See trachea.

C A S E   S T U D Y

Breathing Emergencies

The emergency department at Midvale Central Hospital often sees patients who complain of breathing problems. The physicians on duty are trained to listen to sounds with a stethoscope to determine the immediate needs of the patient. Many of the patients at Midvale are elderly. Respiratory problems are the number-one reason for seeking emergency help. Some of the patients have emphysema, asthma, COPD, or another respiratory ailment, while others have a cardiovascular problem that exhibits symptoms of respiratory problems.

 Critical Thinking

1. How might an elderly person's weakened muscles affect respiration?

2. Midvale is a retirement community in the South. About six times a year, the state department of environmental protection issues pollution or smog warnings, with suggestions that children, the elderly, and those with chronic illnesses stay indoors, preferably with air conditioning. Polluted air diminishes what gas necessary for respiration?

Structure and Function Exercises

Complete the Picture

3. Label the parts of the respiratory system on the following diagram.

   a._____   c._____

   b._____

Bronchioles

Pharynx

Larynx

c. _____

a. _____

Right and left bronchi

b. _____

Check Your Knowledge

Fill in the blanks.

4. Exchanging air between the body and the outside environment is called _____ _____.

5. Foreign bodies entering the respiratory tract are filtered through _____.

6. The nose is divided into two halves by the _____ _____.

7. Food is prevented from going into the larynx by the _____.

8. A simple technique that has saved many people from choking to death is the _____ _____.

9. At the end of each bronchiole is a small cluster of _____ _____ called _____.

10. The right lung has _____ lobes.

11. The left lung has _____ lobes.

12. A muscle that lowers itself to allow more space when one is breathing in is called a(n)_____.

13. The muscles between the ribs that also aid in breathing are called _____ muscles.

   Circle T for true or F for false.

14. The respiratory tract is the major area involved in internal respiration. T F

15. The throat is a passageway for both air and food. T F

16. The pharynx contains the vocal cords. T F

17. Each bronchi enters one lung. T F

18. The pleura are moist layers of membrane surrounding the lungs. T F

19. Humans must have both lungs to live. T F

20. Only the right lung has a middle lobe. T F

21. The hilum is the topmost portion of the lung. T F

22. The larynx is another name for the windpipe. T F

23. The soft palate is at the bottom of the mouth. T F

Spell It Correctly

Write the correct spelling in the blank to the right of any misspelled words. If the word is already correctly spelled, write C.

24. nasopharyngx _____

25. trachae _____

26. resperation _____

27. alveoli _____

28. diagphram _____

29. epiglottus _____

30. pharinx _____

31. mediastinum _____

32. tonsills _____

33. bronchis _____

Combining Forms and Abbreviations

The lists below include combining forms and abbreviations that relate specifically to the respiratory system. Pronunciations are provided for the examples.

Combining Form	Meaning	Example
adenoid(o)	adenoid, gland	*adenoidectomy* [ĂD-ĕ-nŏy-DĔK-tō-mē], operation for removal of adenoid growths
alveol(o)	alveolus	*alveolitis* [ĂL-vē-ō-LĪ-tĭs], inflammation of the alveoli
bronch(o), bronchi(o)	bronchus	*bronchitis* [brŏng-KĪ-tĭs], inflammation of the lining of the bronchial tubes

Combining Form	Meaning	Example
bronchiol(o)	bronchiole	*bronchiolitis* [brŏng-kē-ō-LĪ-tĭs], inflammation of the bronchioles
capn(o)	carbon dioxide	*capnogram* [KĂP-nō-grăm], a continuous recording of the carbon dioxide in expired air
epiglott(o)	epiglottis	*epiglottitis* [ĔP-ĭ-GLŎT-ĭ-tĭs], inflammation of the epiglottis
laryng(o)	larynx	*laryngoscope* [lă-RĬNG-gō-skōp], device used to examine the larynx through the mouth
lob(o)	lobe of the lung	*lobectomy* [lō-BĔK-tō-mē], removal of a lobe
mediastin(o)	mediastinum	*mediastinitis* [MĒ-dē-ăs-tĭ-NĪ-tĭs], inflammation of the tissue of the mediastinum
nas(o)	nose	*nasogastric* [nā-zō-GĂS-trĭk], of the nasal passages and the stomach
or(o)	mouth	*oropharynx* [ŌR-ō-FĂR-ĭngks], the part of the pharynx that lies behind the mouth
ox(o), oxi-, oxy	oxygen	*oximeter* [ŏk-SĬM-ĕ-tĕr], instrument for measuring oxygen saturation of blood
pharyng(o)	pharynx	*pharyngitis* [făr-ĭn-JĪ-tĭs], inflammation in the pharynx
phon(o)	voice, sound	*phonometer* [fō-NŎM-ĕ-tĕr], instrument for measuring sounds
phren(o)	diaphragm	*phrenitis* [frĕn-Ī-tĭs], inflammation in the diaphragm
pleur(o)	pleura	*pleuritis* [plū-RĪ-tĭs], inflammation of the pleura
pneum(o), pneumon(o)	air, lung	*pneumolith* [NŪ-mō-lĭth], calculus in the lungs
rhin(o)	nose	*rhinitis* [rī-NĪ-tĭs], inflammation of the nose
spir(o)	breathing	*spirometer* [spī-RŎM-ĕ-tĕr], instrument used to measure respiratory gases
steth(o)	chest	*stethoscope* [STĔTH-ō-skōp], instrument for listening to sounds in the chest
thorac(o)	thorax, chest	*thoracotomy* [thōr-ă-KŎT-ō-mē], incision into the chest wall

Combining Form	Meaning	Example
tonsill(o)	tonsils	*tonsillectomy* [TŎN-sĭ-LĔK-tō-mē], removal of one entire tonsil or of both tonsils
trache(o)	trachea	*tracheoscopy* [trā-kē-ŎS-kō-pē], inspection of the interior of the trachea

Abbreviation	Meaning
ABG	arterial blood gases
AFB	acid-fast bacillus (causes tuberculosis)
A&P	auscultation and percussion
AP	anteroposterior
ARD	acute respiratory disease
ARDS	adult respiratory distress syndrome
ARF	acute respiratory failure
BS	breath sounds
COLD	chronic obstructive lung disease
COPD	chronic obstructive pulmonary disease
CPR	cardiopulmonary resuscitation
CTA	clear to auscultation
CXR	chest x-ray
DOE	dyspnea on exertion
DPT	diphtheria, pertussis, tetanus (combined vaccination)
ENT	ear, nose, and throat
ET tube	endotracheal intubation tube
FEF	forced expiratory flow
FEV	forced expiratory volume
FVC	forced vital capacity
HBOT	hyperbaric oxygen therapy
IMV	intermittent mandatory ventilation
IPPB	intermittent positive pressure breathing
IRDS	infant respiratory distress syndrome
IRV	inspiratory reserve volume
LLL	left lower lobe [of the lungs]

Abbreviation	Meaning
LUL	left upper lobe [of the lungs]
MBC	maximal breathing capacity
MDI	metered dose inhaler
PA	posteroanterior
PCP	pneumocystis carinii pneumonia (a type of pneumonia to which AIDS patients are susceptible)
PEEP	positive end expiratory pressure
PFT	pulmonary function tests
PND	paroxysmal nocturnal dyspnea; postnasal drip
RD	respiratory disease
RDS	respiratory distress syndrome
RLL	right lower lobe [of the lungs]
RUL	right upper lobe [of the lungs]
SIDS	sudden infant death syndrome
SOB	shortness of breath
T&A	tonsillectomy and adenoidectomy
TB	tuberculosis
TLC	total lung capacity
TPR	temperature, pulse, and respiration
URI	upper respiratory infection
VC	vital capacity
V/Q scan	ventilation/perfusion scan

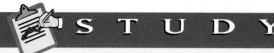

C A S E   S T U D Y

Coping with COPD

The emergency room nurse admitted Mr. DiGiorno, a patient from a nursing home. He was having difficulty breathing and complained of chest pains. The nurse checked his record and found that he has been positive for COPD for five years. This patient has had four hospital admissions in the last six months. He is overweight, smokes, and is sedentary. He takes medications for his COPD.

Critical Thinking

34. What is COPD? What lifestyle factors might play a role in Mr. DiGiorno's disease?

35. Mr. DiGiorno's chest pains may indicate cardiovascular disease. How might this affect internal respiration?

Combining Forms and Abbreviations Exercises

Build Your Medical Vocabulary

Complete the words by putting a combining form in the blank.

36. Removal of the adenoids: _____ectomy.

37. Surgical puncture of the thoracic cavity: _____centesis.

38. Ear, nose, and throat doctor:_____logist.

39. Inflammation of the tonsils: _____itis.

40. Inflammation of the pericardium and surrounding mediastinal tissue: _____pericarditis.

41. Suture of the lung: _____rrhaphy.

42. Relating to the nose and mouth: _____nasal.

43. Inflammation of the pharynx: _____itis.

44. Disease of the vocal cords affecting speech: _____pathy.

45. Record of carbon dioxide in expired air: _____gram.

46. Bronchial inflammation: _____itis.

47. Inflammation of tissue surrounding the bronchi: peri_____itis.

48. Relating to the pericardium and pleural cavity: pericardio_____.

49. Incision into a lobe: ____otomy.

50. Measurement of oxygen in blood: _____metry.

51. Compound of oxygen and a chloride: _____chloride.

52. Swelling in the bronchial area: _____edema.

53. Destruction of the alveolus: _____clasia.

54. Chest pain: _____algia.

55. Incision into the sinus: _____tomy.

Match the Root

Match the respiratory combining forms in the list on the right with the definitions in the list on the left.

56. pain arising in air sacs in the lungs   a. broncho

57. instrument to study vocal folds   b. capno

58. record of heart sounds   c. lob

59. nasal obstruction   d. alveol(o)

60. contraction of the bronchus   e. pharyngo

61. abnormally dilated windpipe   f. laryngo

62. repair of the pharynx   g. phono

63. fissure of the chest wall   h. thoraco

64. inflammation of a lobe   i. rhino

65. instrument for graphing carbon dioxide   j. tracheo

Diagnostic, Procedural, and Laboratory Terms

Disorders of the respiratory system can be diagnosed in several ways. First, a physician usually listens to the lungs with a stethoscope, a process called **auscultation.** Next, the respiratory rate is determined by counting the number of respirations per minute. One inhalation and one exhalation equal a single respiration. Adult respirations normally range from 15 to 20 per minute. The physician may use **percussion,** tapping over the lung area, to see if the lungs are clear (a hollow sound) or filled with fluid (a dull sound). Sputum can be observed for its color. Pus in sputum usually causes a greenish or yellowish color and indicates infection. Blood in the sputum may indicate tuberculosis.

Auscultation is from a Latin verb, *ausculto,* to listen to.

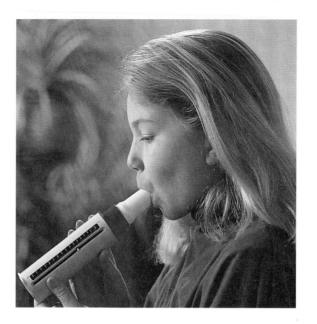

Figure 7-5 **A peak flow meter measures the capacity of breathing.**

Pulmonary function tests measure the mechanics of breathing. Breathing may be tested by a **peak flow meter** (Figure 7-5). Asthmatics often use this type of measuring device to check breathing capacity; they can then take medicine if an attack seems imminent. A **spirometer** is a pulmonary function testing machine that measures the lungs' volume and capacity (*spirometry*). This machine measures the *forced vital capacity (FVC)*, or highest breathing capacity, of the lungs when the patient takes the deepest breath possible. Other breathing measurements such as *forced expiratory volume (FEV)* show capacity at different parts of the respiration cycle.

Tuberculosis is a disease of the respiratory system. Tests for tuberculosis were discussed in Chapter 4, The Integumentary System, because reactions on the surface of the skin indicate a positive result for a tuberculosis test.

Visual images of the chest and parts of the respiratory system play an important role in diagnosing respiratory ailments. Chest x-rays, MRIs, and lung scans can detect abnormalities, such as masses and restricted blood flow within the lungs. A **bronchography** provides a radiological picture of the trachea and bronchi (Figure 7-6). A thoracic CT scan shows a cross-sectional view of the chest that can reveal tissue masses. A *pulmonary angiography* is an x-ray of the blood vessels of the lungs taken after dye is injected into a blood vessel. A *lung scan* or *V/Q perfusion scan* is a recording of radioactive material, injected or inhaled, to show air flow and blood supply in the lungs.

Parts of the respiratory system can also be observed by *endoscopy*, insertion of an **endoscope** (a viewing tube) into a body cavity. A **bronchoscope** is used for *bronchoscopy*, which is performed to examine airways or retrieve specimens, such as fluid retrieved in **bronchial alveolar lavage** or material for biopsy that is retrieved by **bronchial brushing** (a brush inserted through the bronchoscope). In **nasopharyngoscopy,** a flexible endoscope is used to examine nasal passages and the pharynx. **Laryngoscopy** is the procedure for examining the mouth and larynx, and **mediastinoscopy** for examining the mediastinum area and all the organs within it. Such diagnostic testing can reveal structural abnormalities, tumors, and irritations.

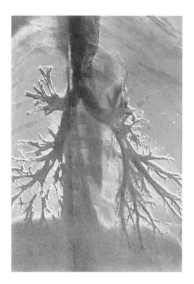

Figure 7-6 **Bronchography displays an image of the lung. The trachea is at the top and the bronchi are the network of tree-like structures inside the lungs.**

Laboratory Tests

Throat cultures are commonly used to diagnose streptococcal infections. A swab is passed over a portion of the throat, and the swab is then put in contact with a culture. If a strep infection is present, the culture will show certain bacteria. A **sputum sample** or **culture** may be taken and cultured to identify any disease-causing organisms. **Arterial blood gases** (ABGs) measure the levels of pressure of oxygen (O_2) and carbon dioxide (CO_2) in arterial

Throat cultures can be done quickly in the doctor's office. However, if it is suspected that the culture is not accurate, the bacteria are cultured overnight.

blood. These measurements help diagnose heart and lung functions. A **sweat test** measures the amount of salt in sweat and is used to confirm cystic fibrosis.

Vocabulary Review

In the previous section, you learned terms relating to diagnosis, clinical procedures, and laboratory tests. Before going on to the exercises, review the terms below and refer to the previous section if you have any questions.

Term	Word Analysis	Definition
arterial blood gases		Laboratory test that measures the levels of oxygen and carbon dioxide in arterial blood.
auscultation	[ăws-kŭl-TĀ-shŭn]	Listening to internal sounds with a stethoscope.
bronchial alveolar lavage		Retrieval of fluid for examination through a bronchoscope.
bronchial brushing		Retrieval of material for biopsy by insertion of a brush through a bronchoscope.
bronchography	[brŏng-KŎG-ră-fē] broncho-, bronchus + -graphy, a recording	Radiological picture of the trachea and bronchi.
bronchoscope	[BRŎNG-kō-skōp] broncho- + -scope, device for viewing	Device used to examine airways.
endoscope	[ĔN-dō-skōp] endo-, within + -scope	Tube used to view a body cavity.
laryngoscopy	[LĂR-ĭng-GŎS-kŏ-pē] laryngo-, larynx + -scopy, a viewing	Visual examination of the mouth and larynx using an endoscope.
mediastinoscopy	[MĒ-dē-ăs-tĭ-NŎS-kō-pē] mediastino-, mediastinum + -scopy	Visual examination of the mediastinum and all the organs within it using an endoscope.

Term	Word Analysis	Definition
nasopharyngoscopy	[NĀ-zō-fă-rǐng-GŎS-kō-pē] naso-, nose + pharyngo-, pharynx + -scopy	Examination of the nasal passages and the pharynx using an endoscope.
peak flow meter		Device for measuring breathing capacity.
percussion	[pěr-KŬSH-ŭn]	Tapping on the surface of the body to see if lungs are clear.
pulmonary function tests		Tests that measure the mechanics of breathing.
spirometer	[spī-RŎM-ě-těr] spiro-, breathing + -meter	Testing machine that measures the lungs' volume and capacity.
sputum culture	[SPŪ-tŭm]	Culture of material that is expectorated (or brought back up as mucus).
sweat test		Test for cystic fibrosis that measures the amount of salt in sweat.
throat culture		Test for streptococcal or other infections in which a swab taken on the surface of the throat is placed in a culture to see if certain bacteria grow.

C A S E S T U D Y

Laboratory Testing

Mr. DiGiorno was admitted to Midvale Hospital from the emergency room. His radiological/laboratory data read as follows:

A chest x-ray showed a pneumonic infiltrate in the left lower lobe with some parapneumonic effusion. Follow-up chest x-rays showed progression of infiltrate and then slight clearing. Serial ECGs showed the development of T-wave inversions anterolaterally compatible with ischemia or a pericardial process. The WBC was 10,000; HCT, 37; platelets, 425,000; PT and PTT were normal. DIG level was 1.4 at discharge. Blood gases showed a pH of 7.43, PCO_2 37, PO_2 71. Sputum culture could not be obtained.

 Critical Thinking

66. Why do you think blood gas tests were ordered for Mr. DiGiorno?

67. What part of his blood was measured at 10,000?

Midvale Hospital Emergency Room: 5/4/XX   **Physician on Duty:** Nina Shaefer, M.D.

Patient Name: Joseph DiGiorno   **Patient No.:** 023456

A chest x-ray showed a pneumonic infiltrate in the left lower lobe with some parapneumonic effusion. Follow-up chest x-rays showed progression of infiltrate and then slight clearing. Serial ECGs showed the development of T-wave inversions anterolaterally compatible with ischemia or a pericardial process. The WBC was 10,000; HCT, 37; platelets, 425,000; PT, PTT were normal. DIG level was 1.4 at discharge. Blood gases showed a pH of 7.43. PCO_2 37, PO_2 71. Sputum culture could not be obtained.

Diagnostic, Procedural, and Laboratory Terms Exercises

Check Your Knowledge

Fill in the blanks.

68. The mechanics of breathing are measured by _____ _____ tests.

69. A test that can confirm the presence of cystic fibrosis is called a(n) _____ _____.

70. A tube for viewing a body cavity is called a(n) _____.

71. The highest breathing capacity is called the _____ _____ capacity.

72. A stethoscope is necessary for _____, listening to the lungs.

73. Streptococcal infections can be detected in a _____ _____.

74. Tapping the skin over the lung area to check whether the lungs are clear is called _____.

75. Asthmatics often use a _____ _____ _____ to check breathing capacity.

76. Disease-causing organisms in sputum can be identified in a(n) _____ _____.

77. A device that measures the lung volume and capacity is called a(n) _____.

Root Out the Meaning

Add the appropriate combining form from the list in this chapter.

78. _____scopy means viewing of the pharynx.

79. _____gram means measure of carbon dioxide in expired air

80. _____ectomy means removal of the larynx.

81. _____itis mean inflammation of a lobe.

82. _____plegia means paralysis of the larynx.

Pathological Terms

The respiratory system is the site for many inflammations, disorders, and infections. This system must contend with foreign material coming into the body from outside, as well as internal problems that may affect any of its parts. Each of its parts may become inflamed.

adenoiditis: inflammation of the adenoids

bronchitis: inflammation of the bronchi, sometimes leading to **chronic bronchitis,** bronchitis that recurs chronically. Bronchitis includes increases in secretions from the mucous membranes of the bronchi, which obstructs breathing. Allergies, dust, infections, and pollution can cause bronchitis.

epiglottitis: inflammation of the epiglottis

laryngitis: inflammation of the larynx

laryngotracheobronchitis: inflammation of the larynx, trachea, and bronchi

nasopharyngitis: inflammation of the nose and pharynx

pansinusitis: inflammation of all sinuses

pharyngitis: inflammation of the pharynx

pleuritis or **pleurisy:** inflammation of the pleura

pneumonitis: inflammation of the lung

rhinitis: inflammation of the nose

sinusitis: inflammation of the sinuses

tonsillitis: inflammation of the tonsils

tracheitis: inflammation of the trachea

Normal breathing (**eupnea**) may become affected by diseases or conditions and change to **bradypnea,** slow breathing; **tachypnea,** fast breathing; **hypopnea,** shallow breathing; **hyperpnea,** abnormally deep breathing; **dyspnea,** difficult breathing; **apnea,** inability to breathe; or **orthopnea,** difficulty in breathing, especially while lying down. Physicians determine the degree of orthopnea by the number of pillows required to allow the patient to breathe easily (i.e., two-pillow orthopnea).

Other irregular breathing patterns may indicate various conditions. **Cheyne-Stokes respiration,** for example, is an irregular breathing pattern with a period of apnea followed by deep, labored breathing that becomes shallow, then apneic. Irregular sounds usually indicate specific disorders—**crackles** or **rales** are popping sounds heard in lung collapse and other conditions, such as congestive heart failure and pneumonia. **Wheezes** or **rhonchi** occur during attacks of asthma or emphysema; **stridor** is a high-pitched crowing sound; and **dysphonia** is hoarseness, often associated with laryngitis. **Singultus** or hiccuping can become uncomfortable if not stopped. **Hyperventilation,** excessive breathing in and out, may be caused by anxiety or overexertion. **Hypoventilation,** abnormally low movement of air in and out of the lungs, may cause excessive buildup of carbon dioxide in the lungs, or **hypercapnia. Hypoxemia** is a deficient amount of oxygen in the blood, and **hypoxia** is a deficient amount of oxygen in tissue.

Upper respiratory infection is a term that covers an infection of some or all of the upper respiratory tract. Other disorders of the upper respiratory tract include **croup,** acute respiratory syndrome in children and infants, and **diphtheria,** acute infection of the throat and upper respiratory tract caused by Corynebacterium diphtheriae bacteria. **Nosebleed** or **epistaxis** results from a trauma to, or a spontaneous rupture of, blood vessels in the nose; **rhinorrhea** is nasal discharge usually caused by an inflammation or infection; and **whoop-**

Cheyne-Stokes respiration is named after John Cheyne (1777–1836), a Scottish physician, and William Stokes (1804–1878), an Irish physician.

ing cough or **pertussis** is a severe infection of the pharynx, larynx, and trachea caused by the Bordetella pertussis bacteria. Diphtheria and pertussis have virtually disappeared in the United States since the regular administration of DPT (diphtheria, pertussis, tetanus) vaccines to most infants.

Chronic obstructive pulmonary disease (COPD) is a term for any disease with chronic obstruction of the bronchial tubes and lungs. Chronic bronchitis and emphysema are two COPD disease processes. In addition to bronchitis, the bronchial tubes can be the site of **asthma,** a condition of bronchial airway obstruction causing **paroxysmal** dyspnea, a sudden breathing difficulty accompanied by wheezing and coughing (Figure 7-7). An asthma attack may be caused by allergy, infection, or anxiety. **Hemoptysis** is a lung or bronchial hemorrhage that results in the spitting of blood. **Cystic fibrosis,** chronic airway obstruction caused by disease of the exocrine glands, also affects the bronchial tubes. The predominant characteristic of cystic fibrosis is the secretion of abnormally thick mucus in various places in the body, causing chronic bronchitis, emphysema, and recurrent pneumonia, along with other ailments. Carcinomas, frequently caused by smoking, can also be found in the respiratory system.

Some disorders in newborns, such as *hyaline membrane disease* or *respiratory distress syndrome*, occur most frequently in premature babies and are often the result of underdeveloped lungs. *Adult respiratory distress syndrome (ARDS)* may have a number of causes, especially injury to the lung. Lung disorders may occur in the alveoli; for example, **atelectasis,** a collapsed lung or part of a lung; **emphysema,** hyperinflation of the air sacs often caused by smoking; and **pneumonia,** acute infection of the alveoli. Pneumonia is a term for a number of infections. Such infections typically affect bedridden and frail people whose internal respiration is compromised. Table 7-1 details several types of pneumonia. **Tuberculosis** is a highly infectious disease caused by bacteria called **bacilli,** which invade the lungs and cause small swellings and inflammation. Many forms of tuberculosis have become drug resistant. A **pulmonary abscess** is a large collection of pus in the lungs, and **pulmonary edema** is a buildup of fluid in the air sacs and bronchioles, usually caused by failure of the heart to pump enough blood to and from the lungs. A **pulmonary embolism** is a clot in the lungs.

Several environmental agents cause **pneumoconiosis,** a lung condition caused by dust in the lungs. **Black lung** or **anthracosis** (Figure 7-8) is caused

Normal bronchiole

Asthmatic bronchiole, showing constriction

Figure 7-7 Asthma causes a narrowing of the bronchi. This airway obstruction can cause sudden breathing difficulty.

For approximately the latter half of the twentieth century, tuberculosis was kept under control using various medications. Previously, tuberculosis was known as *consumption*, a disease that was often fatal. In the 1990s, tuberculosis began to spread again because of new drug-resistant strains and because of the close contact of some infected people with others, particularly in the inner city.

The part *anthraco* in anthracosis means coal.

Table 7-1 Some Types of Pneumonia

Type of Pneumonia	Location	Cause
bacterial pneumonia	lungs	usually streptococcus bacteria
bronchial pneumonia, bronchopneumonia	walls of the smaller bronchial tubes	may be postoperative or from tuberculosis
chronic pneumonia	lungs	any recurrent inflammation or infection
double pneumonia	both lungs at the same time	bacterial infection
Pneumocystis carinii pneumonia	lungs	usually seen in AIDS patients
viral pneumonia	lungs	caused by viral infection

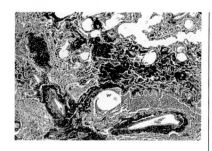

Figure 7-8 The black material in the lung consists of coal particles and dust that were inhaled over many years. Anthracosis is a potentially fatal disease.

by coal dust and is, therefore, a threat to coal miners; **asbestosis** is caused by asbestos particles released during construction of ships and buildings; **silicosis** is caused by the silica dust from grinding rocks or glass, and other manufacturing materials, such as pipe, building, and roofing products.

Disorders of the pleura, other than pleuritis, include **pneumothorax,** an accumulation of air or gas in the pleural cavity; **empyema,** pus in the pleural cavity; **hemothorax,** blood in the pleural cavity; **pleural effusion,** an escape of fluid into the pleural cavity; and, rarely, **mesothelioma,** a cancer associated with asbestosis.

The respiratory system may be disturbed by spasms that cause coughing or constriction. When severe, these spasms can be life-threatening. **Bronchospasms** occur in the bronchi, and **laryngospasms** occur in the larynx.

Vocabulary Review

In the previous section, you learned terms relating to pathology. Before going on to the exercises, review the terms below and refer to the previous section if you have questions.

Term	Word Analysis	Definition
adenoiditis	[ĂD-ĕ-nŏy-DĪ-tĭs] adenoid-, adenoids + -itis, inflammation	Inflammation of the adenoids.
anthracosis	[ăn-thră-KŌ-sĭs] anthrac-, coal + -osis, condition	Lung disease caused by long-term inhalation of coal dust; black lung disease.
apnea	[ĂP-nē-ă] Greek *apnoia,* want of breath	Cessation of breathing.
asbestosis	[ăs-bĕs-TŌ-sĭs] asbest(os) + -osis	Lung disorder caused by long-term inhalation of asbestos (as in construction work).
asthma	[ĂZ-mă] Greek, difficult breathing	Chronic condition with obstruction or narrowing of the bronchial airways.
atelectasis	[ăt-ĕ-LĔK-tă-sĕs]	Collapse of a lung or part of a lung.
bacilli	[bă-SĬL-ī]	A type of bacteria.
black lung		*See* anthracosis.
bradypnea	[brăd-ĭp-NĒ-ă] brady-, slow + -pnea, breathing	Abnormally slow breathing.
bronchitis	[brŏng-KĪ-tĭs] bronch-, bronchus + -itis	Inflammation of the bronchi.

Term	Word Analysis	Definition
bronchospasm	[BRŎNG-kō-spăzm] broncho-, bronchus + -spasm, contraction	Sudden contraction in the bronchi that causes coughing.
Cheyne-Stokes respiration	[chān stōks rĕs-pĭ-RĀ-shŭn]	Irregular breathing pattern with a period of apnea followed by deep, labored breathing that becomes shallow, then apneic.
chronic bronchitis		Recurring or long-lasting bouts of bronchitis.
chronic obstructive pulmonary disease		Disease of the bronchial tubes or lungs with chronic obstruction.
crackles	[KRĂK-ls]	Popping sounds heard in lung collapse or other conditions; rales.
croup	[krūp]	Acute respiratory syndrome in children or infants accompanied by seal-like coughing.
cystic fibrosis	[SĬS-tĭk fĭ-BRŌ-sĭs]	Disease that causes chronic airway obstruction and also affects the bronchial tubes.
diphtheria	[dĭf-THĒR-ē-ă] Greek diphthera, leather	Acute infection of the throat and upper respiratory tract caused by bacteria.
dysphonia	[dĭs-FŌ-nē-ă] dys-, abnormal + Greek phone, voice	Hoarseness usually caused by laryngitis.
dyspnea	[dĭsp-NĒ-ă] Greek dyspnoia, bad breathing	Difficult breathing.
emphysema	[ĕm-fĭ-SĒ-mă] Greek, inflation of the stomach	Chronic condition of hyperinflation of the air sacs; often caused by prolonged smoking.
empyema	[ĕm-pī-Ē-mă] Greek, formation of pus	Pus in the pleural cavity.
epiglottitis	[ĕp-ĭ-glŏt-Ī-tĭs] epiglott(is) + -itis	Inflammation of the epiglottis.
epistaxis	[ĔP-ĭ-STĂK-sĭs] Greek, nosebleed	Bleeding from the nose, usually caused by trauma or a sudden rupture of the blood vessels of the nose.
eupnea	[yūp-NĒ-ă] Greek eupnoia, good breath	Normal breathing.

Term	Word Analysis	Definition
hemoptysis	[hē-MŎP-tĭ-sĭs] hemo-, blood + Greek *ptysis*, spitting	Lung or bronchial hemorrhage resulting in the spitting of blood.
hemothorax	[hē-mō-THŌR-ĭks] hemo- + thorax	Blood in the pleural cavity.
hypercapnia	[hī-pĕr-KĂP-nē-ă] hyper-, excessive + Greek *kapnos*, smoke	Excessive buildup of carbon dioxide in lungs, usually associated with hypoventilation.
hyperpnea	[hī-pĕrp-NĒ-ă] hyper- + -pnea, breathing	Abnormally deep breathing.
hyperventilation	[HĪ-pĕr-vĕn-tĭ-LĀ-shŭn] hyper- + ventilation	Abnormally fast breathing in and out, often associated with anxiety.
hypopnea	[hī-PŎP-nē-ă] hypo-, below normal + -pnea	Shallow breathing.
hypoventilation	[HĪ-pō-vĕn-tĭ-LĀ-shŭn] hypo- + ventilation	Abnormally low movement of air in and out of the lungs.
hypoxemia	[hī-pŏk-SĒ-mē-ă] hyp-, below normal + ox(ygen) + -emia, blood	Deficient amount of oxygen in the blood.
hypoxia	[hī-PŎK-sē-ă] hyp- + ox(ygen) + -ia, condition	Deficient amount of oxygen in tissue.
laryngitis	[lăr-ĭn-JĪ-tĭs] laryng-, larynx + -itis	Inflammation of the larynx.
laryngospasm	[lă-RĬNG-gō-spăsm] laryngo-, larynx + -spasm	Sudden contraction of the larynx, which may cause coughing and may restrict breathing.
laryngotracheobronchitis	[lă-RĬNG-gō-TRĀ-kē-ō-brŏng-KĪ-tĭs] laryngo- + tracheo-, trachea + bronch- + -itis	Inflammation of the larynx, trachea, and bronchi.
mesothelioma	[MĔZ-ō-thē-lē-Ō-mă] mesotheli(um), layer of cells as in the pleura + -oma, tumor	Rare cancer of the lungs associated with asbestosis.

Term	Word Analysis	Definition
nasopharyngitis	[NĀ-zō-fă-rĭn-JĪ-tĭs] naso- + pharyng-, pharynx + -itis	Inflammation of the nose and pharynx.
nosebleed		*See* epistaxis.
orthopnea	[ōr-thŏp-NĒ-ă, ōr-THŎP-nē-ă] ortho-, straight + -pnea	Difficulty in breathing, especially while lying down.
pansinusitis	[păn-sī-nŭ-SĪ-tĭs] pan-, all + sinusitis	Inflammation of all the sinuses.
paroxysmal	[păr-ŏk-SĬZ-măl] Greek *paroxysmos*, spasm	Sudden, as a spasm or convulsion.
pertussis	[pĕr-TŬS-ĭs] Latin *per*, intensive + *tussis*, cough	Severe infection of the pharynx, larynx, and trachea caused by bacteria; whooping cough.
pharyngitis	[făr-ĭn-JĪ-tĭs] pharyng- + -itis	Inflammation of the pharynx.
pleural effusion	[PLŪR-ăl ĕ-FYŪ-zhŭn]	Escape of fluid into the pleural cavity.
pleuritis, pleurisy	[plū-RĪ-tĭs, PLŪR-ĭ-sē] pleur-, pleura + -itis	Inflammation of the pleura.
pneumoconiosis	[NŪ-mō-kō-nē-Ō-sĭs] pneumo-, lung + Greek *konis*, dust + -osis	Lung condition caused by inhaling dust.
pneumonia	[nū-MŌ-nē-ă] Greek, lung condition	Acute infection of the alveoli.
pneumonitis	[nū-mō-NĪ-tĭs] pneumon-, lung + -itis	Inflammation of the lung.
pneumothorax	[nū-mō-THŌR-ăks] pneumo- + thorax	Accumulation of air or gas in the pleural cavity.
pulmonary abscess	[PŬL-mō-nār-ē ĂB-sĕs]	Large collection of pus in the lungs.
pulmonary edema	[PŬL-mō-nār-ē ĕ-DĒ-mă]	Fluid in the air sacs and bronchioles usually caused by failure of the heart to pump enough blood to and from lungs.
pulmonary embolism	[PŬL-mō-nār-ē ĔM-bō-lĭzm]	Clot in the lungs.

Term	Word Analysis	Definition
rales	[răhlz]	*See* crackles.
rhinitis	[rĭ-NĪ-tĭs] rhin-, nose + -itis	Nasal inflammation.
rhinorrhea	[rĭn-nō-RĒ-ă] rhino-, nose + -rrhea, discharge	Nasal discharge.
rhonchi	[RŎNG-kī]	*See* wheezes.
silicosis	[sĭl-ĭ-KŌ-sĭs]	Lung condition caused by silica dust from grinding rocks or glass or other materials used in manufacturing.
singultus	[sĭng-GŬL-tŭs]	Hiccuping.
sinusitis	[sī-nŭ-SĪ-tĭs] sinus + -itis	Inflammation of the sinuses.
stridor	[STRĪ-dōr]	High-pitched crowing sound heard in certain respiratory conditions.
tachypnea	[tăk-ĭp-NĒ-ă] tachy-, fast + -pnea	Abnormally fast breathing.
tonsillitis	[TŎN-sĭ-LĪ-tĭs] tonsill-, tonsils + -itis	Inflammation of the tonsils.
tracheitis	[trā-kē-Ī-tĭs] trache-, trachea + -itis	Inflammation of the trachea.
tuberculosis	[tū-bĕr-kyū-LŌ-sĭs] Latin *tuberculum*, small nodule + -osis	Acute infectious disease caused by bacteria called bacilli.
upper respiratory infection		Infection of all or part of upper portion of respiratory tract.
wheezes	[hwēz-ĕz]	Whistling sounds heard on inspiration in certain breathing disorders, especially asthma.
whooping cough	[HŎOP-ĭng kăwf]	*See* pertussis.

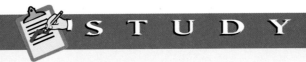

CASE STUDY

X-rays for Pneumonia

Many of the elderly patients admitted to the hospital through the emergency room are suffering from pneumonia. Their chest x-rays will show evidence of the disease. Usually, after a course of antibiotics, the patients are x-rayed again. If the x-rays are not clear a second time, some other underlying problem, such as an abnormal growth or latent disease, may be suspected. Elderly patients, particularly those who are bedridden, are particularly susceptible to pneumonia.

Critical Thinking

83. Why is a bedridden person more susceptible to pneu-monia than a patient who is ambulatory?

84. Patients with any kind of respiratory infection often have breathing problems when lying down, even for weeks after the infection has begun to subside. Why can lying down cause breathing problems?

Pathological Terms Exercises

Match the Condition

Match the words in the column on the left with the definition in the column on the right.

85. pleurisy, pleuritis

86. epistaxis

87. dysphonia

88. hypoxemia

89. hypercapnia

90. anthracosis

91. pleural effusion

92. pertussis

93. tachypnea

94. apnea

a. whooping cough

b. deficient oxygen in blood

c. black lung

d. pleural inflammation

e. hoarseness

f. inability to breathe

g. nosebleed

h. fast breathing

i. too much carbon dioxide

j. fluid in the pleural cavity

Check Your Knowledge

Circle T for true or F for false.

95. Foreign material comes into the body during internal respiration. T F

96. Dysphonia is associated with laryngitis. T F

97. Diphtheria, pertussis, and tuberculosis are all caused by bacteria. T F

98. A pleural effusion is a type of cancer. T F

99. Respiratory spasms may cause uncontrollable coughing. T F

100. A pulmonary edema is a clot in the lungs. T F

101. Tuberculosis cannot be passed from one person to another. T F

102. Atelectasis is another name for a nosebleed . T F

103. Inflammation of the voice box is called laryngitis. T F

104. Hypopnea is abnormally deep breathing. T F

Fill in the blanks

105. Inflammation of the throat is called _____.

106. Any lung condition caused by dust is called _____.

107. Chronic bronchial airway obstruction is a symptom of _____.

108. The sounds heard in atelectasis are _____ or _____.

109. Many respiratory conditions are caused or made worse by _____, an addictive habit.

Surgical Terms

When breathing is disrupted or chronic infections of the respiratory tract occur, surgical procedures can provide relief. Ear, nose, and throat (ENT) doctors or **otorhinolaryngologists** specialize in disorders of the upper respiratory tract. Sometimes it is necessary to remove parts of the respiratory system, either to relieve constant infections or to remove abnormal growths. A **tonsillectomy** is excision of the tonsils (often to stop recurrent tonsillitis). An **adenoidectomy** is removal of the adenoids; a **laryngectomy** removes the larynx (usually to stop cancerous growth); a **pneumonectomy** is the excision of a lung; and a **lobectomy** is the excision of a lobe of a lung (as when cancer is present).

Surgical repair can relieve respiratory problems caused by trauma, abnormalities, growths, or infections. A **bronchoplasty** is the repair of a bronchus;

laryngoplasty is the repair of the larynx; **rhinoplasty** is surgical repair of the nose; **septoplasty** is surgical repair of the nasal septum; and **tracheoplasty** is the repair of the trachea.

Incisions into parts of the respiratory system are sometimes necessary. **Thoracic surgeons** are the specialists who usually perform such procedures. A **laryngotracheotomy** is an incision of the larynx and trachea; **pneumobronchotomy** is an incision of the lung and bronchus; **septostomy** is an incision of the nasal septum; **sinusotomy** is an incision of a sinus; **thoracotomy** is an incision into the chest cavity; **thoracostomy** is establishment of an opening in the chest cavity to drain fluid; and **tracheotomy** is incision into the trachea, usually to provide an airway (Figure 7-9). Surgical punctures provide a means to aspirate or remove fluid. **Laryngocentesis** is a surgical puncture of the larynx; **pleurocentesis** is a surgical puncture of pleural space; and **thoracocentesis** is surgical puncture of the chest cavity.

Artificial openings into the respiratory tract may allow for alternative airways as in a **tracheostomy** (artificial tracheal opening) or a **laryngostomy** (artificial laryngeal opening). An **endotracheal intubation** is the insertion of a tube through the nose or mouth, pharynx, and larynx and into the trachea to establish an airway. A **pleuropexy** is performed to fix the pleura in place surgically, usually in case of injury or deterioration.

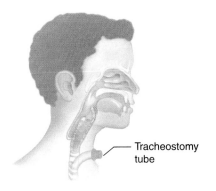

Tracheostomy tube

Figure 7-9 A tracheotomy provides an emergency airway.

Vocabulary Review

In the previous section, you learned terms relating to surgery. Before going on to the exercises, review the terms below and refer to the previous section if you have questions.

Term	Word Analysis	Definition
adenoidectomy	[ĂD-ĕ-nŏy-DĚK-tō-mē] adenoid-, adenoids + -ectomy, removal	Removal of the adenoids.
bronchoplasty	[BRŎNG-kō-plăs-tē] broncho-, bronchus + -plasty, repair	Surgical repair of a bronchus.
endotracheal intubation (ET)	[ĔN-dō-TRĀ-kē-ăl in-tū-BĀ-shŭn] endo-within + trache-, trachea +-al, pertaining to	Insertion of a tube through the nose or mouth, pharynx, and larynx and into the trachea to establish an airway.
laryngectomy	[LĂR-in-JĔK-tō-mē] laryng-, larynx + -ectomy	Removal of the larynx.
laryngocentesis	[lă-RĬNG-gō-sĕn-TĒ-sĭs] laryngo-, larynx + -centesis, puncture	Surgical puncture of the larynx.
laryngoplasty	[lă-RĬNG-gō-plăs-tē] laryngo- + -plasty	Repair of the larynx.

Term	Word Analysis	Definition
laryngostomy	[LĂR-ĭng-GŎS-tō-mē] laryngo- + -stomy, mouth	Creation of an artificial opening in the larynx.
laryngotracheotomy	[lă-RĬNG-gō-trā-kē-ŎT-ō-mē] laryngo- + tracheo-, trachea + -tomy, cutting	Incision into the larynx and trachea.
lobectomy	[lō-BĔK-tō-mē] lob-, lobe + -ectomy	Removal of one of the lobes of a lung.
otorhinolaryngologist	[ō-tō-RĪ-nō-lăr-ĭng-GŎL-ō-jĭst] oto-, ear + rhino-, nose + laryngo- + -logist, specialist	Medical doctor who diagnoses and treats disorders of the ear, nose, and throat.
pleurocentesis	[PLŪR-ō-sĕn-TĒ-sĭs] pleuro-, pleura + -centesis	Surgical puncture of pleural space.
pleuropexy	[PLŪR-ō-PĔK-sē] pleuro- + -pexy, a fixing	Fixing in place of the pleura surgically, usually in case of injury or deterioration.
pneumobronchotomy	[NŪ-mō-brŏng-KŎT-ō-mē] pneumo-, lung + broncho- + -tomy	Incision of the lung and bronchus.
pneumonectomy	[NŪ-mō-NĔK-tō-mē] pneumon-, lung + -ectomy	Removal of a lung.
rhinoplasty	[RĪ-nō-plăs-tē] rhino-, nose + -plasty	Surgical repair of the nose.
septoplasty	[SĔP-tō-plăs-tē] sept(um) + -plasty	Surgical repair of the nasal septum.
septostomy	[sĕp-TŎS-tō-mē] sept(um) + -stomy	Incision of the nasal septum.
sinusotomy	[sĭn-ū-SŎT-ō-mē] sinus + -tomy	Incision of a sinus.
thoracic surgeon	[thō-RĂS-ĭk]	Surgeon who specializes in surgery of the thorax.

Term	Word Analysis	Definition
thoracocentesis	[THŌR-ă-kō-sĕn-TĒ-sĭs] thoraco-, thorax + -centesis	Surgical puncture of the chest cavity.
thoracostomy	[thōr-ă-KŎS-tō-mē] thoraco- + -stomy	Establishment of an opening in the chest cavity.
thoracotomy	[thōr-ă-KŎT-ō-mē] thoraco- + -tomy	Incision into the chest cavity.
tonsillectomy	[TŎN-sĭ-LĔK-tō-mē] tonsill-, tonsils + -ectomy	Removal of the tonsils.
tracheoplasty	[TRĀ-kē-ō-PLĂS-tē] tracheo-, trachea + -plasty	Repair of the trachea.
tracheostomy	[TRĀ-kē-ŎS-tō-mē] tracheo- + -stomy	Creation of an artificial opening in the trachea.
tracheotomy	[trā-kē-ŎT-ō-mē] tracheo- + -tomy	Incision into the trachea.

C A S E S T U D Y

Asthma Emergencies

Emergency rooms are also visited frequently by people with asthma. A severe asthmatic attack requires medication and close monitoring or it can be fatal. Once the patient is stabilized, various tests may be necessary to determine the pathology in the lungs.

June Lytel is a 10-year-old who has asthma. Recently she has had tonsillitis. Four months ago, another case of tonsillitis caused inflammation of her upper respiratory tract. She had two emergency room visits for asthma attacks during the URI. Her physician, an ENT, is also a surgeon.

 Critical Thinking

110. Why is it important that her doctor is a surgeon?

111. How might surgery help avoid future URIs?

Surgical Terms Exercises

Check Your Knowledge

Match the terms in the left column with the definitions in the right column.

112. rhinoplasty   a. artificial laryngeal opening

113. pleuropexy   b. removal of a lobe of the lung

114. adenoidectomy   c. puncture of the pleura

115. tracheostomy   d. incision into the septum

116. tracheotomy   e. incision into the trachea

117. laryngectomy   f. removal of the adenoids

118. lobectomy   g. repair of the nose

119. laryngostomy   h. attaching of the pleura

120. pleurocentesis   i. removal of the larynx

121. septostomy   j. artificial tracheal opening

Fill in the blanks.

122. An incision into the chest cavity is a _____.

123. An airway can be provided by an emergency _____.

124. Cancer of the lung may require a _____.

125. Surgical fixing of the pleura in place is called _____.

126. The nasal septum is repaired during _____.

Pharmacological Terms

Antibiotics, antihistamines, and anticoagulants are used for respiratory system disorders just as with other system disorders. Specific to respiratory problems are **bronchodilators** (Figure 7-10), drugs that dilate the walls of the bronchi (as during an asthmatic attack), and **expectorants,** drugs that promote coughing and the expulsion of mucus. Table 7-2 lists some medications commonly prescribed for respiratory disorders.

Two mechanical devices aid in respiration. Mechanical **ventilators** actually serve as a breathing substitute for patients who cannot breathe on their own. **Nebulizers** deliver medication through the nose or mouth to ease breathing problems. Some nebulizers are MDI (metered dose inhalers) that deliver a specific amount of spray with each puff of the inhaler.

Recently, new medications have become available to control asthma attacks. Traditionally, asthmatics used ventilators or nebulizers to control the occurrence or intensity of attacks. Now it is possible to take medication in pill form to avoid most attacks.

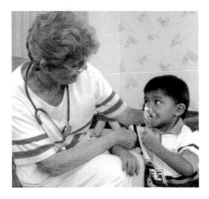

Figure 7-10 **Bronchodilators provide a fine spray to loosen restricted bronchi. These medications are usually delivered via an inhaler or a nebulizer.**

Table 7-2 Some Common Agents Used to Treat the Respiratory System

Drug Class	Purpose	Generic	Trade Name
antitussives	to relieve coughing	codeine dextromethorphan diphenhydramine	none except in combination Benylin, Pertussin, Robitussin, and others Allermax, Benadryl, and many others
bronchodilators	to dilate the walls of the bronchi and prevent spasms	albuterol ephedrine epinephrine terbutaline	Ventolin, Proventil Bronkaid caplets Bronkaid, Primatene Mist Brethaire, Brethine
decongestants	to lower and prevent mucus buildup	pseudoephedrine phenylpropanolamine	Drixoral, Sudafed, and others Contac
expectorants	to promote coughing and expelling of mucus	guaifenesin	Humbid, Deconsal, Mytussin, Robitussin

Vocabulary Review

In the previous section, you learned terms relating to pharmacology. Before going on to the exercises, review the terms below and refer to the previous section if you have any questions.

Term	Word Analysis	Definition
antitussives	[ăn-tē-TŬS-sĭvs] anti-, against + Latin *tussis*, cough	Agents that control coughing.
bronchodilators	[brŏng-kō-dĭ-LĀ-těrs] broncho- + dilator, agent that dilates	Agents that dilate the walls of the bronchi.

Term	Word Analysis	Definition
expectorants	[ĕk-SPĔK-tō-rănts] ex-, out of + Latin *pectus*, chest	Agents that promote the coughing and expelling of mucus.
nebulizer	[NĔB-yū-līz-ĕr]	Device that delivers medication through the nose or mouth in a fine spray to the respiratory tract.
ventilator	[VĔN-tĭ-lā-tōr]	Mechanical breathing device.

C A S E S T U D Y

Mechanical Breathing Apparatus

Missy Ruiz, a 24-year-old mother of two, was admitted to Midvale's trauma center after a serious car accident. Missy could not breathe on her own. A tracheotomy was performed so that Missy could be connected to a ventilator. Brain scans showed little activity, and doctors gave her only a slight chance for recovery. With intravenous feeding and the ventilator, Missy could survive in a vegetative state for a long time.

Critical Thinking

127. Missy cannot breathe unassisted. What organ directs the breathing process? Why is Missy's breathing process interrupted?

128. Missy is bedridden. What respiratory disease might she contract?

Pharmacological Terms Exercises

Check Your Knowledge

Fill in the blanks.

129. Coughing can be controlled with _____.

130. Insufficiently dilated bronchi can be treated with _____.

131. Productive coughing is helped with _____.

132. Medication is delivered in a fine spray by means of a _____.

133. A person who cannot breathe on his or her own may be kept alive on a _____.

The following chest x-ray report is from a patient who received x-rays during an emergency room visit.

CHEST: 11/6/XXXX

PA and lateral views of the chest show evidence of patchy alveolar density in the right mid-lung field, inferior to minor fissure on PA view. It appears to be located in the lateral segment of the right middle lobe, which may represent infiltrate. However, the possibility of a pulmonary neoplasm cannot be excluded. Suggest follow-up chest x-ray after 1 to 2 weeks to confirm its resolution. Remainder of right and left lung are free of any acute pathology. The cardiovascular silhouette shows normal heart size with normal pulmonary vasculature. Both hemidiaphragms

Challenge Section Exercises

Critical Thinking

134. This patient currently has a high fever and chest tightness. He will be treated for infection. What else did the radiologist suggest as a possible cause of his pulmonary problems?

135. Why do you think a follow-up chest x-ray is necessary?

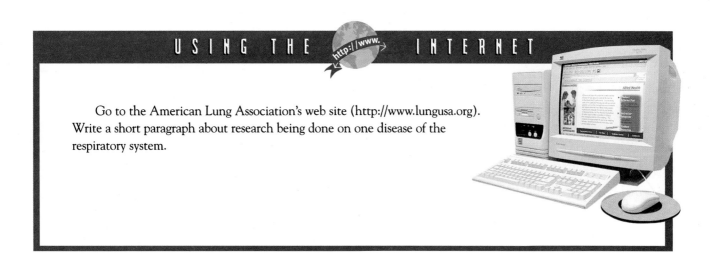

USING THE INTERNET

Go to the American Lung Association's web site (http://www.lungusa.org). Write a short paragraph about research being done on one disease of the respiratory system.

CHAPTER REVIEW

Definitions

Define the following terms and combining forms. Review the chapter before starting. Make sure you know how to pronounce each term as you define it.

Word	Definition
Adam's apple	
adenoid(o)	
adenoidectomy [ĂD-ĕ-nŏy-DĔK-tō-mē]	
adenoiditis [ĂD-ĕ-nŏy-DĪ-tĭs]	
adenoids [ĂD-ĕ-nŏydz]	
alveol(o)	
alveolus (pl. alveoli) [ăl-VĒ-ō-lŭs (ăl-VĒ-ō-lī)]	
anthracosis [ăn-thră-KŌ-sĭs]	
antitussives [ăn-tē-TŬS-sĭvs]	
apex [Ā-pĕks]	
apnea [ĂP-nē-ă]	
arterial blood gases	
asbestosis [ăs-bĕs-TŌ-sĭs]	
asthma [ĂZ-mă]	
atelectasis [ăt-ĕ-LĔK-tă-sĭs]	
auscultation [ăws-kŭl-TĀ-shŭn]	
bacilli [bă-SĬL-ī]	
base [băs]	
black lung	
bradypnea [brăd-ĭp-NĒ-ă]	
bronch(o), bronchi(o)	
bronchial alveolar lavage	
bronchial brushing	
bronchiol(o)	
bronchiole [BRŎNG-kē-ōl]	

Word	Definition
bronchitis [brŏng-KĪ-tĭs]	
bronchodilators [brŏng-kō-dī-LĀ-tĕrs]	
bronchography [brŏng-KŎG-ră-fē]	
bronchoplasty [BRŎNG-kō-plăs-tē]	
bronchoscope [BRŎNG-kō-skōp]	
bronchospasm [BRŎNG-kō-spăzm]	
bronchus (pl. bronchi) [BRŎNG-kŭs (BRŎNG-kī)]	
capn(o)	
Cheyne-Stokes respiration [chān stōks rĕs-pĭ-RĀ-shŭn]	
chronic bronchitis	
chronic obstructive pulmonary disease	
cilia [SĬL-ē-ă]	
crackles [KRĂK-ls]	
croup [krūp]	
cystic fibrosis [SĬS-tĭk fī-BRŌ-sĭs]	
diaphragm [DĪ-ă-frăm]	
diphtheria [dĭf-THĒR-ē-ă]	
dysphonia [dĭs-FŌ-nē-ă]	
dyspnea [dĭsp-NĒ-ă]	
emphysema [ĕm-fĭ-SĒ-mă]	
empyema [ĕm-pī-Ē-mă]	
endoscope [ĔN-dō-skōp]	
endotracheal intubation [ĕn-dō-TRĀ-kē-ăl ĭn-tū-BĀ-shŭn] (ET)	
epiglott(o)	
epiglottis [ĔP-ĭ-GLŎT-ĭs]	
epiglottitis [ĕp-ĭ-glŏt-Ī-tĭs]	
epistaxis [ĔP-ĭ-STĂK-sĭs]	
eupnea [yūp-NĒ-ă]	
exhalation [ĕks-hă-LĀ-shŭn]	
expectorants [ĕk-SPĔK-tō-rănts]	
expiration [ĕks-pĭ-RĀ-shŭn]	

Word	Definition
external nares [ĕks-TĔR-năl NĀR-ēz]	
external respiration	
glottis [GLŎT-ĭs]	
Heimlich [HĪM-lĭk] maneuver	
hemoptysis [hē-MŎP-tĭ-sĭs]	
hemothorax [hē-mō-THŌ-răks]	
hilum (also hilus) [HĪ-lŭm (HĪ-lŭs)]	
hypercapnia [hī-pĕr-KĂP-nē-ă]	
hyperpnea [hī-pĕrp-NĒ-ă]	
hyperventilation [HĪ-pĕr-vĕn-tĭ-LĀ-shŭn]	
hypopharynx [HĪ-pō-FĂR-ĭnks]	
hypopnea [hī-PŎP-nē-ă]	
hypoventilation [HĪ-pō-vĕn-tĭ-LĀ-shŭn]	
hypoxemia [hī-pŏk-SĒ-mē-ă]	
hypoxia [hī-PŎK-sē-ă]	
inferior lobe [ĭn-FĒ-rē-ōr lŏb]	
inhalation [ĭn-hă-LĀ-shŭn]	
inspiration [ĭn-spĭ-RĀ-shŭn]	
intercostal muscles [ĭn-tĕr-KŎS-tăl MŬS-ĕlz]	
internal respiration	
laryng(o)	
laryngectomy [LĂR-ĭn-JĔK-tō-mē]	
laryngitis [lăr-ĕn-JĪ-tĭs]	
laryngocentesis [lă-rĭng-gō-sĕn-TĒ-sĭs]	
laryngopharynx [lă-RĬNG-gō-făr-ĭnks]	
laryngoplasty [lă-RĬNG-gō-plăs-tē]	
laryngoscopy [LĂR-ĭng-GŎS-kŏ-pē]	
laryngospasm [lă-RĬNG-gō-spăsm]	
laryngostomy [LĂR-ĭng-GŎS-tō-mē]	
laryngotracheobronchitis [lă-RĬNG-gō-TRĀ-kē-ō-brŏng-KĪ-tĭs]	

Word	Definition
laryngotracheotomy [lă-RĬNG-gō-trā-kē-ŎT-ō-mē]	
larynx [LĂR-ĭngks]	
lob(o)	
lobectomy [lō-BĔK-tō-mē]	
lung [lŭng]	
mediastin(o)	
mediastinoscopy [MĒ-dē-ăs-tĭ-NŎS-kō-pē]	
mediastinum [MĒ-dē-ăs-TĪ-nŭm]	
mesothelioma [MĔZ-ō-thē-lē-Ō-mă]	
middle lobe	
nas(o)	
nasal cavity	
nasal septum [NĀ-zăl SĔP-tŭm]	
nasopharyngitis [NĀ-zō-fă-rĭn-JĪ-tĭs]	
nasopharyngoscopy [NĀ-zō-fă-rĭng-GŎS-kō-pē]	
nasopharynx [NĀ-zō-FĂR-ĭngks]	
nebulizer [NĔB-yū-lĭz-ĕr]	
nose [nŏz]	
nosebleed	
nostrils [NŎS-trĭls]	
or(o)	
oropharynx [ŌR-ō-FĂR-ĭngks]	
orthopnea [ōr-thŏp-NĒ-ă, ōr-THŎP-nē-ă]	
otorhinolaryngologist [ō-tō-RĪ-nō-lăr-rĭn-GŎL-ō-jĭst]	
ox(o), oxi, oxy	
pansinusitis [păn-sĭ-nŭ-SĪ-tĭs]	
paranasal sinuses [păr-ă-NĀ-săl SĪ-nŭs-ĕz]	
parietal pleura [pă-RĪ-ĕ-tăl PLŪR-ă]	
paroxysmal [păr-ŏk-SĬZ-măl]	

Word	Definition
peak flow meter	
percussion [pěr-KŬSH-ŭn]	
pertussis [pěr-TŬS-ĭs]	
pharyng(o)	
pharyngeal tonsils [fă-RĬN-jē-ăl TŎN-sĭls]	
pharyngitis [făr-ĭn-JĪ-tĭs]	
pharynx [FĂR-ĭngks]	
phon(o)	
phren(o)	
pleur(o)	
pleura (pl. pleurae) [PLŪR-ă (PLŪR-ē)]	
pleural cavity [PLŪR-ăl KĂV-ĭ-tē]	
pleural effusion [PLŪR-ăl ē-FYŪ-zhŭn]	
pleuritis, pleurisy [plū-RĪ-tĭs, PLŪR-ĭ-sē]	
pleurocentesis [PLŪR-ō-sěn-TĒ-sĭs]	
pleuropexy [PLŪR-ō-PĔK-sē]	
pneum(o), pneumon(o)	
pneumobronchotomy [NŪ-mō-brŏng-KŎT-ō-mē]	
pneumoconiosis [NŪ-mō-kō-nē-Ō-sĭs]	
pneumonectomy [NŪ-mō-NĔK-tō-mē]	
pneumonia [nū-MŌ-nē-ă]	
pneumonitis [nū-mō-NĪ-tĭs]	
pneumothorax [nū-mō-THŌR-ăks]	
pulmonary abscess [PŬL-mō-nār-ē ĂB-sěs]	
pulmonary edema [PŬL-mō-nār-ē ě-DĒ-mă]	
pulmonary embolism [PŬL-mō-nār-ē ĔM-bō-lĭzm]	
pulmonary function tests	
rales [răhlz]	

Word	Definition
respiratory [RĔS-pǐ-ră-tōr-ē, rĕ-SPĪR-ă-tōr-ē] tract	
rhin(o)	
rhinitis [rī-NĪ-tǐs]	
rhinoplasty [RĪ-nō-plăs-tē]	
rhinorrhea [rǐ-nō-RĒ-ă]	
rhonchi [RŎNG-kī]	
septoplasty [SĔP-tō-plăs-tē]	
septostomy [sĕp-TŎS-tō-mē]	
septum [SĔP-tŭm]	
silicosis [sǐl-ǐ-KŌ-sǐs]	
singultus [sǐng-GŬL-tŭs]	
sinusitis [sī-nŭ-SĪ-tǐs]	
sinusotomy [sīn-ū-SŎT-ō-mē]	
soft palate [sǒft PĂL-ăt]	
spir(o)	
spirometer [spī-RŎM-ĕ-tĕr]	
sputum [SPŬ-tūm] sample or culture	
steth(o)	
stridor [STRĪ-dōr]	
superior lobe	
sweat test	
tachypnea [tăk-ǐp-NĒ-ă]	
thorac(o)	
thoracic [thō-RĂS-ǐk] surgeon	
thoracocentesis [THŌR-ă-kō-sĕn-TĒ-sǐs]	
thoracostomy [thōr-ă-KŎS-tō-mē]	
thoracotomy [thōr-ă-KŎT-ō-mē]	
thorax [THŌ-răks]	
throat [thrōt]	
throat culture	
thyroid cartilage	
tonsill(o)	
tonsillectomy [TŎN-sǐ-LĔK-tō-mē]	

Word	Definition
tonsillitis [TŎN-sĭ-LĪ-tĭs]	
trache(o)	
trachea [TRĀ-kē-ă]	
tracheitis [trā-kē-Ī-tĭs]	
tracheoplasty [TRĀ-kē-ō-PLĂS-tē]	
tracheostomy [TRĀ-kē-ŎS-tō-mē]	
tracheotomy [trā-kē-ŎT-ō-mē]	
tuberculosis [tū-bĕr-kyū-LŌ-sĭs]	
upper respiratory infection	
ventilator [VĔN-tĭ-lā-tōr]	
visceral pleura [VĬS-ĕr-ăl PLŪR-ă]	
vocal cords	
voice box	
wheezes [HWĒZ-ĕz]	
whooping cough [HŎOP-ĭng kăwf]	
windpipe	

Abbreviations

Write the full meaning of each abbreviation.

Abbreviation	Meaning
ABG	
AFB	
A&P	
AP	
ARD	
ARDS	
ARF	
BS	
COLD	
COPD	
CPR	
CTA	
CXR	

Abbreviation	Meaning
DOE	
DPT	
ENT	
ET tube	
FEF	
FEV	
FVC	
HBOT	
IMV	
IPPB	
IRDS	
IRV	
LLL	
LUL	
MBC	
MDI	
PA	
PCP	
PEEP	
PFT	
PND	
RD	
RDS	
RLL	
RUL	
SIDS	
SOB	
T&A	
TB	
TLC	
TPR	
URI	
VC	
V/Q scan	

Answers to Chapter Exercises

1. Muscles in the diaphragm control the amount of air inhaled and exhaled. Weakened muscles may lead to shallow breathing.
2. Oxygen.
3. a. trachea; b. lungs; c. alveoli
4. external respiration
5. cilia
6. nasal septum
7. epiglottis
8. Heimlich maneuver
9. air sacs / alveoli
10. three
11. two
12. diaphragm
13. intercostal
14. F
15. T
16. F
17. T
18. T
19. F
20. T
21. F
22. F
23. F
24. nasopharynx
25. trachea
26. respiration
27. C
28. diaphragm
29. epiglottis
30. pharynx
31. C
32. tonsils
33. bronchus
34. Chronic obstructive pulmonary disease, smoking, heart disease, age.
35. Internal respiration is the exchange of oxygen and carbon dioxide between the blood and the cells. The heart pumps oxygenated blood throughout the body, and internal respiration requires an efficient cardiovascular system.
36. adenoidectomy
37. thoracocentesis
38. otorhinolaryngologist
39. tonsillitis
40. mediastinopericarditis
41. pneumonorrhaphy
42. oronasal
43. pharyngitis
44. phonopathy
45. capnogram
46. bronchitis
47. peribronchitis
48. pericardiopleural
49. lobotomy
50. oximetry
51. oxychloride
52. bronchoedema
53. alveoloclasia
54. thoracalgia
55. sinusotomy
56. d
57. f
58. g
59. i
60. a
61. j
62. e
63. h
64. c
65. b
66. Mr. DiGiorno has both cardiovascular and respiratory problems. Blood gas tests show how his internal respiration is working.
67. WBC or white blood count
68. pulmonary function
69. sweat test
70. endoscope
71. forced vital
72. auscultation
73. throat culture
74. percussion
75. peak flow meter
76. sputum sample
77. spirometer
78. pharyngo
79. capno
80. laryng
81. lob
82. laryngo
83. The bedridden person's muscles are weaker; breathing is shallower; there is reduced fresh air.
84. Fluids from the infection may still reside in the respiratory system. Lying down causes them to collect rather than to be expelled.
85. d
86. g
87. e
88. b
89. i
90. c
91. j
92. a
93. h
94. f
95. F
96. T
97. T
98. F
99. T
100. F
101. F
102. F
103. T
104. F
105. pharyngitis
106. pneumonoconiosis
107. asthma
108. crackles/rales
109. smoking
110. She may need a tonsillectomy.
111. If the tonsils are removed, they cannot spread infection.
112. g
113. h
114. f
115. j
116. e
117. i
118. b
119. a
120. c
121. d
122. thoracotomy
123. tracheotomy
124. lobectomy or pneumonectomy
125. pleuropexy
126. septoplasty
127. brain; Missy's brain trauma

affects her breathing process.

128. Pneumonia infections may result from long periods spent in bed and not exercising one's muscles and lungs.

129. antitussives
130. bronchodilators
131. expectorants
132. nebulizer

133. ventilator
134. possible tumor
135. to confirm disappearance or presence of tumor

8

The Nervous System

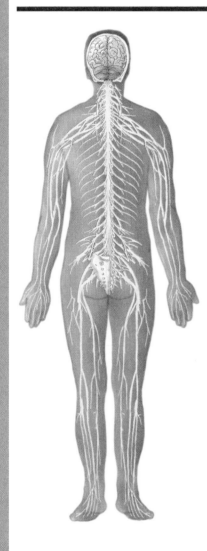

After studying this chapter, you will be able to:

♦ Name the parts of the nervous system and discuss the function of each part

♦ Define the combining forms used in building words that relate to the nervous system

♦ Identify the meaning of related abbreviations

♦ Name the common diagnoses, laboratory tests, and clinical procedures used in testing and treating disorders of the nervous system

♦ Define the major pathological conditions of the nervous system

♦ Define surgical terms related to the nervous system

♦ Recognize common pharmacological agents used in treating disorders of the nervous system

Structure And Function

The nervous system directs the function of all the human body systems (Figure 8-1a and b). Every activity, whether voluntary or involuntary, is controlled by some of the more than 100 billion nerve cells throughout the body. The nervous system is divided into two subsystems: the central nervous system and the peripheral nervous system.

A **nerve cell** or **neuron** is the basic element of the nervous system. Neurons are highly specialized types of cells and vary greatly in function, shape, and size. All neurons have three parts: the **cell body, dendrites,** and an **axon.** The cell body may take several different shapes, but all neuron cell bodies have branches or fibers that reach out to send or receive impulses. The dendrites are thin branching extensions of the cell body. They conduct nerve impulses *toward* the cell body. The axon, which conducts nerve impulses *away* from the cell body, is generally a single branch covered by fatty tissue called the **myelin sheath.** Outside the myelin sheath is a membranous covering called the **neurilemma.** At the end of the axon, there are **terminal end fibers** through which pass the impulses leaving the neuron. The nerve impulse then jumps from one neuron to the next over a space called a **synapse.** The nerve impulse is stimulated to jump over the synapse by a **neurotransmitter,** any of various substances located in tiny sacs at the end of the terminal end fibers. Table 8-1 lists some common neurotransmitters.

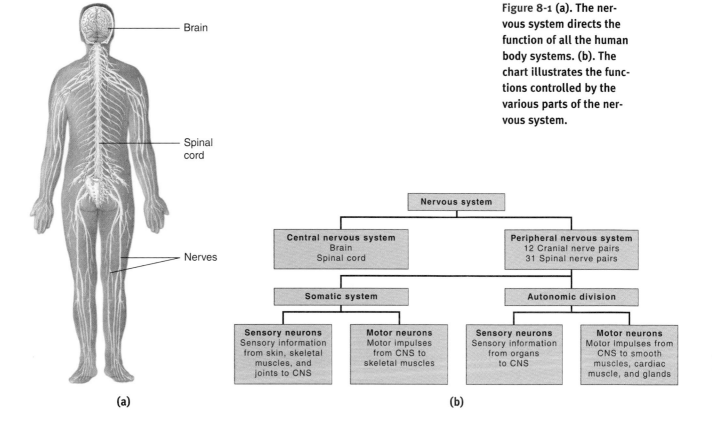

Figure 8-1 (a). The nervous system directs the function of all the human body systems. (b). The chart illustrates the functions controlled by the various parts of the nervous system.

(a)

(b)

Table 8-1 Some Common Neurotransmitters

Neutotransmitter Group	Compounds in Neurotransmitter	Probable Nervous System Functions
acetylcholine	acetylcholine (ACh)	excites and inhibits muscular and glandular activity; affects memory
amino acids	gamma-aminobutyric acid (GABA)	inhibits certain brain activity
	glutamic acid	excites certain brain activity
	aspartic acid	excites certain brain activity
	glycine	inhibits certain spin cord activity
monoamines	dopamine	involved in brain and motor activity
	histamine	involved in brain activity
	norepinephrine (NE)	involved in heat regulation, arousal, motor activity, reproduction; acts as hormone in bloodstream
	serotonin	involved in sleep, mood, appetite, and pain
neuropeptides	somatostatin	involved in secretion of growth hormone
	endorphins	has pain-relieving properties

All neurons also have two basic properties—**excitability,** the ability to respond to a **stimulus** (anything that arouses a response), and **conductivity,** the ability to transmit a signal. The three types of neurons are **efferent (motor) neurons,** which convey information to the muscles and glands from the central nervous system; **afferent (sensory) neurons,** which carry information from sensory receptors to the central nervous system; and **interneurons,** which carry and process sensory information. Some nerves contain combinations of at least two types of neurons. Figure 8-2 shows a neuron.

Neurons are microscopic entities that form bundles called **nerves,** the bearers of electrical messages to the organs and muscles of the body. The body's cells contain stored electrical energy that is released when the cells receive outside stimuli or when internal chemicals (for example, **acetylcholine**) stimulate the cells. The released energy passes through the nerve cell, causing a **nerve impulse.** Nerve impulses are received or transmitted by tissue or organs called **receptors.** These impulses are then transmitted to other receptors throughout the body.

In addition to nerve cells, other cells in the nervous system support, connect, protect, and remove debris from the system. These cells, **neuroglia** or **neuroglial cells,** do not transmit impulses. Each of the three types of neuroglia serves different purposes. Star-shaped **astroglia (astrocytes)** maintain nutrient and chemical levels in neurons. **Oligodendroglia** produce myelin and help in supporting neurons. **Microglia** are phagocytes—cells that remove debris. Certain neuroglia, along with the almost solid walls of the brain's capillaries, form what is known as the *blood-brain barrier,* the barrier that permits some chemical substances to reach the brain's neurons, but blocks most others. Figure 8-3 shows neuroglia.

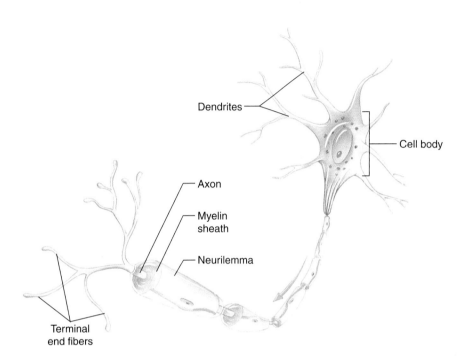

Dendrites

Cell body

Axon

Myelin sheath

Neurilemma

Terminal end fibers

Figure 8-2 Parts of a neuron

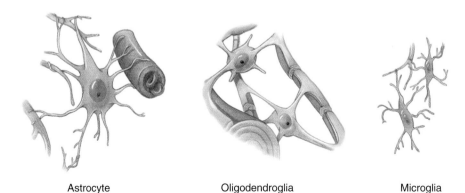

Astrocyte

Oligodendroglia

Microglia

Figure 8-3 The three types of neuroglia shown here perform different functions in the nervous system.

Central Nervous System

The **central nervous system** consists of the brain and spinal cord. The word *central* is the key to the purpose of this subsystem. It is the center of control, receiving and interpreting all stimuli and sending nerve impulses to instruct muscles and glands to take or respond to certain actions. Designated actions throughout the body include both voluntary and involuntary movement, sight, hearing, thinking, secretion of hormones, memory, and responses to outside stimuli. The meninges (described later) are a covering crucial to the protection of the brain and spinal cord.

Brain

The human adult **brain** weighs about three pounds, is 75 percent water, has the consistency of gelatin, contains over 100 billion neurons, and is responsible for controlling the body's many functions and interactions with the outside world. The brain has four major divisions—the brainstem, the cerebellum, the cerebrum, and the diencephalon. Figure 8-4 illustrates the brain.

MORE ABOUT...

the Blood-Brain Barrier

For many years, pharmaceutical researchers have known that the key to curing some brain ailments is to be able to deliver medication to the site of a specific disorder. The goal is to overcome the defenses of the blood-brain barrier without opening it to potentially harmful substances. Penetrating the blood-brain barrier will allow safer, nonsurgical treatment of some brain disorders.

Water-soluble substances are held back by the blood-brain barrier, while fat-soluble substances are generally allowed to pass through. Penicillin is water soluble and cannot get through easily, whereas fat-soluble substances such as alcohol, nicotine, and caffeine pass through easily. Two surgical approaches have been refined to penetrate the barrier. The first one involves two injections: one to cause the brain's capillaries to shrink temporarily, followed by a second injection of a drug that can pass between the shrunken capillaries. The other approach is to implant a disk into the brain that releases chemotherapeutic drugs near the site of a tumor. Both surgical methods are high-risk and costly. Now scientists are exploring substances that pass normally through the barrier. They can sometimes piggyback certain drug molecules to a fat-soluble substance that passes through the barrier and trick the capillaries into letting them through. Some combinations of synthetic substances are also able to penetrate the barrier. This is hopeful news for people with inoperable brain tumors, severe neurological conditions, and certain other diseases.

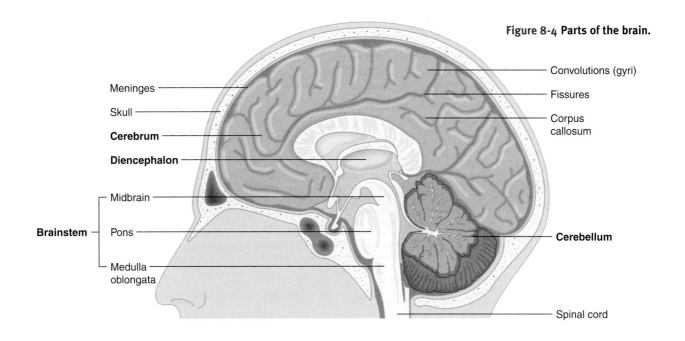

Figure 8-4 Parts of the brain.

Meninges
Skull
Cerebrum
Diencephalon
Midbrain
Brainstem — Pons
Medulla oblongata

Convolutions (gyri)
Fissures
Corpus callosum
Cerebellum
Spinal cord

- The **brainstem** is made up of the **midbrain** (involved with visual reflexes), the **pons** (controls certain respiratory functions), and the **medulla oblongata** (contains centers that regulate heart and lung functions, swallowing, vomiting, coughing, and sneezing). The midbrain connects the pons beneath it with the cerebellum and cerebrum above. The pons lies between the midbrain and the medulla oblongata, which connects the pons to the spinal cord.

- The **cerebellum** is the area that coordinates musculoskeletal movement to maintain posture, balance, and muscle tone.

- Above the cerebellum lies the **cerebrum,** the third major brain structure. The cerebrum has two hemispheres, with an outer portion called the **cerebral cortex** (area of conscious decision making). The cerebral cortex has many **fissures** (also called **sulci**) and **convolutions** (also called **gyri**) and is composed of gray matter (substance in the brain composed mainly of nerve cells and dendrites). Below the cerebral cortex are white matter (substance in the brain composed mainly of nerve fibers) and masses of gray matter called the **basal ganglia** (involved with musculoskeletal movement). The left and right lobes of the cerebrum are each divided into four parts or lobes. The **frontal lobe** controls voluntary motor movements, emotional expression, and moral behavior. The **parietal lobe** controls and interprets the senses and taste. The **temporal lobe** controls memory, equilibrium, emotion, and hearing. The **occipital lobe** controls vision and various forms of expression. The two hemispheres of the cerebrum are connected by the **corpus callosum,** a bridge of nerve fibers that relay information between the two hemispheres.

- The **diencephalon** is the deep portion of the brain containing the **thalamus, hypothalamus, epithalamus,** and the **ventral thalamus.** These parts of the diencephalon serve as relay centers for sensations. They also integrate with the autonomic nervous system in the control of heart rate, blood pressure, temperature regulation, water and electrolyte balance, digestive functions, behavioral responses, and glandular activities.

The brain sits inside the cranium, a strong bony structure that protects it. The area between the brain and the cranium is filled with **cerebrospinal fluid (CSF),** a watery fluid that contains various compounds and flows throughout the brain and around the spinal cord. This watery fluid cradles and cushions the brain. **Ventricles** or cavities in the brain also contain this fluid. The meninges (described below) also protect the brain.

Spinal Cord

The **spinal cord** extends from the medulla oblongata of the brain to the area around the first lumbar vertebra in the lower back. The spinal cord is contained within the vertebral column. The space that contains the spinal column is called the vertebral canal. The spinal cord is protected by the bony structure of the vertebral column, by the cerebrospinal fluid that surrounds it, and by the spinal meninges. Figure 8-5 illustrates a section of the spinal cord. Extending out from the spinal cord are the nerves of the peripheral nervous system.

Meninges

The **meninges** (Figure 8-6) are three layers of membranes that cover the brain and spinal cord. The outer layer, the **dura mater** (from Latin, "hard mother"), is a tough, fibrous membrane that covers the entire length of the

Severe spinal cord injuries usually result in some type of paralysis. Research is under way to grow replacement cells for injured nerves. It is expected that some types of paralysis will be cured by 2010.

spinal cord and contains channels for blood to enter brain tissue. The middle layer, the **arachnoid,** is a weblike structure that runs across the space (called the **subdural space**) containing cerebrospinal fluid. The **pia mater** (Latin, "tender mother"), the innermost layer of meninges, is a thin membrane containing many blood vessels that nourish the spinal cord. The space between the pia mater and the bones of the spinal cord is called the **epidural space.** It contains blood vessels and some fat. It is the space into which anesthetics may be injected to dull pain (as during childbirth and some pelvic operations) or contrast material for certain diagnostic procedures.

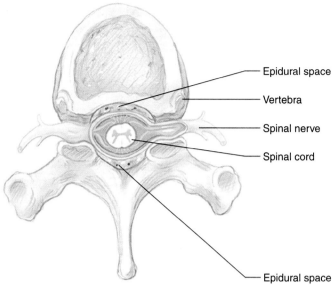

Epidural space

Vertebra

Spinal nerve

Spinal cord

Epidural space

Figure 8-5 A section of the spinal column showing a verterbra.

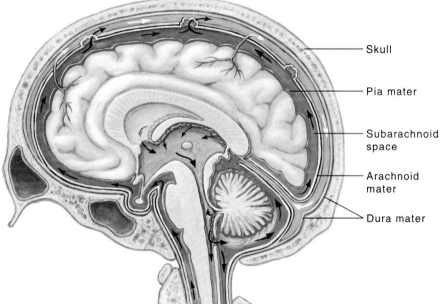

Skull

Pia mater

Subarachnoid space

Arachnoid mater

Dura mater

Figure 8-6 The brain and spinal cord are protected by the meninges.

Peripheral Nervous System

The peripheral nervous system includes the 12 pairs of **cranial nerves** that carry impulses to and from the brain and the 31 pairs of **spinal nerves** that carry messages to and from the spinal cord and the torso and extremities of the body. Table 8-2 on page 274 lists the cranial nerves and their functions.

The 31 pairs of spinal nerves are grouped according to the segments of the spinal cord out of which they extend. Table 8-3 on page 274 lists those groups and the regions served by the nerves of each group. The peripheral nerves are further divided into two subsystems—the somatic and autonomic nervous systems—according to their function.

Somatic Nervous System

Nerves of the **somatic nervous system** receive and process sensory input from the skin, muscles, tendons, joints, eyes, tongue, nose, and ears. They also excite the voluntary contraction of skeletal muscles.

Table 8-2 The Twelve Pairs of Cranial Nerves and Their Function

Pair of Cranial Nerves	Primary Type of Nerve	Function
I olfactory	sensory	involved in sense of smell
II optic	sensory	involved in sense of vision
III oculomotor	motor	involved in movement of eyes, controlling both the exterior and interior parts
IV trochlear	motor	involved in muscles that move the eyes
V trigeminal	sensory and motor	involved in eyes, tear glands, scalp, forehead, teeth, gums, lips, and muscles of the mouth
VI abducens	motor	involved with muscle conditioning
VII facial	sensory and motor	involved with taste, facial expressions, tear and salivary glands
VIII vestibulocochlear	sensory	involved in equilibrium and hearing
IX glossopharyngeal	sensory and motor	involved in pharynx, tonsils, tongue, and carotid arteries; stimulates salivary glands
X vagus	sensory and motor	involved in speech, swallowing, heart muscles, smooth muscles, and certain glands
XI accessory (cranial and spinal)	motor	involved in muscles of the soft palate, pharynx, larynx, neck, and back
XII hypoglossal	motor	involved in muscles that move the tongue

Table 8-3 Major Spinal Nerve Divisions and Their Functions

Region of Spinal Cord	Location	Functions of Nerves
cervical	neck	involved in muscles of the back of the head and neck and in the diaphragm
brachial	lower neck, axilla	involved in the muscles and skin of the neck, shoulder, arm, and hand
lumbar	posterior abdominal wall	involved in abdominal skin and muscles
sacral	posterior pelvic wall	involved in the muscles of the buttocks, thighs, feet, legs, and voluntary sphincters
coccygeal	coccyx and surrounding area	skin in coccyx region

Autonomic Nervous System

Nerves of the **autonomic nervous system** carry impulses from the central nervous system to glands, various smooth (involuntary) muscles, cardiac muscle, and various membranes. The autonomic nervous system stimulates organs, glands, and senses by stimulating secretions of various substances. The autonomic nerves are further divided into the **sympathetic** division and the

parasympathetic division. In general, the two divisions play opposite roles. The sympathetic division operates when the body is under stress. It helps to activate responses necessary to react in dangerous or abnormal situations. The parasympathetic division, on the other hand, operates to keep the body in homeostasis or balance under normal conditions.

Vocabulary Review

In the previous section, you learned terms relating to the nervous system. Before going on to the exercises, review the terms below and refer to the previous section if you have any questions.

Term	Word Analysis	Definition
acetylcholine	[ăs-ē-tĭl-KŌ-lēn]	Chemical that stimulates cells.
afferent (sensory) neuron	[ĂF-ĕr-ĕnt]	Neuron that carries information from the sensory receptors to the central nervous system.
arachnoid	[ă-RĂK-nŏyd] Greek *arachne*, spider + -oid, resembling	Middle layer of meninges.
astrocyte, astroglia	[ĂS-trō-sīt], [ăs-TRŎG-lē-ă] Greek *astron*, star + -cyte, cell	A type of neuroglia that maintains nutrient and chemical levels in neurons.
autonomic nervous system	[ăw-tō-NŎM-ĭk] auto-, self + Greek *nomos*, law	Part of the peripheral nervous system that carries impulses from the central nervous system to glands, smooth muscles, cardiac muscle, and various membranes.
axon	[ĂK-sōn] Greek, axis	Part of a nerve cell that conducts nerve impulses away from the cell body.
basal ganglia	[BĀ-săl GĂNG-glē-ă]	Large masses of gray matter within the cerebrum.
brain	[brān] Old English *braegen*	Body organ responsible for controlling the body's functions and interactions with outside stimuli.
brainstem		One of the four major divisions of the brain; division that controls certain heart, lung, and visual functions.
cell body		Part of a nerve cell that has branches or fibers that reach out to send or receive impulses.
central nervous system		Body system consisting of the brain, spinal cord, and meninges.

Term	Word Analysis	Definition
cerebellum	[sĕr-ĕ-BĔL-ŭm] Latin, little brain	One of the four major divisions of the brain; division that coordinates musculoskeletal movement.
cerebral cortex	[SĔR-ē-brăl KŎR-tĕks]	Outer portion of the cerebrum.
cerebrospinal fluid (CSF)	[SĔR-ē-brō-spī-năl] cerebro-, cerebrum + spinal	Watery fluid that flows throughout the brain and around the spinal cord.
cerebrum	[SĔR-ē-brŭm, sĕ-RĒ-brŭm] Latin, brain	One of the four major divisions of the brain; division involved with emotions, memory, conscious thought, moral behavior, sensory interpretations, and certain bodily movement.
conductivity	[kŏn-dŭk-TĬV-ĭ-tē]	Ability to transmit a signal.
convolution	[kŏn-vō-LŪ-shŭn]	Folds in the cerebral cortex; gyri.
corpus callosum	[KŎR-pŭs kă-LŌ-sŭm] Latin, body with a thick skin	Bridge of nerve fibers that connects the two hemispheres of the cerebrum.
cranial nerves	[KRĀ-nē-ĂL]	Any of 12 pairs of nerves that carry impulses to and from the brain.
dendrite	[DĔN-drīt]	A thin branching extension of a nerve cell that conducts nerve impulses toward the cell body.
diencephalon	[dī-ĕn-SĔF-ă-lŏn] di-, separated + Greek *enkephalos*, brain	One of the four major structures of the brain; it is the deep portion of the brain and contains the thalamus.
dura mater	[DŪ-ră MĀ-tĕr] Latin, hard mother	Outermost layer of meninges.
efferent (motor) neuron	[ĔF-ĕr-ĕnt]	Neuron that carries information to the muscles and glands from the central nervous system.
epidural space	[ĕp-ĭ-DŪ-răl] epi-, upon + dur(a mater)	Area between the pia mater and the bones of the spinal cord.
epithalamus	[ĔP-ĭ-THĂL-ă-mŭs] epi- + thalamus	One of the parts of the diencephalon; serves as a sensory relay station.
excitability	[ĕk-SĪ-tă-BĬL-ĭ-tē]	Ability to respond to stimuli.
fissure	[FĬSH-ŭr]	One of many indentations of the cerebrum; sulci.

Term	Word Analysis	Definition
frontal lobe		One of the four parts of each hemisphere of the cerebrum.
gyrus (pl. gyri)	[JĪ-rŭs (JĪ-rī)]	*See* convolution.
hypothalamus	[HĪ-pō-THĂL-ă-mŭs] hypo-, below + thalamus	One of the parts of the diencephalon; serves as a sensory relay station.
interneuron	[ĬN-tĕr-NŪ-rŏn] inter-, between + neuron	Neuron that carries and processes sensory information.
medulla oblongata	[mĕ-DŪL-ă ŏb-lŏng-GĂ-tă] Latin, long marrow	Part of the brain stem that regulates heart and lung functions, swallowing, vomiting, coughing, and sneezing.
meninges (sing. meninx)	[mĕ-NĬN-jēz (MĚ-nĭnks)] Greek, plural of *meninx*, membrane	Three layers of membranes that cover and protect the brain and spinal cord.
microglia	[mī-KRŎG-lē-ă] micro-, small + Greek *glia*, glue	A type of neuroglia that removes debris.
midbrain	mid-, middle + brain	Part of the brainstem involved with visual reflexes.
myelin sheath	[MĪ-ĕ-lĭn shēth]	Fatty tissue that covers axons.
nerve	[nĕrv]	Bundle of neurons that bear electrical messages to the organs and muscles of the body.
nerve cell		Basic cell of the nervous system having three parts: cell body, dendrite, and axon; neuron.
nerve impulse		Released energy that is received or transmitted by tissue or organs and that usually provokes a response.
neurilemma	[nūr-ĭ-LĔM-ă] neuri-, nerve + Greek *lemma*, husk	Membranous covering that protects the myelin sheath.
neuroglia, neuroglial cell	[nū-RŎG-lē-ă], [nū-RŎG-lē-ăl] neuro-, nerve + Greek *glia*, glue	Cell of the nervous system that does not transmit impulses.
neuron	[NŪR-ŏn] Greek, nerve	Basic cell of the nervous system having three parts; nerve cell.

Term	Word Analysis	Definition
neurotransmitters	[NŬR-ō-trăns-MĬT-ĕr] neuro- + transmitter	Various substances located in tiny sacs at the end of the axon.
occipital lobe	[ŏk-SĬP-ĭ-tăl lōb]	One of the four parts of each hemisphere of the cerebrum.
oligodendroglia	[ŌL-ĭ-gō-dĕn-DRŎG-lē-ă] oligo-, few + Greek *dendron*, tree + *glia*, glue	A type of neuroglia that produces myelin and helps to support neurons.
parasympathetic nervous system	[păr-ă-sĭm-pă-THĔT-ĭk] para-, beside -+ sympathetic	Part of the autonomic nervous system that operates when the body is in a normal state.
parietal lobe	[pă-RĪ-ĕ-tăl lōb]	One of the four parts of each hemisphere of the cerebrum.
pia mater	[PĪ-ă, PĒ-ă MĀ-tĕr, MĂH-tĕr] Latin, tender mother	Innermost layer of meninges.
pons	[pŏnz] Latin, bridge	Part of the brainstem that controls certain respiratory functions.
receptor	[rē-SĔP-tŏr]	Tissue or organ that receives nerve impulses.
somatic nervous system	[sō-MĂT-ĭk]	Part of the peripheral nervous system that receives and processes sensory input from various parts of the body.
spinal cord		Ropelike tissue that sits inside the vertebral column and from which spinal nerves extend.
spinal nerves		Any of 31 pairs of nerves that carry messages to and from the spinal cord and the torso and extremities.
stimulus (pl. stimuli)	[STĬM-yū-lŭs (STĬM-yū-lī)]	Anything that arouses a response.
subdural space	[sŭb-DŪR-ăl] sub-, under + dur(a mater)	Area between the dura mater and the pia mater across which the arachnoid runs.
sulcus (pl. sulci)	[SŬL-kŭs (SŬL-sī)]	*See* fissure.
sympathetic nervous system	[sĭm-pă-THĔT-ĭk]	Of the part of the autonomic nervous system that operates when the body is under stress.

Term	Word Analysis	Definition
synapse	[SĬN-ăps]	Space over which nerve impulses jump from one neuron to another.
temporal lobe	[TĔM-pŏ-răl lōb]	One of the four parts of each hemisphere of the cerebrum.
terminal end fibers		Group of fibers at the end of an axon that passes the impulses leaving the neuron to the next neuron.
thalamus	[THĂL-ă-mŭs]	One of the four parts of the diencephalon; serves as a sensory relay station.
ventral thalamus		One of the four parts of the diencephalon; serves as a sensory relay station.
ventricle	[VĔN-trĭ-kl]	Cavity in the brain for cerebrospinal fluid.

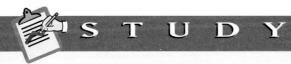

A Neurological Problem

Jose Gutierrez is a patient of Dr. Marla Chin, an internist. He is scheduled for his six-month checkup and medication review. Mr. Gutierrez has a history of heart disease and skin carcinoma. In the past few months he has been having trouble buttoning his shirts and remembering things. He has also developed a limp. Dr. Chin orders some tests.

 Critical Thinking

1. Mr. Gutierrez has some new problems. According to his symptoms, what areas of the brain might have been affected by some disorder?

2. Dr. Chin does a thorough checkup and asks both Mr. Gutierrez and his wife many questions about such things as respiratory function, sleep habits, and so on. How will the answers to the questions help Dr. Chin determine the next steps to take?

Structure and Function Exercises

Know the Position

3. The brain and spinal cord are protected by three layers of meninges. Name the three layers in order from inside the skull to the brain and describe the structure of each.

a. _____

b. _____

c. _____

Find a Match

Match the definition in the right-hand column to the word in the left-hand column.

4. neuroglia
5. meninges
6. neuron
7. acetylcholine
8. excitability
9. ventricle
10. basal ganglia
11. sulci
12. arachnoid
13. epidural space

a. gray matter
b. weblike meningeal layer
c. internal chemical
d. cell that does not transmit impulses
e. fissures
f. area between pia mater and spinal bones
g. responsiveness to stimuli
h. protective membranes
i. cell that transmits impulses
j. cavity for fluid

Complete the Thought

Fill in the blanks.

14. Organs that receive [or transmit] nerve impulses are called _____.

15. Each axon is covered by a _____ _____.

16. Neuron structures that conduct nerve impulses toward the cell body are called _____.

17. Neuron structures that conduct nerve impulses away from the cell body are called

_____.

18. The spinal cord connects to the brain at the _____ _____.

19. The part of the brain with two hemispheres is called the _____.

20. The part of the brainstem that controls certain respiratory functions is called the _____.

21. The bony structure protecting the brain is the _____.

22. Ventricles hold _____ _____.

23. The deep portion of the brain is called the _____.

Spell It Correctly

Write the correct spelling in the blank to the right of each word. If the word is already correctly spelled, write C.

24. meninxes _____

25. thalomus _____

26. ganoglia _____

27. gyri _____

28. synapse _____

29. axen _____

30. neurilemma _____

31. acetycholine _____

32. neurglia _____

33. cerebrellum _____

Combining Forms And Abbreviations

The lists below include combining forms and abbreviations that relate specifically to the circulatory system. Pronunciations are provided for the examples.

Combining Form	Meaning	Example
cerebell(o)	cerebellum	*cerebellitis* [sĕr-ĕ-bĭl-Ī-tĭs], inflammation of the cerebellum
cerebr(o), cerebri	cerebrum	*cerebralgia* [sĕr-ĕ-BRĂL-jē-ă], pain in the head
crani(o)	cranium	*craniofacial* [KRĀ-nē-ō-FĀ-shăl], relating to the face and the cranium
encephal(o)	brain	*encephalitis* [ĕn-sĕf-ă-LĪ-tĭs], inflammation of the brain
gangli(o)	ganglion	*gangliform* [GĂNG-glē-fŏrm], having the shape of a ganglion
gli(o)	neuroglia	*gliomatosis* [glī-ō-mă-TŌ-sĭs], abnormal growth of neuroglia in the brain or spinal cord
mening(o), meningi(o)	meninges	*meningitis* [mĕn-ĭn-JĪ-tĭs], inflammation of the meninges
myel(o)	bone marrow, spinal cord	*myelomalacia* [MĪ-ĕ-lō-mă-LĀ-shē-ă], softening of the spinal cord
neur(o), neuri	nerve	*neuritis* [nū-RĪ-tĭs], inflammation of a nerve
spin(o)	spine	*spinoneural* [spī-nō-NŪ-răl], relating to the spine and the nerves that extend from it

Combining Form	Meaning	Example
thalam(o)	thalamus	*thalamotomy* [thăl-ă-MŎT-ō-mē], incision into the thalamus to destroy a portion causing or transmitting sensations of pain
vag(o)	vagus nerve	*vagectomy* [vā-JĔK-tō-mē], surgical removal of a portion of the vagus nerve
ventricul(o)	ventricle	*ventriculitis* [věn-trĭk-yū-LĪ-tĭs], inflammation of the ventricles of the brain

Abbreviation	Meaning	Abbreviation	Meaning
Ach	acetylcholine	EEG	electroencephalogram
ALS	amyotrophic lateral sclerosis	ICP	intracranial pressure
BBB	blood-brain barrier	LP	lumbar puncture
CNS	central nervous system	MRA	magnetic resonance angiography
CP	cerebral palsy	MRI	magnetic resonance imaging
CSF	cerebrospinal fluid	MS	multiple sclerosis
CT or CAT scan	computerized (axial) tomography	SAH	subarachnoid hemorrhage
CVA	cerebrovascular accident	TIA	transient ischemic attack
CVD	cerebrovascular disease		

C A S E S T U D Y

Referral to a Neurologist

Dr. Chin takes some blood tests and decides to send Mr. Gutierrez to a neurologist, Dr. Martin Stanley, for an evaluation. Dr. Stanley reviews Dr. Chin's notes and finds that Mr. Gutierrez has no history of CVA, but is experiencing numbness in his fingers and difficulty walking. Dr. Stanley will test for CVA, but since Mr. Gutierrez has a history of normal blood pressure, he suspects another disorder.

Critical Thinking

34. Why is Mr. Gutierrez referred to a neurologist?

35. What nerves might affect Mr. Gutierrez's walking?

Combining Forms and Abbreviations Exercises

Root Out the Meaning

Find at least two nervous system combining forms in each word. Write the combining forms and their definitions in the space provided.

36. encephalomyelitis: _____

37. craniomeningocele: _____

38. glioneuroma: _____

39. cerebromeningitis: _____

40. spinoneural: _____

41. neuroencephalomyelopathy: _____

Trace the Root

Add the combining form that completes the word.

42. Acting upon the vagus nerve: _____tropic.

43. Tumor consisting of ganglionic neurons: ganglio_____oma.

44. Myxoma containing glial cells: _____myxoma.

45. Relating to nerves and meninges: neuro_____eal.

In each word, find the combining form that relates to the nervous system and give its definition.

46. parencephalia _____

47. angioneurectomy _____

48. cephalomegaly _____

49. myelitis _____

50. meningocyte _____

51. neurocyte _____

52. craniomalacia _____

53. vagotropic _____

54. glioblast _____

55. cerebrosclerosis _____

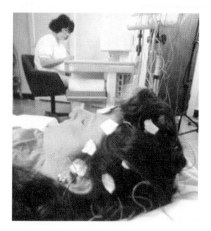

Figure 8-7 An electroencephalogram (EEG) records the brain's impulses. The impulses are collected from electrodes placed around the patient's head.

Diagnostic, Procedural, and Laboratory Terms

Many of the diagnostic tests used to examine the nervous system include electrodiagnostic procedures. An **electroencephalogram (EEG)** is a record of the electrical impulses of the brain (Figure 8-7). This record can detect abnormalities that signal certain neurological conditions. **Evoked potentials** are electrical waves observed in an electroencephalogram. Abnormal wave patterns can help in the diagnosis of auditory, visual, and sensory disorders. Peripheral nervous system diseases can sometimes be detected by shocking the peripheral nerves and timing the conductivity of the shock. This procedure is called **nerve conduction velocity.** **Polysomnography (PSG)** is a recording of electrical and movement patterns during sleep to diagnose sleep disorders, such as *sleep apnea,* a dangerous breathing disorder.

Various types of imaging are used to visualize the structures of the brain and spinal cord. *Magnetic resonance imaging (MRI)* is the use of magnetic fields and radio waves to visualize structures. *Magnetic resonance angiography (MRA)* is the imaging of blood vessels to detect various abnormalities. *Intracranial MRA* is the visualizing of the head to check for aneurysms and other abnormalities. *Extracranial MRA* is the imaging of the neck to check the carotid artery for abnormalities. **SPECT (single photon emission computed tomography) brain scan** is a procedure that produces brain images using radioactive isotopes. **PET (positron emission tomography)** is a procedure that produces brain images using radioactive isotopes and tomography. It gives highly accurate images of the brain structures and physiology and can provide diagnoses of various brain disorders. **Computerized (axial) tomography (CT or CAT) scans** use tomography to show cross-sectional radiographic images.

X-rays are used to diagnose specific malformations or disorders. A **myelogram** is an x-ray of the spinal cord after a contrast medium is injected. A **cerebral angiogram** is an x-ray of the brain's blood vessels after a contrast medium is injected. *Encephalography* is the radiographic study of the ventricles of the brain. The record made by this study is called an **encephalogram.** Sound waves are used to create brain images in a **transcranial sonogram** for diagnosing and managing head and stroke trauma. Ultrasound is also used in *echoencephalography,* encephalography using ultrasound waves.

Reflexes are involuntary muscular contractions in response to a stimulus. Reflex testing can aid in the diagnosis of certain nervous system disorders. **Babinski's reflex** is a reflex on the plantar surface of the foot. In most physical examinations, the reflex of each knee is tested for responsiveness (Figure 8-8).

Cerebrospinal fluid that has been withdrawn from between two lumbar vertebrae during a **lumbar (spinal) puncture** can be studied for the presence of various substances, which may indicate certain diseases.

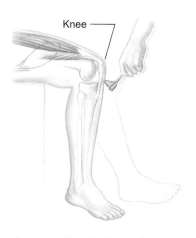

Knee

Figure 8-8 Tapping just below the knee usually causes a reflex reaction similar to the one shown here.

Vocabulary Review

In the previous section, you learned terms relating to diagnosis, clinical procedures, and laboratory tests. Before going on to the exercises, review the terms below and refer to the previous section if you have any questions.

Term	Word Analysis	Definition
Babinski's reflex	[bă-BĬN-skēs] After Joseph F. Babinski, French neurologist (1857–1932)	Reflex on the plantar surface of the foot.
cerebral angiogram		X-ray of the brain's blood vessels after a dye is injected.
computerized (axial) tomography (CT or CAT) scan		Radiographic imaging that produces cross-sectional images.
electroencephalogram (EEG)	[ē-LĔK-trō-ĕn-SĔF-ă-lō-grăm] electro-, electrical + encephalo-, brain + -gram, a recording	Record of the electrical impulses of the brain.
encephalogram	[ĕn-SĔF-ă-lō-grăm] encephalo- + -gram	Record of the radiographic study of the ventricles of the brain.
evoked potentials	[ē-VŌKT pō-TĔN-shăls]	Record of the electrical wave patterns observed in an EEG.
lumbar (spinal) puncture	[LŬM-băr]	Withdrawal of cerebrospinal fluid from between two lumbar vertebrae.
myelogram	[MĪ-ĕ-lō-grăm] myelo-, spinal cord + -gram	X-ray of the spinal cord after a contrast medium has been injected.
nerve conduction velocity		Timing of the conductivity of an electrical shock administered to peripheral nerves.
PET (positron emission tomography)		Imaging of the brain using radioactive isotopes and tomography.
polysomnography (PSG)	[PŎL-ē-sŏm-NŎG-ră-fē] poly-, many + somno-, sleep + -graphy, recording	Recording of electrical and movement patterns during sleep.
reflex	[RĒ-flĕks]	Involuntary muscular contraction in response to a stimulus.
SPECT (single photon emission computed tomography) brain scan		Brain image produced by the use of radioactive isotopes.

Term	Word Analysis	Definition
transcranial sonogram	[trăns-KRĀ-nē-ăl SŎN-ō-grăm] trans-, across + cranial	Brain images produced by the use of sound waves.

C A S E S T U D Y

Ordering Treatment

Dr. Stanley orders an electroencephalogram of Mr. Gutierrez's brain. He also orders some additional blood tests. Dr. Stanley performs a number of reflex tests. The abnormalities present confirm Dr. Stanley's initial suspicion of Parkinson's disease. He prescribes several medications and schedules a visit for Mr. Gutierrez in three weeks to discuss his progress. He asks Mr. Gutierrez to keep a daily log of his walking ability, any vision changes, his speech, and tremors for the three weeks until his appointment.

 Critical Thinking

56. Why does Dr. Stanley want Mr. Gutierrez to keep a log?

57. What might Mr. Gutierrez's abnormal reflex tests indicate?

Diagnostic, Procedural, and Laboratory Terms Exercises

Check Your Knowledge

Circle T for true and F for false.

58. Extracranial MRA is imaging of the spinal cord. T F

59. Reflexes are voluntary muscular contractions. T F

60. An encephalogram is a record of a study of the ventricles of the brain. T F

61. A lumbar puncture removes blood. T F

62. PET is an extremely accurate imaging system. T F

63. Evoked potentials are electrical waves. T F

64. A myelogram and an angiogram are both taken after injection of a contrast medium. T F

65. PSG is taken during waking hours. T F

66. Encephalography uses sound waves to produce brain images. T F

Pathological Terms

Bones, cerebrospinal fluid, and the meninges protect the nervous system from most types of external trauma, but not all. A **concussion** is an injury to the brain from an impact with an object. Cerebral concussions usually clear within 24 hours. A severe concussion can lead to **coma,** abnormally deep sleep with little or no response to stimuli. Coma may also result from other causes, such as stroke. A more serious trauma than concussion is a **brain contusion,** a bruising of the surface of the brain without penetration into the brain. Traumatic injury, as during a car accident, may also cause the brain to hit the skull and then to rebound to the other side of the skull. This is called a *closed head trauma,* because there is no penetration of the skull. *Shaken baby syndrome* is a severe form of closed head trauma in which a young child experiences head trauma (as a result of falling, being shaken, or other trauma), causing the brain to hit the sides of the skull and causing potentially fatal damage. A *subdural hematoma* (between the dura mater and the arachnoid or at the base of the dura mater) is a tumorlike collection of blood often caused by trauma. Other types of cranial hematomas are *epidural hematomas* (located on the dura mater) and *intracerebral hematomas* (within the cerebrum).

In addition, neurological disorders and diseases may be congenital or degenerative or may be caused by infection, inflammation, tumor growth, or vascular problems. Congenital diseases of the brain or spinal cord can be devastating and cause an impact on the activities of daily living. **Spina bifida** is a defect in the spinal column. *Spina bifida occulta* is a covered lesion of the vertebra that is generally visible only by x-ray. This is the least severe form of spina bifida. *Spina bifida cystica* is a more severe form of the condition, usually with a **meningocele** (protrusion of the spinal meninges above the surface of the skin) or a **meningomyelocele** (protrusion of the meninges and spinal cord). Figure 8-9 depicts an infant with spina bifida. **Tay-Sachs** is a hereditary disease found primarily in the descendants of Eastern European Jews. It is a genetic disease characterized by an enzyme deficiency that causes deterioration in the central nervous system's cells. **Hydrocephalus** is an overproduction of fluid in the brain. It usually occurs at birth (although it can occur in adults with infections or tumors) and is treated with a shunt placed from the ventricle of the brain to the peritoneal space to relieve pressure by draining fluid. Figure 8-10 illustrates an infant with a shunt for relief of the pressure of hydrocephalus.

Comas can last for many years. During that time, coma patients are usually fed via a feeding tube. For many people, the issue of keeping people alive for so many years when they might have died naturally is a controversial issue.

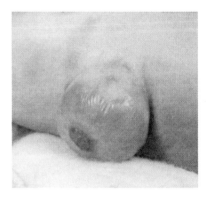

Figure 8-9 **The back of an infant with spina bifida cystica. A meningomyelocele is protruding out of the spinal cord.**

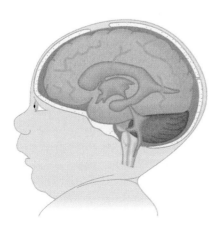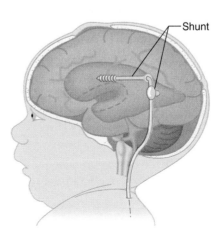

Shunt

Figure 8-10 **A shunt relieves the brain pressure of newborns with hydrocephalus.**

Degenerative diseases of the central nervous system can affect almost any part of the body. Deterioration in mental capacity is found in **dementia** and **Alzheimer's disease,** a progressive degeneration of neurons in the brain, eventually leading to death. Some symptoms that worsen as Alzheimer's disease progresses are **amnesia** (loss of memory), **apraxia** (inability to properly use familiar objects), and **agnosia** (inability to receive and understand outside stimuli). **Amyotrophic lateral sclerosis (ALS)** is a degenerative disease of the motor neurons leading to loss of muscular control and death. It is also known as **Lou Gehrig's disease.** Several other degenerative diseases are not necessarily fatal. **Huntington's chorea** is a hereditary disease with uncontrollable, jerking movements and progressive loss of neural control. **Multiple sclerosis (MS)** is the destruction of the myelin sheath (**demyelination**) leading to muscle weakness, unsteady **gait** (walking), paresthesias, extreme fatigue, and some paralysis. **Myasthenia gravis,** a disease with muscle weakness, can be treated to avoid the overproduction of antibodies that block neurotransmitters from sending proper nerve impulses to skeletal muscles. **Parkinson's disease,** a degeneration of nerves in the brain, causes tremors, weakness of muscles, and difficulty in walking. It is treated with drugs that increase the levels of **dopamine** in the brain. Treatment helps relieve symptoms but does not cure the disease.

Severe neurological disorders cause paralysis, convulsions, and other symptoms, but are not usually degenerative. **Palsy** is partial or complete paralysis. **Cerebral palsy** includes lack of motor coordination from cerebral damage during gestation or birth. **Bell's palsy** is paralysis of one side of the face. It usually disappears after treatment. **Ataxia** is lack of voluntary muscle coordination resulting from disorders of the cerebellum or spinal cord. **Epilepsy** is chronic, recurrent seizure activity. Epilepsy has been known since ancient times, when victims were thought to be under the influence of outside forces. Now it is understood that this disease occurs because of abnormal conditions in the brain that cause sudden excessive electrical activity. The seizures caused by this activity can be preceded by an **aura,** a collection of symptoms felt just before the actual seizure. Seizures may be mild or intense. **Absence seizures (petit mal seizures)** are mild and usually include only a momentary disorientation with the environment. **Tonic-clonic seizures (grand mal seizures)** are much more severe and include loss of consciousness, convulsions, and twitching of limbs.

Tourette syndrome is a neurological disorder that causes uncontrollable sounds and twitching (**tics**). Some drugs are helpful in controlling symptoms and allowing sufferers to lead normal lives.

Infectious disorders of the nervous system include **shingles** and **meningitis.** Shingles is a viral disease caused by the herpes zoster virus. Its symptoms include pain in the peripheral nerves and blisters on the skin. Several types of meningitis, inflammation of the meninges, can be infectious. **Pyrogenic meningitis** (also

MORE ABOUT...

Tourette Syndrome

Medications for Tourette syndrome do not always work. People who have Tourette syndrome may not be able to function in social and work environments because of their inability to control sounds, often scatalogical in nature, and twitching, often extreme and repetitive. The National Tourette Syndrome Association publicizes information about the syndrome, holds conventions for people with the syndrome, and provides information and support to its members. This large support group holds social events where members feel comfortable with their fellow sufferers. More information is available from the Association's website (http://neuro-www2.mgh.harvard.edu/tsa/tsamain.nclk) or from conducting a search for the word *tourette*.

called **bacterial meningitis**) is caused by bacteria and includes such symptoms as fever, headache, and stiff neck. It is usually treated with antibiotics. In some severe cases, it can be fatal. **Viral meningitis** is caused by viruses and, although it has the same symptoms as pyrogenic meningitis, it is usually allowed to run its course. Medication can be given for some of the more uncomfortable symptoms (fever, headache). Inflammation can also occur in the nerves (**neuritis**), the spinal cord (**myelitis**), the brain (**encephalitis**), the cerebellum (**cerebellitis**), the dura mater (**duritis**), the ganglion (**gangliitis**), or the spinal nerve roots (**radiculitis**). Some specific nerve inflammations, such as **sciatica**, cause pain in the area served by the nerve.

Abnormal growths in the nervous system usually occur in the brain or the meninges. About one-third of all brain tumors are growths that spread from cancers in other parts of the body (lungs, breasts, skin, and so on). The remaining tumors can be benign or malignant. In either case, the pressure and distortion of the brain caused by a tumor may result in many other neurological symptoms. **Gliomas** (tumors that arise from neuroglia) and **meningiomas** (tumors that arise from the meninges) can be either benign or malignant. Both may be removed surgically. **Astrocytoma, oligodendroglioma,** and **glioblastoma multiforme** are all types of gliomas, with the latter being the most malignant. Tumors can be treated surgically if they have not infiltrated or affected certain essential areas of the brain. Radiation and medication may be used to try to reduce tumor growth. Some nontumorous growths can cause pain from pressure on nerves. A **ganglion** is any group of nerve cells bunched together to form a growth or a cyst, usually arising from a wrist tendon.

Vascular problems, such as *arteriosclerosis*, may cause a disruption in the normal blood supply to the brain (**cerebrovascular accident** or **CVA**). Various types of **strokes (cerebral infarctions)** result from this disruption. A **thrombus** (blood clot) may cause **occlusion** (blocking of a blood vessel), which in turn may cause a **thrombotic stroke.** As the blockage grows, the person may experience milder symptoms before a major stroke. These short incidents are known as **transient ischemic attacks (TIAs).** An **embolic stroke** is caused by an **embolus,** a clot that travels from somewhere in the body to the cerebral arteries and blocks a small vessel, causing a sudden stroke. A **hemorrhagic stroke** is caused by blood escaping from a damaged cerebral artery. It may be caused by sudden trauma or an **aneurysm,** bursting of the wall of an artery after abnormal widening. Strokes can be mild and result in complete recovery, or they can range from mild to severe, with symptoms that remain permanently. Common symptoms are thought disorders, speech difficulty (**dysphasia**), loss of speech (**aphasia**), loss of muscular control, some paralysis, and disorientation.

Some states of consciousness are changed by lack of oxygen or brain abnormalities that affect the flow of blood and oxygen to the brain. **Fainting** or **syncope** is caused by lack of oxygen to the brain. **Somnolence** (extreme sleepiness), **somnambulism** (sleepwalking), and **narcolepsy** (uncontrollable, sudden lapses into deep sleep) are all altered states of consciousness.

Vocabulary Review

In the previous section, you learned terms relating to pathology. Before going on to the exercises, review the terms below and refer to the previous section if you have questions.

Term	Word Analysis	Definition
absence seizure		Mild epileptic seizure consisting of brief disorientation with the environment.
agnosia	[ăg-NŌ-zē-ă] Greek, ignorance	Inability to receive and understand outside stimuli.
Alzheimer's disease	[ĂLTS-hī-měrz] After Alois Alzheimer, German neurologist (1864–1915)	Any of a variety of degenerative brain diseases causing thought disorders, gradual loss of muscle control, and, eventually, death.
amnesia	[ăm-NĒ-zē-ă] Greek, forgetfulness	Loss of memory.
amyotrophic lateral sclerosis (ALS)	[ă-mī-ō-TRŌ-fĭk LĂT-ěr-ăl sklě-RŌ-sĭs]	Degenerative disease of the motor neurons leading to loss of muscular control and death.
aneurysm	[ĂN-yū-rĭzm] Greek *aneurysma*, dilation	Abnormal widening of an artery wall that bursts and releases blood.
aphasia	[ă-FĀ-zē-ă] a-, without + -phasia, speech	Loss of speech.
apraxia	[ă-PRĂK-sē-ā] a- + Greek *pratto*, to do	Inability to properly use familiar objects.
astrocytoma	[ĂS-trō-sĭ-TŌ-mă] Greek *astron*, star + cyt-, cell + -oma, tumor	Type of glioma formed from astrocytes.
ataxia	[ă-TĂK-sē-ă] a- + Greek *taxis*, order	Condition with uncoordinated voluntary muscular movement, usually resulting from disorders of the cerebellum or spinal cord.
aura	[ĂW-ră] Latin, breeze	Group of symptoms that precede a seizure.
bacterial meningitis	[měn-ĭn-JĪ-tĭs]	Meningitis caused by a bacteria; pyrogenic meningitis.
Bell's palsy	[PĂWL-zē] After Sir Charles Bell, Scottish surgeon (1774–1842)	Paralysis of one side of the face; usually temporary.
brain contusion	[kŏn-TŪ-shŭn]	Bruising of the surface of the brain without penetration.

Term	Word Analysis	Definition
cerebellitis	[sĕr-ĕ-bĕl-Ī-tĭs] cerebell-, cerebellum + -itis, inflammation	Inflammation of the cerebellum.
cerebral infarction	[SĔR-ĕ-brăl ĭn-FĂRK-shŭn]	*See* cerebrovascular infarction.
cerebral palsy	[SĔR-ĕ-brăl PĂWL-zē]	Congenital disease caused by damage to the cerebrum during gestation or birth and resulting in lack of motor coordination.
cerebrovascular accident (CVA)	[SĔR-ĕ-brō-VĂS-kyū-lăr] cerebro-, brain + vascular	Neurological incident caused by disruption in the normal blood supply to the brain; stroke.
coma	[KŌ-mă] Greek *koma*, trance	Abnormally deep sleep with little or no response to stimuli.
concussion	[kŏn-KŬSH-ŭn]	Brain injury due to trauma.
dementia	[dē-MĔN-shē-ă]	Deterioration in mental capacity, usually in the elderly.
demyelination	[dē-MĪ-ĕ-lĭ-NĀ-shŭn]	Destruction of myelin sheath, particularly in MS.
dopamine	[DŌ-pă-mēn]	Substance in the brain or manufactured substance that helps relieve symptoms of Parkinson's disease.
duritis	[dū-RĪ-tĭs] dur(a mater) + -itis	Inflammation of the dura mater.
dysphasia	[dĭs-FĀ-zē-ă] dys-, difficult + -phasia	Speech difficulty.
embolic stroke	[ĕm-BŎL-ĭk]	Sudden stroke caused by an embolus.
embolus	[ĔM-bō-lŭs]	Clot from somewhere in the body that blocks a small blood vessel in the brain.
encephalitis	[ĕn-sĕf-ă-LĪ-tĭs] encephal-, brain + -itis	Inflammation of the brain.
epilepsy	[ĔP-ĭ-LĔP-sē]	Chronic recurrent seizure activity.
fainting		*See* syncope.
gait	[gāt]	Manner of walking.
gangliitis	[găng-glē-Ī-tĭs] gangli(on) + -itis	Inflammation of a ganglion.

Term	Word Analysis	Definition
ganglion (pl. ganglia, ganglions)	[GĂNG-glē-ŏn (-ă-ŏns)]	Any group of nerve cell bodies forming a mass or a cyst in the peripheral nervous system; usually forms in the wrist.
glioblastoma multiforme	[GLĪ-ō-blăs-TŌ-mă MŬL-tĭ-fŏrm]	Most malignant type of glioma.
glioma	[glī-Ō-mă] Greek *glia*, glue + -oma	Tumor that arises from neuroglia.
grand mal seizure	[măhl]	*See* tonic-clonic seizure.
hemorrhagic stroke	[hĕm-ō-RĂJ-ĭk]	Stroke caused by blood escaping from a damaged cerebral artery.
Huntington's chorea	[kōr-Ē-ă] After George Huntington, U.S. physician (1850–1916)	Hereditary disorder with uncontrollable, jerking movements.
hydrocephalus	[hī-drō-SĔF-ă-lŭs] hydro-, water + Greek *kephale*, head	Overproduction of fluid in the brain.
Lou Gehrig's disease		*See* amyotrophic lateral sclerosis.
meningioma	[mĕ-NĬN-jē-Ō-mă] meningi-, meninges + -oma, tumor	Tumor that arises from the meninges.
meningitis	[mĕn-in-JĪ-tĭs] mening-, meninges + -itis	Inflammation of the meninges.
meningocele	[mĕ-NĬNG-gō-sēl] meningo-, meninges + -cele, hernia	In spina bifida cystica, protrusion of the spinal meninges above the surface of the skin.
meningomyelocele	[mĕ-nĭn-gō-MĪ-ĕ-lō-sēl] meningo- + myelo-, spinal cord + -cele	In spina bifida cystica, protrusion of the meninges and spinal cord above the surface of the skin.
multiple sclerosis (MS)	[MŬL-tĕ-pŭl sklĕ-RŌ-sĭs]	Degenerative disease with loss of myelin, resulting in muscle weakness, extreme fatigue, and some paralysis.
myasthenia gravis	[mī-ăs-THĒ-nē-ă GRĂV-ĭs]	Disease involving overproduction of antibodies that block certain neurotransmitters; causes muscle weakness.
myelitis	[mī-ĕ-LĪ-tĭs] myel-, spinal cord + -itis	Inflammation of the spinal cord.

Term	Word Analysis	Definition
narcolepsy	[NĂR-kō-lĕp-sē] narco-, sleep + -lepsy, condition with seizures	Nervous system disorder that causes uncontrollable, sudden lapses into deep sleep.
neuritis	[nū-RĪ-tĭs] neur-, nerve + -itis	Inflammation of the nerves.
occlusion		Blocking of a blood vessel.
oligodendroglioma	[ŎL-ĭ-gō-DĔN-drŏ-glĭ-Ō-mă] oligodendrogli(a) + -oma	Type of glioma formed from oligodendroglia.
palsy	[PĂWL-zē]	Partial or complete paralysis.
Parkinson's disease	[PĂR-kĕn-sŏnz] After James Parkinson, British physician (1755–1824)	Degeneration of nerves in the brain caused by lack of sufficient dopamine.
petit mal seizure	[PĔ-tē măhl]	*See* absence seizure.
pyrogenic meningitis	[pī-rō-JĔN-ĭk] pyro-, fever + -genic, producing	Meningitis caused by bacteria; can be fatal; bacterial meningitis.
radiculitis	[ră-dĭk-yū-LĪ-tĭs] radicul-, root + -itis	Inflammation of the spinal nerve roots.
sciatica	[sī-ĂT-ĭ-kă]	Inflammation of the sciatic nerve.
shingles		Viral disease affecting the peripheral nerves.
somnambulism	[sŏm-NĂM-byū-lĭzm] somno-, sleep + Latin *ambulo*, to walk	Sleepwalking.
somnolence	[SŎM-nō-lĕns] Latin, sleepiness	Extreme sleepiness caused by a neurological disorder.
spina bifida	[SPĪ-nă BĬF-ĭ-dă] Latin, cleft spine	Congenital defect of the spinal column.
stroke	[strōk]	*See* cerebrovascular accident (CVA).
syncope	[SĬN-kŏ-pē]	Loss of consciousness due to a sudden lack of oxygen in the brain.
Tay-Sachs disease	[TĀ-săks]	Hereditary disease that causes deterioration in the central nervous system and, eventually, death.

Term	Word Analysis	Definition
thrombotic stroke	[thrŏm-BŎT-ĭk]	Stroke caused by a thrombus.
thrombus	[THRŎM-bŭs]	Blood clot.
tics		Twitching movements that accompany some neurological disorders.
tonic-clonic seizure		Severe epileptic seizure accompanied by convulsions, twitching, and loss of consciousness.
Tourette syndrome	[tū-RĔT] After Gilles de la Tourette, French physician (1857–1904)	Neurological disorder that causes uncontrollable speech sounds and tics.
transient ischemic	[ĭs-KĒ-mĭk] attāck	Short neurological incident usually not resulting in permanent injury, but usually signaling that a larger stroke may occur.
viral meningitis		Meningitis caused by a virus and not as severe as pyrogenic meningitis.

C A S E S T U D Y

Adjusting the Dosage

When Mr. Gutierrez returns to Dr. Stanley's office after three weeks, he reports that he can button his shirt again and that his walking has improved. He complains, however, that some of his cognitive symptoms have not improved. Dr. Stanley is encour-

aged that some of the physical symptoms have begun to improve. He will increase the dosage of the anti-Parkinson's medication he has prescribed. He is confident that Mr. Gutierrez will stabilize and possibly even gain strength.

 Critical Thinking

67. Many medications cure the symptoms, but not the disease. How might exercise help Mr. Gutierrez regain mobility?

68. What compound does Mr. Gutierrez's medication contain?

Pathological Terms Exercises

Check Your Knowledge

Fill in the blanks.

69. Palsy is partial or complete _____.

70. Dopamine sometimes helps the symptoms of _____ disease.

71. Inflammation of the spinal nerve roots is called _____.

72. A stationary blood clot is called a(n) _____.

73. A blood clot that moves is called a(n) _____

74. Abnormally deep sleep with lack of responsiveness is a(n) _____.

75. A mild stroke that may be a signal that a larger stroke will occur is called a(n) _____

    _____.

76. _____ seizures are milder than _____ seizures.

77. Multiple sclerosis is usually associated with loss of _____, a covering for nerves.

78. ALS is a disease of the _____ neurons.

Make a Match

Match the definition in the right-hand column with the correct word in the left-hand column.

79. coma	a. speech difficulty
80. shaken baby syndrome	b. fainting
81. glioma	c. disruption in brain's blood supply
82. duritis	d. loss of speech
83. aphasia	e. short, mild stroke
84. CVA	f. congenital spinal cord disorder
85. spina bifida	g. abnormally deep sleep
86. TIA	h. brain damage caused by rough handling
87. syncope	i. neurological tumor
88. dysphasia	j. meningeal inflammation

Lobotomy is rarely used; however, certain seizure disorders that do not respond to medication require removal of part of the brain. In many cases, the remaining brain tissue takes over the functions of the removed part.

Surgical Terms

Neurosurgeons are the specialists who perform surgery on the brain and spinal cord. Neurosurgery is considered high risk because the potential for permanent injury is great. When some brain diseases, such as epilepsy, do not respond well to drugs, they may, in extreme cases, require surgery. A **lobectomy** is removal of a portion of the brain to treat epilepsy and other disorders, such as brain cancer. A **lobotomy,** severing of nerves in the frontal lobe of the brain, was once considered a primary method for treating mental illness. Now it is rarely used. Laser surgery to destroy damaged parts of the brain is also used to treat some neurological disorders.

When it is necessary to operate directly on the brain (as in the case of a tumor), a **craniectomy,** removal of part of the skull, or a **craniotomy,** incision into the skull, may be performed. **Trephination** is a circular opening into the skull to operate on the brain or to relieve pressure when there is fluid buildup. **Stereotaxy** or **stereotactic surgery** is the destruction of deep-seated brain structures using three-dimensional coordinates to locate the structures.

Neuroplasty is the surgical repair of a nerve. **Neurectomy** is the surgical removal of a nerve. A **neurotomy** is the dissection of a nerve. A **neurorrhaphy** is the suturing of a severed nerve. A **vagotomy** is the cutting off of the vagus nerve to relieve pain. **Cordotomy** is an operation to resect part of the spinal cord.

Vocabulary Review

In the previous section, you learned terms relating to surgery. Before going on to the exercises, review the terms below and refer to the previous section if you have questions.

Term	Word Analysis	Definition
cordotomy	[kŏr-DŎT-ō-mē] Greek *chorde*, cord + -tomy, a cutting	Resectioning of a part of the spinal cord.
craniectomy	[krā-nē-ĔK-tō-mē] crani-, cranium + -ectomy, removal	Removal of a part of the skull.
craniotomy	[KRĀ-nē-ŎT-ō-mē] cranio-, cranium + -tomy	Incision into the skull.
lobectomy	[lō-BĔK-tō-mē] lob-, lobe + -ectomy	Removal of a portion of the brain to treat certain disorders.
lobotomy	[lō-BŎT-ō-mē] lobo-, lobe + -tomy	Removal of the frontal lobe of the brain.
neurectomy	[nū-RĔK-tō-mē] neur-, nerve + -ectomy	Surgical removal of a nerve.

Term	Word Analysis	Definition
neuroplasty	[NŪR-ō-PLĂS-tē] neuro-, nerve + -plasty, repair	Surgical repair of a nerve.
neurorrhaphy	[nūr-ŎR-ă-fē] neuro- + -rrhaphy, a suturing	Suturing of a severed nerve.
neurosurgeon	[nūr-ō-SĔR-jŭn] neuro- + surgeon	Medical specialist who performs surgery on the brain and spinal cord.
neurotomy	[nū-RŎT-ō-mē] neuro- + -tomy	Dissection of a nerve.
stereotaxy or stereotactic surgery	[stēr-ē-ō-TĂK-sē] Greek *stereos*, solid + *taxis*, orderly arrangement	Destruction of deep-seated brain structures using three-dimensional coordinates to locate the structures.
trephination	[trĕf-ĭ-NĀ-shŭn]	Circular incision into the skull.
vagotomy	[vā-GŎT-ō-mē] vag-, vagus nerve + -tomy	Surgical cutting off of the vagus nerve.

CASE STUDY

Repairing a Neurological Injury

Later in the year, Mr. Gutierrez was seriously injured in a car accident. He experienced some nerve damage in his leg. A neurosurgeon was called in to see if she could repair enough of the leg nerves to allow Mr. Gutierrez to walk. She operated, and the results were mixed. The trauma of the accident seemed to worsen some of the symptoms of Parkinson's disease, but Mr. Gutierrez experienced improvement with his walking after undergoing physical therapy. The neurologist decided not to increase Mr. Gutierrez's medication and to give him time to overcome the trauma.

 Critical Thinking

89. The damaged leg nerves could actually be a result of an injury elsewhere in the body. What particular nerves or areas might the neurosurgeon examine before determining exactly where to operate?

90. Traumas can temporarily change body chemistry. The body produces dopamine naturally. Why did the doctor not increase the dosage?

Check Your Knowledge

Fill in the blanks.

91. An incision into the skull is a(n) _____.

92. Removal of a portion of the skull is a(n) _____.

93. A circular skull incision is _____.

94. The removal of a frontal lobe is called a(n) _____.

95. The removal of a portion of the brain is called a(n)_____.

96. Suturing of a severed nerve is _____.

97. Removal of a nerve is _____.

98. Repair of a nerve is _____.

99. Vagotomy is cutting off of the _____ nerve.

100. Sectioning of a part of the spinal cord is a _____.

Pharmacological Terms

The nervous system can be the site of severe pain. **Analgesics** relieve pain. Other problems of the nervous system may be associated with diseases such as epilepsy. **Anticonvulsants** are often used to treat epilepsy and other disorders to lessen or prevent convulsions. **Narcotics** relieve pain by inducing a stuporous or euphoric state. **Sedatives** and **hypnotics** relax the nerves and sometimes induce sleep. **Anesthetics** block feelings or sensation and are used in surgery. Anesthetics can be given *locally* (to numb sensation to one section of the body) or *generally* (to numb sensation to the entire body). Table 8-4 lists some of the common pharmacological agents prescribed for the nervous system.

Table 8-4 Medications for the Nervous System

Drug Class	Purpose	Generic	Trade Name
analgesic	relieves or eliminates pain	methotrimeprazine	Levoprome, Nozinan
		salicylates (aspirin)	various
		acetaminophen	various
		NSAIDS	various
			(continued on next page)

Table 8-4 continued

Drug Class	Purpose	Generic	Trade Name
local anesthetic	causes loss of sensation in a localized area of the body	lidocaine	Anestacon, L-caine, Xylocaine
general anesthetic	causes loss of sensation over the whole body	propofol midazolam pentobarbital	Disoprofol, Diprivan Versed Nembutol, Pentogen
anticonvulsant	lessens or prevents convulsions	phenobarbital clonazepam carbamazeprine phenytoin	Luminal, Phenobarbital, Solfoton Klonopin, Rivotril Tegetrol, Mazeprine Dilantin, Diphenylan
sedative/hypnotic	relieves feeling of agitation; induces sleepiness	triazolam promethazine	Apo-Triazo, Halcion Phenazine, Phenergen, Promethazine HCL

Vocabulary Review

In the previous section, you learned terms relating to pharmacology. Before going on to the exercises, review the terms below and refer to the previous section if you have questions.

Term	Word Analysis	Definition
analgesic	[ăn-ăl-JĒ-zĭk] Greek *analgesia*, insensibility	Agent that relieves or eliminates pain.
anesthetic	[ăn-ĕs-THĔT-ĭk] Greek *anaisthesia*, without sensation	Agent that causes loss of feeling or sensation.
anticonvulsant	[ĂN-tē-kŏn-VŬL-sănt] anti-, against + convulsant	Agent that lessens or prevents convulsions.
hypnotic	[hĭp-NŎT-ĭk] Greek *hypnotikos*, inducing sleep	Agent that induces sleep.
narcotic	[năr-KŎT-ĭk] Greek *narkotikos*, numbing	Agent that relieves pain by inducing a stuporous or euphoric state.
sedative	[SĔD-ă-tĭv] Latin *sedativus*	Agent that relieves feeling of agitation.

C A S E 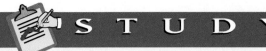 S T U D Y

Easing Pain with Medication

Mr. Gutierrez's internist, Dr. Chin, visited him in the hospital daily. She reconsidered all his medications in light of his trauma. She checked all the medications for any side effects that might be harmful and for any possible interactions among the medications. She ordered a sedative and a mild painkiller, to be taken as needed. Dr. Chin also made notes for the nutritionist, now that Mr. Gutierrez will have to stay in the hospital for at least three more weeks.

 Critical Thinking

101. Pain management is a delicate art. Physicians have to consider the addictive nature and strong side effects of many painkillers while at the same time making the patient comfortable enough to recover. Many physicians and medical ethicists have endorsed the unlimited use of pain medication for those with terminal diseases. What might explain the reluctance of some practitioners to allow unlimited painkillers?

102. What might Dr. Chin ask the nutritionist to consider for Mr. Gutierrez in the next three weeks?

Pharmacological Terms Exercises

Check Your Knowledge

Fill in the blanks.

103. An agent that induces sleep is called a(n) _____.

104. An agent that causes loss of feeling is called a(n) _____.

105. An agent that relieves nervousness is called a(n) _____.

106. A drug prescribed for epilepsy is probably a(n) _____.

107. Pain is relieved with _____.

108. A pain reliever that induces a euphoric state is a _____.

C H A L L E N G E S E C T I O N

Dr. Stanley has a patient whose diagnosis of a sleep disorder does not fit with some of the symptoms she is now experiencing. Dr. Stanley gives the patient, Mary Carpenter, a full physical exam and records notes on her chart.

The patient has had sleep difficulties since her CABG (coronary artery bypass graft) in 1993. She falls asleep easily but awakens 1 to 2 hours later and then sleeps little through the night. In the last two years she has noted increased difficulty in remembering names, numbers, and how to do things. She has gotten lost driving, and her family wishes her to surrender her license. She has had intermittent numbness in her fingers and legs and seems more unsteady on her feet.

Vitals: Wt. 160 P 56 BP 112/72 R 16 Temp. 97.3

Objective:

  Chest: Clear to percussion and auscultation

  Generally very slow and wobbly gait.

  Sense: Normal vibratory sense.

  Cereb: F-F. H-K doing well.

  Motor: Symmetric strength and tone.

  Reflex: Symmetric.

  Gave date.

  Cannot spell easy words backwards.

Challenge Section Exercises

109. Dr. Stanley tested physical and cognitive functions. He noted that Mary's family wanted her license surrendered and seemed to be legitimately worried about her ability to concentrate. What disease might Dr. Stanley be considering as a diagnosis?

110. Does the sleep disorder affect cognitive functioning?

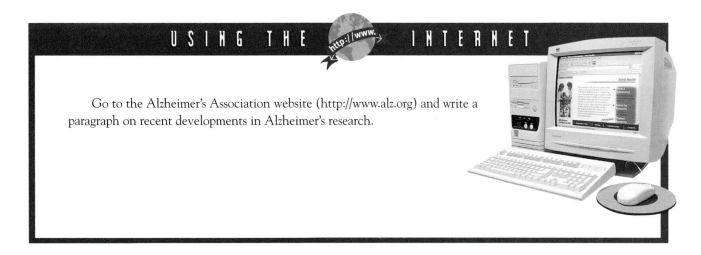

USING THE INTERNET

Go to the Alzheimer's Association website (http://www.alz.org) and write a paragraph on recent developments in Alzheimer's research.

CHAPTER REVIEW

Definition

Write the definition in the space provided.

Word	Definition
absence seizure	
acetylcholine [ăs-ē-tĭl-KŌ-lēn]	
afferent [ĂF-ĕr-ĕnt] (sensory) neuron	
agnosia [ăg-NŌ-zē-ă]	
Alzheimer's [ĂLTS-hī-mĕrz] disease	
amnesia [ăm-NĒ-zē-ă]	
amyotrophic lateral sclerosis [ă-mī-ō-TRŌ-fĕk LĂT-ĕr-ăl sklĕ-RŌ-sĭs] (ALS)	
analgesic [ăn-ăl-JĒ-zĭk]	
anesthetic [ăn-ĕs-THĔT-ĭk]	
aneurysm [ĂN-yū-rĭzm]	
anticonvulsant [ĂN-tē-kŏn-VŬL-sănt]	
aphasia [ā-FĀ-zē-ă]	
apraxia [ă-PRĂK-sē-ā]	
arachnoid [ă-RĂK-nŏyd]	
astrocyte [ĂS-trō-sīt], astroglia [ăs-TRŎG-lē-ă]	
astrocytoma[ĂS-trō-sī-TŌ-mă]	
ataxia [ā-TĂK-sē-ă]	
aura [ĂW-ră]	
autonomic [ăw-tō-NŌM-ĭk] nervous system	
axon [ĂK-sōn]	
bacterial meningitis [mĕn-ĭn-JĪ-tĭs]	
Babinski's [bă-BĬN-skēs] reflex	
basal ganglia [BĀ-săl GĂNG-glē-ă]	
Bell's palsy [PĂWL-zē]	

Word	Definition
brain [brān]	
brain contusion [kŏn-TŪ-shŭn]	
brainstem	
cell body	
central nervous system	
cerebell(o)	
cerebellitis [sĕr-ĕ-bĭl-Ī-tĭs]	
cerebellum [sĕr-ē-BĔL-ŭm]	
cerebr(o), cerebri	
cerebral angiogram	
cerebral cortex [SĔR-ē-brăl KŎR-tĕks]	
cerebral infarction [SĔR-ē-brăl ĭn-FĂRK-shŭn]	
cerebral palsy [SĔR-ē-brăl PĂWL-zē]	
cerebrospinal [SĔR-ē-brō-spī-năl] fluid (CSF)	
cerebrovascular [SĔR-ē-brō-VĂS-kyū-lăr] accident (CVA)	
cerebrum [SĔR-ē-brŭm, sĕ-RĒ-brŭm]	
coma [KŌ-mă]	
computerized (axial) tomography (CT or CAT) scan	
concussion [kŏn-KŬSH-ŭn]	
conductivity [kŏn-dŭk-TĬV-ĭ-tē]	
convolution [kŏn-vō-LŪ-shŭn]	
cordotomy [kŏr-DŎT-ō-mē]	
corpus callosum [KŎR-pŭs kă-LŌ-sŭm]	
crani(o)	
cranial [KRĀ-nē-ăl] nerves	
craniectomy [krā-nē-ĔK-tō-mē]	
craniotomy [krā-nē-ŎT-ō-mē]	
dementia [dē-MĔN-shē-ă]	
demyelination [dē-MĪ-ĕ-lĭ-NĀ-shŭn]	
dendrite [DĔN-drīt]	
diencephalon [dī-ĕn-SĔF-ă-lŏn]	

Word	Definition
dopamine [DŌ-pă-mēn]	
dura mater [DŪ-ră MĀ-tĕr]	
duritis [dū-RĪ-tĭs]	
dysphasia [dĭs-FĀ-zē-ă]	
efferent [ĔF-ĕr-ĕnt] (motor) neuron	
electroencephalogram (EEG) [ē-LĔK-trō-ĕn-SĔF-ă-lō-grăm]	
embolic [ĕm-BŌL-ĭk] stroke	
embolus [ĔM-bō-lŭs]	
encephal(o)	
encephalitis [ĕn-sĕf-ă-LĪ-tĭs]	
encephalogram [ĕn-SĔF-ă-lō-grăm]	
epidural [ĕp-ĭ-DŪR-ăl] space	
epilepsy [ĔP-ĭ-LĔP-sē]	
epithalamus [ĔP-ĭ-THĂL-ă-mŭs]	
evoked potentials [ē-VŌKT pō-TĔN-shăls]	
excitability [ĕk-SĪ-tă-BĬL-ĭ-tē]	
fainting	
fissure [FĬSH-ŭr]	
frontal lobe	
gait [gāt]	
gangli(o)	
gangliitis [găng-glē-Ī-tĭs]	
ganglion [GĂNG-glē-ŏn]	
gli(o)	
glioblastoma multiforme [GLĪ-ō-blăs-TŌ-mă MŬL-tĭ-fŏrm]	
glioma [glī-Ō-mă]	
grand mal [măhl] seizure	
gyrus (pl. gyri) [JĪ-rŭs (JĪ-rī)]	
hemorrhagic [hĕm-ō-RĂJ-ĭk] stroke	
Huntington's chorea [kōr-Ē-ă]	
hydrocephalus [hī-drō-SĔF-ă-lŭs]	
hypnotic [hĭp-NŎT-ĭk]	

Word	Definition
hypothalamus [HĪ-pō-THĂL-ă-mŭs]	
interneuron [ĬN-tĕr-NŪ-rŏn]	
lobectomy [lō-BĔK-tō-mē]	
lobotomy [lō-BŎT-ō-mē]	
Lou Gehrig's disease	
lumbar [LŬM-băr] (spinal) puncture	
medulla oblongata [mĕ-DŪL-ă ŏb-lŏng-GĂ-tă]	
mening(o), meningi(o)	
meninges (sing. meninx) [mĕ-NĬN-jēz (MĒ-nĭnks)]	
meningioma [mē-NĬN-jē-Ō-mă]	
meningitis [mĕn-ĭn-JĪ-tĭs]	
meningocele [mĕ-NĬNG-gō-sēl]	
meningomyelocele [mĕ-nĭn-jō-MĪ-ĕ-lō-sĕl]	
microglia [mī-KRŎG-lē-ă]	
midbrain	
multiple sclerosis [MŬL-tĕ-pŭl skĕl-RŌ-sĭs] (MS)	
myasthenia gravis [mī-ăs-THĒ-nē-ă GRĂV-ĭs]	
myel(o)	
myelin sheath [MĪ-ĕ-lĭn shēth]	
myelitis [mī-ĕ-LĪ-tĭs]	
myelogram [MĪ-ĕ-lō-grăm]	
narcolepsy [NĂR-kō-lĕp-sē]	
narcotic [năr-KŎT-ĭk]	
nerve [nĕrv]	
nerve cell	
nerve conduction velocity	
nerve impulse	
neur(o), neuri	
neurectomy [nū-RĔK-tō-mē]	
neurilemma [nūr-ĭ-LĔM-ă]	

Word	Definition
neuritis [nū-RĬ-tĭs]	
neuroglia [nū-RŎG-lē-ă], neuroglial [nū-RŎG-lē-ăl] cell	
neuron [NŪR-ŏn]	
neuroplasty [NŪR-ō-PLĂS-tē]	
neurorrhaphy [nūr-ŎR-ā-fē]	
neurosurgeon [nūr-ō-SĔR-jŭn]	
neurotomy [nū-RŎT-ō-mē]	
neurotransmitter [NŪR-ō-trăns-MĬT-ĕr]	
occipital lobe [ŏk-SĬP-ĭ-tăl lōb]	
occlusion	
oligodendroglia [ŌL-ĭ-gō-dĕn-DRŎG-lē-ă]	
oligodendroglioma [ŎL-ĭ-gō-DĔN-drŏ-glī-Ō-mă]	
palsy [PĂWL-zē]	
parasympathetic [păr-ă-sĭm-pă-THĔT-ĭk] nervous system	
parietal lobe [pă-RĬ-ĕ-tăl lōb]	
Parkinson's [PĂR-kĕn-sŏnz] disease	
PET (positron emission tomography)	
petit mal [PĔ-tē măhl] seizure	
pia mater [PĬ-ă, PĒ-ă MĀ-tĕr, MĂH-tĕr)]	
polysomnography (PSG)[PŎL-ē-sŏm-NŎG-ră-fē]	
pons [pŏnz]	
pyrogenic [pī-rō-JĔN-ĭk] meningitis	
radiculitis [ră-dĭk-yū-LĬ-tĭs]	
receptor [rē-SĔP-tŏr]	
reflex [RĒ-flĕks]	
sciatica [sī-ĂT-ĭ-kă]	
sedative [SĔD-ă-tĭv]	
shingles	
somatic [sō-MĂT-ĭk] nervous system	

Word	Definition
somnambulism [sŏm-NĂM-byū-lĭzm]	
somnolence [SŎM-nō-lĕns]	
SPECT (single photon emission computed tomography) brain scan	
spin(o)	
spina bifida [SPĪ-nă BĬF-ĭ-dă]	
spinal cord	
spinal nerves	
stereotaxy [stēr-ē-ō-TĂK-sē]	
stimulus (pl. stimuli) [STĬM-yū-lŭs (STĬM-yū-lī)]	
stroke [strōk]	
subdural [sŭb-DŪR-ăl] space	
sulcus (pl. sulci) [SŬL-kŭs (SŬL-sī)]	
sympathetic [sĭm-pă-THĔT-ĭk] nervous system	
synapse [SĬN-ăps]	
syncope [SĬN-kō-pē]	
Tay-Sachs [TĀ-săks] disease	
temporal lobe [TĔM-pŏ-răl lōb]	
terminal end fibers	
thalam(o)	
thalamus [THĂL-ă-mŭs]	
thrombotic [thrŏm-BŎT-ĭk] stroke	
thrombus [THRŎM-bŭs]	
tics	
tonic-clonic seizure	
transcranial sonogram [trăns-KRĀ-nē-ăl SŎN-ō-grăm]	
trephination [trĕf-ĭ-NĀ-shŭn]	
Tourette [tū-RĔT] syndrome	
transient ischemic [ĭs-KĒ-mĭk] attack	
vag(o)	
vagotomy [vā-GŎT-ō-mē]	
ventral thalamus	

Word	Definition
ventricle [VĔN-trĭ-kl]	
ventricul(o)	
viral meningitis	

Abbreviation

Write the full meaning of each abbreviation.

Abbreviation	Meaning
Ach	
ALS	
BBB	
CNS	
CP	
CSF	
CT or CAT scan	
CVA	
CVD	
EEG	
ICP	
LP	
MRA	
MRI	
MS	
SAH	
TIA	

1. brainstem, frontal lobe, temporal lobe
2. symptoms may point to one or two specific disorders
3. a. dura mater, tough fibrous membrane
   b. arachnoid, weblike structure across a space.
   c. pia mater, thin membrane containing blood vessels
4. d
5. h
6. i
7. c
8. g
9. j
10. a
11. e
12. b
13. f
14. receptors
15. myelin sheath
16. dendrites
17. axon
18. medulla oblongata
19. cerebrum
20. pons
21. cranium
22. cerebrospinal fluid
23. diencephalon
24. meninges
25. thalamus
26. ganglia
27. c
28. c
29. axon
30. c
31. acetylcholine
32. neuroglia
33. cerebellum
34. Mr. Gutierrez has normal blood pressure and no history of CVA. He does, however, have neurological impairments and may well have a neurological disorder.
35. sciatic, spinal, leg
36. encephalo-, brain; myelo-, spinal cord

37. cranio-, brain; meningo-, meninges
38. glio-, neuroglia; neuro-, nerve
39. cerebro-, cerebrum; meningo-, meninges
40. spino-, spine; neur-, nerve
41. neuro-, nerve, encephalo-, brain, myelo-, spinal cord
42. vago-
43. neur-
44. glio-
45. mening-
46. encephal-, brain
47. neur-, nerve
48. cephalo-, head
49. myel-, spinal cord
50. meningo-, meninges
51. neuro-, nerve
52. cranio-, cranium
53. vago-, vagus nerve
54. glio-, neuroglia
55. cerebro-, cerebrum
56. to see how the medicine is helping improve symptoms and to adjust the dosage as necessary
57. weakened reflexes, particularly in the legs and hands
58. F
59. F
60. T
61. F
62. T
63. T
64. T
65. F
66. F
67. Once the weakness symptoms are relieved, exercise can strengthen muscles in the legs and arms.
68. dopamine
69. paralysis
70. Parkinson's
71. radiculitis
72. thrombus
73. embolus
74. coma

75. transient ischemic attack
76. absence, tonic- clonic
77. myelin
78. motor
79. g
80. h
81. I
82. j
83. d
84. c
85. f
86. e
87. b
88. a
89. spinal, brainstem
90. because Mr. Gutierrez may normalize within a short time and an overdose might cause other problems
91. craniotomy
92. craniectomy
93. trephination
94. lobotomy
95. lobectomy
96. neurorrhaphy
97. neurectomy
98. neuroplasty
99. vagus
100. cordotomy
101. Some physicians feel that the addictive nature of painkillers and the strong side effects change the patient's ability to relate normally to family.
102. a lower-calorie diet because of his lack of exercise
103. hypnotic
104. anesthetic
105. sedative
106. anticonvulsant
107. analgesics
108. narcotic
109. Alzheimer's disease
110. probably; exhaustion clouds cognitive functioning

CHAPTER 9

The Urinary System

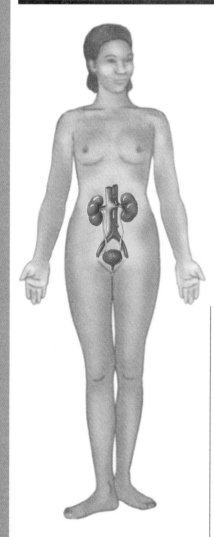

After studying this chapter, you will be able to:

- ◆ Name the parts of the urinary system and discuss the function of each part

- ◆ Define combining forms used in building words that relate to the urinary system

- ◆ Identify the meaning of related abbreviations

- ◆ Name the common diagnoses, clinical procedures, and laboratory tests used in treating disorders of the urinary system

- ◆ List and define the major pathological conditions of the urinary system

- ◆ Explain the meaning of surgical terms related to the urinary system

- ◆ Recognize common pharmacological agents used in treating the urinary system

Structure and Function

The **urinary system** (also called the *renal system* or *excretory system*) maintains the proper amount of water in the body and removes waste products from the blood by excreting them in the urine. The urinary system consists of two **kidneys,** organs that remove dissolved waste and other substances from the blood and urine; two **ureters,** tubes that transport urine from the kidneys to the bladder; the **bladder,** the organ that stores urine; and the **urethra,** a tubular structure that transports urine through the **meatus,** the external opening of a canal, to the outside of the body. Figure 9-1a shows the urinary system, and Figure 9-1b diagrams the path of urine through the system.

Kidneys

Each kidney is a bean-shaped organ about the size of a human fist, weighs about 4 to 6 ounces, and is about 12 centimeters long, 6 centimeters wide, and 3 centimeters thick. The kidneys are located in the **retroperitoneal** (posterior to the peritoneum) portion of the abdominal cavity on either side of the vertebral column. The kidneys sit against the deep muscles of the back surrounded by fatty and connective tissue. The left kidney is usually slightly higher than the right one.

The kidneys serve two functions—to form urine for excretion and to retain essential substances the body needs in the process called **reabsorption.**

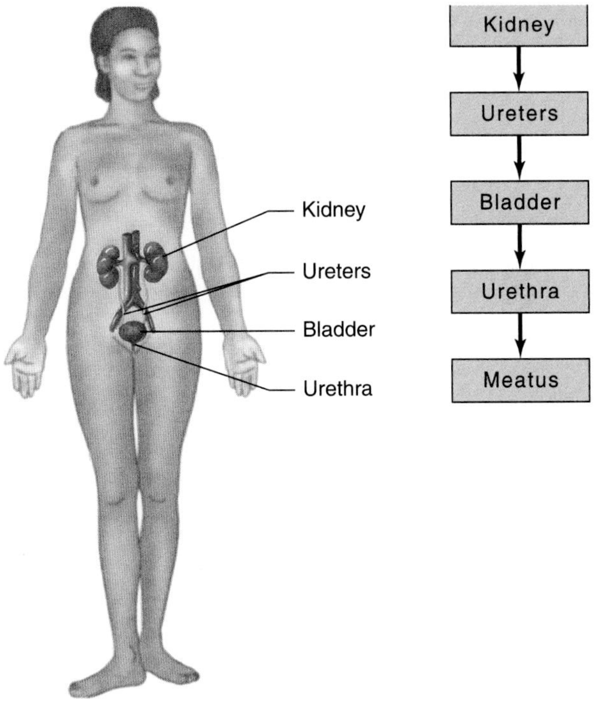

Urine is produced by **filtration** of water, salts, sugar, **urea,** and other waste materials such as **creatine** (and its component **creatinine**) and **uric acid.** Kidneys in the average adult filter about 1700 liters of blood per day.

The kidneys have an outer protective portion, the **cortex,** and an inner soft portion, the **medulla,** which is a term used for the inner, soft portion of any organ. In the middle of the concave side of the kidney is a depression, the **hilum,** through which the blood vessels, the nerves, and the ureters enter and leave. Each kidney contains about one million **nephrons.** These are units in which the kidney functions are performed. Each kidney contains more nephrons than one person needs. That is why people can live a normal life with only one kidney.

Blood enters each kidney through the *renal artery* and leaves through the *renal vein.* Once inside the kidney, the renal artery branches into smaller arteries called *arterioles.* Each arteriole leads into a nephron. Each nephron contains a *renal corpuscle* made up of a group of capillaries called a **glomerulus** (Figure 9-2). The glomerulus filters fluid from the blood and is the first place where urine is formed in the kidney. Each nephron also contains a *renal tubule,* which carries urine to ducts in the kidney's cortex. Blood flows through the kidneys at a constant rate. If the blood flow is decreased, the kidney automatically produces **renin,** a substance that causes an increase in the blood pressure in order to maintain the filtration rate of blood. The wall of each glomerulus is thin enough to allow water, salts, sugars, urea, and certain wastes to pass through. Each glomerulus is surrounded by a capsule, **Bowman's capsule,** where this fluid collects and then passes into a renal tubule. Figure 9-3 indicates the flow of blood and urine through a kidney.

The renal tubule is surrounded by tiny capillaries that allow most of the water and sugars and some of the salts to be reabsorbed back into

Kidney

Ureters

Bladder

Urethra

Meatus

Kidney

Ureters

Bladder

Urethra

Figure 9-1a The urinary system helps to maintain fluid balance in the body.

Figure 9-1b The path of urine through the system.

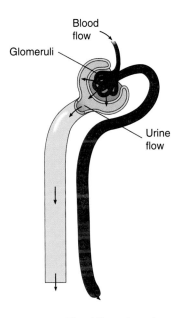

Blood flow

Glomeruli

Urine flow

Figure 9-2 Blood flows into the glomeruli where urine is excreted and moved to the kidney's cortex.

M O R E   A B O U T...

Blood Pressure and the Kidneys

The kidneys have mechanisms to maintain *homeostasis,* equilibrium, in the filtration rate of the glomeruli. The constant flow of water and its substances back into the bloodstream and the flow of water and waste substances into the renal tubule maintain the body's balance of water, salts (the most common salt in the body is sodium chloride), sugars (the most common sugar in the body is glucose), and other substances. To do this, the kidneys have two lines of defense. The first is the automatic dilating and constricting of the arterioles as needed to increase or decrease the flow of blood into the glomeruli. The second is to release renin to increase the blood pressure and the filtration rate of blood to maintain a constant supply. Maintaining homeostasis affects blood pressure either by lowering it when blood is flowing too quickly or by increasing it when blood is flowing too slowly. Some forms of high blood pressure result from the effort of poorly functioning kidneys to maintain homeostasis.

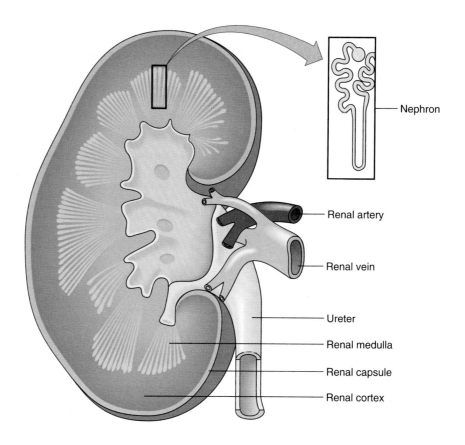

- Nephron
- Renal artery
- Renal vein
- Ureter
- Renal medulla
- Renal capsule
- Renal cortex

Latin *urina* and Greek *ouron* both mean urine. Greek *oureter,* urinary canal, is the source of the word *ureter.*

the bloodstream. The remaining fluid, **urine,** contains water, salts, some urea, and uric acid. It travels to the **renal pelvis,** a collecting area in the center of the kidney. *Pelvis* is a general term for the collecting area of an organ or system. The renal pelvis contains small cuplike structures called **calices** that collect urine before passing it into the ureter.

Ureters

Attached to each kidney is a *ureter,* a tube (usually 6 to 7 inches [about 16 to 18 centimeters] long) that transports urine from the renal pelvis to the urinary bladder. The two ureters are made up of three layers of tissue—smooth muscle, fibrous tissue, and a mucous layer. *Peristalsis,* a rhythmic contraction of the smooth muscle, helps to move urine into the urinary bladder. It travels in waves similar to the progression of digested food through the intestines.

Bladder

The **urinary bladder** is a hollow, muscular organ that stores urine until it is ready to be excreted from the body. *Bladder* is a general term meaning a receptacle. Urine is pumped into the bladder every few seconds. The *sphincter muscles,* muscles that encircle a duct to contract or expand the duct, hold the urine in place. Control of urination has to be taught to young children (usually between the ages of one and three), while in adults it is usually easily controlled. The bladder can hold from 300 to 400 milliliters of urine before emptying. The bladder's walls contain epithelial tissue that can stretch and allow the bladder to hold twice as much as it does when normally full. The walls also contain three layers of muscle that help in the emptying process. The base of the bladder contains a triangular area, the **trigone,** where the ureters enter the bladder and the urethra exits it. Figure 9-4 shows the bladder with ureters entering and the urethra exiting.

Urethra

Urine is excreted outside the body through the *urethra*, a tube of smooth muscle with a mucous lining. The female urethra is only about 1.5 inches long. It opens through the meatus, which is located at the distal end of the urethra between the clitoris and the vagina. The male urethra is about 8 inches long and passes through three different regions. The first region is the **prostate,** a gland where the urethra and the ejaculatory duct meet. Thus, the urethra in the male is part of the urinary system as well as part of the reproductive system. The second region is a membranous portion, after which urine passes into the third part, the penis, and is excreted through the meatus at the distal end of the penis. Excreting urine is called *voiding* or *micturition*.

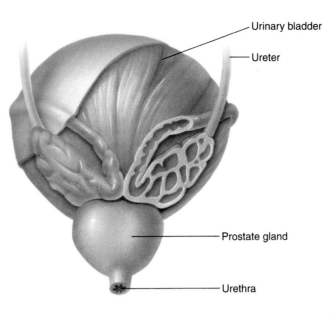

Urinary bladder
Ureter
Prostate gland
Urethra

Figure 9-4 **Both the male and female urinary bladders store urine to be released into the urethra to exit the body.**

Vocabulary Review

In the previous section, you learned terms relating to the urinary system. Before going on to the exercises, review the terms below and refer to the previous section if you have any questions.

Terms	Word Analysis	Definition
bladder	[BLĂD-ĕr] Old English blaedre	Organ where urine collects before being excreted from the body.
Bowman's capsule	After Sir William Bowman (1816–1892), English anatomist.	Capsule surrounding a glomerulus and serving as a collection site for urine.
calices, calyces (sing. calix, calyx)	[KĂL-ĭ-sēz (KĂ-lĭks)] From Greek *kalyx*, cup of a flower	Cup-shaped structures in the renal pelvis for the collection of urine.
cortex	[KŌR-tĕks] Latin, bark	Outer portion of the kidney.
creatine	[KRĒ-ă-tēn] From Greek *kreas*, flesh	Substance found in urine; elevated levels may indicate muscular dystrophy.

Terms	Word Analysis	Definition
creatinine	[krē-ĂT-ĭ-nēn]	A component of creatine.
filtration	[fĭl-TRĀ-shŭn]	Process of separating solids from a liquid by passing it through a porous substance.
glomerulus (pl. glomeruli)	[glō-MĂR-yū-lŭs (glō-MĂR-yū-lĭ)] From Latin *glomus*, ball of yarn	Group of capillaries in a nephron.
hilum	[HĪ-lŭm] Latin, a small bit	Portion of the kidney where blood vessels and nerves enter and exit.
kidney	[KĬD-nē]	Organ that forms urine and reabsorbs essential substances back into the bloodstream.
meatus	[mē-Ă-tŭs] Latin, passage	External opening of a canal, such as the urethra.
medulla	[mě-DŪL-ă] Latin, marrow	Soft, central portion of the kidney.
nephron	[NĚF-rŏn] From Greek *nephros*, kidney	Functional unit of a kidney.
prostate	[PRŎS-tāt] Greek *prostates*, one that protects	Gland surrounding the urethra in the male; active in ejaculation of semen.
reabsorption	[rē-ăb-SŎRB-shŭn] re-, again + absorption	Process of returning essential elements to the bloodstream after filtration.
renal pelvis		Collecting area for urine in the center of the kidney.
renin	[RĚ-nĭn] Latin *ren*, kidney	Enzyme produced in the kidneys to regulate the filtration rate of blood by increasing blood pressure as necessary.
retroperitoneal	[RĚ-trō-PĚR-ĭ-tō-nē-ăl] retro-, behind + peritoneal	Posterior to the peritoneum.
trigone	[TRĪ-gōn] Latin *trigonum*, triangle	Triangular area at the base of the bladder through which the ureters enter and the urethra exits the bladder.
urea	[yū-RĒ-ă] Greek *ouron*, urine	Waste product of nitrogen metabolism excreted in normal adult urine.

Terms	Word Analysis	Definition
ureter	[yū-RĒ-tĕr] Greek *oureter*, urinary canal	One of two tubes that conducts urine from the kidney to the bladder.
urethra	[yū-RĒ-thră] Greek *ourethra*	Tube through which urine is transported from the bladder to the exterior of the body.
uric acid	[YŪR-ĭk] ur-, urine + -ic, pertaining to	Nitrogenous waste excreted in the urine.
urinary bladder	[YŪR-ĭ-nār-ē]	*See* bladder.
urinary system		Body system that forms and excretes urine and helps in the reabsorption of essential substances.
urine	[YŪR-ĭn] Greek *ouron*, urine	Fluid excreted by the urinary system.

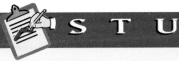

CASE STUDY

Visiting a Clinic

Central Valley HMO is located in a large medical office building next to a hospital complex. The first floor is a large clinic where patients are evaluated first. Later, they may be referred to specialists located in the same building.

Three of the morning patients complained of problems relating to the urinary system. The first, Mr. Delgado, was having difficulty urinating. The second, Ms. Margolis, showed blood in her urine, and the third, Ms. Jones, complained of frequent, painful urination. All three were seen by Dr. Chorzik, a family practitioner employed by the HMO.

 Critical Thinking

1. Is blood normally seen in the urine? Why or why not?

2. Does the fact that Mr. Delgado and Ms. Jones are of different sexes make the diagnosis of their urinary problems different?

Structure and Function Exercises

Check Your Knowledge

Fill in the blanks.

3. Urine is transported within the urinary system via the _____.

4. Urine is transported to the outside of the body via the _____.

5. Each kidney has about one million _____.

6. The renal corpuscle contains a mass of capillaries termed a _____.

7. The collecting area in the center of the kidney is called the _____ _____.

8. The return of essential substances to the bloodstream is called _____.

9. The urethra draws urine from the _____.

10. Two words meaning excreting urine are _____ and _____.

11. A fluid collection site in a nephron is called a _____ _____.

12. A triangular area at the base of the bladder is called a _____.

Check Your Accuracy

Circle T for true or F for false.

13. The loss of one kidney is fatal. T F

14. The urethra transports urine from the kidney to the bladder. T F

15. Most of the water and sugar filtered in the kidney are reabsorbed. T F

16. Renin increases blood flow through the kidneys. T F

17. Two fluid collection sites within the kidney are the calices and the Bowman's capsule. T F

18. The female urethra is longer than the male urethra. T F

19. The female urethra opens into the vagina. T F

20. The prostrate gland ejects semen into the male urethra. T F

21. The left kidney is usually slightly higher than the right one. T F

22. Blood flows through the kidney at varying intervals. T F

Go with the Flow

Put the following steps, which describe the flow of urine, in order by placing the letters a–h in the space provided.

23. Urine flows from the ureters into the bladder.___

24. Fluid collects in the Bowman's capsule.___

25. Urine flows through the renal tubules to ducts in the kidney. ___

26. Urine exits the body. ___

27. Urine flows from the bladder to the urethra. ___

28. Urine flows from the kidneys into the ureter. ___

29. Fluid flows from the glomerulus to the renal tubule. ___

Combining Forms and Abbreviations

The lists below include combining forms and abbreviations that relate specifically to the urinary system. Pronunciations are provided for the examples.

Combining Forms	Meaning	Examples
cali(o), calic(o)	calix	*calioplasty* [KĂ-lē-ō-plăs-tē], surgical reconstruction of a calix
cyst(o)	bladder	*cystitis* [sĭs-TĪ-tĭs], bladder inflammation.
glomerul(o)	glomerulus	*glomerulitis* [glō-MĀR-yū-LĪ-tĭs], inflammation of the glomeruli
meato	meatus	*meatotomy* [mē-ă-TŎT-ō-mē], surgical enlargement of the meatus
nephr(o)	kidney	*nephritis* [nĕ-FRĪ-tĭs], kidney inflammation
pyel(o)	renal pelvis	*pyeloplasty* [PĪ-ĕ-lō-plăs-tē], surgical repair of the renal pelvis
ren(o)	kidney	*renomegaly* [RĒ-nō-MĔG-ă-lē], enlargement of the kidney
trigon(o)	trigone	*trigonitis* [TRĪ-gō-NĪ-tĭs], inflammation of the trigone of the bladder
ur(o), urin(o)	urine	*uremia* [yū-RĒ-mē-ă], excess of urea and other wastes in the blood
ureter(o)	ureter	*ureterostenosis* [yū-RĒ-tĕr-ō-stĕ-NŌ-sĭs], narrowing of a ureter
urethr(o)	urethra	*urethrorrhea* [yū-rē-thrō-RĒ-ă], abnormal discharge from the urethra
vesic(o)	bladder	*vesicoabdominal* [VĔS-ĭ-kō-ăb-DŎM-ĭ-năl], relating to the urinary bladder and the abdominal wall

Abbreviation	Meaning	Abbreviation	Meaning
ADH	antidiuretic hormone	ARF	acute renal failure
A/G	albumin/globulin	ATN	acute tubular necrosis
AGN	acute glomerulonephritis	BNO	bladder neck obstruction

Abbreviation	Meaning	Abbreviation	Meaning
BUN	blood urea nitrogen	K+	potassium
CAPD	continuous ambulatory peritoneal dialysis	KUB	kidney, ureter, bladder
Cath	catheter	Na+	sodium
Cl	chlorine	pH	power of hydrogen concentration
CRF	chronic renal failure	PKU	phenylketonuria
cysto	cystoscopy	RP	retrograde pyelogram
ESRD	end-stage renal disease	SG	specific gravity
ESWL	extracorporeal shock wave lithotripsy	UA	urinalysis
HD	hemodialysis	UTI	urinary tract infection
IVP	intravenous pyelogram	VCU, VCUG	voiding cystourethrogram

C A S E   S T U D Y

Using Tests for Diagnosis

Dr. Chorzik ordered a urinalysis for each of the three patients. The results give some clues to a possible diagnosis.

 Critical Thinking

30. Whose tests had the most abnormal readings?

31. Spell out at least three of the items being tested for.

Meadow Health Systems, Inc.
1420 Glen Road
Meadowvale, OK 44444

Run Date: 09/22/XX
Run Time: 1507
111-222-3333

Page 1
Specimen Report

Patient: James Carlton
Reg Dr: S. Anders, M.D.

Acct #: A994584732
Age/Sx: 55/M
Status: Reg ER

Loc: ED
Room:
Bed:

U #:
Reg: 09/22/XX
Des:

Spec #: 0922 : U0009A

Coll: 09/22/XX
Recd.: 09/22/XX

Status: Comp
Subm Dr:

Req #: 77744444

Entered: 09/22/XX–0841
Ordered: UA with micro
Comments: Urine Description: Clean catch urine

Other Dr:

Test	Result	Flag	Reference
Urinalysis			
UA with micro			
COLOR	YELLOW		
APPEARANCE	HAZY	**	
SP GRAVITY	1.018		1.001-1.030
GLUCOSE	NORMAL		NORMAL mg/dl
BILIRUBIN	NEGATIVE		NEG
KETONE	NEGATIVE		NEG mg/dl
BLOOD	2+	**	NEG
PH	5.0		4.5-8.0
PROTEIN	TRACE	**	NEG mg/dl
UROBILINOGEN	NORMAL		NORMAL-1.0 mg/dl
NITRITES	NEGATIVE		NEG
LEUKOCYTES	2+	**	NEG
WBC	20-50	**	0-5 /HPF
RBC	2-5		0-5 /HPF
EPI CELLS	20-50		/HPF
BACTERIA	2+	**	
MUCUS			

Patient 1

Meadow Health Systems, Inc.
1420 Glen Road

Run Date: 09/22/XX   Meadowvale, OK 44444   Page 1
Run Time: 1507   111-222-3333   Specimen Report

Patient: Sarah Haupt	Acct #: E005792849	Loc:	U #:
Reg Dr: S. Anders, M.D.	Age/Sx: 45/F	Room:	Reg: 09/22/XX
	Status: Reg ER	Bed:	Des:

Spec #: 0922 : U00010R	Coll: 09/22/XX	Status: Comp	Req #: 00704181
	Recd.: 09/22/XX	Subm Dr:	

Entered: 09/22/XX–0936
Other Dr:
Ordered: UA with micro
Comments: Urine Description: Clean catch urine

Test	Result	Flag	Reference
Urinalysis			
UA with micro			
COLOR	YELLOW		
APPEARANCE	CLEAR		
SP GRAVITY	1.017		1.001-1.030
GLUCOSE	NORMAL		NORMAL mg/dl
BILIRUBIN	NEGATIVE		NEG
KETONE	NEGATIVE		NEG mg/dl
BLOOD	TRACE	**	NEG
PH	5.0		4.5-8.0
PROTEIN	NEGATIVE		NEG mg/dl
UROBILINOGEN	NORMAL		NORMAL-1.0 mg/dl
NITRITES	NEGATIVE		NEG
LEUKOCYTES	NEGATIVE		NEG
WBC	NO CELLS		0-5 /HPF
RBC	2-5		0-5 /HPF
EPI CELLS	0-2		/HPF
MUCUS	1+		

Patient 2

Meadow Health Systems, Inc.
1420 Glen Road

Run Date: 09/22/XX   Meadowvale, OK 44444   Page 1
Run Time: 1507   111-222-3333   Specimen Report

Patient: Consuela Diaz	Acct #: F009435543	Loc:	U #:
Reg Dr: S. Anders, M.D.	Age/Sx: 35/F	Room:	Reg: 09/22/XX
	Status: Reg ER	Bed:	Des:

Spec #: 0922 : U0008A	Coll: 09/22/XX	Status: Comp	Req #: 00704876
	Recd.: 09/22/XX	Subm Dr:	

Entered: 09/22/XX–0925
Other Dr:
Ordered: UA with micro
Comments: Urine Description: Clean catch urine

Test	Result	Flag	Reference
Urinalysis			
UA with micro			
COLOR	YELLOW		
APPEARANCE	CLEAR		
SP GRAVITY	1.017		1.001-1.030
GLUCOSE	NORMAL		NORMAL mg/dl
BILIRUBIN	NEGATIVE		NEG
KETONE	NEGATIVE		NEG mg/dl
BLOOD	NEGATIVE		NEG
PH	5.0		4.5-8.0
PROTEIN	NEGATIVE		NEG mg/dl
UROBILINOGEN	NORMAL		NORMAL-1.0 mg/dl
NITRITES	NEGATIVE		NEG
LEUKOCYTES	NEGATIVE		NEG
WBC	NO CELLS		0-5 /HPF
RBC	2-5		0-5 /HPF
EPI CELLS	0-2		/HPF
MUCUS	1+		

Patient 3

Combining Forms and Abbreviations Exercises

Build Your Medical Vocabulary

Complete the words by adding combining forms, suffixes, or prefixes you have learned in this chapter and in Chapters 2 and 3.

32. Lack of urination: _____uresis

33. Inflammation of the renal pelvis: _____itis

34. Excessive urination: _____uria

35. Kidney disease: _____pathy

36. Scanty urination: olig_____

37. Bladder paralysis: _____plegia

38. Lipids in the urine: lip_____

39. Abnormally large bladder: mega_____

40. Relating to the bladder and the urethra: vesico_____al

41. Kidney enlargement: reno_____

42. Inflammation of the tissues surrounding the bladder: _____cystitis

43. Medical specialty concerned with kidney disease: _____logy

44. Inflammation of the renal pelvis and other kidney parts: pyelo_____itis

45. Suturing of a calix: calio_____

46. Between the two kidneys: inter_____

47. Abnormal urethral discharge: urethro_____

48. Hemorrhage from a ureter: _____rrhagia

49. Softening of the kidneys: nephro_____

50. Within the urinary bladder: _____cystic

51. Removal of a kidney stone: _____litho_____

52. Imaging of the kidney: _____graphy

53. Kidney-shaped: reni____

Root Out the Meaning

Divide the following words into parts. Write the urinary combining forms in the space at the right and define the word shown.

54. glomerulonephritis _____

55. nephrocystosis _____

56. urethrostenosis _____

57. ureterovesicostomy _____

58. urocyanosis _____

59. urolithology _____

60. pyeloureterecstasis _____

61. calicotomy _____

62. cystolithotomy _____

63. nephroma _____

64. meatorrhaphy _____

65. nephrosclerosis _____

66. renopulmonary _____

67. trigonitis _____

Find the Right Words

Define the following abbreviations.

68. ADH

69. pH

70. CAPD

71. VCU

72. HD

73. PKU

74. BUN

75. KUB

76. ESWL

77. UTI

78. RP

Diagnostic, Procedural, and Laboratory Terms

Specialists in the urinary system are *urologists*, who specialize in disorders of the male and female urinary tracts and the male reproductive system, and *nephrologists*, who specialize in disorders of the kidneys. **Urinalysis** is the most common diagnostic and laboratory test of the urinary system. It involves the examination of urine for the presence of normal or abnormal amounts of various elements. Substances in the urine are a prime factor in the diagnosis of diseases of the urinary system as well as of other body systems. In addition, various imaging and blood tests help diagnose conditions or diseases.

Urinalysis

Urinalysis is the examination of urine for its physical and chemical properties (Figure 9-5). Urine is gathered from clients who fill a specimen bottle by themselves or whose urine is obtained by *urinary catheterization*, the insertion of a flexible tube through the meatus and into the urinary bladder. Some patients do not have bladder control or may have certain conditions that require catheters to aid in urination. A **Foley catheter** (Figure 9-6) is

Many employers routinely require all job applicants to undergo drug testing. The most common test is a urinalysis to detect the presence of illegal substances.

Figure 9-5 Urinalysis is a crucial diagnostic test. Dissolved wastes in the urine may reveal any of a number of diseases. For example, in the test results shown here, the patient's glucose is higher than normal, indicating possible diabetes.

	Meadow Health Systems, Inc.		
	1420 Glen Road		
Run Date: 02/22/XX	Meadowvale, OK 44444		Page 1
Run Time: 1632	111-222-3333		Specimen Report

Patient: Maria Bozutti	Acct #: C038642	Loc:	U #:
Reg Dr: S. Anders, M.D.	Age/Sx: 28/F	Room:	Reg: 02/22/XX
	Status: Reg ER	Bed:	Des:

Spec #: 0222 : U00022	Coll: 02/22/XX	Status: Comp	Req #: 77744590
	Recd.: 02/22/XX	Subm Dr:	

Entered: 02/22/XX–0841   Other Dr:
Ordered: UA with micro
Comments: Urine Description: Clean catch urine

Test	Result	Flag	Reference
Urinalysis			
UA with micro			
COLOR	YELLOW		
APPEARANCE	HAZY		
SP GRAVITY	1.018		1.001-1.030
GLUCOSE	NORMAL		NORMAL mg/dl
BILIRUBIN	NEGATIVE		NEG
KETONE	NEGATIVE		NEG mg/dl
BLOOD	NEGATIVE		NEG
PH	5.0		4.5-8.0
PROTEIN	NEGATIVE		NEG mg/dl
UROBILINOGEN	NORMAL		NORMAL-1.0 mg/dl
NITRITES	NEGATIVE		NEG
LEUKOCYTES	NEGATIVE		NEG
WBC	3		0-5 /HPF
RBC	3.5		0-5 /HPF
EPI CELLS	20-50		/HPF
BACTERIA	NEGATIVE		
MUCUS			

indwelling (left in the bladder) and is held in place by a balloon inflated in the bladder. Foley catheters are also known as *retention catheters*. Other types of catheters may be disposable units. **Condom catheters** (also called *Texas catheters, external urinary drainage [EUD] catheters,* or *latex catheters*) are changed at least once a day (Figure 9-7). A condom catheter consists of a rubber sheath placed over the penis with tubing connected to a drainage or leg bag where the urine collects.

Various properties of urine help in diagnosing certain conditions. The color, odor, and clarity of urine give certain diagnostic clues. Normal urine is straw-colored and clear. Blood in the urine may darken it, or show up clearly as blood. Pus or infection may make the urine cloudy. The normal **pH** range of urine is from 4.5 to 8.0. A reading above 7 indicates alkaline urine; a reading below 7 indicates acid urine. Alkaline urine may indicate the presence of a bladder infection. Also examined in urine are **casts,** which are formed when protein accumulates in the urine. This may indicate the presence of kidney disease. The casts are often composed of pus or fats. The amount of wastes, minerals, and solids in urine is measured as the **specific gravity.** Low specific gravity may indicate kidney disease, and high specific gravity may indicate diabetes. High uric acid may indicate gout, a metabolic disorder. Appendix C gives the chemical analyses and ranges commonly used in urinalysis.

In addition, tests of urine are designed to detect various substances indicative of specific conditions. The presence of high quantities of **acetones** usually occurs in diabetes. **Ketones** in the urine may indicate starvation or diabetes. Ketones in the urine can lead to dangerously high levels of acid in the blood, a potential cause of coma and/or death. The presence of the serum protein **albumin** in urine may indicate a leakage of protein from the blood. **Glucose** in the urine usually indicates diabetes. Pus in the urine makes the urine cloudy and indicates an infection or inflammation in the urinary system. Bacteria in the urine indicates a specific bacterial infection. Blood in the urine usually indicates bleeding in the urinary tract. Calcium in the urine is abnormal and indicates one of several conditions, such as rickets. **Bilirubin** in the urine indicates liver disease, such as obstructive disease of the biliary tract and liver cancer. **Phenylketones (PKU)** in the urine show a lack of an important enzyme that can lead to mental retardation in infants unless a strict diet is followed into adulthood. Infants are routinely tested for this deficiency at birth by taking a blood sample (using a heel stick), which is analyzed for presence of the enzyme.

Blood Tests

Two important blood tests of kidney function are the *blood urea nitrogen (BUN)* and the *creatinine clearance test.* The presence of high amounts of urea or creatinine in the kidney shows that the kidney is not filtering these substances properly. If this is not treated and kidney failure persists, death may result.

Imaging Tests

Various tests are used to visually diagnose stones, growths, obstructions, or abnormalities in the urinary system. A *cystoscopy* is the insertion of a tubular instrument (a **cystoscope**) to examine the bladder with a light (Figure 9-8). An *intravenous pyelogram (IVP)* and an *intravenous urogram* are x-rays of the urinary tract after a contrast medium is injected into the bloodstream. A **kidney,**

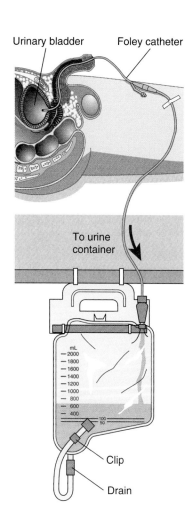

Figure 9-6 A Foley catheter remains in place; the collection bag is drained and cleaned.

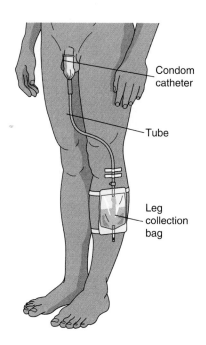

Figure 9-7 A condom catheter is changed daily.

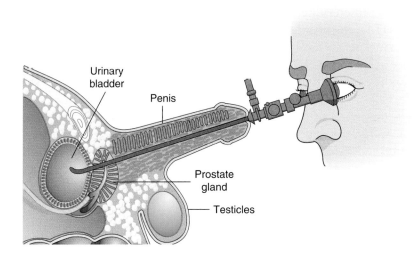

ureter, bladder (**KUB**) is an x-ray of three parts of the urinary tract. A *renal angiogram* is an x-ray of the renal artery after a contrast medium is injected into the artery. A **retrograde pyelogram (RP)** is an x-ray of the kidney, bladder, and ureters taken after a cystoscope is used to introduce a contrast medium. A **voiding (urinating) cystourethrogram (VCU, VCUG)** is an x-ray taken during urination to examine the flow of urine through the system. An *abdominal sonogram* is the production of an image of the urinary tract using sound waves.

Radioactive imaging is also used to diagnose kidney disorders via a *renal scan*. A **renogram** is used to study kidney function.

Urinary Tract Procedures

Certain procedures, particularly **dialysis,** can mechanically maintain kidney or renal function when kidney failure occurs. **Hemodialysis** is the process of filtering blood outside the body in an artificial kidney machine and returning it to the body after filtering (Figure 9-9). **Peritoneal dialysis** is the insertion and removal of a dialysis solution into the peritoneal cavity (Figure 9-10).

Figure 9-9 **Hemodialysis is the removal of waste from the bloodstream by passing blood through a filtering machine.**

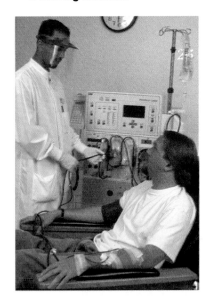

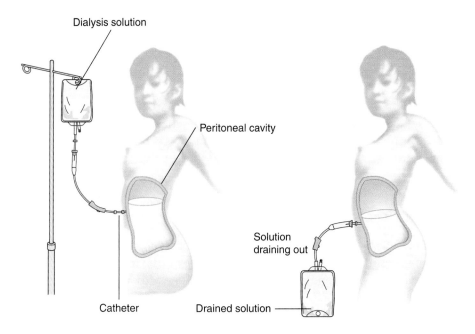

Figure 9-10 **In peritoneal dialysis, the inserted fluid stays in the peritoneal cavity for about 6 hours until it is drained out through the opening in the peritoneum.**

The action of this type of dialysis causes the wastes in the capillaries of the peritoneum to be released and drained out of the body. Peritoneal dialysis is used for patients who are able to have dialysis while ambulatory. The patient attaches a bag containing the dialysis solution to an opening in the peritoneum and fills the peritoneal cavity. Once empty, the bag is removed and replaced by a drainage bag into which the solution flows gradually.

Extracorporeal shock wave lithotripsy (ESWL) is the breaking up of urinary stones by using shock waves from outside the body. Figure 9-11 shows a patient undergoing this procedure. The stones are broken into fragments that can then pass through the urine. This procedure is often used for kidney stones.

Figure 9-11 ESWL is the use of shock waves to break up urinary stones.

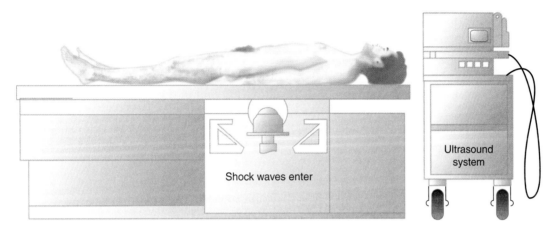

Shock waves enter

Ultrasound system

Vocabulary Review

In the previous section, you learned terms relating to diagnosis, clinical procedures, and laboratory tests. Before going on to the exercises, review the terms below and refer to the previous section if you have any questions.

Terms	Word Analysis	Definition
acetone	[ĂS-ĕ-tōn]	Type of ketone normally found in urine in small quantities; found in larger quantities in diabetic urine.
albumin	[ăl-BYŪ-mǐn] Latin *albumen*, egg white	Simple protein; when leaked into urine, may indicate a kidney problem.
bilirubin	[bǐl-ǐ-RŪ-bǐn] bil(e) + Latin *ruber*, red	Substance produced in the liver; elevated levels may indicate liver disease or hepatitis when found in urine.
casts		materials formed in urine when protein accumulates; may indicate renal disease.
condom catheter	[KĂTH-ĕ-tĕr]	Disposable catheter for urinary sample collection or incontinence.

Terms	Word Analysis	Definition
cystoscope	[SĬS-tō-skōp] cysto-, bladder + -scope, instrument for viewing	Tubular instrument for examining the interior of the bladder.
dialysis	[dī-ĂL-ĭ-sĭs] Greek, a separation	Method of filtration used when kidneys fail.
extracorporeal shock wave lithotripsy (ESWL)		Breaking of kidney stones by using shock waves from outside the body.
Foley catheter	After F. E. B. Foley (1891–1966), American urologist	Indwelling catheter held in place by a balloon that inflates inside the bladder.
glucose	[GLŪ-kōs] Greek *gleukos*, sweetness	Form of sugar found in the blood; may indicate diabetes when found in the urine.
hemodialysis	[HĒ-mō-dī-ĂL-ĭ-sĭs] hemo-, blood + dialysis	Dialysis performed by passing blood through a filter outside the body and returning filtered blood to the body.
indwelling	[ĬN-dwĕ-lĭng] in + dwelling	Of a type of catheter inserted into the body.
ketone	[KĒ-tōn]	Substance that results from the breakdown of fat; indicates diabetes or starvation when present in the urine.
kidney, ureter, bladder (KUB)		X-ray of three parts of the urinary system.
peritoneal dialysis	[PĔR-ĭ-tō-NĒ-ăl]	Type of dialysis in which liquid that extracts substances from blood is inserted into the peritoneal cavity and emptied outside the body.
pH		Measurement of the acidity or alkalinity of a solution such as urine.
phenylketones	[FĔN-ĭl-KĒ-tōns]	Substances that, if accumulated in the urine of infants, indicate phenylketonuria, a disease treated by diet.
renogram	[RĒ-nō-grăm] reno-, kidney + -gram, a recording	Radioactive imaging of kidney function after introduction of a substance that is filtered through the kidney while it is observed.
retrograde pyelogram (RP)	[RĔT-rō-grād PĪ-ĕl-ō-grăm]	X-ray of the bladder and ureters after a contrast medium is injected into the bladder.

Terms	Word Analysis	Definition
specific gravity		Measurement of the concentration of wastes, minerals, and solids in urine.
urinalysis	[yū-rĭ-NĂL-ĭ-sĭs] urin-, urine + (an)alysis	Examination of the properties of urine.
voiding (urinating) cystourethrogram (VCU, VCUG)	[sĭs-tō-yū-RĒ-thrō-grăm]	X-ray image made after introduction of a contrast medium and while urination is taking place.

C A S E   S T U D Y

Examining the Symptoms

Ms. Jones is a 77-year-old female who complained to Dr. Chorzik of painful, scanty, and frequent urination for the past two days. She says that she normally drinks 7 to 8 glasses of water a day, but lately has cut down because of the frequent urination. Her urine was cloudy with a strong odor.

Critical Thinking

79. What did the cloudy urine most likely indicate?

80. What might be present in cloudy urine to indicate infection?

Diagnostic, Procedural, and Laboratory Terms Exercises

Find the Test

In the space provided, put Y for those properties or substances tested for in urinalysis and N for those substances that are not tested for in urinalysis.

81. glucose _____

82. sodium _____

83. albumin _____

84. cholesterol _____

85. protein _____

86. lipids _____

87. specific gravity _____

88. pH _____

89. bilirubin _____

90. acetone _____

91. phenylketones _____

92. ketones _____

93. homocysteine _____

Finish the Thought

Fill in the blanks.

94. Removing wastes from the blood outside the body is called _____.

95. Removing wastes from the peritoneal cavity using a portable apparatus is called _____ _____.

96. A type of indwelling catheter is (a) _____ catheter.

97. A catheter changed at least once a day is called a(n)_____ catheter.

98. Two substances found in the urine that may indicate diabetes are _____ and _____.

99. Lithotripsy is used to break up _____ that have formed.

100. Solids found in urine are called _____.

101. Dialysis is a method of _____ used in _____ failure.

102. Kidney disorders may be diagnosed by blood tests such as the _____ _____ _____ or

_____ _____ _____.

103. An x-ray image taken during urination is a(n) ____ _____.

Pathological Terms

Infections can occur anywhere in the urinary tract. A **urinary tract infection (UTI)** commonly refers to a bladder or urethra infection. Symptoms include painful and frequent urination and a general feeling of malaise (general discomfort). Treatment generally includes antibiotics. Fully emptying the bladder during urination, adequate water intake, and careful maintenance of cleanliness around the urethra can help in preventing UTIs.

Hardened lumps of matter (*calculi* or *stones*) tend to form in the kidneys and other parts of the urinary system. If possible, the stones are allowed to pass into the urine. The patient's urine is then filtered through something (such as gauze) that retains the solid material. The solid material is analyzed for content, and a diet or medication is prescribed to prevent the occurrence of further stones. Kidney stones are also known as *nephrolithiasis.*

Nephritis is the general term for inflammation of the kidney. **Glomerulonephritis** refers to a kidney inflammation located in the glomerulus. This inflammation, known as **Bright's disease,** can be acute, as after a systemic infection, or may become chronic. When chronic, high blood pressure, kidney failure, and other conditions can result. *Interstitial nephritis* is an inflammation of the connective tissue between the renal tubules. **Pyelitis** is an inflammation of the renal pelvis. *Pyelonephritis* is a bacterial infection in the renal pelvis with abscesses. **Nephrosis** or *nephrotic syndrome* is a group of symptoms usually following or related to another illness that causes protein loss in the urine (**proteinuria**). **Edema** (swelling) may result from this syndrome (Figure 9-12). Such swelling may adversely affect blood pressure. **Hydronephrosis** is the collection of urine in the kidneys without release due to a blockage. **Polycystic kidney disease** is a progressive, hereditary condition in which numerous kidney cysts form that can cause other conditions in adults, such as high blood pressure and excess blood and waste in the urine. *Renal hypertension* may result from other kidney or systemic diseases. **Kidney** *(renal)* **failure,** the loss of kidney function, may result from other conditions—some chronic, such as diabetes, and some acute, such as a kidney infection. Kidney failure can be treated with dialysis and medications. **Uremia** and **azotemia,** excesses of urea and other wastes in the blood, may result from kidney failure. **End-stage renal disease (ESRD)** is severe, and fatal if not treated. *Renal cell carcinoma* or kidney cancer is usually treated by surgery. **Wilms' tumor** or a **nephroblastoma** is a malignant tumor of the kidneys found primarily in children. It is usually treated with surgery, radiation, and chemotherapy. A **nephroma** is any renal tumor.

Cystitis is an inflammation of the bladder. Aside from urinary tract infections, the bladder may be the site of **bladder cancer.** Various tumors can be removed or treated. In cases of extensive malignancy, the bladder may need to be surgically removed. Other bladder problems include a **cystocele,** a hernia of the bladder, and a **cystolith,** a stone in the bladder.

Inflammations can also occur in the urethra (*urethritis*), the urethra and bladder together (*urethrocystitis*), or the ureters (*ureteritis*). *Urethral stenosis* is a narrowing of the urethra that causes voiding difficulties.

Difficulties in urination are often a symptom of another systemic disease, such as diabetes, or a localized infection (UTI). Such difficulties can include no urine output (**anuresis** or *urinary retention,* **anuria**), painful urination (**dysuria**), lack of bladder control (**enuresis,** including *nocturnal enuresis,* nighttime bed-wetting), frequent nighttime urination (**nocturia**), scanty urination (**oliguria**), excessive urination (**polyuria**), or urination during sneezing or coughing (*stress incontinence*). The general term **incontinence** refers to the involuntary discharge of urine or feces.

Abnormal substances or specific levels of substances in the urine indicate either urinary tract disorders or

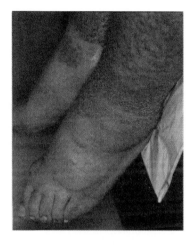

Figure 9-12 **Edema is swelling caused by fluid retention.**

M O R E   A B O U T...

Bed-wetting

Some children, particularly boys, may wet their beds at night (a condition called *nocturnal enuresis*) up to their teenage years. For years, parents have tried everything from humiliation, restricting fluids, and waking children in the middle of the night, to some sort of shock therapy, such as awakening with a loud sound when wetting occurs. Most of these methods have not worked. Usually the problem resolves by itself by the teenage years or earlier. In most cases, the children are found to have immature development of the urinary tract, allergies, or such sound sleep habits that they are unable to awaken.

systemic disorders. Some can be minor infections or major problems. **Albuminuria** or *proteinuria* indicates the presence of albumin in the urine; **hematuria** indicates the presence of blood in the urine. **Ketonuria** indicates the presence of ketone bodies in the urine. **Pyuria** indicates the presence of pus and white blood cells in the urine.

Diabetes is a name for several metabolic diseases that both affect, and are diagnosed in part, through observation of the urinary system. Diabetes is covered in detail in Chapter 15, The Endocrine System.

Many congenital problems can occur in the urinary system. Surgery can correct many of these. Hypospadias is a congenital problem and is discussed in Chapters 10 and 11. It is a defect in which the urinary meatus opens at a place other than the distal end of the penis in males or between the clitoris and vagina in females. **Atresia** (narrowing) of the ureters or urethra may also be present at birth.

Vocabulary Review

In the previous section, you learned terms relating to pathology. Before going on to the exercises, review the terms below and refer to the previous section if you have any questions.

Terms	Word Analysis	Definition
albuminuria	[ăl-byū-mĭ-NŪ-rē-ă] albumin + -uria, urine	Presence of albumin in urine, usually indicative of disease.
anuresis	[ăn-yū-RĒ-sĭs] an-, without + Greek *ouresis*, urination	Abnormal retention of urine.
anuria	[ăn-YŪ-rē-ă] an- + -uria	Lack of urine formation.
atresia	[ă-TRĒ-zē-ă] a-, without + Greek *tresis*, hole	Abnormal narrowing, as of the ureters or urethra.
azotemia	[ăz-ō-TĒ-mē-ă] French *azote*, nitrogen + -emia, blood	*See* uremia.
bladder cancer		Malignancy of the bladder.
Bright's disease	After Richard Bright (1789–1858), English internist	Inflammation of the glomeruli that can result in kidney failure.
cystitis	[sĭs-TĪ-tĭs] cyst-, bladder + -itis, inflammation	Inflammation of the bladder.

Terms	Word Analysis	Definition
cystocele	[SĬS-tō-sēl] cysto-, bladder + -cele, hernia	Hernia of the bladder.
cystolith	[SĬS-tō-lǐth] cysto- + -lith, stone	Bladder stone.
dysuria	[dǐs-YŪ-rē-ǎ] dys-, difficult + -uria	Painful urination.
edema	[ĕ-DĒ-mǎ] Greek *oidema*, a swelling	Retention of water in cells, tissues, and cavities, sometimes due to kidney disease.
end-stage renal disease (ESRD)		The last stages of kidney failure.
enuresis	[ĕn-yū-RĒ-sǐs] Greek *enoureo*, to urinate in	Urinary incontinence.
glomerulonephritis	[glō-MĂR-yū-lō-nĕf-RĪ-tǐs] glomerulo-, glomerulus + nephr-, kidney + -itis	Inflammation of the glomeruli of the kidneys.
hematuria	[hē-mǎ-TŪ-rē-ǎ] hemat-, blood + -uria	Blood in the urine.
hydronephrosis	[HĪ-drō-nĕ-FRŌ-sǐs] hydro-, water + nephr- + -osis, condition	Abnormal collection of urine in the kidneys due to a blockage.
incontinence	[ǐn-KŎN-tǐ-nĕns] From in-, not + Latin *contineo*, to hold together	Inability to prevent excretion of urine or feces.
ketonuria	[kē-tō-NŪ-rē-ǎ] keton(e) + -uria	Increased urinary excretion of ketones, usually indicative of diabetes or starvation.
kidney failure		Loss of kidney function.
nephritis	[nĕ-FRĪ-tǐs] nephr- + -itis	Inflammation of the kidneys.
nephroblastoma	[NĔF-rō-blǎs-TŌ-mǎ] nephro-, kidney + blastoma	*See* Wilms' tumor.

Terms	Word Analysis	Definition
nephroma	[nĕ-FRŌ-mă] nephr- + -oma, tumor	Any renal tumor.
nephrosis	[nĕ-FRŌ-sĭs] nephr- + -osis	Disorder caused by loss of protein in the urine.
nocturia	[nŏk-TŪ-rē-ă] noct-, night + -uria	Nighttime urination.
oliguria	[ŏl-ĭ-GŪ-rē-ă] olig-, scant + -uria	Scanty urine production.
polycystic kidney disease	[pŏl-ē-SĬS-tĭk]	Condition with many cysts on and within the kidneys.
polyuria	[pŏl-ē-ŪR-ē-ă] poly-, much + -uria	Excessive urination.
proteinuria	[prō-tē-NŪ-rē-ă] protein + -uria	Abnormal presence of protein in the urine.
pyelitis	[pī-ĕ-LĪ-tĭs] pyel-, pelvis + -itis	Inflammation of the renal pelvis.
pyuria	[pī-YŪ-rē-ă] py-, pus + -uria	Pus in the urine.
uremia	[yū-RĒ-mē-ă] ur-, urine + -emia, blood	Excess of urea and other wastes in the blood.
urinary tract infection (UTI)		Infection of the urinary tract.
Wilms' tumor	After Max Wilms (1867–1918), German surgeon	Malignant kidney tumor found primarily in young children; nephroblastoma.

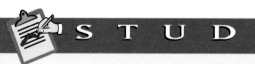

CASE STUDY

Seeing a Specialist

Ms. Jones had pus in her urine, and it was cloudy. She had complained about painful, scanty, and excessive urination at various times. Dr. Chorzik concluded that she had a urinary tract infection. Mr. Delgado had a fairly normal urinalysis, but restricted urination indicated some other urinary tract problem. Dr. Chorzik referred Mr. Delgado to a urologist. Ms. Margolis had blood in her urine and some signs of infection.

CASE STUDY (continued)

 Critical Thinking

104. What are the medical terms for the symptoms Ms. Jones experienced?

105. What course of treatment was prescribed for Ms. Jones?

Pathological Terms Exercises

Build Your Medical Vocabulary

Using the combining forms in this chapter, complete the names of the disorders.

106. Inflammation of the urethra: _____itis

107. Inflammation of the ureter: _____itis

108. Inflammation of the bladder and urethra:_____itis

109. Inflammation of the kidneys: _____itis

110. Tumor in the kidneys: _____oma

Spell It Correctly

Check the spelling of the following words. Write C if the spelling is correct. If it is incorrect, write the correct spelling in the space provided.

111. ureteritis_____

112. cystitis_____

113. dysuria_____

114. uretheritis_____

115. cytorrhaphy____

Check Your Knowledge

Circle T for true or F for false.

116. Wilms' tumor is found only in middle-aged adults. T F

117. Urine collects in the renal pelvis. T F

118. Edema is swelling that may be due to kidney disease. T F

119. Oliguria is abnormally high production of urine. T F

120. Anuresis means the same as enuresis. T F

Surgical Terms

Urology is the practice of medicine specializing in the urinary tract. The practitioner is called a *urologist*. Urologists diagnose, treat, and perform surgery on the urinary system in the female and on the urinary and reproductive system in the male.

Parts of the urinary system may be surgically removed. A person can live with only one kidney, so a diseased kidney may be removed in a **nephrectomy.** Diseased kidneys are removed before a *kidney* or *renal transplant*. Other surgical procedures on the kidney include **nephrolysis,** the removal of adhesions in the kidney; **nephrostomy,** the creation of an opening in the kidney leading to the outside of the body; **nephrolithotomy,** surgical removal of a kidney stone; **nephropexy,** surgical fixing in place of a floating kidney; and **nephrorrhaphy,** suturing of a damaged kidney.

An incision into the renal pelvis is called a **pyelotomy.** A **pyeloplasty** is the surgical repair of the renal pelvis. Surgical repair of a ureter is **ureteroplasty. Ureterorrhaphy** is the suture of a damaged ureter. **Ureterectomy** is the surgical removal of a diseased ureter.

The urinary bladder can be the site of stones, which are removed during a **lithotomy.** A **cystectomy** is the removal of the bladder (usually when cancer is present). Surgical fixing of the bladder to the abdominal wall is **cystopexy,** an operation to help correct urinary incontinence. **Cystoplasty** is the surgical repair of a bladder and **cystorrhaphy** is the suturing of a damaged bladder.

The urethra may also need surgical repair (**urethroplasty**), surgical fixation (**urethropexy**), or suturing (**urethrorrhaphy**). A **urethrostomy** is the surgical creation of an opening between the urethra and the skin, while a **meatotomy** is the surgical enlargement of the opening of the meatus. Either of these operations may be necessary when certain birth defects are present. A narrowing in the urethra may require a **urethrotomy,** a surgical incision to enlarge the narrowed area.

Sometimes an opening is made to bypass diseased parts of the urinary tract. A **urostomy** is the creation of an artificial opening in the abdomen through which urine exits the body. **Intracorporeal electrohydraulic lithotripsy** is the use of an endoscope, an instrument for examining an interior canal or cavity, to break up stones in the urinary tract. A **resectoscope** is an endoscope used to cut and remove lesions in parts of the urinary system.

There is a worldwide shortage of kidneys available for transplant. Patients with kidney disease often have to wait years, undergoing painful dialysis, before a compatible kidney is found.

Vocabulary Review

In the previous section, you learned terms relating to surgery. Before going on to the exercises, review the terms below and refer to the previous section if you have any questions.

Terms	Word Analysis	Definition
cystectomy	[sĭs-TĔK-tō-mē] cyst-, bladder + -ectomy, removal	Surgical removal of the bladder.
cystopexy	[SĬS-tō-pĕk-sē] cysto-, bladder + -pexy, fixing	Surgical fixing of the bladder to the abdominal wall.
cystoplasty	[SĬS-tō-plăs-tē] cysto- + -plasty, repair	Surgical repair of the bladder.
cystorrhaphy	[sĭs-TŌR-ă-fē] cysto- + -rrhaphy, suturing	Suturing of a damaged bladder.
intracorporeal electro-hydraulic lithotripsy	[ĬN-tră-kōr-PŌ-rē-ăl ē-LĔK-trō-hī-DRŌ-lĭk LĬTH-ō-trĭp-sē]	Use of an endoscope to break up stones.
lithotomy	[lĭ-THŎT-ō-mē] litho-, stone + -tomy, a cutting	Surgical removal of bladder stones.
meatotomy	[mē-ă-TŎT-ō-mē] meat(us) + -tomy	Surgical enlargement of the meatus.
nephrectomy	[nĕ-FRĔC-tō-mē] nephr-, kidney + -ectomy	Removal of a kidney.
nephrolithotomy	[NĔF-rō-lĭ-THŎT-ō-mē] nephro-, kidney + litho- + -tomy	Surgical removal of a kidney stone.
nephrolysis	[nĕ-FRŎL-ĭ-sĭs] nephro- + -lysis, dissolving	Removal of kidney adhesions.
nephropexy	[NĔF-rō-pĕk-sē] nephro- + -pexy	Surgical fixing of a kidney to the abdominal wall.
nephrorrhaphy	[nĕf-RŌR-ă-fē] nephro- + -rrhaphy	Suturing of a damaged kidney.
nephrostomy	[nĕ-FRŎS-tō-mē] nephro- + -stomy, opening	Establishment of an opening from the renal pelvis to the outside of the body.

Terms	Word Analysis	Definition
pyeloplasty	[PĪ-ĕ-lō-PLĂS-tē] pyelo-, pelvis + -plasty	Surgical repair of the renal pelvis.
pyelotomy	[pī-ĕ-LŎT-ō-mē] pyelo- + -tomy	Incision into the renal pelvis.
resectoscope	[rē-SĔK-tō-skōp] Latin *reseco*, to cut off + -scope, instrument for viewing	Type of endoscope for removal of lesions.
ureterectomy	[yū-rē-tĕr-ĔK-tō-mē] ureter + -ectomy	Surgical removal of all or some of a ureter.
ureteroplasty	[yū-RĒ-tĕr-ō-PLĂS-tē] uretero-, ureter + -plasty	Surgical repair of a ureter.
ureterorrhaphy	[yū-rē-tĕr-ŌR-ă-fē] uretero- + -rrhaphy	Suturing of a ureter.
urethropexy	[yū-RĒ-thrō-pĕk-sē] urethro-, urethra + -pexy	Surgical fixing of the urethra.
urethroplasty	[yū-RĒ-thrō-PLĂS-tē] urethro- + -plasty	Surgical repair of the urethra.
urethrorrhaphy	[yū-rē-THRŎR-ă-fē] urethro- + -rrhaphy	Suturing of the urethra.
urethrostomy	[yū-rē-THRŎS-tō-mē] urethro- + -stomy	Establishment of an opening between the urethra and the exterior of the body.
urethrotomy	[yū-rē-THRŎT-ō-mē] urethro- + -tomy	Surgical incision of a narrowing in the urethra.
urology	[yū-RŎL-ō-jē] uro-, urine + -logy, study of	Medical specialty that diagnoses and treats the urinary system and the male reproductive system.
urostomy	[yū-RŎS-tō-mē] uro- + -stomy	Establishment of an opening in the abdomen to the exterior of the body for the release of urine.

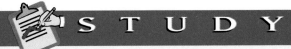

C A S E S T U D Y

Getting the Diagnosis

Patient #1. Ms. Margolis, a 69-year-old female, had additional tests and was found to have serious kidney disease in one kidney. A nephrectomy was performed, and eventually her symptoms subsided.

Patient #2. Mr. Delgado's appointment with the urologist was scheduled for the next day. During a physical examination, the urologist noticed some swelling in the prostate gland, but did not think this was enough to cause Mr. Delgado's difficulties. The urologist ordered a blood test (PSA) to determine if there were another possible cause. The PSA results were normal. The urologist then ordered imaging tests. One test showed a narrowing of the urethra.

Critical Thinking

121. Ms. Margolis had one kidney removed. The other one is healthy. Does Ms. Margolis need dialysis?

122. What procedure might relieve Mr. Delgado's symptoms?

Surgical Terms Exercises

Build Your Medical Vocabulary

Complete the name of the operation by adding one or more combining forms.

123. Removal of kidney stones: _____tomy

124. Removal of kidney adhesions: _____lysis

125. Removal of a kidney: _____ectomy

126. Removal of a ureter:_____ectomy

127. Creation of an artificial opening in the urinary tract: _____stomy

Check Your Knowledge

Circle T for true or F for false.

128. Surgical repair of the urethra is ureteroplasty. T F

129. Several organs and structures in the urinary system may need surgical fixing to be held in position. T F

130. A resectoscope is an instrument used to remove lesions. T F

131. A urethrostomy and a urostomy serve the same function. T F

132. A cystopexy can help urinary incontinence. T F

Pharmacological Terms

Medications for the urinary tract can relieve pain (*analgesics*), relieve spasms (**antispasmodics**), or inhibit the growth of microorganisms (*antibiotics*). They may also increase (**diuretics**) or decrease (*antidiuretics*) the secretion of urine. Table 9-1 shows some common medications prescribed for urinary tract disorders.

Table 9-1 Some Common Medications Used to Treat the Urinary System

Drug Class	Purpose	Generic	Trade Name
analgesic	to relieve pain	phenazopyridine	Azo-Standard, Phenazodine, Pyridium, Urodine, Urogesic, Viridium
antibiotic	to treat infections (especially UTIs) including ones with a fungal cause	penicillin, tetracycline	Sumycin, Tetralan
antidiuretic	to control secretion of urine	vasopressin	Pitressin, Pressyn
antispasmodic	to relax muscles so as to relieve pain and decrease urgency to urinate	oxybutynin	Ditropan
diuretic	to increase urination	bethanecol	Duvoid, Urecholine

Vocabulary Review

In the previous section, you learned terms relating to pharmacology. Before going on to the exercises, review the terms below and refer to the previous section if you have any questions.

Agent	Word Analysis	Purpose
antispasmodic	[ĂN-tē-spăz-MŎD-ĭk] anti-, against + spasmodic	Pharmacological agent that relieves spasms; also decreases frequency of urination.
diuretic	[dī-yū-RĔT-ĭk] From Greek *dia-*, through + *ouresis*, urine	Pharmacological agent that increases urination.

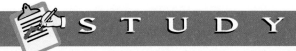

CASE STUDY

Receiving Treatment

Ms. Jones recovered from her urinary tract infection but came in a few months later with swollen feet and high blood pressure. She was given a prescription, a list of dietary changes she should observe, and a course of mild, daily exercise to follow.

💡 **Critical Thinking**

133. What type of medication do you think was prescribed for Ms. Jones?

134. How might diet help reduce swelling?

Pharmacological Terms Exercises

Know the Right Medication

Fill in the blanks.

135. To help relieve edema, a(n) _____ may be prescribed.

136. For dysuria, a(n) _____ may be prescribed.

137. For cystitis a(n) _____ may be prescribed.

138. Sudden contractions may lead to urinary incontinence and, therefore, a(n) _____ may be prescribed.

Review the following doctor's notes and test results for a patient hospitalized with a high fever, dysuria, and general malaise.

	Meadow Health Systems, Inc.		
Run Date: 09/22/XX	1420 Glen Road		Page 1
Run Time: 1507	Meadowvale, OK 44444		Specimen Report
	111-222-3333		

Patient: Dexter Judge	Acct #: E115592848	Loc:	U #:
Reg Dr: S. Anders, M.D.	Age/Sx: 40/M	Room:	Reg: 06/10/XX
	Status: Reg ER	Bed:	Des:

Spec #: 0922 : U00010R	Coll: 09/22/XX	Status: Comp	Req #: 00704181
	Recd.: 09/22/XX	Subm Dr:	

Entered: 06/10/XX–0936   Other Dr:
Ordered: UA with micro
Comments: Urine Description: Clean catch urine

Test	Result	Flag	Reference
Urinalysis			
UA with micro			
COLOR	YELLOW		
APPEARANCE	CLEAR		
SP GRAVITY	1.017		1.001-1.030
GLUCOSE	4.7	**	NEG
BILIRUBIN	NEGATIVE		NEG
KETONE	NEGATIVE		NEG mg/dl
BLOOD	NEGATIVE		NEG
PH	5.0		4.5-8.0
PROTEIN	NEGATIVE		NEG mg/dl
UROBILINOGEN	NORMAL		NORMAL-1.0 mg/dl
NITRITES	NEGATIVE		NEG
LEUKOCYTES	NEGATIVE		NEG
WBC	8-10	**	0-5 /HPF
RBC	2-5		0-5 /HPF
EPI CELLS	0-2		/HPF
MUCUS	1+		

Patient 4

MEDICAL RECORD	PROGRESS NOTES
DATE 6/10/XX	*Patient is a forty-year-old male admitted yesterday with symptoms including high fever and dysuria. Blood pressure normal; lungs clear. Urinalysis positive for glucose and white blood count. Test for infection. Talk to patient about high glucose reading. —Steve Anders, M.D.*

PATIENT'S IDENTIFICATION *(For typed or written entries give: Name—last, first, middle; grade; rank; hospital or medical facility)*	REGISTER NO.	WARD NO.
Judge, Dexter *000-000-000*	**PROGRESS NOTES** STANDARD FORM 509	

139. What do some of the abnormal results of the urinalysis indicate?

140. What other tests might be necessary to reach a diagnosis?

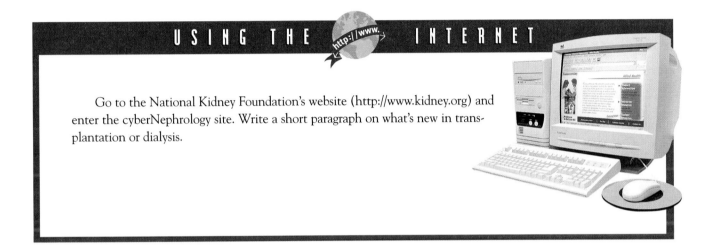

USING THE http://www. INTERNET

Go to the National Kidney Foundation's website (http://www.kidney.org) and enter the cyberNephrology site. Write a short paragraph on what's new in transplantation or dialysis.

CHAPTER REVIEW

Definitions

Define the following terms and combining forms. Review the chapter before starting. Make sure you know how to pronounce each term as you define it.

Word	Definition
acetone [ĂS-ĕ-tōn]	
albumin [ăl-BYŪ-mĭn]	
albuminuria [ăl-byū-mĭ-NŪ-rē-ă]	
antispasmodic [ĂN-tē-spăz-MŎD-ĭk]	
anuresis [ăn-yū-RĒ-sĭs]	
anuria [ăn-YŪ-rē-ă]	
atresia [ā-TRĒ-zē-ă]	
azotemia [ăz-ō-TĒ-mē-ă]	
bilirubin [bĭl-ĭ-RŪ-bĭn]	
bladder [BLĂD-ēr]	
bladder cancer	
Bowman's capsule	
Bright's disease	
cali(o), calic(o)	
calices, calyces (sing. calix, calyx) [KĂL-ĭ-sēz (KĂ-lĭks)]	
casts	
condom catheter [KĂTH-ĕ-tĕr]	
cortex [KŌR-tĕks]	
creatine [KRĒ-ă-tēn]	
creatinine [krē-ĂT-ĭ-nēn]	
cyst(o)	
cystectomy [sĭs-TĔK-tō-mē]	
cystitis [sĭs-TĪ-tĭs]	
cystocele [SĬS-tō-sēl]	
cystolith [SĬS-tō-lĭth]	

Word	Definition
cystopexy [SĬS-tō-pěk-sē]	
cystoplasty [SĬS-tō-plăs-tē]	
cystorrhaphy [sĭs-TŌR-ă-fē]	
cystoscope [SĬS-tō-skōp]	
cystoscopy [sis-TOS-ko-pe]	
dialysis [dī-ĂL-ĭ-sĭs]	
diuretic [dī-yū-RĒT-ĭk]	
dysuria [dĭs-YŪ-rē-ă]	
edema [ě-DĒ-mă]	
end-stage renal disease (ESRD)	
enuresis [ěn-yū-RĒ-sĭs]	
extracorporeal shock wave lithotripsy (ESWL)	
filtration [fĭl-TRĀ-shŭn]	
Foley catheter	
glomerul(o)	
glomerulonephritis [glō-MĀR-yū-lō-něf-RĬ-tĭs]	
glomerulus (pl. glomuleri) [glō-MĀR-yū-lŭs (glō-MĀR-yū-lĭ)]	
glucose [GLŪ-kōs]	
hematuria [mē-mā-TŪ-rē-ă]	
hemodialysis [HĒ-mō-dī-ĂL-ĭ-sĭs]	
hilum [HĪ-lŭm]	
hydronephrosis [HĪ-drō-ně-FRŌ-sĭs]	
incontinence [ĭn-KŎN-tĭ-něns]	
indwelling [ĬN-dwě-lĭng]	
intracorporeal electrohydraulic lithotripsy [ĬN-tră-kōr-PŌ-rē-ăl ē-LĚK-trō-hī-DRŌ-lĭk LĬTH-ō-trĭp-sē]	
ketone [KĒ-tōn]	
ketonuria [kē-tō-NŪ-rē-ă]	
kidney [KĬD-nē]	
kidney failure	
kidney, ureter, bladder (KUB)	

Word	Definition
lithotomy [lĭ-THŎT-ō-mē]	
meato	
meatotomy [mē-ă-TŎT-ō-mē]	
meatus [mē-Ā-tŭs]	
medulla [mĕ-DŪL-ă]	
nephrectomy [nĕ-FRĔC-tō-mē]	
nephritis [nĕ-FRĪ-tĭs]	
nephro(o)	
nephroblastoma [NĔF-rō-blăs-TŌ-mă]	
nephrolithotomy [NĔF-rō-lĭ-THŎT-ō-mē]	
nephrolysis [nĕ-FRŎL-ĭ-sĭs]	
nephroma [nĕ-FRO-mă]	
nephron [NĔF-rŏn]	
nephropexy [NĔF-rō-pĕk-sē]	
nephrorrhaphy [nĕf-RŌR-ă-fē]	
nephrosis [nĕ-FRŌ-sĭs]	
nephrostomy [nĕ-FRŎS-tō-mē]	
nocturia [nŏk-TŪ-rē-ă]	
oliguria [ŏl-ĭ-GŪ-rē-ă]	
peritoneal [PĔR-ĭ-tō-NĒ-ăl] dialysis	
pH	
phenylketones [FĔN-ĭl-KĒ-tōns]	
polycystic [pŏl-ē-SĬS-tĭk] kidney disease	
polyuria [pŏl-ē-ŬR-ē-ă]	
prostate [PRŎS-tāt]	
proteinuria [prō-tē-NŪ-rē-ă]	
pyel(o)	
pyelitis [pī-ĕ-LĪ-tĭs]	
pyeloplasty [PĪ-ĕ-lō-PLĂS-tē]	
pyelotomy [pī-ĕ-LŎT-ō-mē]	
pyuria [pī-YŪ-rē-ă]	
reabsorption [rē-ăb-SŎRB-shŭn]	
ren(o)	

Word	Definition
renal pelvis	
renin [RĔ-nĭn]	
renogram [RĒ-nō-grăm]	
resectoscope [rē-SĔK-tō-skōp]	
retrograde pyelogram (RP) [RĔT-rō-grād PĪ-ĕl-ō-grăm]	
retroperitoneal [RĔ-trō-PĔR-ĭ-tō-nē-ăl]	
specific gravity	
trigon(o)	
trigone [TRĪ-gōn]	
ur(o), urin (o)	
urea [yū-RĒ-ă]	
uremia [yū-RĒ-mē-ă]	
ureter(o)	
ureter [yū-RĒ-tĕr]	
ureterectomy [yū-rē-tĕr-ĔK-tō-mē]	
ureteroplasty [yū-RĒ-tĕr-ō-plăs-tē]	
ureterorrhaphy [yū-rē-tĕr-ŌR-ă-fē]	
urethr(o)	
urethra [yū-RĒ-thră]	
urethropexy [yū-RĒ-thrō-pĕx-ē]	
urethroplasty [yū-RĒ-thrō-plăs-tē]	
urethrorrhaphy [yū-rē-THRŎR-ă-fē]	
urethrostomy [yū-rē-THRŎS-tō-mē]	
urethrotomy [yū-rē-THRŎT-ō-mē]	
uric [YŪR-ĭk] acid	
urinalysis [yū-rĭ-NĂL-ĭ-sĭs]	
urinary [YŪR-ĭ-nār-ē] bladder	
urinary system	
urinary tract infection (UTI)	
urine [YŪR-ĭn]	
urology [yū-RŎL-ō-jē]	
urostomy [yū-RŎS-tō-mē]	
vesic(o)	

Word	Definition
voiding (urinating) cystourethrogram (VCU, VCUG) [sĭs-tō-yū-RĒ-thrō-grăm]	
Wilms' tumor	

Abbreviations

Write the full meaning of each abbreviation.

Abbreviation	Meaning
ADH	
A/G	
AGN	
ARF	
ATN	
BNO	
BUN	
CAPD	
Cath	
Cl	
CRF	
cysto	
ESRD	
ESWL	
HD	
IVP	
K+	
KUB	
Na+	
pH	
PKU	
RP	
SG	
UA	
UTI	
VCU, VCUG	

1. No, blood is normally filtered in the kidneys and returned to the bloodstream.
2. Yes, males have prostates, external urethral exits, and other anatomical features different from females, whose urethras are shorter than those of males.
3. ureters
4. urethra
5. nephrons
6. glomerulus
7. renal pelvis
8. reabsorption
9. bladder
10. voiding and micturition
11. Bowman's capsule
12. trigone
13. F
14. F
15. T
16. T
17. T
18. F
19. F
20. F
21. T
22. F
23. e
24. a
25. c
26. g
27. f
28. d
29. c
30. Patient 1
31. sample answer: white blood count, red blood count
32. anuresis
33. pyelitis
34. polyuria
35. nephropathy
36. oliguria
37. cystoplegia
38. lipuria
39. megacystis
40. vesicourethral
41. renomegaly
42. pericystitis
43. nephrology
44. pyelonephritis
45. caliorrhaphy
46. interrenal
47. urethrorrhea
48. ureterorrhagia
49. nephromalacia
50. intracystic
51. nephrolithotomy
52. nephrography
53. reniform
54. glomulero-, glomulerus; nephro-, kidney; kidney disease located in the glomulerus
55. nephro-, kidney; condition with cysts in the kidneys
56. urethro-, urethra; condition with narrowing of the urethra
57. uretero-, ureter, vesico-, bladder; surgical connection of the ureter to the bladder
58. uro-, urine; condition with bluish color in the urine
59. uro-, urine; study of stones in the urinary system
60. pyelo-, renal pelvis; ureter-, ureter; dilation of the renal pelvis and ureter
61. calico-, calix; removal of a calix
62. cysto-, bladder; removal of stones in the bladder
63. nephro-, kidney; kidney tumor
64. meato-, meatus; suture of the meatus
65. nephro-, kidney; hardening of kidney tissue
66. reno-, kidney; pertaining to the kidneys and lungs
67. trigon-, trigone; inflammation of the trigone
68. antidiuretic hormone
69. power of hydrogen concentration
70. continuous ambulatory peritoneal dialysis
71. voiding cystourethrogram
72. hemodialysis
73. phenylketonuria
74. blood urea nitrogen
75. kidney, ureter, bladder
76. extracorporeal shock wave lithotripsy
77. urinary tract infection
78. retrograde pyelogram
79. infection
80. pus
81. Y
82. Y
83. Y
84. N
85. Y
86. N
87. Y
88. Y
89. Y
90. Y
91. Y
92. Y
94. hemodialysis
95. peritoneal dialysis
96. Foley
97. condom
98. glucose and ketones
99. stones
100. casts
101. filtration, kidney
102. blood urea nitrogen, creatinine clearance test
103. voiding cystourethrogram
104. dysuria, oliguria, polyuria
105. antibiotics.
106. urethritis
107. ureteritis
108. urethrocystitis
109. nephritis
110. nephroma
111. c
112. c
113. c
114. urethritis
115. cystorrhaphy
116. F
117. T
118. T
119. F
120. F
121. No. One kidney can filter the blood for the whole body.
122. urethrotomy
123. F
124. T
125. T
126. T
127. T
128. nephrolithotomy
129. nephrolysis
130. nephrectomy
131. ureterectomy
132. urostomy
133. diuretic
134. Limiting salt in the diet can relieve swelling
135. diuretic
136. analgesic
137. antibiotic
138. antispasmodic
139. High glucose and high white blood count—possible diabetes and infection
140. Blood tests

CHAPTER 10

Female Reproductive System

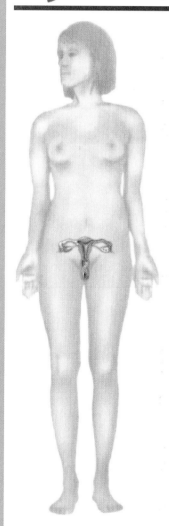

After studying this chapter, you will be able to:

◆ Name the parts of the female reproductive system and discuss the function of each part

◆ Define combining forms used in building words that relate to the female reproductive system

◆ Identify the meaning of related abbreviations

◆ Name the common diagnoses, clinical procedures, and laboratory tests used in treating the female reproductive system

◆ List and define the major pathological conditions of the female reproductive system

◆ Explain the meaning of surgical terms related to the female reproductive system

◆ Recognize common pharmacological agents used in treating the female reproductive system

◆ Explain the meaning of surgical terms related to the urinary system

◆ Recognize common pharmacological agents used in treating the urinary system

Structure and Function

The female reproductive system is a group of organs and glands that produce female *sex cells* (**ova** or *egg cells*), move them to the site of fertilization, and, if they are fertilized by a male sex cell (sperm), nurture them until birth (Figure 10-1a). Sex cells are also called **gametes** and are manufactured in the female **gonads** or **ovaries.** The ovaries release the eggs cyclically (as part of the *ovarian cycle*) from the **graafian follicle** to the **uterine** or **fallopian tubes** (Figure 10-1b). If fertilized, the egg is transported to the **uterus,** where it develops into an embryo and then into a fetus. At the end of gestation, the infant is born through the **vagina** in a routine delivery or surgically through the abdomen in a Caesarean delivery. The organs and structures described form the basic reproductive structure. The female breast, the **mammary gland**

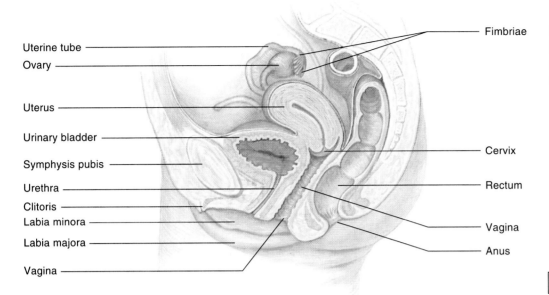

Figure 10-1a **The female reproductive system has cycles that determine fertility.**

Uterine tube
Ovary

Uterus

Urinary bladder

Symphysis pubis

Urethra
Clitoris
Labia minora
Labia majora

Vagina

Fimbriae

Cervix

Rectum

Vagina

Anus

(Figure 10-2), is also part of the female reproductive system as an *accessory organ*, providing milk to nurse the infant (**lactation**) after birth. In addition to fertilization, female reproduction is controlled by hormones, such as estrogen and progesterone.

Ovary

Egg

Uterine tube

Uterus

If not fertilized

If fertilized

Expulsion through menstruation

Implantation

Figure 10-1b **The path of an egg in the ovarian cycle.**

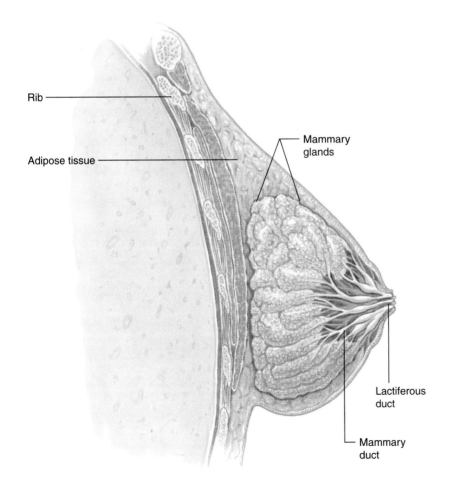

Rib

Adipose tissue

Mammary glands

Lactiferous duct

Mammary duct

Figure 10-2 **The female breast has mammary glands and ducts through which nourishment is provided to the infant.**

Reproductive Organs

The gonads or ovaries are two small, solid oval structures in the pelvic cavity that produce ova and secrete female hormones. The ovaries lie on either side of the uterus and, in the monthly cycle of egg production, they usually release (**ovulation**) only one mature ova. In rare cases, more eggs are released. In some females, the monthly cycle alternates between the two ovaries. In others, the cycle does not alternate in a repeated pattern. The production of sex cells in most females follows a monthly pattern. In males, the production of sex cells is not cyclical.

At birth, most females have from 200,000 to 400,000 immature ova (**oocytes**) in each ovary. Many of these disintegrate before the female reaches **puberty,** the stage at which ovulation and **menarche** (first menstruation) and the **menstruation** cycle occur (usually between 10 and 14 years of age). **Menopause** signals the end of the ovulation/menstruation cycle and, therefore, the end of the childbearing years. The period of hormonal changes leading up to menopause is called the **climacteric.** The three to five years of decreasing estrogen levels prior to menopause is called **perimenopause.**

After release, the ovum next enters the uterine or fallopian tubes, which have hairlike ends, **fimbriae,** to sweep the ovum into one of the fallopian tubes where it may be fertilized by a sperm. Fertilized or not, the ovum moves by contractions of the tube to the uterus (Figure 10-3). The uterus is about three inches long and wider at the top than at the bottom, where it attaches to the vagina. Once inside the uterus, a fertilized ovum attaches to the uterine wall, where it will be nourished for about 40 weeks of development (**gestation**). The upper portion of the uterus, the **fundus,** is where a nutrient-rich organ (the **placenta**) grows in the uterine wall. An ovum that has not been fertilized is released along with the lining of the uterus (endometrium) during menstruation.

The middle portion of the uterus is called the **body.** It leads to a narrow region, the **isthmus,** which opens into the **cervix.** The cervix is a protective

For women who do not ovulate normally or men who do not produce enough live sperm, alternative methods of conception exist. Infertility clinics regularly fertilize either a woman's own egg or a donor egg with her husband's or a donor's sperm.

Figure 10-3 Movement of an oocyte during the female cycle.

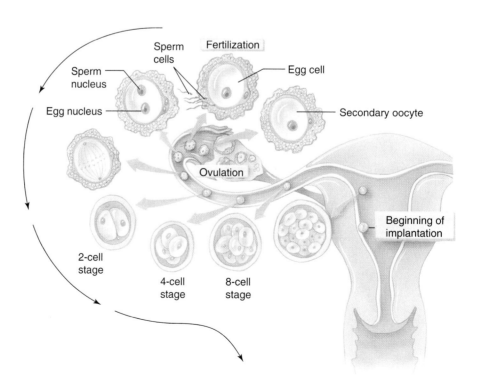

body with glands that secrete mucous substances into the vagina. The vagina can expand to accommodate an erect penis during intercourse or the passage of a baby during childbirth. A fold of mucous membranes, the **hymen,** covers the external opening (**introitus**) of the vagina. It is usually ruptured during the female's first sexual intercourse, but may be broken earlier during physical activity or because of use of a tampon. It may also be congenitally absent.

The uterus is made up of three layers of tissue—the **perimetrium,** the outer layer; the **myometrium,** the middle layer; and the **endometrium,** the inner mucous layer. The outer layer is a protective layer of membranous tissue. The middle layer is really three layers of smooth muscle that move in strong downward motions. This middle layer stretches during pregnancy. The endometrium is deep and velvety, has an abundant supply of blood vessels and glands, and is built up and broken down during the ovulation/menstruation cycle.

The external genitalia (Figure 10-4), collectively known as the **vulva,** consist of a mound of soft tissue, the **mons pubis,** which is covered by pubic hair after puberty. Two folds of skin below the mons pubis, the **labia majora,** form the borders of the vulva. Between the labia majora lie two smaller skin folds, the **labia minora,** which merge at the top to form the **foreskin** of the **clitoris,** the primary female organ of sexual stimulation. The space between the labia minora contains the **Bartholin's glands,** which secrete fluid into the vagina, and the openings for the vagina and urethra.

The space between the bottom of the labia majora and the anus is called the **perineum.** During childbirth, it is possible for the perineum to become torn. A surgical procedure (episiotomy) is commonly done before childbirth to avoid tearing the perineum, because an even surgical incision is easier to repair.

The mammary glands or breasts are full of glandular tissue that is stimulated by hormones after puberty to grow and respond to the cycles of menstruation and birth. During pregnancy, hormones stimulate the **lactiferous** (milk-producing) ducts and **sinuses** that transport milk to the **nipple** (or *mammary papilla*). The dark-pigmented area surrounding the nipple is called the **areola.** After birth (**parturition**), the mammary glands experience a *let-down reflex*, which allows milk to flow through the nipples when the infant suckles (lactation).

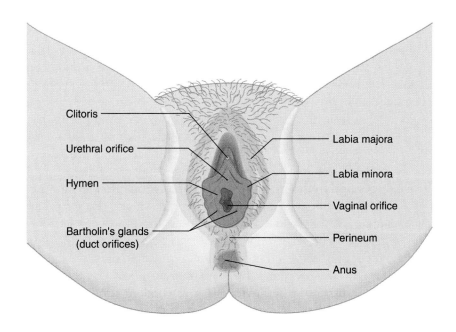

Figure 10-4 External female genitalia.

Clitoris

Urethral orifice

Hymen

Bartholin's glands (duct orifices)

Labia majora

Labia minora

Vaginal orifice

Perineum

Anus

Hormones and Cycles

The ovaries secrete **estrogen** and **progesterone,** the primary female **hormones.** In the stages before and during puberty, estrogen and progesterone play an important role in the development of mature genitalia and of secondary sex characteristics, such as pubic hair and breasts. Other hormones help in childbirth and milk production. Table 10-1 lists the major reproductive hormones and their functions. In the chapter on the endocrine system (Chapter 15), hormones that stimulate glands in the female reproductive system are discussed.

Table 10-1 Major Reproductive Hormones

Hormone	Purpose	Source
estrogen	stimulates development of female sex characteristics and uterine wall thickening; inhibits FSH and increases LH	ovarian follicle; corpus luteum
progesterone	stimulates uterine wall thickening and formation of mammary ducts	corpus luteum
prolactin	promotes lactation	pituitary gland
oxytocin	stimulates labor and lactation	pituitary gland
FSH (follicle-stimulating hormone)	stimulates oocyte maturation; increases estrogen	pituitary
HCG (human chorionic gonadotropin)	stimulates estrogen and progesterone from corpus luteum	placenta, embryo
LH (luteinizing hormone)	stimulates oocyte maturation; increases progesterone	pituitary

Ovulation and menstruation are contained within the average 28-day female cycle (Figure 10-5). At puberty, the first menstruation (menarche) begins. Although the timing of cycles may vary, the average female cycle is divided into four phases. Menstruation takes place during the first five days. The next seven days sees the repair of the endometrial lining that has been passed out of the body during menstruation. The next two days, approximately two weeks after the beginning of menstruation, is the time of ovulation or the egg's release from the graafian follicle and the beginning of its trip down the fallopian tube. Meanwhile, the graafian follicle fills with a yellow substance that secretes estrogen and progesterone. This secreting structure is known as the **corpus luteum.** The secreted hormones encourage the uterus to prepare for a pregnancy. In the second 14 days of the cycle, either fertilization occurs or the built-up endometrium starts to break down and the symptoms (bloating, cramps, nervousness, and depression) of the hormonal changes during the phase leading to menstruation (*premenstrual syndrome [PMS]*) appear.

It is at the point of ovulation that fertilization can occur or be prevented. Prevention of fertilization is accomplished with **contraception.** Contraceptive devices include the **intrauterine device (IUD), condom** (both male and female), **spermicide, diaphragm,** or **sponge.** Some forms of hormone interac-

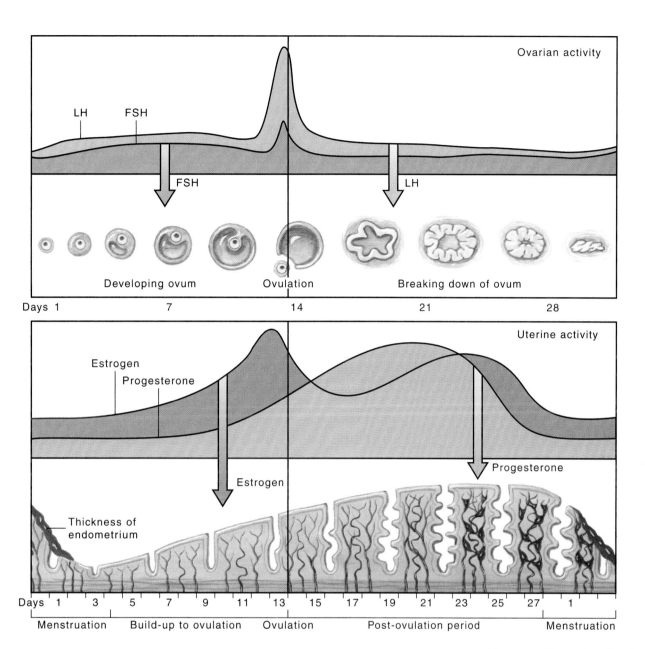

Figure 10-5 The cycles of ovulation and menstruation are parts of the overall female cycle.

tion will also prevent fertilization. High doses of estrogen and progesterone shut off production of **follicle-stimulating hormone (FSH)** and **luteinizing hormone (LH)**, without which ovulation cannot occur. These doses are taken in pill form, by injection, or through the use of an implant just beneath the skin. The *rhythm method* is another method that may be used. It involves knowing one's cycle carefully and abstaining from intercourse for a few days before, during, and after the time of ovulation—about 2 days.

Other female hormones, such as oxytocin, aid in the birth process by intensifying contractions of the uterus. Release of hormones is a function of the endocrine system, discussed in Chapter 15.

Pregnancy

As a result of sexual intercourse (**coitus, copulation**), fertilization may occur. If so, implantation in the uterus takes place, the placenta forms, and pregnancy begins. A pregnant woman is known as a **gravida,** with gravida I being the first pregnancy, gravida II being the second, and so on. An **umbilical cord** connects the placenta to the navel of the fetus so that the mother's blood and the fetal blood do not mix, but nutrients are exchanged through the umbilical cord. The fetus develops in a sac containing the **chorion,** the outermost membrane covering the fetus, and the **amnion,** the innermost membrane next to the fluid surrounding the fetus (**amniotic fluid**). The birth process usually begins when the sac breaks naturally or is broken by medical intervention.

The placenta separates from the uterus after delivery and is expelled from the body as the **afterbirth.** The umbilical cord is then severed and tied so that the infant is physically separated from its mother. At the end of this process, the woman is known as a **para** (one who has borne at least one viable infant). Para I equals the first child, para II the second, and so on.

Vocabulary Review

In the previous section, you learned terms relating to the female reproductive system. Before going on to the exercises, review the terms below and refer to the previous section if you have any questions.

Term	Word Analysis	Definition
afterbirth	[ĂF-tĕr-bĕrth] after + birth	Placenta and membranes that are expelled from the uterus after birth.
amnion	[ĂM-nē-ŏn] From Greek *amnios,* lamb	Innermost membrane of the sac surrounding the fetus during gestation.
amniotic fluid	[ăm-nē-ŎT-ĭk]	Fluid surrounding the fetus and held by the amnion.
areola	[ă-RĒ-ō-lă] Latin, small area	Darkish area surrounding the nipple on a breast.
Bartholin's gland	[BĂR-thō-lĕnz] After Casper Bartholin (1655–1738), Danish anatomist	One of two glands on either side of the vagina that secrete fluid into the vagina.
body		Middle portion of the uterus.
cervix	[SĔR-vĭks] Latin, neck	Protective part of uterus, located at the bottom and protruding through the vaginal wall; contains glands that secrete fluid into the vagina.
chorion	[KŌ-rē-ŏn] Greek, membrane covering fetus	Outermost membrane of the sac surrounding the fetus during gestation.

Term	Word Analysis	Definition
climacteric	[klĭ-MĂK-tēr-ĭk, klĭ-măk-TĔR-ĭk] Greek *klimakter*, the rung of a ladder	Period of hormonal changes just prior to menopause.
clitoris	[KLĬT-ō-rĭs] Greek *kleitoris*	Primary organ of female sexual stimulation, located at the top of the labia minora.
coitus	[KŌ-ĭ-tŭs] Latin	Sexual intercourse.
condom	[KŎN-dŏm]	Contraceptive device consisting of a rubber or vinyl sheath placed over the penis or as a lining that covers the vaginal canal that blocks contact between the sperm and the female sex organs.
contraception	[kŏn-tră-SĔP-shŭn] contra-, against + conceptive, able to conceive	Method of controlling conception by blocking access or interrupting reproductive cycles; birth control.
copulation	[kŏp-yū-LĀ-shŭn] Latin *copulatio*, a joining	Sexual intercourse.
corpus luteum	[KŌR-pŭs LŪ-tē-ŭm] Latin, yellow body	Structure formed after the graafian follicle fills with a yellow substance that secretes estrogen and progesterone.
diaphragm	[DĪ-ă-frăm] Greek *diaphragma*, partition	Contraceptive device that covers the cervix and blocks sperm from entering; used in conjunction with spermicide.
endometrium	[ĔN-dō-MĒ-trē-ŭm] endo-, within + Greek *metra*, uterus	Inner mucous layer of the uterus.
estrogen	[ĔS-trō-jĕn] estr(us), sexual cycle phase in female animals + -gen, producing	One of the primary female hormones produced by the ovaries.
fallopian tube	[fă-LŌ-pē-ăn] After Gabriele Fallopio (1523–1562), Italian anatomist	One of the two tubes that lead from the ovaries to the uterus; uterine tube.
fimbriae	[FĬM-brē-ē] Latin, fringes	Hairlike ends of the uterine tubes that sweep the ovum into the uterus.

Term	Word Analysis	Definition
follicle-stimulating hormone (FSH)		Hormone necessary for maturation of oocytes and ovulation.
foreskin	[FŌR-skĭn] fore-, in front + skin	Fold of skin at the top of the labia minora.
fundus	[FŬN-dŭs] Latin, bottom	Top portion of the uterus.
gamete	[GĂM-ēt] Greek *gamete*, wife or *gametes*, husband	Sex cell; *see* ovum.
gestation	[jĕs-TĀ-shŭn] Latin *gestatio*	Period of fetal development in the uterus; usually about 40 weeks.
gonad	[GŌ-năd] From Greek *gone*, seed	Male or female sex organ; *see* ovary.
graafian follicle	[gră-FĒ-ĕn FŎL-ĭ-kl] After Reijnier de Graaf (1641–1673), Dutch physiologist	Follicle in the ovary that holds an oocyte during development and then releases it.
gravida	[GRĂV-ĭ-dă] Latin, from *gravis*, heavy	Pregnant woman.
hormone	[HŌR-mōn] Greek *hormon*, one that rouses	Chemical secretion from glands such as the ovaries.
hymen	[HĪ-mĕn] Greek, membrane	Fold of mucous membranes covering the vagina of a young female; usually ruptures during first intercourse.
intrauterine device (IUD)	[ĬN-tră-YŪ-tĕr-ĭn] intra-, within + uterine	Contraceptive device consisting of a coil placed in the uterus to block implantation of a fertilized ovum.
introitus	[ĭn-TRŌ-ĭ-tŭs] Latin, entrance	External opening or entrance to a hollow organ, such as a vagina.
isthmus	[ĬS-mŭs] Greek *isthmus*, narrow area	Narrow region at the bottom of the uterus opening into the cervix.
labia majora	[LĀ-bē-ă mă-JŌR-ă] Latin, larger lips	Two folds of skin that form the borders of the vulva.
labia minora	[mă-NŌR-ă] Latin, smaller lips	Two folds of skin between the labia majora.

Term	Word Analysis	Definition
lactation	[lăk-TĀ-shŭn] Latin *lactatio*, to nurse	Production of milk from the breasts following delivery.
lactiferous	[lăk-TĬF-ĕr-ŭs] lacti-, milk + -ferous, bearing	Producing milk.
luteinizing hormone (LH)	[LŪ-tē-ĭn-Ī-zĭng] From Latin luteus, dark yellow	Hormone essential to ovulation.
mammary glands	[MĂM-ă-rē] From Latin *mamma*, breast	Glandular tissue that forms the breasts, which respond to cycles of menstruation and birth.
menarche	[mĕ-NĂR-kē] meno-, menstruation + Greek *arche*, beginning	First menstruation.
menopause	[MĔN-ō-păwz] meno- + pause	Time when menstruation ceases; usually between ages 45 and 55.
menstruation	[mĕn-strū-Ā-shŭn] Latin *menstruo*, to menstruate	Cyclical release of uterine lining through the vagina; usually every 28 days.
mons pubis	[mŏnz pyū-BĬS]	Mound of soft tissue in the external genitalia covered by pubic hair after puberty.
myometrium	[MĪ-ō-MĒ-trē-ŭm] myo-, muscle + Greek *metrium*, uterus	Middle layer of muscle tissue of the uterus.
nipple	[NĬP-l]	Projection at the apex of the breast through which milk flows during lactation.
oocyte	[Ō-ō-sīt] oo-, egg + -cyte, cell	Immature ovum produced in the gonads.
ovary	[Ō-vă-rē] From Latin *ovum*, egg	One of two glands that produce ova.
ovulation	[ŎV-yū-LĀ-shŭn]	Release of an ovum (or rarely, more than one ovum) as part of a monthly cycle that leads to fertilization or menstruation.
ovum (p. ova)	[Ō-vŭm (Ō-vă)] Latin, egg	Mature female sex cell produced by the ovaries, which then travels to the uterus. If fertilized, it implants in the uterus; if not, it is released during menstruation to the outside of the body.

Term	Word Analysis	Definition
para	[PĂ-ră] Latin *pario*, to bring forth	Woman who has given birth to one or more viable infants.
parturition	[păr-tūr-ĬSH-ŭn] Latin *parturitio*	Birth.
perimenopause	[pĕr-ĭ-MĔN-ō-păws] peri-, around + menopause	Three- to five-year period of decreasing estrogen levels prior to menopause.
perimetrium	[pĕr-ĭ-MĒ-trē-ŭm] peri- + Greek *metra*, uterus	Outer layer of the uterus.
perineum	[PĔR-ĭ-NĒ-ŭm]	Space between the labia majora and the anus.
placenta	[plă-SĔN-tă] Latin, flat cake	Nutrient-rich organ that develops in the uterus during pregnancy; supplies nutrients to the fetus.
progesterone	[prō-JĔS-tĕr-ōn] pro-, before + gest(ation)	One of the primary female hormones.
puberty	[PYŪ-bĕr-tē] Latin *pubertas*	Pre-teen or early teen period when secondary sex characteristics develop and menstruation begins.
sinus	[SĪ-nŭs] Latin, cavity	Space between the lactiferous ducts and the nipple.
spermicide	[SPĔR-mĭ-sīd] sperm + -cide, killing	Contraceptive chemical that destroys sperm; usually in cream or jelly form.
sponge	Greek *spongia*, sea sponge	Polyurethane contraceptive device filled with spermicide and placed in vagina near cervix.
umbilical cord	[ŭm-BĬL-ĭ-kăl] From Latin *umbilicus*, navel	Cord that connects the placenta in the mother's uterus to the navel of the fetus during gestation for nourishment of the fetus.
uterine tube	[YŪ-tĕr-ĭn]	One of two tubes through which ova travel from an ovary to the uterus.
uterus	[YŪ-tĕr-ŭs] Latin	Female reproductive organ; site of implantation after fertilization or release of the lining during menstruation.
vagina	[vă-JĪ-nă] Latin	Genital canal leading from the uterus to the vulva.
vulva	[VŬL-vă] Latin	External female genitalia.

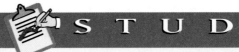

C A S E   S T U D Y

Examining the Patient

D r. Liana Malvern is an internist on the staff of Crestwood HMO. She examined Jane Smits and entered the following notes on Jane's chart.

S: Patient is a 29-year-old female who reports generalized lower abdominal pain for the past three days, which seems to have worsened today. She had trouble sleeping last night because of it. States she threw up one time last night but it was after she coughed. She ate today, had no problems digesting her food. She has been afebrile, not taking any medicines. Patient denies burning upon urination; no appreciable vaginal discharge. Her last menstrual period was eleven days ago.

   Past history—she has had ovarian cysts on the right ovary. The right ovary and right fallopian tube were removed surgically. She states that her appendix was removed ten years ago. She states she has fairly normal periods.

O: Exam shows her to be afebrile. She has bilateral lower quadrant discomfort but no rebound and no remarkable guarding. Pelvic exam done. Normal appearing introitus; cervix is viewed. No remarkable discharge. She is minimally uncomfortable to manipulation of the cervix but does have more discomfort with palpation toward the uterus. Rectal exam is negative.

   Lab: White count: 15,500 with 70 segs. UA: 3-5 red cells, no white cells.

A: Probable pelvic inflammatory infection

P: Prescriptions for Velosef (antibiotic) for infection and recommended ibuprofen for pain. To return to office if any increased symptoms appear such as fever, nausea, vomiting, or increased pain.

 Critical Thinking

1. The patient was afebrile. What does afebrile mean?

2. Patient has normal menstruation, but she has only one ovary. How is that possible?

Structure and Function Exercises

Follow the Path

Using letters a–d, put the following in order according to the path of an ovum from its production to implantation.

3. uterine tube_____

4. ovary_____

5. fimbriae_____

6. uterus_____

Check Your Knowledge

Fill in the blanks.

7. The oocyte is first released from the_____.

8. Implantation usually takes place in the _____.

9. The monthly cycle of egg production is called _____.

10. The release of the uterine lining on a cyclical basis is called _____.

11. The upper portion of the uterus where the placenta usually develops is the _____.

12. The opening at the bottom of the uterus into the vagina is called the _____.

13. The outermost layer of the uterus is the _____.

14. The mammary glands make up the tissue of the _____.

15. The first menstruation is known as _____.

16. The time when menstruation is beginning to cease is called_____.

17. The primary female hormones are _____ and _____.

18. Birth control pills or implants are chemical forms of _____.

19. The fetus gestates in a sac containing the _____, the outermost membrane, and the _____, the innermost membrane.

20. When the placenta is expelled from the body, it is called the _____.

Combining Forms and Abbreviations

The lists below include combining forms and abbreviations that relate specifically to the female reproductive system. Pronunciations are provided for the examples.

Combining Form	Meaning	Example
amni(o)	amnion	*amniocentesis* [ĂM-nē-ō-sĕn-TĒ-sĭs], test of amniotic fluid by insertion of a needle into the amnion
cervic(o)	cervix	*cervicitis* [sĕr-vĭ-SĪ-tĭs], inflammation of the cervix
colp(o)	vagina	*colporrhagia* [kōl-pō-RĀ-jē-ă], vaginal hemorrhage
episi(o)	vulva	*episiotomy* [ĕ-pĭz-ĕ-ŌT-tō-mē] surgical incision into the perineum to prevent tearing during childbirth
galact(o)	milk	*galactopoiesis* [gă-LĂK-tō-pŏy-Ē-sĭs], milk production
gynec(o)	female	*gynecology* [gī-nĕ-KŎL-ō-jē], medical specialty that diagnoses and treats disorders of the female reproductive system.
hyster(o)	uterus	*hysterectomy* [hĭs-tĕr-ĔK-tō-mē], surgical removal of the uterus
lact(o), lacti	milk	*lactogenesis* [lăk-tō-JĔN-ē-sĭs], milk production
mamm(o)	breast	*mammography* [mă-MŎG-ră-fē], imaging of the breast
mast(o)	breast	*mastitis* [măs-TĪ-tĭs], inflammation of the breast
men(o)	menstruation	*menopause* [MĔN-ō-păwz], cessation of menstruation
metr(o)	uterus	*metropathy* [mĕ-TRŎP-ă-thē], disease of the uterus
oo	egg	*oogenesis* [ō-ō-JĔN-ĕ-sĭs], production of eggs
oophor(o)	ovary	*oophoritis* [ō-ŏf-ōr-Ī-tĭs], inflammation of an ovary
ov(i), ov(o)	egg	*ovoid* [Ō-vŏyd], egg-shaped
ovari(o)	ovary	*ovariocele* [ō-VĂR-ē-ō-sēl], hernia of an ovary
perine(o)	perineum	*perineocele* [pĕr-ĭ-NĒ-ō-sēl], hernia in the perineum

Combining Form	Meaning	Example
salping(o)	fallopian tube	*salpingoplasty* [săl-PĬNG-ō-plăs-tē], surgical repair of a fallopian tube
uter(o)	uterus	*uteroplasty* [YŪ-těr-ō-plăs-tē], surgical repair of the uterus
vagin(o)	vagina	*vaginitis* [văj-ĭ-NĪ-tĭs], inflammation of the vagina
vulv(o)	vulva	*vulvitis* [vŭl-VĪ-tĭs], inflammation of the vulva

Abbreviation	Meaning
AB	abortion
AFP	alpha-fetoprotein
AH	abdominal hysterectomy
CIS	carcinoma in situ
CS	caesarean section
C-section	caesarean section
Cx	cervix
D & C	dilation and curettage
DES	diethylstilbestrol
DUB	dysfunctional uterine bleeding
ECC	endocervical curettage
EDC	expected date of confinement
EMB	endometrial biopsy
ERT	estrogen replacement therapy
FHT	fetal heart tones
FSH	follicle-stimulating hormone
G	gravida (pregnancy)
gyn	gynecology
HCG	human chorionic gonadotropin

Abbreviation	Meaning
HRT	hormone replacement therapy
HSG	hysterosalpingography
HSO	hysterosalpingoophorectomy
IUD	intrauterine device
LH	luteinizing hormone
LMP	last menstrual period
multip	multiparous
OB	obstetrics
OCP	oral contraceptive pill
P	para (live births)
Pap smear	Papanicolaou smear
PID	pelvic inflammatory disease
PMP	previous menstrual period
PMS	premenstrual syndrome
primip	primiparous
TAH-BSO	total abdominal hysterectomy with bilateral salpingo-oophorectomy
TSS	toxic shock syndrome
UC	uterine contractions

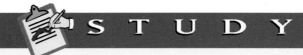
Treating an Unusual Occurrence

Dr. Alvino's next patient, Sarah Messer, was having a heavier than usual menstrual flow. After the visit, her chart read as follows.

 Critical Thinking

21. Did the laboratory tests confirm that the patient was pregnant?

_____

22. What do BP and P mean, and were Sarah Messer's BP and P normal?

S: Patient is a 22-year-old white female who presents with a heavier than usual menstrual flow. Patient states she is using 12-15 pads per day. She states her period started two days ago but is much heavier than usual. Period was about two days late. She is sexually active, no form of birth control, does not think she could be pregnant. She is worried about going to work where she is on her feet all day, and that she seems to flow heavier when she is on her feet. Patient reports cramping. She has had a persistent problem with her right ovary. A previous ultrasound showed problems with the ovary, most likely benign ovarian cysts.

O: Examination shows a young, white female who does not appear in any remarkable distress. She is afebrile. BP 122/70, P 80. Abdomen is soft, no remarkable discomfort, no guarding or rebound present. Pelvic exam was performed. Cervix was closed, significant amount of blood in the cervical vault. There was no remarkable discharge otherwise noted. No discomfort at cervix. No remarkable discomfort or mass in the LLQ on bimanual exam. Lab shows negative serum pregnancy. White count 5500 with 62 segs, HCG 11.5.

A: Menorrhagia. Persistent right ovarian pain.

P: Prescribed Naprosyn 250 mg., one b.i.d. for pain. Provided patient with note to take off work for next two days. Patient to rest and report blood flow tomorrow. Patient to return if problems continue; will monitor HCG.

Combining Forms and Abbreviations Exercises

Build Your Medical Vocabulary

For the following definitions, provide a medical term. Use the combining forms listed in this chapter and in Chapters 2 and 3.

23. narrowing of the vulva _____

24. x-ray of the breast _____

25. production of milk _____

26. hernia of an ovary _____

27. agent that stimulates milk production _____

28. suture of the perineum _____

29. vaginal infection due to a fungus _____

30. uterine pain _____

31. inflammation of the vulva _____

32. vaginal hemorrhage _____

33. formation and development of the egg _____

34. any disease of the breast _____

35. plastic surgery of the uterus _____

36. inflammation of a fallopian tube _____

37. removal of the cervix _____

38. ovarian tumor _____

39. incision into an ovary _____

40. narrowing of the uterine cavity _____

41. resembling a woman _____

42. rupture of the amniotic membrane _____

Make a Match

Match the definition in the right-hand column with the correct term in the left-hand column.

43. episioperineorrhapy

44. galactophoritis

45. ovariorrhexis

46. oviduct

47. colpodynia

48. metritis

49. perineoplasty

50. ookinesis

51. amniorrhea

52. metrosalpingitis

a. rupture of an ovary

b. vaginal pain

c. surgical repair of the perineum

d. egg movement

e. inflammation of the milk ducts

f. escape of amniotic fluid

g. uterine tube

h. inflammation of the uterus and fallopian tubes

i. inflammation of the uterus

j. surgical repair of a tear in the vulva and perineum

Diagnostic, Procedural, and Laboratory Terms

The major function of the female reproductive system is to bear children. There are several basic tests for pregnancy. Diagnosis of fertility problems involves more sophisticated technology. Aside from pregnancy, the health of the female reproductive system is monitored on a regular basis by a **gynecologist,** a physician who diagnoses and treats disorders of the female reproductive system. An **obstetrician** diagnoses and treats both normal and abnormal pregnancies and childbirths.

A routine gynecological exam usually includes a **Papanicolaou (Pap) smear,** a gathering of cells from the cervix to detect cervical or vaginal cancer or other anomalies. The vagina is held open by a *speculum,* a device that holds open any cavity or canal for examination. The cervix and vagina may also be examined by **colposcopy,** use of a lighted instrument (a *colposcope*) for viewing into the vagina. **Hysteroscopy** is the use of a *hysteroscope,* a lighted instrument for examination of the interior of the uterus. **Culdoscopy** is the use of an endoscope to examine the contents of the pelvic cavity. These tests can determine whether masses, tumors, or other abnormalities are present.

Depending on a woman's age, a routine gynecological exam usually includes a prescription for a *mammogram,* a cancer screening test. **Mammography** is an x-ray of the breasts (Figure 10-6). The age recommended for routine mammography differs according to family history, physical condition, and the recommending body. (Recommendations from the American Medical Association, American Cancer Society, and the National Institutes for Health vary.) A mammogram is a cancer screening test that can detect tumors before they can be felt.

A *pregnancy test* is a blood or urine test to detect *human chorionic gonadotropin* (HCG), a hormone that stimulates growth during the first

Figure 10-6 Early breast cancer detection has been increased by mammography, which can locate a cancerous growth up to two years earlier than it can be felt by palpation.

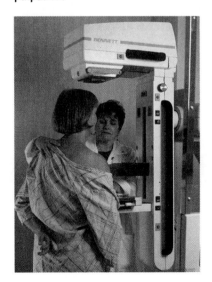

trimester of pregnancy. A pregnancy test may also involve palpation of the uterus during an internal examination by the gynecologist or an obstetrician, a specialist in pregnancy and birth.

Several tests for fertility problems include **hysterosalpingography,** x-ray of the uterus and uterine tubes after a contrast medium is injected; *pelvic ultrasonography,* imaging of the pelvic region using sound waves (used both for detection of tumors and for examination of the fetus); and *transvaginal ultrasound,* also a sound wave image of the pelvic area but done with a probe inserted into the vagina. During pregnancy, the dimensions of the pelvis are measured during **pelvimetry,** an x-ray to see if the pelvis is large enough to allow delivery. *Fetal monitoring* records an infant's heart rate and other functions during labor. Male fertility tests are discussed in Chapter 11.

Vocabulary Review

In the previous section, you learned terms related to diagnosis, clinical procedures, and laboratory tests. Before going on to the exercises, review the terms below and refer to the previous section if you have any questions.

Term	Word Analysis	Definition
colposcopy	[kŏl-PŎS-kō-pē] colpo-, vagina + -scopy, a viewing	Examination of the vagina with a colposcope.
culdoscopy	[kŭl-DŎS-kō-pē] French *cul-d(e-sac)*, bottom of a sack + -scopy	Examination of the pelvic cavity using an endoscope.
gynecologist	[gī-nĕ-KŎL-ō-jĭst] gyneco-, female + -logy, study of	Specialist who diagnoses and treats the processes and disorders of the female reproductive system.
hysterosalpingography	[HĬS-tĕr-ō-săl-pĭng-GŎG-ră-fē] hystero-, uterus + salpingo-, fallopian tube + -graphy, a recording	X-ray of the uterus and uterine tubes after a contrast medium has been injected.
hysteroscopy	[hĭs-tĕr-ŎS-kō-pē] hystero- + -scopy	Examination of the uterus using a hysteroscope.
mammography	[mă-MŎG-ră-fē] mammo-, breast + -graphy	X-ray imaging of the breast as a cancer screening method.
obstetrician	[ŏb-stĕ-TRĬSH-ŭn] Latin *obstetrix*, midwife	Physician who specializes in pregnancy and childbirth care.

Term	Word Analysis	Definition
Papanicolaou (Pap) smear	[pă-pĕ-NĒ-kō-lū] After George N. Papanicolaou (1883– 1962), Greek-American physician	Gathering of cells from the cervix and vagina to observe for abnormalities.
pelvimetry	[pĕl-VĬM-ĕ-trē] pelvi(s) + -metry, measurement	Measurement of the pelvis during pregnancy.

C A S E   S T U D Y

Seeing a Specialist

Jane Smits (patient in the case study on page 359) called two days after her visit to say that the pain in her lower abdomen seemed to have increased. Also, she said that she had had some unusual bleeding from her vagina yesterday. She was told to come in and see Dr. Maurice Alvino, a gynecologist. He discussed her health history, examined her with a colposcope, and scheduled her for x-rays.

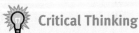 **Critical Thinking**

53. Why did Dr. Alvino use a colposcope?

54. What are some of the specific areas he might want to view on an x-ray?

Diagnostic, Procedural, and Laboratory Terms Exercises

Check Your Knowledge

Fill in the blanks.

55. Viewing of the cervix and vagina may be done with a _____.

56. Viewing of the uterus may be done with a _____.

57. Pap smears and mammograms are both _____ screening tests.

58. A pregnancy test can be performed on _____ or _____.

59. Presence of HCG indicates _____.

Pathological Terms

Pregnancy is a normal process, with gestation taking about 40 weeks and ending in the birth of an infant through the vagina. Some pregnancies are not in themselves normal and spontaneously end in **abortion.** Abortion is a controversial term in public discourse, but in medicine, it simply means the premature end of a pregnancy, whether spontaneously during a **miscarriage,** or surgically. There are several types of abortion, such as *habitual abortion*—three or more consecutive abortions; spontaneous abortions—those that appear to occur for no specific medical reason; and *missed abortion*, an abortion in which the fetus is dead in the womb for two months or more.

Pregnancies can involve many complications. The initial pregnancy can implant abnormally outside the uterus as in an *ectopic pregnancy*, which requires surgery to remove the fetus because it will die due to lack of nourishment. A *tubal pregnancy* is implantation of the fetus within the fallopian tube or partially within the tube and partially within the abdominal cavity or uterus, and also requires immediate surgery to remove the fetus to avoid rupture as the ovum grows. The placenta may break away from the uterine wall (**abruptio placentae**) and require immediate delivery of the infant. **Placenta previa** is a condition in which the placenta blocks the birth canal, and usually requires a caesarean delivery. Even though a pregnancy appears normal, a *stillbirth*, birth of a dead fetus, may occur. The typical pregnancy lasts from 37 to 40 weeks. An infant may be born *prematurely*, before 37 week's gestation. A toxic condition during pregnancy is called **preeclampsia.** Symptoms are sudden hypertension with proteinuria and/or edema. Left untreated, preeclampsia can lead to *eclampsia* or *toxemia*, a life-threatening condition.

Chapter 12 discusses blood types. If untreated, one of the most dangerous conditions in pregnancy occurs when a mother has a different Rh factor from the father. The child may then carry an Rh factor different from the mother's, in which case *Rh incompatibility* or *erythroblastosis fetalis*, a potentially dangerous fetal condition, may occur.

Normal delivery of an infant is with a *cephalic presentation*, in which the head appears first, but a fetus may have to be delivered in *breech presentation*, in which the buttocks or feet appear first.

Fetal birth defects can occur in any of the body's systems. In the reproductive system, abnormalities such as *hypospadias*, a defect in which the urethra opens into the vagina, can occur. Other malformations, such as of the uterus or uterine tubes, may cause fertility problems later in life.

Menstrual abnormalities sometimes occur. **Amenorrhea,** the absence of menstruation, may result from a normal condition (pregnancy or menopause) or an abnormal condition (excessive dieting or extremely strenuous exercise). It may also occur for no apparent reason. **Dysmenorrhea** is painful cramping associated with menstruation. **Menorrhagia** is excessive menstrual bleeding. **Oligomenorrhea** is a scanty menstrual period. **Menometrorrhagia** is irregular and often excessive bleeding during or between menstrual periods. **Metrorrhagia** is uterine bleeding between menstrual periods.

Other abnormal conditions in the female cycle also occur. **Anovulation** is the absence of ovulation. **Oligo-ovulation** is irregular ovulation. **Leukorrhea** is an abnormal vaginal discharge. **Dyspareunia** is painful sexual intercourse, usually due to some condition, such as dryness, inflammation, or other disorder, in the female reproductive system. The uterus normally sits forward over the bladder. Abnormal positioning of the uterus includes **anteflexion,** a bending forward. **Retroflexion** is a bending backward of the uterus, and **retroversion** is a backward turn of the uterus sometimes called a *tipped uterus*. Various inflammations and infections occur in the female reproductive system. **Cervicitis** is an inflammation of the cervix. **Mastitis** is a general term for inflammation of the breast, particularly during lactation. **Salpingitis** is an inflammation of the fallopian tubes. **Vaginitis** is an inflammation of the vagina. *Toxic shock syndrome* is a rare, severe infection that occurs in menstruating women and is usually associated with tampon use. *Pelvic inflammatory disease (PID)* is a bacterial infection anywhere in the female reproductive system.

Organs of the reproductive system may suffer from muscle weakness. A *prolapsed uterus* is a condition where the uterine muscles cause the cervix to protrude into the vaginal opening. Pubic muscles can be strengthened using **Kegel exercises,** alternately contracting and releasing the perineal muscles.

Growths in the female reproductive system are benign or malignant. Benign or malignant growths can cause pain, abnormal bleeding, infertility, and pregnancy complications. *Cervical polyps* usually start out benign, but can become malignant. If accompanying bleeding is troublesome or if there is danger of their becoming malignant, polyps can be removed surgically. A **condyloma** is a growth on the outside of the genitalia that may be a result of a disease such as human papilloma virus. An *ovarian cyst* develops on or in the ovaries. **Fibroids** are common benign tumors found in the uterus or other areas. They may cause pain and bleeding. Some growths occur when normal tissue is found in abnormal areas; for example, **endometriosis** is an abnormal condition in which uterine wall tissue is found in the pelvis or on the abdominal wall. Any symptom that is new or unusual should be watched and checked with a healthcare provider.

Malignant growths are commonly found in the reproductive system. *Cervical cancer* is a potentially fatal disease that is often detected early with Pap smears before having spread (**carcinoma in situ**). *Endometrial cancer* occurs in the endometrium. *Ovarian cancer* is a potentially fatal cancer of the ovary, which is difficult to diagnose in its earliest stages and often spreads to other organs before it is detected. *Breast cancer* can be found locally in one site without spreading (carcinoma in situ) or may require more extensive treatment if it has spread to the lymph nodes. An important chemical test for estrogen receptors (cells that bind to estrogen) indicates whether hormone therapy is an option for the patient.

Sexually transmitted diseases (STDs) are diseases that are transmitted primarily through sexual contact. **Syphilis,** acute infection disease treatable with antibiotics; **gonorrhea,** a contagious infection of the genital mucous membrane; *herpes II,* contagious and recurring infection with lesions on the genitalia; *human papilloma virus (HPV),* contagious infection that causes genital warts; **chlamydia,** a common bacterial agent in sexually transmitted diseases or the disease itself; and *HIV* (which leads to AIDS) are some common sexually transmitted diseases. *Trichomoniasis,* another name for vaginitis or urethritis, may also be transmitted through sexual contact.

MORE ABOUT...
Diagnosing Breast Cancer

Breast cancer is often seen on a mammogram as an unusual growth. The next step is a biopsy to determine whether the growth is malignant or benign. Research is in progress on a number of fronts. Some so-called "breast cancer" genes have been identified. Women who have such a gene are many times more likely to develop breast cancer than those in the general population. Some preventive medications, such as Tamoxifen, have been found to be beneficial. The best outcome results from the earliest possible diagnosis and breast self-examination and mammography are used widely to try and catch breast cancer early.

Vocabulary Review

In the previous section, you learned terms related to pathology. Before going on to the exercises, review the terms below and refer to the previous section if you have any questions.

Term	Word Analysis	Definition
abortion	[ă-BŎR-shŭn] From Latin *abortus*, abortion	Premature ending of a pregnancy.
abruptio placentae	[ăb-RŬP-shē-ō plă-SĔN-tē] Latin, a breaking off of the placenta	Breaking away of the placenta from the uterine wall.
amenorrhea	[ā-mĕn-ō-RĒ-ă] a-, without + meno-, menstruation + -rrhea, flow	Lack of menstruation.
anovulation	[ăn-ŏv-yū-LĀ-shŭn] an-, without + ovulation	Lack of ovulation.
anteflexion	[ăn-tē-FLĔK-shŭn] ante-, before + flexion, a bending	Bending forward, as of the uterus.
carcinoma in situ	[kăr-sĭ-NŌ-mă ĭn SĪ-tū]	Localized malignancy that has not spread.
cervicitis	[sĕr-vĭ-SĪ-tĭs] cervico-, cervix + -itis, inflammation	Inflammation of the cervix.
chlamydia	[klă-MĬD-ē-ă] Greek *chlamys*, cloak	Sexually transmitted bacterial infection affecting various parts of the male or female reproductive systems; the bacterial agent itself.
condyloma	[kŏn-dĭ-LŌ-mă] Greek *kondyloma*, knob	Growth on the external genitalia.
dysmenorrhea	[dĭs-mĕn-ōr-Ē-ă] dys-, abnormal + meno- + -rrhea	Painful menstruation.
dyspareunia	[dĭs-pă-RŪ-nē-ă] dys- + Greek *pareumos*, lying beside	Painful sexual intercourse due to any of various conditions, such as cysts, infection, or dryness, in the vagina.
endometriosis	[ĔN-dō-mē-trē-Ō-sĭs] endometri(um) + -osis, condition	Abnormal condition in which uterine wall tissue is found in the pelvis or on the abdominal wall.

Term	Word Analysis	Definition
fibroid	[FĪ-brŏyd]	Benign tumor commonly found in the uterus.
gonorrhea	[gŏn-ō-RĒ-ă] Greek *gonorrhoia*, from *gone*, seed + -rrhea	Sexually transmitted inflammation of the genital membranes.
Kegel exercises	[KĒ-gĕl] After A. H. Kegel, U. S. gynecologist	Exercises to strengthen pubic muscles.
leukorrhea	[lū-kō-RĒ-ă] leuko-, white + -rrhea	Abnormal vaginal discharge; usually whitish.
mastitis	[măs-TĪ-tĭs] mast-, breast + -itis	Inflammation of the breast.
menometrorrhagia	[MĔN-ō-mĕ-trō-RĀ-jē-ă] meno- + metro-, uterus + -rrhagia, excessive flow	Irregular or excessive bleeding between or during menstruation.
menorrhagia	[mĕn-ō-RĀ-jē-ă] meno- + -rrhagia	Excessive menstrual bleeding.
metrorrhagia	[mĕ-trŏ-RĀ-jē-ă] metro- + -rrhagia	Uterine bleeding between menstrual periods.
miscarriage	[mĭs-KĂR-ĭj]	Spontaneous, premature ending of a pregnancy.
oligomenorrhea	[ŎL-ĭ-gō-mĕn-ō-RĒ-ă] oligo-, scanty + meno- + -rrhea	Scanty menstrual period.
oligo-ovulation	[ŎL-ĭ-gō-ŎV-yū-LĀ-shŭn] oligo- + ovulation	Irregular ovulation.
placenta previa	[plă-SĔN-tă PRĒ-vē-ă] placenta + Latin *prae*, before + *via*, the way	Placement of the placenta so it blocks the birth canal.
preeclampsia	[prē-ĕ-KLĂMP-sē-ă] pre-, before + eclampsia, convulsion	Toxic infection during pregnancy.
retroflexion	[rĕ-trō-FLĔK-shŭn] retro-, toward the back + flexion, a bending	Bending backward of the uterus.
retroversion	[rĕ-trō-VĔR-shŭn] retro- + version, a change of position	Backward turn of the uterus.

Term	Word Analysis	Definition
salpingitis	[săl-pĭn-JĪ-tĭs] salping-, fallopian tube + -itis	Inflammation of the fallopian tubes.
syphilis	[SĬF-ĭ-lĭs]	Sexually transmitted acute infection.
vaginitis	[văj-ĭ-NĪ-tĭs] vagin-, vagina + -itis	Inflammation of the vagina.

C A S E S T U D Y

Finding the Cause

Sarah Messer recovered from menorrhagia and persistent ovarian pain, and was able to return to work after two days off. Six months later, however, Sarah experienced heavy bleeding and painful cramps after missing one menstrual period. She did not think she was pregnant, but Dr. Alvino had her HCG level checked and it showed that she was indeed pregnant. Sarah's bleeding turned out to be an early miscarriage. Dr. Alvino prescribed medication for the pain, and again told Sarah to take two days off from work, during which the bleeding should stop. If not, she was to call him.

Dr. Alvino talked to Sarah about the benefits of birth control. He particularly thought that condoms would be appropriate for now, while Sarah remains sexually active with more than one partner.

 Critical Thinking

60. What diseases might Sarah contract if she does not use condoms?

61. Does the birth control pill protect you from sexually transmitted diseases?

Pathological Terms Exercises

Check Your Knowledge

Fill in the blanks.

62. If an ovum is not fertilized, _____ usually occurs within two weeks.

63. Amenorrhea can result from two normal conditions—_____ and _____.

64. Painful menstruation is called _____.

65. Toxic shock syndrome is a rare infection that usually occurs during _____.

66. Pap smears test for _____ cancer.

67. Benign tumors found in the uterus are _____.

68. Pubic muscles can be strengthened using _____ exercises.

69. Chlamydia is a _____ _____ disease.

70. An abortion is the premature ending of a _____, whether spontaneously or by choice.

71. Scanty menstruation is _____.

72. A toxic infection during pregnancy is _____.

73. AIDS is caused by _____, a sexually transmitted virus.

74. A localized cancer is called a _____ _____ _____.

75. Uterine bleeding other than that associated with menstruation is called _____.

76. Delivery of the buttocks or feet first is known as a _____ _____.

77. Premature birth occurs before _____ weeks of gestation.

Surgical Terms

Surgery of the female reproductive system is performed for a variety of reasons. During pregnancy, it may be necessary to terminate a pregnancy prematurely (*abortion*), to remove a fetus through an abdominal incision (*caesarean birth*), to open and scrape the lining of the uterus (*dilation and curettage [D & C]*), or to puncture the amniotic sac to obtain a sample of the fluid for examination (**amniocentesis**). In **culdocentesis,** a sample of fluid from the base of the pelvic cavity may show if an ectopic pregnancy has ruptured. An ectopic pregnancy can be removed through a **salpingotomy,** an incision into one of the fallopian tubes. Surgery may also be performed as a form of birth control. *Tubal ligation*, a method of female sterilization, blocks the fallopian tubes by cutting or tying and, therefore, blocking the passage of ova. It is usually performed using a *laparoscope*, a thin tube inserted into a woman's navel during **laparoscopy. Cryosurgery** and **cauterization** are two methods of destroying tissue (such as polyps) using cold temperatures in the former and burning in the latter.

Parts of the female reproductive system may have to be removed, usually because of the presence of cancer or benign growths that cause pain or excessive bleeding. A biopsy is usually performed first to determine the spread of cancer. A **conization** is the removal of a cone-shaped section of the cervix for examination. Breast cancer may be diagnosed by **aspiration,** a type of biopsy in which fluid is withdrawn through a needle by suction. A **hysterectomy** is removal of the uterus that may be done through the abdomen (*abdominal hysterectomy*) or through the vagina (*vaginal hysterectomy*). Figure 10-7 shows the two types of hysterectomies. New procedures such as laparascopic hysterectomies are reducing recovery time. A **myomectomy** is the removal of fibroid tumors. An **oophorectomy** is the removal of an ovary. An *ovarian cystectomy* is the removal of an ovarian cyst. A **salpingectomy** is the removal of a fallopian tube. A *salpingo-oophorectomy* is the removal of one ovary and one

Amniocentesis provides information about the genetic makeup and development of a fetus.

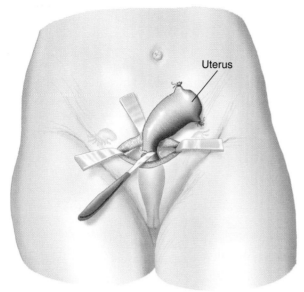

Uterus

Abdominal hysterectomy

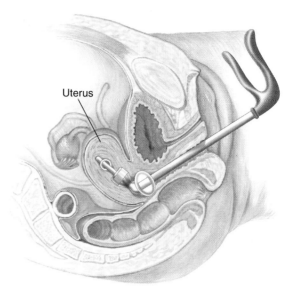

Uterus

Vaginal hysterectomy

Figure 10-7 Hysterectomies can be performed abdominally or vaginally. A surgical instrument is inserted through the cervix in a vaginal hysterectomy.

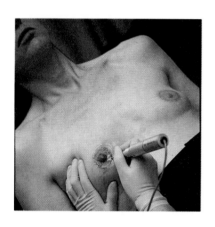

Figure 10-8 Mastectomies can usually be followed by breast reconstruction. Shown here is tattooing of an areola on a reconstructed breast.

fallopian tube. A *bilateral salpingo-oophorectomy* is the removal of the ovaries and both fallopian tubes. A **salpingotomy** is an incision into the fallopian tubes (to remove blockages).

Breast cancer may be treated surgically. A **lumpectomy** is the removal of the tumor itself along with surrounding tissue. A **mastectomy** is the removal of a breast, which may mean the breast and underlying muscle as in a *simple mastectomy*; the breast, underlying muscles, and the lymph nodes, as in a *radical mastectomy*; or removal of the breast and lymph nodes, as in a *modified radical mastectomy*. Figure 10-8 shows one type of mastectomy and reconstruction, rebuilding of the breast after a mastectomy.

Breast surgery may include plastic surgery after mastectomy (**mammoplasty**) or reduction of the size of the breast (*reduction mammoplasty*). Some women have pendulous breast tissue raised (**mastopexy**) or have small breasts augmented by surgical insertion of implants (*augmentation mammoplasty*).

Vocabulary Review

In the previous section, you learned terms relating to surgery. Before going on to the exercises, review the terms below and refer to the previous section if you have any questions.

Term	Word Analysis	Meaning
amniocentesis	[ĂM-nē-ō-sĕn-TĒ-sĭs] amnio-, amnion + -centesis, puncture	Removal of a sample of amniotic fluid through a needle injected in the amniotic sac.

Term	Word Analysis	Meaning
aspiration	[ăs-pĭ-RĀ-shŭn] Latin *aspiratio*, breath	Biopsy in which fluid is withdrawn through a needle by suction.
cauterization	[kăw-tĕr-ĭ-ZĀ-shŭn] From Greek *kauterion*, a branding iron	Removal or destruction of tissue using chemicals or devices, such as laser-guided equipment.
conization	[kō-nĭ-ZĀ-shŭn]	Removal of a cone-shaped section of the cervix for examination.
cryosurgery	[krī-ō-SĔR-jĕr-ē] cryo-, cold + surgery	Removal or destruction of tissue using cold temperatures.
culdocentesis	[KŬL-dō-sĕn-TĒ-sĭs] French *cul-de-sac*, bottom of the sack + -centesis	Taking of a fluid sample from the base of the pelvic cavity to see if an ectopic pregnancy has ruptured.
hysterectomy	[hĭs-tĕr-ĔK-tō-mē] hyster-, uterus + -ectomy, removal	Removal of the uterus.
laparoscopy	[lăp-ă-RŌS-kō-pē] laparo-, loins + -scopy, a viewing	Use of a lighted tubular instrument inserted through a woman's navel to perform a tubal ligation or to examine the fallopian tubes.
lumpectomy	[lŭm-PĔK-tō-mē] lump + -ectomy	Removal of a breast tumor.
mammoplasty	[MĂM-ō-plăs-tē] mammo-, breast + -plasty, repair	Plastic surgery to reconstruct the breast, particularly after a mastectomy.
mastectomy	[măs-TĔK-tō-mē] mast-, breast + -ectomy	Removal of a breast.
mastopexy	[MĂS-tō-pĕk-sē] masto-, breast + -pexy, a fixing	Surgical procedure to attach sagging breasts in a more normal position.
myomectomy	[mī-ō-MĔK-tō-mē] myoma, benign tumor + -ectomy	Removal of fibroids from the uterus.
oophorectomy	[ō-ŏf-ōr-ĔK-tō-mē] oophor-, ovary + -ectomy	Removal of an ovary.

Term	Word Analysis	Meaning
salpingectomy	[săl-pĭn-JĔK-tō-mē] salping-, fallopian tube + -ectomy	Removal of a fallopian tube.
salpingotomy	[săl-pĭng-GŎT-ō-mē] salpingo- + -tomy, a cutting	Incision into the fallopian tubes.

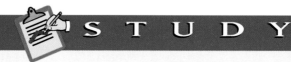

C A S E   S T U D Y

Treating the Problem

Jane Smits learned in her next exam that she now has some cysts on her left ovary. Her right ovary had been removed earlier because of cysts. Jane wants to have a child and expresses her concern to Dr. Alvino.

 Critical Thinking

78. Jane had a surgery in which one ovary and one fallopian tube were removed. What is the medical term for this surgery ?

79. Jane wants to have children. How might her current condition present a problem?

Surgical Terms Exercises

Know the Parts

Refer to Figure 10-1(a) on page 349. In the following list, write the name of the part(s) to be removed or altered in the surgery indicated.

80. salpingectomy _____

81. hysterectomy _____

82. bilateral salpingo-oophorectomy _____

83. tubal ligation _____

Pharmacological Terms

Various forms of birth control are pharmacological agents. Spermicides destroy sperm in the vagina; **birth control pills** and **implants** control the flow of hormones to block ovulation; and **abortifacients** or **morning-after pills** prevent implantation of an ovum. **Hormone replacement therapy (HRT)** is used during and after menopause to alleviate symptoms, such as hot flashes. **Oxytocin,** another hormone, is used to induce labor. A **tocolytic agent** stops labor contractions. Table 10-2 lists common pharmacological agents used for the female reproductive system.

Table 10-2 Some Common Medications Used in Providing Birth Control and in Treating Disorders of the Female Reproductive System.

Drug Class	Purpose	Generic	Trade Name
abortifacient or morning-after pill	to prevent implantation of an ovum		RU-486
hormone replacement therapy (HRT)	to normalize hormone levels in the body	estrogen progesterone	Estratab, Premarin Cycrin, Fematrone, Progestilin
hormones related to birth	to induce labor to stop labor	oxytocin tocolytic	Pitocin, Syntocin

Vocabulary Review

In the previous section, you learned terms related to pharmacology. Before going on to the exercises, review the terms below and refer to the previous section if you have any questions.

Agent	Word Analysis	Purpose
abortifacient	[ă-bōr-tǐ-FĀ-shĕnt] Latin *abortus*, abortion + *faceo*, to make	Medication to prevent implantation of an ovum.
birth control pills or implants		Medication that controls the flow of hormones to block ovulation.
hormone replacement therapy (HRT)		Treatment with hormones when the body stops or decreases the production of hormones by itself.
morning-after pill		*See* abortifacient.
oxytocin	[ŏk-sē-TŌ-sǐn] Greek *okytokos*, quick birth	Hormone given to induce labor.
tocolytic agent	[tō-kō-LĬT-ǐk] Greek *tokos*, birth + -lytic, loosening	Hormone given to stop labor.

CASE STUDY

Removing a Malignancy

Jane Smits, who had several check-ups over the next few months, eventually required a hysterectomy. Some abnormal cells on her latest pap smear turned out to be malignant. The cancer was contained, so her prognosis for recovery is excellent.

Critical Thinking

84. Jane, 30 years old at the time of her hysterectomy, was given estrogen and progesterone following her surgery. What is this treatment called?

85. Is it necessary for Jane and her husband to use birth control?

Pharmacological Terms Exercises

Check Your Knowledge

Circle T for true or F for false.

86. An abortifacient is a birth control medication. T F

87. Hormone replacement therapy is generally used around menopause. T F

88. It is never proper to induce labor. T F

89. Birth control pills are used to control hormones. T F

90. Tocolytic agents stop labor. T F

CHALLENGE SECTION

Dr. Maya Lundgren, an obstetrician at the HMO, examined Elisa Mayaguez, who is 26 years old. Dr. Lundgren entered the following notes on Elisa's chart.

Patient is a 26-year old, gravida 2, para 1, seen in the office today with symptoms of preterm labor at 30 weeks' gestation.

Patient reports an uncomplicated prenatal course until two weeks ago. Patient stated that she had some break-through bleeding, which seemed to improve following bed rest. Patient reports mild, regular contractions starting yesterday but diminishing today. Patient reports only mild "twinges" today. No cramping or back pain. She had preterm labor with her first gestation. Her first child was born at 32-week's gestation.

Physical exam was essentially normal. BP 130/80, P 100. HEENT: PERRLA. Lungs were clear to auscultation. Pelvic exam consistent with gestational dates. Cervix is dilated 2 cm. No edema noted. Her membranes are intact. Fetal heart tones 150's with increases noted to 170's. Baby active.

Patient was placed on strict bed rest. She was prescribed oral terbutaline to suppress labor. Patient to return to office in one week.

Challenge Section Exercises

91. The patient's first child was born at 32-week's gestation. What is the period of normal gestation? Was her first child born pre-term or post-term?

92. The patient is gravida 2, para 1. This means_____

_____

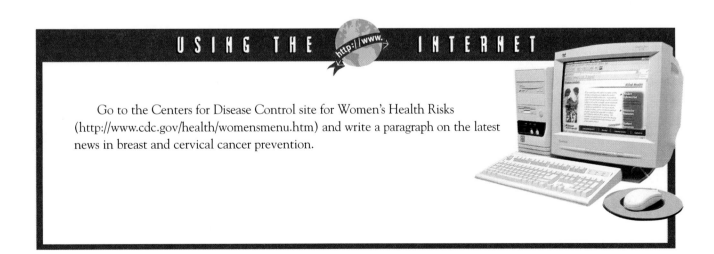

USING THE INTERNET

Go to the Centers for Disease Control site for Women's Health Risks (http://www.cdc.gov/health/womensmenu.htm) and write a paragraph on the latest news in breast and cervical cancer prevention.

CHAPTER REVIEW

Definitions

Define the following terms and combining forms. Review the chapter before starting. Make sure you know how to pronounce each term as you define it.

Word	Definition
abortion [ă-BŎR-shŭn]	
abortifacient [ă-bŏr-tĭ-FĀ-shĕnt]	
abruptio placentae [ăb-RŬP-shē-ō plă-SĔN-tē]	
afterbirth [ĂF-tĕr-bĕrth]	
amenorrhea [ā-mĕn-ō-RĒ-ă]	
amni(o)	
amniocentesis [ĂM-nē-ō-sĕn-TĒ-sĭs]	
amnion [ĂM-nē-ŏn]	
amniotic [ăm-nē-ŎT-ĭk] fluid	
anovulation [ăn-ŏv-yū-LĀ-shŭn]	
anteflexion [ăn-tē-FLĔK-shŭn]	
areola [ă-RĒ-ō-lă]	
aspiration [ăs-pĭ-RĀ-shŭn]	
Bartholin's [BĂR-thō-lĕnz] gland	
birth control pills or implants	
body	
carcinoma in situ [kăr-sĭ-NŌ-mă ĭn SĪ-tū]	
cauterization [kăw-tĕr-ĭ-ZĀ-shŭn]	
cervic(o)	
cervicitis [sĕr-vĭ-SĪ-tĭs]	
cervix [SĔR-vĭks]	
chlamydia [klă-MĬD-ē-ă]	
chorion [KŌ-rē-ŏn]	
climacteric [klĭ-MĂK-tēr-ĭk, klĭ-măk-TĔR-ĭk]	

Word	Definition
clitoris [KLĬT-ō-rĭs]	
coitus [KŌ-ĭ-tŭs]	
colp(o)	
colposcopy [kŏl-PŎS-kō-pē]	
condom [KŎN-dŏm]	
condyloma [kŏn-dĭ-LŌ-mă]	
conization [kō-nĭ-ZĀ-shŭn]	
contraception [kŏn-tră-SĔP-shŭn]	
copulation [kŏp-yū-LĀ-shŭn]	
corpus luteum [KŌR-pŭs LŪ-tē-ŭm]	
cryosurgery [krī-ō-SĔR-jĕr-ē]	
culdocentesis [KŬL-dō-sĕn-tē-sĭs]	
culdoscopy [kŭl-DŎS-kō-pē]	
diaphragm [DĪ-ă-frăm]	
dysmenorrhea [dĭs-mĕn-ōr-Ē-ă]	
dyspareunia [dĭs-pă-RŪ-nē-ă]	
endometriosis [ĔN-dŏ-mē-trē-Ō-sĭs]	
endometrium [ĔN-dō-MĒ-trē-ŭm]	
episi(o)	
estrogen [ĔS-trō-jĕn]	
fallopian [fă-LŌ-pē-ăn] tube	
fibroid [FĪ-brŏyd]	
fimbriae [FĬM-brē-ē]	
follicle-stimulating hormone (FSH)	
foreskin [FŌR-skĭn]	
fundus [FŬN-dŭs]	
galact(o)	
gamete [GĂM-ēt]	
gestation [jĕs-TĀ-shŭn]	
gonad [GŌ-năd]	
gonorrhea [gŏn-ō-RĒ-ă]	
graafian follicle [gră-FĒ-ĕn FŎL-Ĭ-kl]	
gravida [GRĂV-Ĭ-dă]	
gynec(o)	

Word	Definition
gynecologist [gī-nĕ-KŎL-ō-jĭst]	
hormone [HŌR-mōn]	
hormone replacement therapy (HRT)	
hymen [HĪ-mĕn]	
hyster(o)	
hysterectomy [hĭs-tĕr-ĔK-tō-mē]	
hysterosalpingography [HĬS-tĕr-ō-săl-pĭng-GŎG-rĕ-fē]	
hysteroscopy [hĭs-tĕr-ŎS-kō-pē]	
intrauterine [ĬN-tră-YŪ-tĕr-ĭn] device (IUD)	
introitus [ĭn-TRŌ-ĭ-tŭs]	
isthmus [ĬS-mŭs]	
Kegel [KĒ-gĕl] exercises	
labia majora [LĀ-bē-ă mă-JŌR-ă]	
labia minora [mă-NŌR-ă]	
lact(o), lacti	
lactation [lăk-TĀ-shŭn]	
lactiferous [lăk-TĬF-ĕr-ŭs]	
laparoscopy [lăp-ă-RŎS-kō-pē]	
leukorrhea [lū-kō-RĒ-ă]	
lumpectomy [lŭm-PĔK-tō-mē]	
luteinizing [LŪ-tē-ĭn-Ī-zĭng] hormone (LH)	
mamm(o)	
mammary [MĂM-ă-rē] glands	
mammography [mă-MŎG-ră-fē]	
mammoplasty [MĂM-ō-plăs-tē]	
mast(o)	
mastectomy [măs-TĔK-tō-mē]	
mastitis [măs-TĪ-tĭs]	
mastopexy [MĂS-tō-pĕk-sē]	
men(o)	
menarche [mĕ-NĂR-kē]	

Word	Definition
menometrorrhagia [MĔN-ō-mĕ-trō-RĀ-jē-ă]	
menopause [MĔN-ō-păwz]	
menorrhagia [mĕn-ō-RĀ-jē-ă]	
menstruation [mĕn-strū-Ā-shŭn]	
metr(o)	
metrorrhagia [mĕ-trŏ-RĀ-jē-ă]	
miscarriage [mĭs-KĂR-ĭj]	
mons pubis [mŏnz pyū-BĬS]	
morning-after pill	
myomectomy [mī-ō-MĔK-tō-mē]	
myometrium [MĪ-ō-MĒ-trē-ŭm]	
nipple [NĬP-l]	
oo	
obstetrician [ŏb-stĕ-TRĬSH-ŭn]	
oligomenorrhea [ŎL-ĭ-gō-mĕn-ō-RĒ-ă]	
oligo-ovulation [ŎL-ĭ-gō-ŎV-yū-LĀ-shŭn]	
oocyte [Ō-ō-sīt]	
oophor(o)	
oophorectomy [ō-ŏf-ōr-ĔK-tō-mē]	
ov(i), ov(o)	
ovari(o)	
ovary [Ō-vă-rē]	
ovulation [ŎV-yū-LĀ-shŭn]	
ovum (p. ova) [Ō-vŭm (Ō-vă)]	
oxytocin [ŏk-sē-TŌ-sĭn]	
Papanicolaou (Pap) [pă-pĕ-NĒ-kō-lū] smear	
para [PĂ-ră]	
parturition [păr-tūr-ĬSH-ŭn]	
pelvimetry [pĕl-VĬM-ĕ-trē]	
perimenopause [pĕr-ĭ-MĔN-ō-păws]	
perimetrium [pĕr-ĭ-MĒ-trē-ŭm]	

Word	Definition
perine(o)	
perineum [PĚR-ĭ-NĒ-ŭm]	
placenta [plă-SĚN-tă]	
placenta previa [plă-SĚN-tă PRĒ-vē-ă]	
preeclampsia [prē-ĕ-KLĂMP-sē-ă]	
progesterone [prō-JĚS-tĕr-ōn]	
puberty [PYŪ-bĕr-tē]	
retroflexion [rĕ-trō-FLĚK-shŭn]	
retroversion [rĕ-trō-VĚR-shŭn]	
salping(o)	
salpingectomy [săl-pĭn-JĚK-tō-mē]	
salpingitis [săl-pĭn-JĪ-tĭs]	
salpingotomy [săl-pĭng-GŎT-ō-mē]	
sinus [SĪ-nŭs]	
spermicide [SPĚR-mĭ-sīd]	
sponge	
syphilis [SĬF-ĭ-lĭs]	
tocolytic [tō-kō-LĬT-ĭk] agent	
umbilical [ŭm-BĬL-ĭ-kăl] cord	
uter(o)	
uterine [YŪ-tĕr-ĭn] tube	
uterus [YŪ-tĕr-ŭs]	
vagin(o)	
vagina [vă-JĪ-nă]	
vaginitis [văj-ĭ-NĬ-tĭs]	
vulv(o)	
vulva [VŬL-vă]	

Abbreviations

Write the full meaning of each abbreviation.

Abbreviation	Meaning
AB	
AFP	
AH	

Abbreviation	Meaning
CIS	
CS	
C-section	
Cx	
D & C	
DES	
DUB	
ECC	
EDC	
EMB	
ERT	
FHT	
FSH	
G	
gyn	
HCG	
HRT	
HSG	
HSO	
IUD	
LH	
LMP	
multip	
OB	
OCP	
P	
Pap smear	
PID	
PMP	
PMS	
primip	
TAH-BSO	
TSS	
UC	

Answers to Chapter Exercises

1. Without fever.
2. Ovaries do not always alternate ovulation by months. Her single ovary has taken over the function of both.
3. c
4. a
5. b
6. d
7. ovary
8. uterus
9. ovulation
10. menstruation
11. fundus
12. cervix
13. perimetrium
14. breasts
15. menarche
16. menopause
17. estrogen, progesterone
18. contraception
19. chorion, amnion
20. afterbirth
21. no
22. blood pressure, pulse, yes
23. episiostenosis
24. mammogram
25. galactopoiesis
26. ovariocele
27. lactogen
28. perineorrhaphy
29. vaginomycosis
30. metralgia, metrodynia
31. vulvitis
32. colporrhagia
33. oogenesis
34. mastopathy
35. uteroplasty

36. salpingitis
37. cervicectomy
38. oophoroma
39. ovariotomy
40. metrostenosis
41. gynecoid
42. amniorrhexis
43. j
44. e
45. a
46. g
47. b
48. i
49. c
50. d
51. f
52. h
53. Jane's suggested diagnosis was pelvic inflammatory disease (PID). Examination of the vagina is a first step to confirming the diagnosis and seeing if there is an additional problem.
54. uterus, ovaries, fallopian tubes
55. colposcope
56. hysteroscope
57. cancer
58. blood, urine
59. pregnancy
60. a sexually transmitted disease, such as HIV, gonorrhea, herpes II, HPV, chlamydia
61. No; it does not block fluid-to-fluid contact.
62. menstruation

63. pregnancy, menopause
64. dysmenorrhea
65. menstruation
66. cervical
67. fibroids
68. Kegel
69. sexually transmitted
70. pregnancy
71. oligomenorrhea
72. preeclampsia
73. HIV
74. carcinoma in situ
75. metrorrhagia
76. breech birth
77. 37
78. salpingo-oophorectomy
79. If her left ovary needs to be removed, Jane will not be able to have children.
80. uterine tube
81. uterus
82. uterine tubes and ovaries
83. uterine tubes
84. hormone replacement therapy
85. No, a hysterectomy means that pregnancy is not possible.
86. T
87. T
88. F
89. T
90. T
91. 37-40 weeks; pre-term
92. She is in her second pregnancy and has one other child.

11

The Male Reproductive System

After studying this chapter, you will be able to

* Name the parts of the male reproductive system and discuss the function of each part

* Define combining forms used in building words that relate to the male reproductive system

* Identify the meaning of related abbreviations

* Name the common diagnoses, clinical procedures, and laboratory tests used in treating the male reproductive system

* List and define the major pathological conditions of the male reproductive system

* Explain the meaning of surgical terms related to the male reproductive system

* Recognize common pharmacological agents used in treating the male reproductive system

Structure And Function

The sex cell or **spermatozoon** (plural **spermatozoa**) or **sperm** is produced in the male gonads or **testes.** The testes are also called **testicles** and are contained within the **scrotum,** a sac outside the body. The development of sperm (**spermatogenesis**) takes place in the scrotum, where the temperature is lower than inside the body. The lower temperature is necessary for the safe development of sperm. Inside the testes are cells that manufacture the sperm cells. These cells are contained in *seminiferous tubules*. Between the seminiferous tubules lie endocrine cells that produce **testosterone,** the most important male hormone that is thought to decrease during a stage of life sometimes referred to as "male menopause." Table 11-1 lists the male reproductive hormones and their purpose. At the top part of each testis is the **epididymis,** a group of ducts for storing sperm. The sperm develop to maturity and become *motile* (able to move) in the epididymis. They leave the epididymis and enter a narrow tube called the **vas deferens.** The sperm then travel to the *seminal*

Table 11-1 Male Reproductive Hormones

Hormone	Purpose	Source
testosterone	stimulates development of male sex characteristics; increases sperm; inhibits LH	testes
FSH (follicle-stimulating hormone)	increases testosterone; aids in sperm maturation	pituitary gland
LH	stimulates testosterone secretion	pituitary gland
inhibin	inhibits FSH	testes

vesicles (which secrete material to help the sperm move) and to the *ejaculatory duct* leading to the **prostate gland** and the urethra. The prostate gland also secretes a fluid, **semen** (a mixture of sperm and secretions from the seminal vesicles, Cowper's glands, and prostate), that helps the sperm move. The gland then contracts its muscular tissue during ejaculation to help the sperm exit the body. Just below the prostate are the two **bulbourethral glands (Cowper's glands)** that also secrete a fluid that lubricates the inside of the urethra to help the semen move easily. The urethra passes through the **penis** to the outside of the body. The tip of the penis is called the **glans penis,** a sensitive area covered at birth by the **foreskin** (*prepuce*). Between the penis and the anus is the area called the **perineum.** Figure 11-1a shows the male reproductive system. Figure 11-1b is a diagram of the path of sperm through the system.

Figure 11-1a. The male reproductive system usually maintains fertility well into old age.

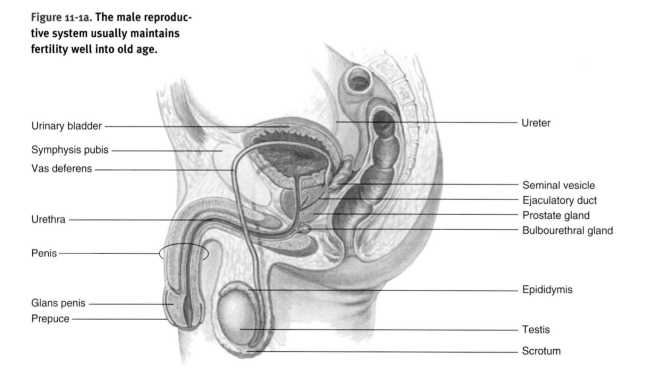

Urinary bladder

Symphysis pubis

Vas deferens

Urethra

Penis

Glans penis

Prepuce

Ureter

Seminal vesicle

Ejaculatory duct

Prostate gland

Bulbourethral gland

Epididymis

Testis

Scrotum

Male Hormones

Traditionally, the term *menopause* has referred to women only. In recent years, some researchers have studied the hormonal cycle of males. While males do not experience menstruation and its ultimate cessation, they do seem to experience reduced hormone production, particularly testosterone. This can cause symptoms similar to those of female menopause, including mood swings, decreased libido, and increased fatigue. Some men require treatment with hormonal therapy.

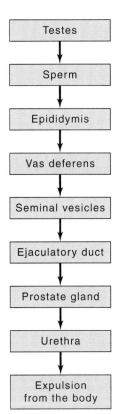

Figure 11-1b. A diagram of the path that sperm travel.

The spermatozoon is a microscopic cell, much smaller than an ovum. It has a head region that carries genetic material (*chromosomes*) and a tail (**flagellum**) that propels the sperm forward (Figure 11-2). During **ejaculation,** hundreds of millions of sperm are released. Usually only one sperm can fertilize a single ovum. In rare instances, two or more ova are fertilized at a single time, resulting in twins, triplets, quadruplets, and so on. *Identical twins* are the result of one ovum's splitting after it has been fertilized by a single sperm. *Fraternal twins* are the result of two sperm fertilizing two ova.

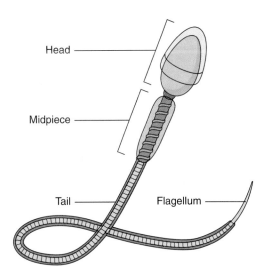

Figure 11-2. Spermatozoa have a flagellum to help propel them forward.

Vocabulary Review

In the previous section, you learned terms relating to the male reproductive system. Before going on to the exercises, review the terms below and refer to the previous section if you have any questions.

Term	Word Analysis	Definition
bulbourethral gland	[BŬL-bō-yū-RĒ-thrăl] bulbo-, bulb + urethra	*See* Cowper's gland.
Cowper's gland	[KŎW-pĕrs] After William Cowper (1666–1709), English anatomist	One of two glands below the prostate that secrete a fluid to lubricate the inside of the urethra.

Term	Word Analysis	Definition
ejaculation	[ē-jăk-yū-LĀ-shŭn] Latin *e-iaculo*, to shoot out	Expulsion of semen outside the body.
epididymis	[ĕp-ĭ-DĬD-ĭ-mĭs] Greek, on twins (testes)	Group of ducts at the top of the testis where sperm are stored.
flagellum	[flă-JĔL-ŭm] Latin, little whip	Tail at the end of a sperm that helps it move.
foreskin	[FŌR-skĭn] fore-, in front + skin	Flap of skin covering the glans penis; removed by circumcision in many cultures.
glans penis	[glănz PĒ-nĭs] Latin *glans*, acorn	Sensitive area at the tip of the penis.
penis	[PĒ-nĭs]	Male reproductive part that covers the urethra on the outside of the body.
perineum	[PĔR-ĭ-NĒ-ŭm] Greek *perineon*	Area between the penis and the anus.
prostate gland	[PRŎS-tāt] Greek *prostates*, one that protects	Gland surrounding the urethra that emits a fluid to help the sperm move and contracts its muscular tissue during ejaculation to help the sperm exit the body.
scrotum	[SKRŌ-tŭm] Latin, sac	Sac outside the body containing the testicles.
semen	[SĒ-mĕn] Latin, seed	Thick, whitish fluid containing spermatozoa and secretions from the seminal vesicles, Cowper's glands, and prostate; ejaculated from the penis.
sperm	[spĕrm] Greek *sperma*, seed	Male sex cell that contains chromosomes.
spermatogenesis	[SPĔR-mă-tō-JĔN-ĕ-sĭs] spermato-, sperm + -genesis	Production of sperm.
spermatozoon (pl. spermatozoa)	[SPĔR-mă-tō-ZŌ-ŏn (SPĔR-mă-tō-ZŌ-ă)] spermato- + Greek *zoon*, animal	*See* sperm.
testicle	[TĔS-tĭ-kl] Latin *testiculus*, small testis	*See* testis.

Term	Word Analysis	Definition
testis (pl. testes)	[TĔS-tĭs (TĔS-tēz)] Latin	Male organ that produces sperm and is contained in the scrotum.
testosterone	[tĕs-TŎS-tĕ-rōn]	Primary male hormone.
vas deferens	[vǎs DĔF-ĕr-ĕns] Latin, vessel that carries away	Narrow tube through which sperm leave the epididymis and travel to the seminal vesicles and into the urethra.

C A S E S T U D Y

Getting Help

Marta and Luis Consalvo have been trying to have a baby for two years. They are both young and healthy. Recently, Marta's obstetrician-gynecologist referred the couple to an infertility clinic. They found nothing in Marta that would cause infertility. They found, however, that Luis had a low sperm count. Marta's ob-gyn referred Luis to a urologist, Dr. Medina, for an examination.

Critical Thinking

1. Why did Marta's ob-gyn refer Luis to a urologist?

2. What parts of the male reproductive system might Dr. Medina examine for the cause of Luis's low sperm count?

Structure and Function Exercises

Check Your Knowledge

Choose answer a, b, or c to identify each of the following parts of the reproductive system.

a. only in males   b. only in females   c. in both males and females

3. sex cell _____

4. prostate gland _____

5. perineum _____

6. foreskin _____

7. scrotum _____

8. epididymis _____

9. fallopian tube _____

10. gamete _____

11. ova _____

12. spermatozoa _____

Follow the Path

Put in order the following sites through which sperm travel, starting with the letter a.

13. epididymis ____

14. seminal vesicles ____

15. testes ____

16. ejaculatory ducts ____

17. vas deferens ____

18. urethra ____

Check Your Understanding

Circle T for true or F for false.

19. Urine is stored in the prostate gland. T F

20. Fluid from the seminal vesicles helps the sperm move. T F

21. During ejaculation, about three thousand sperm are released. T F

22. Cowper's gland is another name for the prostate gland. T F

23. Identical twins result from two sperm and one ovum. T F

24. Male genetic material is called testosterone. T F

25. In many cultures, the glans penis is removed during circumcision. T F

Combining Forms and Abbreviations

The lists below include combining forms and abbreviations that relate specifically to the male reproductive system. Pronunciations are provided for the examples.

Combining Form	Meaning	Example
andr(o)	men	*andropathy* [ăn-DRŎP-ă-thē], any disease peculiar to men
balan(o)	glans penis	*balanitis* [băl-ă-NĪ-tĭs], inflammation of the glans penis
epididym(o)	epididymis	*epididymoplasty* [ĕp-ĭ-DĬD-ĭ-mō-plăs-tē], surgical repair of the epididymis
orch(o), orchi(o), orchid(o)	testes	*orchitis* [ōr-KĪ-tĭs], inflammation of the testis
prostat(o)	prostate gland	*prostatitis* [prŏs-tă-TĪ-tĭs], inflammation of the prostate
sperm(o), spermat(o)	sperm	*spermatogenesis* [SPĔR-mă-tō-JĔN-ĕ-sĭs], sperm production

Abbreviation	Meaning
AIH	artificial insemination homologous
BPH	benign prostatic hypertrophy
PED	penile erectile dysfunction
PSA	prostate-specific antigen
SPP	suprapubic prostatectomy
TURP	transurethral resection of the prostate

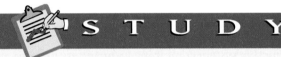

C A S E   S T U D Y

Achieving Results

Dr. Medina was able to help Luis by giving him prescription medication and telling him about certain techniques that can increase sperm count. Within six months, Marta was pregnant.

As a urologist, Dr. Medina treats both the reproductive and urinary systems of males. Men who have fertility problems account for a small percentage of Dr. Medina's practice. A slightly larger group sees Dr. Medina about difficulties in sexual functioning (PED, ED). Most of Dr. Medina's patients are much older than Luis. Middle-aged and elderly men tend to have urinary tract problems more frequently than younger men.

Bernard McCoy, who is 58 years old, called for an appointment. The receptionist scheduled a visit for 10:00 a.m. on November 15. She told Mr. McCoy to come in 10 minutes early to fill out a new patient information form.

Mr. McCoy arrived at 9:50 a.m. on November 15. After filling out the form, Mr. McCoy was escorted to the examining room where she made notes on the chart about his complaints. The doctor examined Mr. McCoy, and the examination included a digital rectal examination. The doctor added his notes to the patient's chart and ordered several tests. The patient was sent to the lab and told that Dr. Medina would speak to him as soon as the lab results come in. Dr. Medina adds his diagnosis on 11/22/XX.

Critical Thinking

26. What part of the urinary tract is tested for by a PSA test?

27. What condition does Dr. Medina think Mr. McCoy has?

11/15/XX TW: Bernard McCoy, age 58, complains of frequent urination, small stream, and stop and start urine flow; inability to achieve erection. RM: Lab: CBC, chem screen panel, PSA. Preliminary diagnosis: BPH. A. Medina, M. D.

Combining Forms and Abbreviations Exercises

Build Your Medical Vocabulary

Build words for the following definitions using at least one combining form from this chapter. You can refer to Chapters 2 and 3 for general combining forms.

28. Morbid fear of men: _____

29. Surgical reconstruction of the glans penis: _____

30. Killer of sperm: _____

31. Incision into a testis: _____

32. Abnormal discharge of prostate fluid: _____

Put the reproductive system combining form and its meaning in the space following the sentence.

33. A prostatectomy is usually performed only in cases of cancer.

_____

34. Androgens cause the development of male secondary sex characteristics.

_____

35. An orchiectomy is done in cases of cancer.

_____

36. Balanoplasty may be necessary in cases of injury.

_____

Diagnostic, Procedural, and Laboratory Terms

A normal male medical checkup may include a *digital rectal exam (DRE)*, the insertion of a finger into the rectum to check the rectum and prostate for abnormalities, and a **prostate-specific antigen (PSA) test,** a blood test to screen for prostate cancer. If a couple is having fertility problems, a **semen analysis** is done to determine the quantity and quality of the male partner's sperm.

X-ray or imaging procedures are used to further test for abnormalities or blockages. A **urethrogram** is an x-ray of the urethra and prostate. A sonogram may be used when needle biopsies are taken, as of the testicles or prostate. If cancer is present, surgery, chemotherapy, or radiation may be used. Hormone replacement therapy is given to males who have a deficiency of male hormones. Men who have erectile dysfunction may be treated chemically or with a *penile prosthesis*, a device implanted in the penis to treat impotence.

A positive PSA test may not mean that treatment is required. Some types of prostate cancer are slow to develop or occur in old age and are likely to remain contained. Other types of prostate cancer metastasize quickly and can be fatal.

Vocabulary Review

In the previous section, you learned terms relating to diagnosis, clinical procedures, and laboratory tests. Before going on to the exercises, review the following terms and refer to the previous section if you have any questions.

Term	Word Analysis	Definition
prostate-specific antigen (PSA) test		Blood test for prostate cancer.
semen analysis		Observation of semen for viability of sperm.
urethrogram	[yū-RĒ-thrō-grăm] urethro-, urethra + gram, a recording	X-ray of the urethra and prostate.

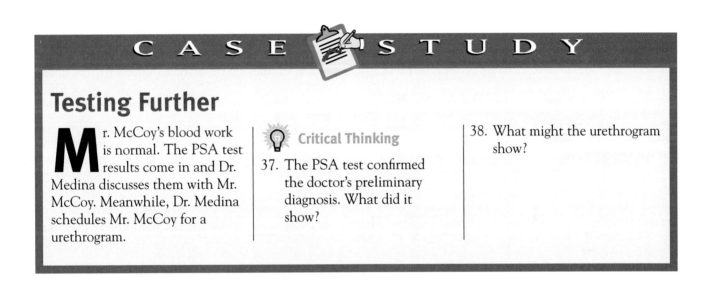

C A S E   S T U D Y

Testing Further

Mr. McCoy's blood work is normal. The PSA test results come in and Dr. Medina discusses them with Mr. McCoy. Meanwhile, Dr. Medina schedules Mr. McCoy for a urethrogram.

💡 **Critical Thinking**

37. The PSA test confirmed the doctor's preliminary diagnosis. What did it show?

38. What might the urethrogram show?

Diagnostic, Procedural, and Laboratory Terms Exercises

Check Your Knowledge

Fill in the blanks.

39. A semen analysis examines the _____ and _____ of sperm.

40. A DRE is for finding any abnormalities in the _____ and _____.

41. A PSA tests for _____ cancer.

42. Both males and females may need _____ _____ therapy.

43. Erectile problems may be treated chemically or with a _____ _____.

Pathological Terms

Birth or developmental defects affect the functioning of the reproductive system. An *undescended testicle* (**cryptorchism**) means that the normal descending of the testicle to the scrotal sac does not take place during gestation and requires surgery to place it properly (Figure 11-3). **Anorchism** or **anorchia** is the lack of one or both testes. **Hypospadias** is an abnormal opening of the urethra on the underside of the penis. **Epispadias** is an abnormal opening on the top side of the penis. Figure 11-4 shows these two abnormal conditions of the urinary meatus. **Phimosis** is an abnormal narrowing of the foreskin over the glans penis (only in uncircumsized males). These conditions are also repaired by surgery (circumcision), in which the foreskin is removed. As the male matures, infections and various other medical conditions may cause **infertility,** an inability to produce enough viable sperm to fertilize an ovum or an inability to deliver sperm to the proper location in the vagina. Several levels of sperm production may be involved in infertility. **Aspermia** is the inability to produce sperm; **azoospermia** is semen without living sperm; and **oligospermia** is the scanty production of sperm. Medical or psychological conditions may cause **impotence** (*penile erectile dysfunction*), inability to maintain an erection for ejaculation. **Priapism** is a persistent, painful erection, usually related to other medical conditions. **Hernias,** abnormal protrusions of part of a tissue or an organ out of its normal space through a barrier, may occur in the male reproductive system. A **hydrocele** is a fluid-containing hernia in a testicle (Figure 11-5); a **varicocele** is a group of herniated veins near the testes.

Various inflammations occur in the male reproductive system. **Prostatitis** is any inflammation of the prostate; **balanitis** is an inflammation of the glans penis; and **epididymitis** is an inflammation of the epididymis. Likewise, some diseases and conditions affect the function of the reproductive system. *Benign prostatic hypertrophy* or *hyperplasia (BPH)* is enlargement of the prostate gland not involving cancer but causing some obstruction of the urinary tract. **Peyronie's disease** is a disorder with curvature of the penis caused by some hardening in the interior structure of the penis. *Prostate cancer* and *testicular cancer* are fairly common malignancies. A common tumor of the testicle is a **seminoma.**

Figure 11-3. Cryptorchism is also known as an undescended testicle.

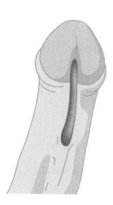

Undescended testis

Figure 11-4. Hypospadias and epispadias are two congenital urethral abnormalities.

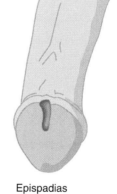

Hypospadias   Epispadias

Male infertility can be treated hormonally. Simple fertility techniques, such as waiting a certain number of days between ejaculation, can increase the number and viability of sperm in some cases.

Sexually transmitted diseases are the same for the male as for the female (see Chapters 10, 12, and 13), with males being more susceptible to **chancroids,** venereal sores caused by a bacterial infection on the penis, urethra, or anus.

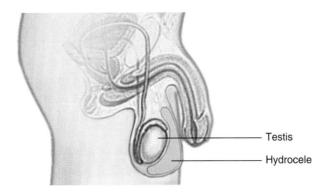

Figure 11-5. Hydroceles commonly occur in the scrotal sac.

Testis

Hydrocele

Vocabulary Review

In the previous section, you learned terms relating to pathology. Before going on to the exercises, review the terms below and refer to the previous section if you have any questions.

Term	Word Analysis	Definition
anorchism, anorchia	[ăn-ŌR-kĭzm, -kē-ă] an-, without + orch-, testicle + -ism, state of being	Congenital absence of one or both testicles.
aspermia	[ā-SPĔR-mē-ă] a-, without + sperm + -ia, condition	Inability to produce sperm.
azoospermia	[ā-zō-ō-SPĔR-mē-ă] a- + zoo-, life + sperm + -ia	Semen without living sperm.
balanitis	[băl-ă-NĪ-tĭs] Greek *balanos*, acorn + -itis, inflammation	Inflammation of the glans penis.
chancroids	[SHĂNG-krŏyds] chancr(e) + -oid, like	Bacterial infection that can be sexually transmitted; results in sores on the penis, urethra, or anus.
cryptorchism	[krĭp-TŌR-kĭzm] crypto-, hidden + orch- + -ism	Birth defect with the failure of one or both of the testicles to descend in to the scrotal sac.
epididymitis	[ĕp-ĭ-dĭd-ĭ-MĪ-tĭs] epididym(is) + -itis	Inflammation of the epididymis.

Term	Word Analysis	Definition
epispadias	[ĕp-ĭ-SPĀ-dē-ăs] epi-, upon + Greek *spadon*, a ripping or tearing	Birth defect with abnormal opening of the urethra on the top side of the penis.
hernia	[HĔR-nē-ă] Latin, rupture	Abnormal protrusion of tissue through muscle that contains it.
hydrocele	[HĪ-drō-sēl] hydro-, water + -cele, hernia	Fluid-containing hernia of the testis.
hypospadias	[HĪ-pō-SPĀ-dē-ăs] hypo-, under + Greek *spadon*, a ripping or tearing	Birth defect with abnormal opening of the urethra on the bottom side of the penis.
impotence	[ĬM-pō-tĕns] Latin *impotentia*, inability	Inability to maintain an erection for ejaculation.
infertility	[ĭn-fĕr-TĬL-ĭ-tē] in-, not + fertility	Inability to fertilize ova.
oligospermia	[ŏl-ĭ-gō-SPĔR-mē-ă] oligo-, few + sperm + -ia	Scanty production of sperm.
Peyronie's disease	[pā-RŌN-ēs] After Francois de la Peyronie (1678–1747), French surgeon	Abnormal curvature of the penis caused by hardening in the interior of the penis.
phimosis	[fĭ-MŌ-sĭs] Greek, a muzzling	Abnormal narrowing of the opening of the foreskin.
priapism	[PRĪ-ă-pĭzm] After Priapus, god of creation	Persistent, painful erection of the penis.
prostatitis	[prŏs-tă-TĪ-tĭs] prostat-, prostate + -itis	Inflammation of the prostate.
seminoma	[sĕm-ĭ-NŌ-mă] Latin *semen*, seed + -oma, tumor	Malignant tumor of the testicle.
varicocele	[VĂR-ĭ-kō-sēl] varico(se) + -cele	Enlargement of veins of the spermatic cord.

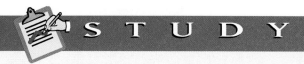

C A S E   S T U D Y

Resolving Problems

Marta and Luis Consalvo's baby, an 8-pound boy, was healthy except for hypospadias. Dr. Medina told the Consalvos that an operation to properly place the urethral opening would be needed, but as long as the baby remained in diapers, they could wait until he was a bit older for the surgery. The parents were also told to delay circumcision, so that any excess skin might be used to repair the penis.

After the Consalvo family left, Dr. Medina checked the results of several lab tests he had ordered in the last two weeks. Mr. McCoy, another of Dr. Medina's patients, had a PSA test that came back negative. Because Mr. McCoy had a swollen prostate, Dr. Medina called him to schedule an appointment. He planned to reexamine Mr. McCoy's prostate and to treat his condition if it still persisted.

Critical Thinking

44. Why might hypospadias cause urination problems once the baby is out of diapers and trained to use a toilet?

45. Hypospadias, if left untreated, may cause fertility problems later in life. How?

Pathological Terms Exercises

Find a Match

Match the definitions in the right-hand column with the terms in the left-hand column.

46. anorchism

47. aspermia

48. seminoma

49. balinitis

50. hydrocele

51. impotence

52. infertility

53. hypospadias

54. cryptorchism

55. azoospermia

a. inflammation of the glans penis

b. hernia in the testes

c. inability to maintain an erection

d. inability to fertilize an ovum

e. undescended testicle

f. lacking sperm

g. abnormal urethral opening

h. lacking testicles

i. having no living sperm

j. testicular tumor

Surgical Terms

The most common surgery of the male reproductive system is **circumcision,** the removal of the foreskin or prepuce (Figure 11-6). Various cultures and religions have rituals associated with this removal. Some parents prefer to have

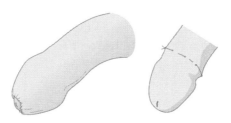

it done in the hospital immediately after birth. Other surgeries are to prevent or enhance the possibility of conception, diagnose or remove cancerous tumors, remove or reduce blockages, and remove or repair parts of the system.

Biopsies are commonly taken of the testicles and prostate when cancer is suspected. Various operations to remove cancerous or infected parts of the reproductive system are an **epididymectomy,** removal of an epididymis; an **orchiectomy** or **orchidectomy,** removal of a testicle; a **prostatectomy,** removal of the prostate gland, which may be done through the perineum or above the pubic bone; and a *transurethral resection of the prostate (TURP),* removal of a portion of the prostate through the urethra (Figure 11-7). A **vasectomy** is the removal of part of the vas deferens as a method of birth control. A **vasovasostomy** is the reversing of a vasectomy so the male regains fertility. **Castration** is the removal of the testicles in the male.

Figure 11-6. Circumcision is usually determined by cultural preference.

Figure 11-7. A TURP (transurethral resection of the prostate) is the removal of some prostate tissue through the urethra.

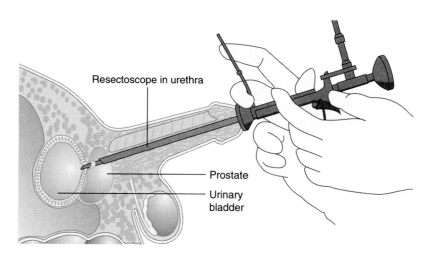

Resectoscope in urethra

Prostate

Urinary bladder

M O R E   A B O U T...
Birth Control

An operation is not necessary for male birth control. Other options available to males are a *condom,* a sheath worn over the penis to collect the semen after ejaculation, *coitus interruptus,* removal of the penis from the vagina before ejaculation, and a *male birth control pill,* which blocks the production of sperm.

In the previous section, you learned terms relating to pathology. Before going on to the exercises, review the terms below and refer to the previous section if you have any questions.

Term	Word Analysis	Definition
castration	[kăs-TRĀ-shŭn] Latin *castro*, to deprive of power	Removal of the testicles.
circumcision	[sĕr-kŭm-SĬZH-ŭn] Latin *circumcido*, to cut around	Removal of the foreskin.
epididymectomy	[ĔP-ĭ-dĭd-ĭ-MĔK-tō-mē] epididym(is) + -ectomy, removal	Removal of an epididymis.
orchidectomy	[ōr-kĭ-DĔK-tō-mē] orchid-, testicle + -ectomy	Removal of a testicle.
orchiectomy	[ōr-kē-ĔK-tō-mē] orchi-, testicle + -ectomy	Removal of a testicle.
prostatectomy	[prŏs-tă-TĔK-tō-mē] prostat- + -ectomy	Removal of the prostate.
vasectomy	[vā-SĔK-tō-mē] Latin *vas*, vessel + -ectomy	Removal of part of the vas deferens to prevent conception.
vasovasostomy	[VĀ-sō-vă-SŎS-tō-mē] vaso-, vessel + vaso- + -stomy, creation of a hole	Reversal of a vasectomy.

C A S E   S T U D Y

Surgical Relief

D r. Medina checked the results of Mr. McCoy's urethrogram. There did not seem to be any abnormalities other than in the prostate. He scheduled Mr. McCoy for a TURP, which is done as cryogenic surgery (surgery using cold to numb an area prior to

CASE STUDY (continued)

operating). The procedure is done on an outpatient basis, and one week later, Mr. McCoy is improving rapidly. Dr. Medina wants to wait a while to see if the TURP also helps improve erectile function, before exploring other options. One such option is new medication that can improve erectile function.

 Critical Thinking

56. Why did Dr. Medina schedule Mr. McCoy for a TURP?

57. If medication does not work to improve sexual function, what is another option for men with impaired erectile function?

Surgical Terms Exercises

Check Your Knowledge

Fill in the blanks.

58. Circumcision is removal of the _____ and is commonly practiced in different cultures.

59. An _____ or _____ is removal of a testicle.

60. A prostatectomy is a general term for removal of the _____.

61. A contraceptive operation is a(n) _____.

62. An operation to reverse a previously done contraceptive one is a(n) _____.

Pharmacological Terms

Males are sometimes treated with hormone replacement therapy (usually, testosterone). Such treatment can help with sexual problems and with some of the signs of aging. Medications for impotence may help some men restore sexual function. It may also be treated surgically or with mechanical devices.

Anabolic steroids can help overcome the symptoms of some wasting diseases and build muscle mass. The ability of such drugs to increase muscle mass means that they are important to some athletes. However, the widespread overuse of anabolic steroids by some people has proven to be dangerous, even fatal.

402   Chapter 11 • The Male Reproductive System

CASE STUDY

Trying Medication

About a month later, Mr. McCoy is back for an appointment to discuss his sexual dysfunction. He still is having difficulty sustaining erections. Dr. Medina reviews other medications that Mr. McCoy takes to check for possible interactions, prescribes a drug to treat impotence, and asks Mr. McCoy to call him in about a month. The drug works well for Mr. McCoy.

In recent years, Dr. Medina has seen an increase in the number of patients who cite sexual dysfunction as a problem. Often, people would rather accept the condition rather than talk to a doctor openly about it. Media publicity about impotence has made known some of the available treatments.

 Critical Thinking

63. Mr. McCoy's impotence existed for about ten years before he told a doctor about it. Do you think all the media coverage of the issue of impotence or PED helps people to discuss this issue with their health care practitioners, and why?

64. Dr. Medina tells Mr. McCoy to call him if his internist prescribes any other drugs for him while he is taking his medication for impotence. Why is Dr. Medina concerned?

Pharmacological Terms Exercises

Check Your Knowledge

Fill in the blanks.

65. Male hormone replacement therapy usually involves the hormone _____.

66. Inability to maintain an erection can be treated with _____.

67. Weight trainers and sports figures sometimes illegally use _____ _____.

CHALLENGE SECTION

William Hartman, 30 years old, has a history of orchialgia, which was usually treatable with a mild painkiller. Lately, he tells his internist, the pain is increasing. He is referred to Dr. Medina. His records are sent to Dr. Medina's office for review. Dr. Medina notes that the patient has an encysted hydrocele that has been aspirated and drained once before. Now it is quite large. He suggests removal of the hernia on an outpatient basis. He explains to the patient that its removal may affect the functioning of his left testicle.

Challenge Section Exercises

68. Should William be worried about fertility issues?

69. What is inside a hydrocele that makes it swell?

Go to the WWW Virtual Library: Men's Health Issues (http://www.vix.com/pub/men/health/health.html) and write a short paragraph on recent news about prostate cancer.

CHAPTER REVIEW

Definitions

Define the following terms and combining forms. Review the chapter before starting. Make sure you know how to pronounce each term as you define it.

Word	Definition
anabolic steroids	
andr(o)	
anorchism, anorchia [ăn-ŌR-kĭzm, -kē-ă]	
aspermia [ā-SPĔR-mē-ă]	
azoospermia [ā-zō-ō-SPĔR-mē-ă]	
balan(o)	
balanitis [băl-ă-NĪ-tĭs]	
bulbourethral [BŬL-bō-yū-RĒ-thrăl] gland	
castration [kăs-TRĀ-shŭn]	
chancroids [SHĂNG-krŏyds]	
circumcision [sĕr-kŭm-SĬZH-ŭn]	
Cowper's [KŎW-pĕrs] gland	
cryptorchism [krĭp-TŌR-kĭzm]	
ejaculation [ē-jăk-yū-LĀ-shŭn]	
epididym(o)	
epididymectomy [ĔP-ĭ-dĭd-ĭ-MĔK-tō-mē]	
epididymis [ĕp-ĭ-DĬD-ĭ-mĭs]	
epididymitis [ĕp-ĭ-dĭd-ĭ-MĪ-tĭs]	
epispadias [ĕp-ĭ-SPĀ-dē-ăs]	
flagellum [flă-JĔL-ŭm]	
foreskin [FŌR-skĭn]	
glans penis [glănz PĒ-nĭs]	
hernia [HĔR-nē-ă]	
hydrocele [HĪ-drō-sēl]	

Word	Definition
hypospadias [HĪ-pō-SPĀ-dē-ăs]	
impotence [ĬM-pō-těns]	
infertility [ĭn-fěr-TĬL-ĭ-tē]	
oligospermia [ŏl-ĭ-gō-SPĚR-mē-ă]	
orch(o), orchi(o), orchid(o)	
orchidectomy [ōr-kĭ-DĔK-tō-mē]	
orchiectomy [ōr-kē-ĔK-tō-mē]	
penis [PĒ-nĭs]	
perineum [PĚR-ĭ-NĒ-ŭm]	
Peyronie's [pā-RŌN-ēs] disease	
phimosis [fĭ-MŌ-sĭs]	
priapism [PRĪ-ă-pĭzm]	
prostat(o)	
prostate [PRŎS-tāt] gland	
prostatectomy [prŏs-tă-TĔK-tō-mē]	
prostate-specific antigen (PSA) test	
prostatitis [prŏs-tă-TĪ-tĭs]	
scrotum [SKRŌ-tŭm]	
semen [SĒ-měn]	
semen analysis	
seminoma [sĕm-ĭ-NŌ-mă]	
sperm [spěrm]	
sperm(o), spermat(o)	
spermatogenesis [SPĚR-mă-tō-JĔN-ĕ-sĭs]	
spermatozoon (pl. spermatozoa) [SPĚR-mă-tō-ZŌ-ŏn (SPĚR-mă-tō-ZŌ-ă)]	
testicle [TĔS-tĭ-kl]	
testis (pl. testes) [TĔS-tĭs (TĔS-tēz)]	
testosterone [tĕs-TŎS-tě-rōn]	
urethrogram [yū-RĒ-thrō-grăm]	
varicocele [VĂR-ĭ-kō-sēl]	
vas deferens [văs DĔF-ěr-ěns]	
vasectomy [vă-SĔK-tō-mē]	
vasovasostomy [VĀ-sō-vă-SŎS-tō-mē]	

Abbreviations

Write the full meaning of each abbreviation.

Abbreviation	Meaning
AIH	
BPH	
PED	
PSA	
SPP	
TURP	

Answers to Chapter Exercises

1. Ob-gyns do not treat male infertility.
2. testicles, seminal vesicles, epididymis, prostate, and vas deferens
3. c
4. a
5. c
6. c
7. a
8. a
9. b
10. c
11. b
12. a
13. b
14. d
15. a
16. e
17. c
18. f
19. F
20. T
21. F
22. F
23. F
24. F
25. F
26. prostate
27. benign prostatic hypertrophy

28. androphobia
29. balanoplasty
30. spermicide, spermatocide
31. orchiotomy
32. prostatorrhea
33. prostat-, prostate
34. andro-, male
35. orchi-, testes
36. balano-, glans penis
37. Cancer was not present.
38. growths or other abnormalities in the urethra or prostate
39. quantity/quality
40. rectum/prostate
41. prostate
42. hormone replacement
43. penile prosthesis
44. If the urethra opens on the bottom, the child will urinate straight down and probably find it difficult to keep his urine from splattering.
45. Delivery of sperm to the cervix during male ejaculation usually requires a centered meatus.
46. h
47. f
48. j

49. a
50. b
51. c
52. d
53. g
54. e
55. I
56. The prostate was enlarged and interfering with urination. A TURP removes some prostate tissue.
57. penile prosthesis
58. foreskin
59. orchidectomy/orchiectomy
60. prostate
61. vasectomy
62. vasovasostomy
63. Most people have the opinion that open discussions of sexual dysfunction make it easier to seek and receive medical help.
64. Dr. Medina does not want his patient to experience drug interactions.
65. testosterone
66. medications for impotence
67. anabolic steroids
68. No, his other testis should be fine.
69. fluid

CHAPTER 12

The Blood System

After studying this chapter, you will be able to

- Name the parts of the blood system and discuss the function of each part

- Define combining forms used in building words that relate to the blood system

- Identify the meaning of related abbreviations

- Name the common diagnoses, clinical procedures, and laboratory tests used in treating the blood system

- List and define the major pathological conditions of the blood system

- Explain the meaning of surgical terms related to the blood system

- Recognize common pharmacological agents used in treating the blood system

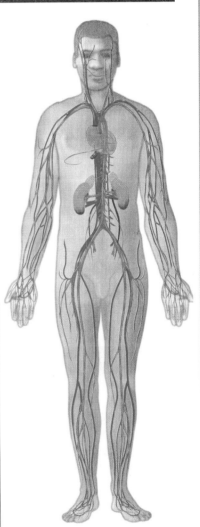

Structure and Function

Blood is a complex mixture of cells, water, and various biochemical agents, such as proteins and sugars. It transports life-sustaining nutrients, oxygen, and hormones to all parts of the body. As a transport medium for waste products from cells of the body, it prevents toxic buildup. It helps maintain the stability of the fluid volume that exists within body tissues (a form of homeostasis, a maintaining of a balance), and it helps regulate body temperature. Without blood, human life is not possible. Figure 12-1a illustrates the blood system, with arteries shown in red and veins shown in blue. Figure 12-1b is a schematic showing the path of blood through the body.

An average adult has about 5 liters of blood circulating within the body. The volume of blood changes with body size, usually equaling about 8 percent of body weight. If a person loses blood, either through bleeding or by donating blood, most of the blood is replaced within 24 hours. If bleeding is extensive, blood transfusions may be necessary.

Blood is a thick liquid made up of a fluid part, **plasma,** and a solid part containing **red blood cells, white blood cells,** and **platelets.** Plasma consists of water, proteins, salts, nutrients, vitamins, and hormones. If some proteins and blood cells are removed from plasma, as happens during *coagulation* (clotting), the resulting fluid is called **serum.** *Serology* is the science that deals with the properties of serum, such as the presence of immunity-provoking agents.

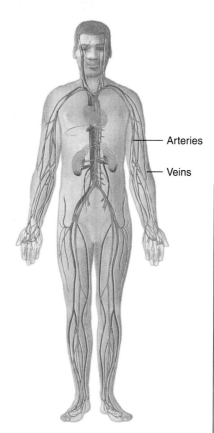

- — Arteries

- — Veins

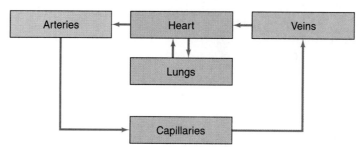

Figure 12-1 (a) The blood system transports life-sustaining nutrients to all parts of the body; (b) A schematic showing the path of blood through the body.

Plasma

When blood is separated, the plasma (about 55 percent of the blood) is the clear liquid made up of 92 percent water and 8 percent organic and inorganic biochemicals. The 8 percent consists of proteins, nutrients, gases, electrolytes, and other substances.

The main groups of plasma proteins are **albumin, globulin, fibrinogen,** and **prothrombin.** Albumin helps regulate water movement between blood and tissue. Plasma proteins cannot pass through capillaries, and, in order to maintain a balance of fluids on both sides of the capillary walls, they create pressure that forces water into the bloodstream. Leakage of water out of the bloodstream can cause edema. An injury can upset the balance of water in the blood and, if too much water is lost, can eventually lead to shock.

Globulins have different functions depending on their type. The *alpha* and *beta globulins*, which are joined in the liver, transport lipids and fat-soluble vitamins. **Gamma globulins** arise in the lymphatic tissues and function as part of the immune system. Globulins can be separated from each other when plasma is placed in a special solution and electrical currents attract the different proteins to move in the direction of the electricity through a process called

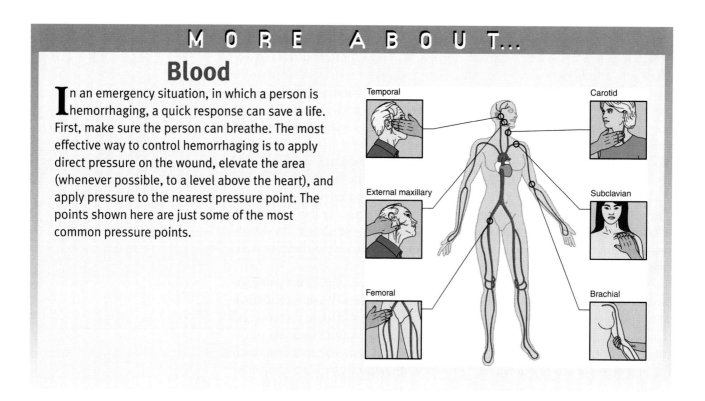

M O R E A B O U T...

Blood

In an emergency situation, in which a person is hemorrhaging, a quick response can save a life. First, make sure the person can breathe. The most effective way to control hemorrhaging is to apply direct pressure on the wound, elevate the area (whenever possible, to a level above the heart), and apply pressure to the nearest pressure point. The points shown here are just some of the most common pressure points.

Temporal

Carotid

External maxillary

Subclavian

Femoral

Brachial

electrophoresis. Blood may also be *centrifuged*, put in a device that separates blood elements by spinning. **Plasmapheresis** is a process that uses centrifuging to take a patient's blood and return only red cells to that patient.

Fibrinogen and prothrombin are essential for blood **coagulation,** the process of *clotting.* The clot is formed by platelets that rush to the site of an injury. They clump at the site and release a protein, **thromboplastin,** which combines with calcium and various clotting factors (I-V and VII-XIII) to form the **fibrin clot** (Figure 12-2). **Thrombin,** an enzyme, helps in formation of the clot. The clot tightens while releasing serum, a clear liquid. Blood clotting at the site of a wound is essential. Without it, one would bleed to death. Blood clotting inside blood vessels, however, can cause major cardiovascular problems. Some elements of the blood, such as **heparin,** prevent clots from forming during normal circulation.

Blood Cells

The solid part of the blood that is suspended in the plasma consists of the red blood cells (RBCs), also called **erythrocytes,** white blood cells (WBCs), also called **leukocytes,** and platelets, also referred to as **thrombocytes.** These cells or the solids in the blood make up about 45 percent of the blood. The measurement of the percentage of packed red blood cells is known as the **hematocrit.** Most blood cells are formed as **stem cells (hematocytoblasts)** or immature blood cells in the bone marrow. Stem cells mature in the bone marrow before entering the bloodstream and becoming *differentiated,* specialized in their purpose. Figure 12-3 shows the stages of blood cell development. The term *differential* refers to the percentage of each type of white blood cell in the bloodstream.

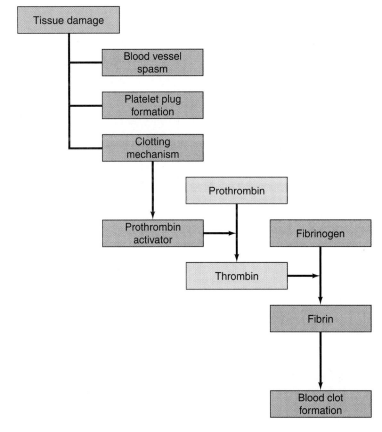

Figure 12-2 A fibrin clot is formed at the site of an injury.

Erythropoietin is used in the treatment of AIDS patients to encourage red blood cell production.

Erythrocytes or Red Blood Cells

A hormone produced in the kidneys, **erythropoietin,** stimulates the production of red blood cells in the bone marrow. When stem cells mature into erythrocytes, they lose their nucleus and become bi-concave.

A protein within red blood cells, **hemoglobin,** aids in the transport of oxygen to the cells of the body. About one-third of each red blood cell is made up of hemoglobin. Hemoglobin is composed of **heme,** a pigment containing iron, and **globin,** a protein. Erythrocytes live for about 120 days. Some are removed from circulation each day to maintain a steady concentration of red blood cells. Macrophages are cells formed from stem cells that consume damaged or aged cells. The average number of red blood cells in a cubic millimeter of blood is 4.6 to 6.4 million for adult males and 4.2 to 5.4 million for adult females. This measurement is known as the **red blood cell count.** Figure 12-4 tracks the life cycle of a red blood cell.

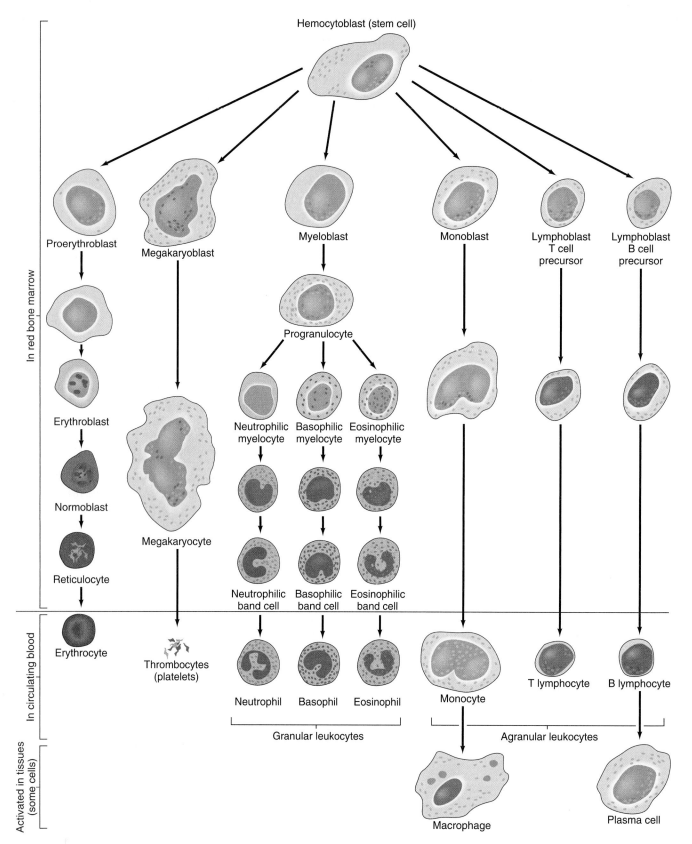

Figure 12-3 Development of blood cells from a hemocytoblast.

Labels in figure:

Hemocytoblast (stem cell)

In red bone marrow

Proerythroblast
Megakaryoblast
Myeloblast
Monoblast
Lymphoblast T cell precursor
Lymphoblast B cell precursor

Erythroblast
Progranulocyte

Normoblast
Neutrophilic myelocyte
Basophilic myelocyte
Eosinophilic myelocyte

Megakaryocyte

Reticulocyte

Neutrophilic band cell
Basophilic band cell
Eosinophilic band cell

In circulating blood

Erythrocyte
Thrombocytes (platelets)

Neutrophil
Basophil
Eosinophil
Monocyte
T lymphocyte
B lymphocyte

Granular leukocytes
Agranular leukocytes

Activated in tissues (some cells)

Macrophage
Plasma cell

Leukocytes

Leukocytes or white blood cells protect against disease in various ways—for example, by destroying foreign substances. Leukocytes are transported in the bloodstream to the site of an infection. There are two main groups of leuko-

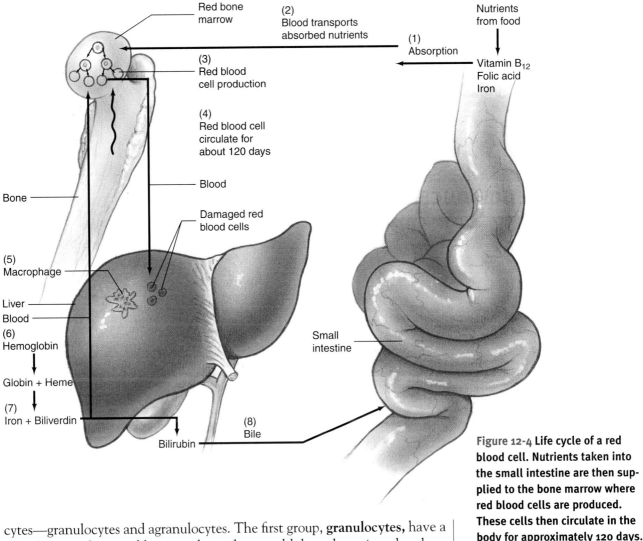

Red bone marrow

(2) Blood transports absorbed nutrients

Nutrients from food

(1) Absorption

Vitamin B$_{12}$
Folic acid
Iron

(3) Red blood cell production

(4) Red blood cell circulate for about 120 days

Blood

Damaged red blood cells

Bone

(5) Macrophage

Liver

Blood

(6) Hemoglobin

Globin + Heme

(7) Iron + Biliverdin

Bilirubin

(8) Bile

Small intestine

Figure 12-4 Life cycle of a red blood cell. Nutrients taken into the small intestine are then supplied to the bone marrow where red blood cells are produced. These cells then circulate in the body for approximately 120 days.

cytes—granulocytes and agranulocytes. The first group, **granulocytes,** have a granular cytoplasm and have nuclei with several lobes when viewed under a microscope and when stain is used. There are three types of granulocytes: neutrophils, eosinophils, and basophils. **Neutrophils** are the most plentiful leukocytes (over half of the white blood cells in the bloodstream). They do not stain distinctly with either an acidic or an alkaline dye. Their purpose is to remove small particles of unwanted material from the bloodstream. **Eosinophils** are only about 1 to 3 percent of the leukocytes in the bloodstream. Their granules stain bright red in the presence of an acidic red dye called *eosin.* Their purpose is to kill parasites and to help control inflammations and allergic reactions. **Basophils** are less than 1 percent of the leukocytes in the bloodstream. Their granules stain dark purple in the presence of alkaline dyes. They release heparin, an anticlotting factor, and **histamine,** a substance involved in allergic reactions.

The second group of leukocytes, **agranulocytes,** have cytoplasm with no granules. Their single nucleus does not have the dark-staining elements of granulocytes. There are two types of agranulocytes: monocytes and lymphocytes. **Monocytes,** the largest blood cells, make up about 3 to 9 percent of the leukocytes in the bloodstream. They destroy large particles of unwanted material (such as old red blood cells) in the bloodstream. **Lymphocytes** make up about 25 to 33 percent of the leukocytes in the bloodstream. They are essential to the immune system (Chapter 13). Table 12-1 lists the types of white blood cells.

Table 12-1 Types of Leukocytes

Leukocytes	Staining Properties	Percentage of Leukocytes in Blood	Function
granulocytes basophils	stains dark purple	minimal—under 1 percent	release heparin and histamine kill parasites and help control inflammations
eosinophils	bright red	minimal—under 3 percent	remove unwanted particles
neutrophils	indistinct	most plentiful—over 50 percent	
agranulocytes lymphocyte	do not stain	plentiful—25 to 33 percent	important to immune system destroy large unwanted particles
monocyte		minimal—3 to 9 percent	

Platelets

Platelets or thrombocytes are fragments that break off from large cells in red bone marrow called **megakaryocytes.** Platelets live for about 10 days and help in blood clotting. Platelets adhere to damaged tissue and to each other and group together to control blood loss from a blood vessel. Figure 12-5 shows platelets clumping together.

Figure 12-5 Platelets clumping together to form a clot.

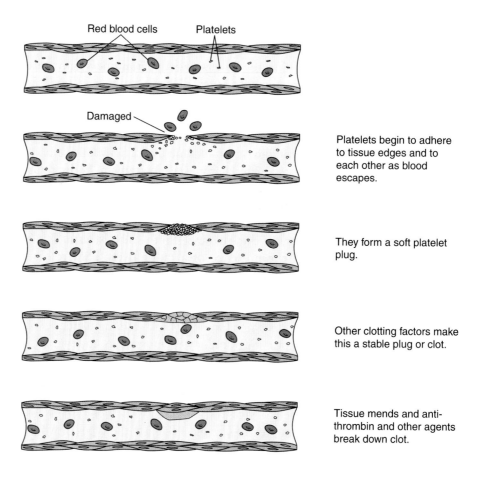

Red blood cells   Platelets

Damaged

Platelets begin to adhere to tissue edges and to each other as blood escapes.

They form a soft platelet plug.

Other clotting factors make this a stable plug or clot.

Tissue mends and anti-thrombin and other agents break down clot.

Blood Types

When blood is needed for **transfusion,** the blood being donated is karyotyped, put into one of four human **blood types** or **groups.** The donated blood must be karyotyped since an incompatible blood type from a donor can cause adverse reactions. Blood typing is based on the antigens (substances that promote an immune response) and antibodies (special proteins in the blood) present in the blood. (Chapter 13 describes the work of antigens and antibodies in the immune system.) The most common types of blood in the population are O, A, B, and AB. Table 12-2 lists the four blood types and their characteristics.

The growth of DNA testing has led to grouping of more blood types based on common genetic characteristics. Eventually, the basic four blood types and factors may be replaced by more exact matching. Some underlying genetic characteristics found in DNA may lead to more useful blood products.

Table 12-2 Blood Types

Blood Type	Antigen	Antibody	Percent of Population with This Type
A	A	Anti-B	41
B	B	Anti-A	10
AB	A and B	Neither anti-A nor anti-B	4
O	Neither A nor B	Both anti-A and anti-B	45

The danger in transfusing blood of a different type is that **agglutination** or clumping of the antigens stops the flow of blood, which can be fatal. People with type O blood have no antigens, so people with type O can donate to all other types and are, therefore, called *universal donors*. People with AB blood are called *universal recipients* because they can receive blood from people with all the other types and not experience clotting.

In addition to the four human blood types, there is a positive or negative element in the blood. **Rh factor** is a type of antigen first identified in rhesus monkeys. **Rh-positive** blood contains this factor and **Rh-negative** blood does not. The factor contains any of more that 30 types of **agglutinogens,** substances that cause agglutination, and can be fatal to anyone who receives blood with a factor different from the donor.

Rh factor is particularly important during pregnancy. The fetus of parents with different Rh factors could be harmed by a fatal disease or a type of anemia if preventive measures are not taken prior to birth. The problem

MORE ABOUT...

Transfusions

Two early scientists attempted various experimental transfusions. Sir Christopher Wren (1632–1723), a famous English architect and scientist, did biological experiments in which he injected fluids into the veins of animals. This process is regarded as an early attempt at blood transfusions. During the same century, a French physician, Jean Baptiste Denis (1643–1704) tried unsuccessfully to transfuse sheep's blood into a human. Later, experiments with transfusing human blood succeeded somewhat, but the majority of people receiving transfusions died, until the advent of blood typing in the twentieth century. Once blood factors and typing became routine, transfusions were widely used in surgery. Later, it was found that some infections (hepatitis, AIDS) were transmitted by blood. Now, donated blood is carefully screened for infections.

arises when the mother is Rh negative and produces antibodies to the father's Rh positive factor present in the fetus. The problem does not arise during a first pregnancy but will arise in each subsequent pregnancy. Treatment with Rho-gam, a gamma globulin, during each pregnancy usually prevents the problem. Figure 12-6 shows how a combination of Rh factors affects pregnancy.

Figure 12-6 How the Rh factor affects pregnancy.

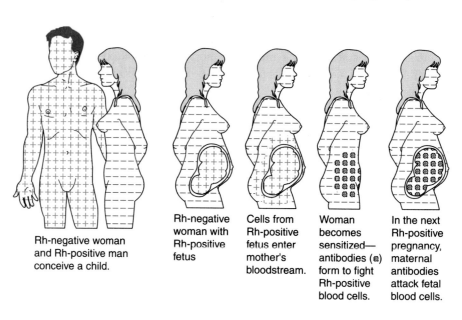

Rh-negative woman and Rh-positive man conceive a child.

Rh-negative woman with Rh-positive fetus

Cells from Rh-positive fetus enter mother's bloodstream.

Woman becomes sensitized—antibodies (●) form to fight Rh-positive blood cells.

In the next Rh-positive pregnancy, maternal antibodies attack fetal blood cells.

Vocabulary Review

In the previous section, you learned terms relating to the blood system. Before going on to the exercises, review the terms below and refer to the previous section if you have any questions.

Term	Word Analysis	Definition
agglutination	[ă-glū-ti-NĀ-shŭn] From Latin *ad-*, to + *gluten*, glue	Clumping of cells and particles in blood.
agglutinogen	[ă-glŭ-TĬN-ō-jĕn]	Substance that causes agglutination.
agranulocyte	[ā-GRĂN-yū-lō-sīt] a-, without + Latin *granulum*, granule + -cyte, cell	Leukocyte with nongranular cytoplasm.
albumin	[ăl-BYŪ-mĭn] Latin *albumen*, egg white	Simple protein found in plasma.
basophil	[BĀ-sō-fĭl] baso-, base + -phil, attraction	Leukocyte containing heparin and histamine and performing a phagocytic function.

Term	Word Analysis	Definition
blood	[blŭd] Old English *blod*	Fluid (containing plasma, red blood cells, white blood cells, and platelets) circulated throughout the arteries, veins, capillaries, and heart.
blood types or groups		Classification of blood according to its antigen and antibody qualities.
coagulation	[kō-ăg-yū-LĀ-shŭn]	Changing of a liquid, especially blood, into a semi-solid.
electrophoresis	[ē-lĕk-trō-FŌR-ē-sĭs] electro-, electricity + -phoresis, carrying	Process of separating particles in a solution by passing electricity through the liquid.
eosinophil	[ē-ō-SĬN-ō-fĭl] eosino-, fluorescent dye + -phil	Type of granulocyte.
erythrocyte	[ĕ-RĬTH-rō-sīt] erythro-, red blood cell + -cyte	Mature red blood cell.
erythropoietin	[ĕ-rĭth-rō-PŎY-ĕ-tĭn] erythro(cyte) + -poiesis, making	Hormone released by the kidneys to stimulate red blood cell production.
fibrin clot	[FĪ-brĭn]	Clot-forming threads formed at the site of an injury during coagulation where platelets clump together with various other substances.
fibrinogen	[fĭ-BRĬN-ō-jĕn] fibrino-, fibrin + -gen, producing	Protein in plasma that aids in clotting.
gamma globulin	[GĂ-mă GLŎB-yū-lĭn]	Globulin that arises in lymphatic tissue and functions as part of the immune system.
globin	[GLŌ-bĭn] From Latin *globus*, ball	Protein molecule; in the blood, a part of hemoglobin.
globulin	[GLŎB-yū-lĭn] From Latin *globulus*, globule	Any of a family of proteins in blood plasma.
granulocyte	[GRĂN-yū-lō-sīt] Latin *granulum*, granule + -cyte	Leukocyte with granular cytoplasm.

Term	Word Analysis	Definition
hematocrit	[HĔ-mă-tō-krĭt, HĔM-ă-tō-krĭt] hemato- + Greek *krino*, to separate	Measure of the percentage of red blood cells in a blood sample.
hematocytoblast	[HĔ-mă-tō-SĪ-tō-blăst] hemato-, blood + -cyto-. cell + -blast, immature cell	Most immature blood cell.
heme	[hēm] Greek *haima*, blood	Pigment containing iron in hemoglobin.
hemoglobin	[hē-mō-GLŌ-bĭn] hemo-, blood + glob(ul)in	Protein in red blood cells essential to the transport of oxygen.
heparin	[HĔP-ă-rĭn] From Greek *hepar*, liver	Substance in blood that prevents clotting.
histamine	[HĬS-tă-mēn]	Substance released by basophils and eosinophils; involved in allergic reactions.
leukocyte	[LŪ-kō-sīt] leuko-, white + -cyte	Mature white blood cell.
lymphocyte	[LĬM-fō-sīt] lympho-, lymph + -cyte	Type of agranulocyte.
megakaryocyte	[mĕg-ă-KĀR-ē-ō-sīt] mega-, large + karyo-, nucleus + -cyte	Large cells in red bone marrow that form platelets.
monocyte	[MŎN-ō-sīt] mono-, one + -cyte	Type of agranulocyte.
neutrophil	[NŪ-trō-fĭl] neutro-, neutral + -phil	Type of leukocyte; granulocyte.
plasma	[PLĂZ-mă] Greek	Liquid portion of unclotted blood.
plasmapheresis	[PLĂZ-mă-fĕ-RĒ-sĭs] plasma + -pheresis, removal	Process of removing blood from a person, centrifuging it, and returning only red blood cells to that person.
platelet	[PLĀT-lĕt] plate + -let, small	Thrombocyte; part of a megakaryocyte that initiates clotting.
prothrombin	[prō-THRŎM-bĭn]	Type of plasma protein that aids in clotting.

Term	Word Analysis	Definition
red blood cell		One of the solid parts of blood formed from stem cells and having hemoglobin within; erythrocyte.
red blood cell count		Measurement of red blood cells in a cubic millimeter of blood.
Rh factor	rh(esus monkey)	Type of antigen in blood that can cause a transfusion reaction.
Rh-negative		Lacking Rh factor on surface of blood cells.
Rh-positive		Having Rh factor on surface of blood cells.
serum	[SĒR-ŭm] Latin, whey	The liquid left after blood has clotted.
stem cell		Immature cell formed in bone marrow that becomes differentiated into either a red or a white blood cell.
thrombin	[THRŎMB-ĭn]	Enzyme that helps in clot formation.
thrombocyte	[THRŎM-bō-sĭt] thrombo-, blood clot + -cyte	Platelet; cell fragment that produces thrombin.
thromboplastin	[thrŏm-bō-PLĂS-tĭn] thrombo- + Greek *plastos*, formed	Protein that aids in forming a fibrin clot.
transfusion	[trăns-FYŪ-zhŭn] From Latin *transfundo*, to pour from one vessel to another	Injection of donor blood into a person needing blood.
white blood cell		One of the solid parts of blood from stem cells that plays a role in defense against disease; leukocyte.

C A S E   S T U D Y

Getting Treatment

John Maynard was admitted to the hospital on April 2, XXXX, complaining of respiratory problems and left-sided lower abdominal pain. The doctor on call ordered blood tests, and Mr. Maynard was found to be anemic. Because of Mr. Maynard's multiple medical problems, a hematologist was called in to consult about the disease and treatment of this patient. The history as written on his chart is as follows:

HISTORY OF PRESENT ILLNESS: John Maynard is an 83-year-old man who was admitted on April 2, XXXX, with acute exacerbation of chronic obstructive pulmonary disease and left-sided lower abdominal pain. He has been admitted in the past with a similar kind of pain but on the right side. He was evaluated by Dr. Evans in the past, but no obvious additional problem was identified. During this present admission, he was also found to be anemic.

On direct interviewing: Mr. Maynard denies any acute blood loss. His stool and urine color are normal. He has a history of a stroke and has not been ambulatory. He lives with his nephew, who takes care of him. He denies any night sweats. He did not notice any new lumps or bruising anywhere. No new bone pain. He feels short of breath with minimal activity. He denies any chest pain or palpitations. He feels dizzy at times.

 Critical Thinking

1. Blood tests can reveal problems almost anywhere in the body. Why are the elements in blood a good measure of many bodily functions?

2. Does Mr. Maynard's blood type (O positive) make him more susceptible to illnesses? Why or why not?

Structure and Function Exercises

Check Your Knowledge

After each of the following, write the letter of the component of blood that is most closely related to either a, b, or c.

    a. red blood cell   b. white blood cell   c. component of plasma

3. albumin ____

4. hemoglobin ____

5. leukocyte ____

6. eosinophils ____

7. gamma globulin ____

8. fibrinogen ____

9. basophils ____

10. beta globulin ____

11. monocyte ____

12. neutrophils ____

13. histamine ____

14. alpha globulin ____

15. lymphocytes ____

Find the Type

Write the correct blood type, A, B, AB, or O, in the space following each phrase.

16. Has A and B antigens ____

17. Has neither A nor B antigens ____

18. Has only B antigens ____

19. Has only A antigens ____

20. Has both anti-A and anti-B antibodies ____

21. Has neither anti-A nor anti-B antibodies ____

22. Has only anti-A antibodies ____

23. Has only anti-B antibodies ____

Find a Match

Match the term in the left column with its correct definition in the right column.

24. coagulation   a. categorize into blood groups

25. heparin   b. a blood protein

26. karyotype   c. clumping of incompatible blood cells

27. albumen   d. process of clotting

28. agglutination   e. antigen

29. Rh factor   f. cell that activates clotting

30. erythrocyte   g. an anticoagulant

31. platelet   h. red blood cell

Combining Forms and Abbreviations

The lists below include combining forms and abbreviations that relate specifically to the blood system. Pronunciations are provided for the examples.

Combining Form	Meaning	Example
agglutin(o)	agglutinin	*agglutinogenic* [ă-GLŪ-tĭn-ō-JĔN-ĭk], causing the production of agglutinin
eosino	eosinophil	*eosinopenia* [Ē-ŏ-sĭn-ō-PĒ-nē-ă], abnormally low count of eosinophils
erythr(o)	red	*erythrocyte* [ĕ-RĬTH-rō-sīt], red blood cell
hemo, hemat(o)	blood	*hemodialysis* [HĒ-mō-dī-ĂL-ĭ-sĭs], dialysis performed by separating solid substances and water from the blood
leuk(o)	white	*leukoblast* [LŪ-kō-blăst], immature white blood cell
phag(o)	eating, devouring	*phagocyte* [FĂG-ō-sīt], cell that consumes other substances, such as bacteria
thromb(o)	blood clot	*thrombocyte* [THRŎM-bō-sīt], cell involved in blood clotting

Abbreviation	Meaning
APTT	activated partial thromboplastin time
baso	basophil
BCP	biochemistry panel
BMT	bone marrow transplant
CBC	complete blood count
diff	differential blood count
eos	eosinophils
ESR	erythrocyte sedimentation rate
G-CSF	granulocyte colony-stimulating factor
GM-CSF	granulocyte macrophage colony-stimulating factor
HCT, Hct	hematocrit
HGB, Hgb, HB	hemoglobin
MCH	mean corpuscular hemoglobin

Abbreviation	Meaning
MCHC	mean corpuscular hemoglobin concentration
MCV	mean corpuscular volume
mono	monocyte
PCV	packed cell volume
PLT	platelet count
PMN, poly	polymorphonuclear neutrophil
PT	prothrombin time
PTT	partial thromboplastin time
RBC	red blood cell count
SR; sed. rate	sedimentation rate
seg	segmented mature white blood cells
WBC	white blood cell count

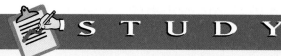

Interpreting Results

The laboratory data on Mr. Maynard's chart is as follows.

April 2, XXXX: PSA 1.8

April 2, XXXX: BUN 6, creatinine .7, calcium 8.3, uric acid 8.7, SGOT 42, SGPT 38, alkaline phosphatase 86, total bilirubin .7.

April 2, XXXX: white blood cell count 5.8, hemoglobin 10.4, HCT 31.1, platelet count 275,000.

December 4, XXXX: vitamin B12 1,230, folate 16.1.

December 6, XXXX: HCT 38.9.

December 10, XXXX: HCT 32.3.

 Critical Thinking

32. What procedure is used to obtain the blood samples needed in Mr. Maynard's case? Is it safe to take several blood samples at once? Why or why not?

33. What is the difference between an RBC and a WBC?

Combining Forms and Abbreviations Exercises

Find a Match

Match the terms on the left that contain blood system combining forms with the correct definition on the right.

34. leukocytolysis

35. hemotoxin

36. thrombogenic

37. hemostasis

38. eosinopenia

39. erythrocytometer

40. hemanalysis

41. thrombolysis

42. erythralgia

43. leukopoiesis

a. development of white blood cells

b. instrument for counting red blood cells

c. destruction of a clot

d. painful skin redness

e. destruction of white blood cells

f. substance that causes blood poisoning

g. causing blood coagulation

h. stoppage of bleeding

i. blood analysis

j. low number of eosinophils

Build Your Medical Vocabulary

Define the following words using the list of blood system combining forms above and the prefixes, suffixes, and combining forms in Chapters 2 and 3.

44. agglutinophilic _____

45. thrombectomy _____

46. erythroblast _____

47. hematopathology _____

48. eosinotaxis _____

49. lymphoblast _____

50. phagosome _____

51. polycythemia _____

52. cytology _____

53. leukocyte _____

54. leukemia _____

55. thrombocytopenia _____

56. hematoma _____

57. erythrocytosis _____

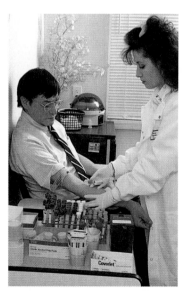

Figure 12-7 **Venipuncture is used in most regular medical examinations to extract blood for analysis.**

Diagnostic, Procedural, and Laboratory Terms

Phlebotomy or **venipuncture,** the withdrawal of blood for examination, is probably the most frequently used diagnostic tool in medicine (Figure 12-7). Various measurements provide a clue as to someone's general health and aid in diagnosing specific conditions. Table 12-3 lists common blood analyses, and Figure 12-8 shows laboratory results for specific blood tests.

Table 12-3 Common Blood Analyses

Test or Procedure	Purpose of Test	Common Diseases/Disorders That May Be Indicated
complete blood count (CBC)	common screen for basic medical checkup (Figure 12-8)	iron deficiency anemia bacterial or viral infection internal bleeding dehydration aplastic anemia impaired renal function liver disease circulatory disorder
blood chemistry	test of plasma for presence of most substances, such as glucose, cholesterol, uric acid, and electrolytes	diabetes hyperlipidemia gout circulatory disorders impaired renal function liver diseases general metabolic disorder
biochemistry panel	group of automated tests for various common diseases or disorders	same as blood chemistry
blood indices	measurement of size, volume, and content of red blood cells	classification of anemias
blood culture	test of a blood specimen in a culture in which microorganisms are observed; test for infections	septicemia bacterial infections
erythrocyte sedimentation rate (ESR); sedimentation rate (SR)	test for rate at which red blood cells fall through plasma; indicator of inflammation and/or tissue injury	infections joint inflammation sickle cell anemia liver and kidney disorders
white blood cell differential and red blood cell morphology	test for number of types of leukocytes and shape of red blood cells	infection anemia leukemia poikilocytosis anisocytosis
platelet count (PLT)	test for number of thrombocytes in a blood sample	hemorrhage infections malignancy hypersplenism aplastic anemia thrombocytopenia *(continued on next page)*

Table 12-3 (continued)

Test or Procedure	Purpose of Test	Common Diseases/Disorders That May Be Indicated
partial thromboplastin time (PTT)	test for coagulation defects	vitamin K deficiency hepatic disease hemophilia hemorrhagic disorders
prothrombin time (PT)	test for coagulation defects	vitamin K deficiency hepatic disease hemorrhagic disorders hemophilia
antiglobulin test; *Coombs' test*	test for antibodies on red blood cells	Rh factor and anemia
white blood count (WBC)	number of white blood cells in a sample (usually done as part of complete blood count)	bacterial or viral infection aplastic anemia leukemia leukocytosis
red blood count (RBC)	number of red blood cells in a sample (usually done as part of complete blood count)	polycythemia dehydration iron deficiency anemia blood loss erythropoiesis
hemoglobin (HGB, Hgb)	level of hemoglobin in blood (usually done as part of complete blood count)	polycythemia dehydration anemia sickle cell anemia recent hemorrhage
hematocrit (HCT, Hct)	measure of packed red blood cells in a sample (usually done as part of complete blood count)	polycythemia dehydration blood loss anemia
mean corpuscular volume (MCV)	volume of individual cells (usually part of blood indices)	microcytic or macrocytic anemia
mean corpuscular hemoglobin (MCH)	weight of hemoglobin in average red blood cell (usually part of blood indices)	classification of anemia
mean corpuscular hemoglobin concentration (MCHC)	concentration of hemoglobin in a red blood cell (usually part of blood indices)	hyperchromic or hypochromic anemia

Elyse Armadian, M.D. 3 South Windsor Street Fairfield, MN 00219 300-546-7890	Laboratory Report Sunview Diagnostics 6712 Adams Drive Fairfield, MN 00220 300-546-7000	
Patient: Janine Josephs Date Collected: 09/30/XXXX Date Received: 09/30/XXXX	Patient ID: 099-00-1200 Time Collected: 16:05 Date Reported: 10/06/XXXX	Date of Birth: 08/07/43 Total Volume: 2000

Test	Result	Flag	Reference
Complete Blood Count			
WBC	4.0		3.9-11.1
RBC	4.11		3.80-5.20
HCT	39.7		34.0-47.0
MCV	96.5		80.0-98.0
MCH	32.9		27.1-34.0
MCHC	34.0		32.0-36.0
MPV	8.6		7.5-11.5
NEUTROPHILS %	45.6		38.0-80.0
NEUTROPHILS ABS.	1.82		1.70-8.50
LYMPHOCYTES %	36.1		15.0-49.0
LYMPHOCYTES ABS.	1.44		1.00-3.50
EOSINOPHILS %	4.5		0.0-8.0
EOSINOPHILS ABS.	0.18		0.03-0.55
BASOPHILS %	0.7		0.0-2.0
BASOPHILS ABS.	0.03		0.000-0.185
PLATELET COUNT	229		150-400
Automated Chemistries			
GLUCOSE	80		65-109
UREA NITROGEN	17		6-30
CREATININE (SERUM)	0.6		0.5-1.3
UREA NITROGEN/CREATININE	28		10-29
SODIUM	140		135-145
POTASSIUM	4.4		3.5-5.3
CHLORIDE	106		96-109
CO_2	28		20-31
ANION GAP	6		3-19
CALCIUM	9.8		8.6-10.4
PHOSPHORUS	3.6		2.2-4.6
AST (SGOT)	28		0-30
ALT (SGPT)	19		0-34
BILIRUBIN, TOTAL	0.5		0.2-1.2
PROTEIN, TOTAL	7.8		6.2-8.2
ALBUMIN	4.3		3.5-5.0
GLOBULIN	3.5		2.1-3.8
URIC ACID	2.4		2.0-7.5
CHOLESTEROL	232	*	120-199
TRIGLYCERIDES	68		40-199
IRON	85		30-150
HDL CHOLESTEROL	73	*	35-59
CHOLESTEROL/HDL RATIO	3.2		3.2-5.7
LDL, CALCULATED	148	*	70-129
T3, UPTAKE	32		24-37
T4, TOTAL	6.9		4.5-12.8

Most of the blood tests described in Table 12-3 are performed in a laboratory. Names of tests may vary according to the region of the country or the practice of a particular doctor. For example, a biochemistry panel is sometimes called a **chemistry profile,** and a blood chemistry is sometimes known as an **SMA (sequential multiple analyzer),** the name of the first machine used to analyze blood chemistries.

Vocabulary Review

In the previous section, you learned diagnostic, procedural, and laboratory terms. Before going on to the exercises, review the terms below and refer to the previous section if you have any questions.

Term	Word Analysis	Definition
antiglobulin test	[ĂN-tē-GLŎB-yū-lĭn] anti(body) + globulin	Test for antibodies on red blood cells.
biochemistry panel		Common group of automated tests run on one blood sample.
blood chemistry		Test of plasma for presence of a particular substance such as glucose.
blood culture		Test of a blood specimen in a culture medium to observe for particular microorganisms.
blood indices	[ĬN-dĭ-sēz]	Measurement of the characteristics of red blood cells.
chemistry profile		*See* blood chemistry.
complete blood count (CBC)		Most common blood test for a number of factors.
erythrocyte sedimentation rate (ESR)		Test for rate at which red blood cells fall through plasma.
partial thromboplastin time (PTT)		Test for ability of blood to coagulate.
phlebotomy	[flĕ-BŎT-ō-mē] phlebo-, vein + -tomy, a cutting	*See* venipuncture.
platelet count (PLT)		Measurement of number of platelets in a blood sample.
prothrombin time (PT)		Test for ability of blood to coagulate.
red blood cell morphology		Observation of shape of red blood cells.
sedimentation rate (SR)		*See* erythrocyte sedimentation rate.
SMA (sequential multiple analyzer)		Original blood chemistry machine; now a synonym for blood chemistry.
venipuncture	[VĔN-ĭ-pŭnk-chŭr, VĒ-nĭ-pŭnk-chŭr] veni-, vein + puncture	Insertion of a needle into a vein, usually for the purpose of extracting a blood sample.

CASE STUDY

Evaluating the Tests

Mr. Maynard's chart has the following notes from the hematologist's evaluation.

ASSESSMENT: Mr. Maynard has multiple medical problems. He has recently been admitted with abdominal discomfort, the etiology of which is unclear at this point. He was also found to have normal MCV anemia. A review of his labora-tory data shows that his hematocrit has been fluctuating between 27 and 38. His hematocrit on December 6, XXXX, was 38.9, but within four days it dropped to 32.3. Since then there have also been several incidences in which his hematocrit dropped further, but then improved. This variation in the hematocrit is suggestive of some ongoing blood loss.

Critical Thinking

58. Other than blood loss, name at least two other conditions the HCT results might indicate.

59. What is the name of a test for leukocytes?

Diagnostic, Procedural, and Laboratory Terms Exercises

Match the Test

Match the name of the test in the column on the left to its correct description in the column on the right.

60. blood culture

61. hematocrit

62. sedimentation rate

63. white blood count

64. antiglobulin test

65. mean corpuscular hemoglobin concentration

66. mean corpuscular volume

67. complete blood count

68. prothrombin time

69. biochemistry panel

a. average red blood cell volume

b. antibodies on red blood cells

c. rate at which red blood cells fall

d. group of automated tests

e. most common blood test

f. clotting factors test

g. number of white blood cells

h. measure of packed red blood cells

i. concentration of hemoglobin in red blood cells

j. growing of microorganisms in a culture

Find the Value

Give the expected (normal) range for each of the following laboratory measurements.

70. cholesterol

71. sodium

72. iron

73. thyroid (T4)

74. MCV

75. PLT

76. HCT

77. RBC

78. WBC

79. MCHC

Pathological Terms

Many diseases and disorders have some effect on the blood, but they are really diseases of other body systems. For example, diabetes is a disorder of the endocrine system, but its diagnosis includes an analysis of blood glucose levels. Actual diseases of the blood are characterized by changes in the supply or characteristics of blood cells, presence of microorganisms affecting the blood, or presence or lack of certain substances in the blood. **Dyscrasia** is a general term for any disease of the blood with abnormal material present.

Anemia is a general term for a condition in which the red blood cells do not transport enough oxygen to the tissues due to a low number or volume of cells or because of a low amount of hemoglobin. The most common types of anemia include *iron-deficiency anemia*, a lack of enough iron in the blood that affects the production of hemoglobin; *aplastic anemia*, a failure of the bone marrow to produce enough red blood cells; *pernicious anemia*, a condition in which the shape and number of the red blood cells changes due to a lack of sufficient vitamin B_{12}; *sickle cell anemia*, a hereditary condition (usually in persons of African-American ancestry) characterized by sickle-shaped red blood cells and a breakdown in red blood cell membranes; *hemolytic anemia*, a disorder characterized by destruction of red blood cells; *posthemorrhagic anemia*, a disorder resulting from a sudden, dramatic loss of blood; and **thalassemia,** an inherited disorder (usually in people of Mediterranean origin) resulting in an inability to produce sufficient hemoglobin (the most severe form of which is *Cooley's anemia*). **Von Willebrand's disease** is a hemorrhagic disorder in which there is a greater tendency to bleed due to the lack of a clotting factor called *Factor VIII.* Common symptoms are bruising and nosebleeds. Figure 12-9 shows blood cell characteristics for some anemias.

Figure 12-9 Characteristics of blood cells in certain anemias.

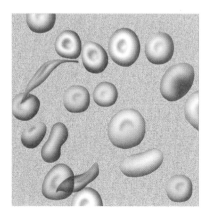

Two other disorders of the blood that involve excessive bleeding are **hemophilia,** a hereditary lack of clotting factor VIII. Hemophiliacs can be treated with medications and transfusions. **Thrombocytopenia** is a bleeding disorder with insufficient platelets to aid in the clotting process. Thrombocytopenia is present in **purpura,** a condition with multiple, tiny hemorrhages under the skin (Figure 12-10). Small, flat, red spots called *petechiae* may indicate a deficiency in the number of platelets.

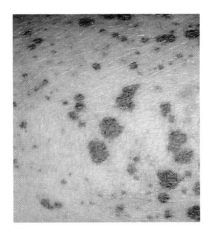

Figure 12-10 Purpura

There are a number of disorders of the blood cells or related substances in the blood. **Pancytopenia** is a condition with a low number of all blood cell components (red blood cells, white blood cells, and thrombocytes). The blood must be supplemented with transfusions. **Erythropenia** (also called *erythrocytopenia*) is a disorder with an abnormally low number of red blood cells. **Hemochromatosis** is a hereditary disorder leading to excessive buildup of iron in the blood. Because excessive iron in the blood can ultimately cause heart failure, people with this disorder have to limit their iron intake. **Polycythemia** is a disease that causes an abnormal increase in red blood cells and hemoglobin. Various forms of the disease are associated with conditions such as hypertension and emphysema. **Anisocytosis** is characterized by red blood cells of differing sizes and shapes, a characteristic that prevents them from functioning normally. **Macrocytosis** is a disorder with abnormally large red blood cells present, and **microcytosis** is a disorder with abnormally small red blood cells present. **Poikilocytosis** is a disorder with irregularly-shaped red blood cells present. **Reticulocytosis** is a disorder with an abnormal number of immature erythrocytes present. **Hemolysis** is a disorder with breakdowns in the red blood cell membrane.

There are also disorders of white blood cells. The major disease involving white blood cells is **leukemia.** Leukemia is a general term for a neoplastic disorder with an excessive increase in white blood cells in the bone marrow and bloodstream. People with leukemia may experience remissions (disappearances of the disease) and relapses (recurrences of the disease). Some leukemias (acute lymphocytic leukemia and chronic lymphocytic leukemia) occur in the lymph system. The two most common leukemias of the bone marrow and bloodstream are AML and CML. *Acute myelogenous leukemia (AML)* is a disorder in which immature granulocytes (or **myeloblasts**) invade the bone marrow. *Chronic myelogenous leukemia (CML)* or *chronic granulocytic leukemia* is a disorder in which mature and immature myeloblasts are present in the bloodstream and marrow. It is usually a slowly developing illness with a reasonably good prognosis. *Acute lymphocytic leukemia (ALL)* is a disorder with an abnormal number of immature lymphocytes. It is usually a disease of childhood and adolescence. The prognosis for recovery is very good. *Chronic lymphocytic leukemia (CLL)* appears mainly in adults and includes an abnormal number of mature lymphocytes.

Another disorder of the white blood cells is **granulocytosis,** an abnormal increase in granulocytes in the bloodstream such as neutrophils during infection. Granulocytosis can also occur in combination with allergic conditions or certain infections, in which case it is called **eosinophilia,** an abnormal increase in eosinophilic granuloctyes. **Basophilia** is an increase in basophilic granuloctyes that is found in some types of leukemia. *Neutropenia* is a disorder with an abnormally low number of neutrophils in the bloodstream. *Neutrophilia* is a disorder with an abnormal increase in neutrophils.

Erythroblastosis fetalis, or Rh factor incompatibility between the mother and a fetus, can cause death to the fetus or a type of fetal anemia. A blood transfusion or treatment with medication can sometimes save the fetus.

Multiple myeloma is a malignant tumor of the bone marrow. It involves overproduction of certain white blood cells that produce immunoglobulins. The myeloma cells then migrate to different areas of the body where they cause tumors and destroy bony structures.

Vocabulary Review

In the previous section, you learned terms relating to pathology. Before going on to the exercises, review the terms below and refer to the previous section if you have any questions.

Terms	Word Analysis	Definition
anemia	[ă-NĒ-mē-ă] Greek *anaimia* from an-, without + *haima*, blood	Condition in which red blood cells do not transport enough oxygen to the tissues.
anisocytosis	[ăn-Ī-sō-sī-TŌ-sĭs] aniso-, unequal + cyt-, cell + -osis, condition	Condition with abnormal variation in the size of red blood cells.
basophilia	[bā-sō-FĬL-ē-ă]	Condition with an increased number of basophils in the blood.
dyscrasia	[dĭs-KRĀ-zē-ă] Greek, bad temperament	Any disease with abnormal particles in the blood.
eosinophilia	[Ē-ō-sĭn-ō-FĬL-ē-ă]	Condition with an abnormal number of eosinophils in the blood.
erythroblastosis fetalis	[ĕ-RĬTH-rō-blăs-TŌ-sĭs fē-TĂL-ĭs]	Incompatibility disorder between a mother with Rh negative and a fetus with Rh positive.
erythropenia	[ĕ-rĭth-rō-PĒ-nē-ă] erythro-, red blood cells + -penia, deficiency	Disorder with abnormally low number of red blood cells.
granulocytosis	[GRĂN-yū-lō-sī-TŌ-sĭs] granulocyt(e) + -osis, condition	Condition with an abnormal number of granulocytes in the bloodstream.
hemochromatosis	[HĒ-mō-krō-mă-TŌ-sĭs] hemo-, blood + chromat-, color + -osis	Hereditary condition with excessive iron buildup in the blood.
hemolysis	[hē-MŎL-ĭ-sĭs] hemo-, blood + -lysis, destruction of	Disorder with breakdown of red blood cell membranes.

Terms	Word Analysis	Definition
hemophilia	[hē-mō-FĬL-ē-ă] hemo-, blood + -philia, attraction	Hereditary disorder with lack of clotting factor in the blood.
leukemia	[lū-KĒ-mē-ă] leuk-, white + -emia, blood	General term for a number of disorders with excessive white blood cells in the bloodstream and bone marrow.
macrocytosis	[MĂK-rō-sī-TŌ-sĭs] macro-, large + cyt + -osis	Disorder with abnormally large red blood cells.
microcytosis	[MĬK-rō-sī-TŌ-sĭs] micro-, small + cyt- + -osis	Disorder with abnormally small red blood cells.
multiple myeloma	[mī-ĕ-LŌ-mă]	Malignant tumor of the bone marrow.
myeloblast	[MĪ-ĕ-lō-blăst] myelo-, marrow + -blast, immature cell	Immature granulocytes.
pancytopenia	[PĂN-sī-tō-PĒ-nē-ă] pan-, all + cyto- + -penia	Condition with a low number of blood components.
poikilocytosis	[PŎY-kĭ-lō-sī-TŌ-sĭs] poikilo-, irregular + cyt- + -osis	Disorder with irregularly shaped red blood cells.
polycythemia	[PŎL-ē-sī-THĒ-mē-ă] poly-, many + cyt- + -emia	Disorder with an abnormal increase in red blood cells and hemoglobin.
purpura	[PŬR-pū-ră] Latin, purple	Condition with multiple, tiny hemorrhages under the skin.
reticulocytosis	[rĕ-TĬK-yū-lō-sī-TŌ-sĭs] recticulo-, fine network + cyt- + -osis	Disorder with an abnormal number of immature erythrocytes.
thalassemia	[thăl-ă-SĒ-mē-ă] Greek thalassa, sea + -emia	Hereditary disorder characterized by inability to produce sufficient hemoglobin.
thrombocytopenia	[THRŎM-bō-sī-tō-PĒ-nē-ă] thrombocyt(e) + -penia	Bleeding condition with insufficient production of platelets.
von Willebrand's disease	[vŏn WĬL-lĕ-brăndz] After E. A. von Willebrand (1870–1949), Finnish physician	Hemorrhagic disorder with tendency to bleed from mucous membranes.

CASE STUDY

Reading the X-Rays

Next, the radiology report is added to Mr. Maynard's chart, and the hematologist adds notes.

RADIOLOGY: Abdomen: Adynamic ileus.

April 2, XXXX: Chest; bibasilar changes compatible with a small pleural effusion. Increased density in the right lung and small localized density because of rotation.

December 4, XXXX: Abdominal ultrasound; normal biliary examination. Bilateral multiple renal cysts. Liver; fatty texture.

In summary, I have initiated more workup for anemia. The possibilities include anemia of chronic disease, myelodysplasia, or chronic blood loss. If his workup is inconclusive, then he might require bone marrow aspiration and biopsy to establish the diagnosis.

Critical Thinking

80. Does a CBC provide enough information for a diagnosis of anemia or chronic blood loss?

81. Is Rh factor important for an 83-year-old man? Why or why not?

Pathological Terms Exercises

Spell It Correctly

The following terms are either spelled correctly or incorrectly. Put C in the space following correctly spelled words. Put the correct spelling in the space following incorrectly spelled words.

82. hemphilia _____

83. pancypenia _____

84. macrocytosis _____

85. anemia _____

86. alplastic anemia _____

87. eosinphilia _____

88. pupura _____

89. reticulocytosis _____

90. thrombocytenia _____

91. poikilocytosis _____

Check Your Knowledge

Circle T for true or F for false.

92. Sickle cell anemia is found primarily in people of Mediterranean origin. T F

93. All red blood cell disorders are inherited. T F

94. A sudden loss of blood can cause anemia. T F

95. Multiple myeloma is a form of cancer. T F

96. Rh factor incompatibility can cause hemochromatosis. T F

97. Pernicious anemia may result from a deficiency of vitamin B12. T F

98. Leukemia and anemia are closely related diseases. T F

99. Too many red blood cells can be a symptom of a disorder. T F

Find the Meaning

Describe the cause of each of the following forms of anemia.

100. aplastic anemia_____

101. iron-deficiency anemia_____

102. pernicious anemia_____

103. thalassemia_____

104. sickle cell anemia_____

Surgical Terms

Surgery is not generally performed on the blood system. Sometimes venipuncture is considered a minor surgical procedure. (In this text, we have classified it as a diagnostic procedure.) The exceptions are **bone marrow biopsy** and **bone marrow transplant.** A needle is introduced into the bone marrow cavity and marrow is extracted for examination. This procedure is used in the diagnosis of various blood disorders, such as anemia and leukemia. A bone marrow transplant is performed for serious ailments, such as leukemia and cancer. In this procedure, a donor's marrow is introduced into the bone marrow of the patient. First, all the diseased cells are killed through extensive radiation and chemotherapy. After the donor's marrow is introduced, successful transplants result in healthy cells taking over the patient's marrow. Unsuccessful transplants may result in rejection of the marrow or a recurrence of the disease.

Vocabulary Review

In the previous section, you learned terms relating to surgery. Before going to the exercises, review the terms below and refer to the previous section if you have any questions.

Term	Word Analysis	Definition
bone marrow biopsy		Extraction of bone marrow, by means of a needle, for observation.
bone marrow transplant		Injection of donor bone marrow into a patient whose diseased cells have been killed through radiation and chemotherapy.

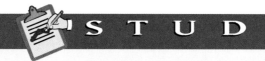

C A S E   S T U D Y

Getting Confirmation

In addition to his other problems, Mr. Maynard has prostate cancer. His PSA has remained normal for a few years, so the cancer is thought to be in remission. However, the cause of the anemia was not confirmed. His diagnosis is also not confirmed, so a bone marrow biopsy is ordered. The bone marrow biopsy confirms aplastic anemia.

 Critical Thinking

105. Describe the abnormality that the bone marrow biopsy reveals.

106. Does Mr. Maynard's condition require treatment before he has any surgery?

Pharmacological Terms

Medications that directly affect the work of the blood system are **anticoagulants** (to prevent blood clotting); **thrombolytics** (to dissolve blood clots); **coagulants** or *clotting agents* (to aid in blood clotting); and **hemostatics** (to stop bleeding, such as vitamin K). Anticoagulants are administered before most types of surgeries to prevent emboli. Blood flow is affected by vasoconstrictors and vasodilators, two medications given for cardiovascular problems.

Chemotherapy, therapy that uses drugs, is used to cause a **remission** (disappearance of the disease) in leukemia. Sometimes more treatment is needed when a **relapse** (recurrence of the disease) occurs. Table 12-4 lists common pharmaceutical agents used in treating blood disorders.

Table 12-4 Some Pharmaceutical Agents Used to Treat Blood Disorders

Drug Class	Purpose	Generic	Trade Name
anticoagulants	to prevent clotting	warfarin	Coumadin, Sofarin
		heparin calcium, heparin sodium	Calciparine, Heparin Sodium
		aspirin	Bayer, Excedrin
clotting agents; coagulants	to aid in clotting	phytonadione, Vitamin K	Mephyton, Konakion
hemostatic	to stop blood flow within vessels	desmopressin	Concentraid, DDAVP
		aminocaproic acid	Amicar
thrombolytic	to dissolve clots	alteplase	Activase
		anistreplase	Eminase
		streptokinase	Streptase, Kabikinase
		urokinase	Abbokinase

Vocabulary Review

In the previous section, you learned terms relating to pharmacology. Before going on to the exercises, review the terms below and refer to the previous section if you have any questions.

Term	Word Analysis	Definition
anticoagulant	[ĂN-tē-kō-ĂG-yū-lănt] anti-, against + coagulant	Agent that prevents formation of blood clots.
coagulant	[kō-ĂG-yū-lănt] Latin coagulo, to curdle	Clotting agent.
hemostatic	[hē-mō-STĂT-ĭk] hemo-, blood + -static, maintaining a state	Agent that stops bleeding.
relapse	[RĒ-lăps] From Latin relabor, to slide back	Recurrence of a disease.
remission	[rē-MĬSH-ŭn] Latin remissio, a relaxation	Disappearance of a disease for a time.
thrombolytic	[thrŏm-bō-LĬT-ĭk] thrombo-, thrombus + -lytic, a loosening	Agent that dissolves blood clots.

Coordinating Prescription Medication

Mr. Maynard's medication list at admission is:

Cardura 4 mg p.o. q.h.s.

Ventolin unit dose t.i.d.

Atrovent unit dose t.i.d.

Ceftin 250 mg b.i.d. prior to admission.

Magnesium citrate b.i.d.

Lactulose 30 cc p.o. b.i.d.

Cardura is for his high blood pressure and prostate problems; Ventolin and Atrovent are prescribed for his respiratory symptoms. Ceftin is an antibiotic for a urinary tract infection. Magnesium citrate and lactulose are laxatives.

💡 **Critical Thinking**

107. Aspirin is known to promote some bleeding. Should Mr. Maynard use aspirin for pain?

108. What vitamin might improve Mr. Maynard's condition?

Pharmacological Terms Exercises

Check Your Knowledge

Fill in the blanks.

109. Hemophiliacs require _____ and _____ to control bleeding.

110. A prescription for someone with coronary artery disease might include an _____.

111. If medication is not taken regularly, a _____ of a disease might occur.

112. Sometimes the temporary disappearance of a disease, called a(n) _____ is unexplained.

CHALLENGE SECTION

The form shown in Figure 12-8 gives results for a patient and expected ranges for lab tests done in a large lab service.

Challenge Section Exercises

113. What tests, if any, are abnormal?

114. The laboratory was instructed to do a T3 and T4 uptake test. What was the patient's physician trying to determine?

USING THE http://www. INTERNET

Go to the site of the Aplastic Anemia Association (www.aplastic.org). Choose one of their online articles and write a paragraph summarizing its content.

CHAPTER REVIEW

Definitions

Define the following terms and combining forms. Review the chapter before starting. Make sure you know how to pronounce each term as you define it.

Term	Definition
agglutin(o)	
agglutination [ă-glū-tĭ-NĀ-shŭn]	
agglutinogen [ă-glŭ-TĬN-ō-jĕn]	
agranulocyte [ā-GRĂN-yū-lō-sīt]	
albumin [ăl-BYŪ-mĭn]	
anemia [ă-NĒ-mē-ă]	
anisocytosis [ăn-Ī-sō-sī-TŌ-sĭs]	
anticoagulant [ĂN-tĕ-kō-ĂG-yū-lănt]	
antiglobulin [ĂN-tē-GLŎB-yū-lĭn] test	
basophil [BĀ-sō-fĭl]	
basophilia [bā-sō-FĬL-ē-ă]	
biochemistry panel	
blood [blŭd]	
blood chemistry	
blood culture	
blood indices [ĬN-dĭ-sēz]	
blood types or groups	
bone marrow biopsy	
bone marrow transplant	
chemistry profile	
coagulant [kō-ĂG-yū-lănt]	
coagulation [kō-ăg-yū-LĀ-shŭn]	
complete blood count (CBC)	
dyscrasia [dĭs-KRĀ-zē-ă]	
electrophoresis [ē-lĕk-trō-FŌR-ē-sĭs]	
eosino	

Term	Definition
eosinophil [ē-ō-SĬN-ō-fĭl]	
eosinophilia [Ē-ō-sĭn-ō-FĬL-ē-ă]	
erythr(o)	
erythroblastosis fetalis [ĕ-RĬTH-rō-blăs-TŌ-sĭs fē-TăL-ĭs]	
erythrocyte [ĕ-RĬTH-rō-sīt]	
erythrocyte sedimentation rate (ESR)	
erythropenia [ĕ-rĭth-rō-PĒ-nē-ă]	
erythropoietin [ĕ-rĭth-rō-PŎY-ĕ-tĭn]	
fibrin [FĪ-brĭn] clot	
fibrinogen [fĭ-BRĬN-ō-jĕn]	
gamma globulin [GĂ-mă GLŎB-yū-lĭn]	
globin [GLŌ-bĭn]	
globulin [GLŎB-yū-lĭn]	
granulocyte [GRĂN-yū-lō-sīt]	
granulocytosis [GRĂN-yū-lō-sī-TŌ-sĭs]	
hematocrit [HĒ-mă-tō-krĭt, HĔM-ă-tō-krĭt]	
hematocytoblast [HĒ-mă-tō-SĪ-tō-blăst]	
heme [hēm]	
hemo, hemat(o)	
hemochromatosis [HĒ-mō-krō-mă-TŌ-sĭs]	
hemoglobin [hē-mō-GLŌ-bĭn]	
hemolysis [hē-MŎL-ĭ-sĭs]	
hemophilia [hē-mō-FĬL-ē-ă]	
hemostatic [hē-mō-STĂT-ĭk]	
heparin [HĔP-ă-rĭn]	
histamine [HĬS-tă-mēn]	
leuk(o)	
leukocyte [LŪ-kō-sīt]	
leukemia [lū-KĒ-mē-ă]	
lymphocyte [LĬM-fō-sīt]	
macrocytosis [MĂK-rō-sī-TŌ-sĭs]	
megakaryocyte [mĕg-ă-KĂR-ē-ō-sīt]	

Term	Definition
microcytosis [MĬK-rō-sī-TŌ-sĭs]	
monocyte [MŎN-ō-sīt]	
multiple myeloma [mī-ĕ-LŌ-mă]	
myeloblast [MĪ-ĕ-lŏ-blăst]	
neutrophil [NŪ-trō-fĭl]	
pancytopenia [PĂN-sī-tō-PĒ-nē-ă]	
partial thromboplastin time (PTT)	
phag(o)	
phlebotomy [flĕ-BŎT-ō-mē]	
plasma [PLĂZ-mă]	
plasmapheresis [PLĂZ-mă-fĕ-RĒ-sĭs]	
platelet [PLĀT-lĕt]	
platelet count (PLT)	
poikilocytosis [PŎY-kĭ-lō-sī-TŌ-sĭs]	
polycythemia [PŎL-ē-sī-THĒ-mē-ă]	
prothrombin [prō-THRŎM-bĭn]	
prothrombin time (PT)	
purpura [PŬR-pū-ră]	
red blood cell	
red blood cell count	
red blood cell morphology	
relapse [RĒ-lăps]	
remission [rē-MĬSH-ŭn]	
reticulocytosis [rĕ-TĬK-yū-lō-sī-TŌ-sĭs]	
Rh factor	
Rh-negative	
Rh-positive	
sedimentation rate (SR)	
serum [SĒR-ŭm]	
SMA (sequential multiple analyzer)	
stem cell	
thalassemia [thăl-ă-SĒ-mē-ă]	
thromb(o)	
thrombin [THRŎMB-ĭn]	

Term	Definition
thrombocyte [THRŎM-bō-sīt]	
thrombocytopenia [THRŎM-bō-sī-tō-PĒ-nē-ă]	
thrombolytic [thrŏm-bō-LĬT-ĭk]	
thromboplastin [thrŏm-bō-PLĂS-tĭn]	
transfusion [trăns-FYŪ-zhŭn]	
venipuncture [VĔN-ĭ-pŭnk-chŭr, VĒ-nĭ-pŭnk-chŭr]	
von Willebrand's [vŏn WĬL-lĕ-brăndz] disease	
white blood cell	

Abbreviation	Meaning
APTT	
baso	
BCP	
BMT	
CBC	
diff	
eos	
ESR	
G-CSF	
GM-CSF	
HCT, Hct	
HGB, Hgb, HB	
MCH	
MCHC	
MCV	
mono	
PCV	
PLT	
PMN, poly	
PT	
PTT	
RBC	

Abbreviation	Meaning
SR; sed. rate	
seg	
WBC	

1. Blood circulates throughout the body and exchanges substances with most of the body's cells.
2. No; blood type does not make one more susceptible.
3. c
4. a
5. b
6. b
7. c
8. c
9. b
10. c
11. b
12. b
13. b
14. c
15. b
16. AB
17. O
18. B
19. A
20. O
21. AB
22. B
23. A
24. d
25. g
26. a
27. b
28. c
29. e
30. h
31. f
32. Venipuncture; Yes; small amounts of blood are replaced within a day or so.
33. RBC measures red blood cells and WBC measures white blood cells.
34. e
35. f
36. g
37. h
38. j
39. b
40. i
41. c
42. d
43. a
44. tending to clump together

45. removal of a thrombus
46. immature red blood cell
47. study of diseases of the blood
48. movement of eosinophils
49. immature white blood cell
50. part of the cell that aids a cell in digesting unwanted particles
51. disease with increased red blood cells
52. study of cells
53. white blood cell
54. disease (type of cancer) with abnormal number of white blood cells
55. abnormally small amount of platelets in the blood
56. blood-filled mass
57. disease with increased red blood cell counts
58. anemia; chronic blood loss; dehydration; polycythemia
59. white blood count (WBC)
60. j
61. h
62. c
63. g
64. b
65. i
66. a
67. e
68. f
69. d
70. 120–199
71. 135–145
72. 30–150
73. 4.5-12.8
74. 80.0–98.0
75. 150–400
76. 34.0–47.0
77. 3.8–5.2
78. 3.9–11.1
79. 32.0–36.0
80. Yes. Anemia and chronic blood loss are indicated by the percentage of red blood cells noted in a CBC.
81. Yes; it is important for everybody who might need a transfusion.
82. hemophilia
83. pancytopenia

84. C
85. C
86. aplastic anemia
87. eosinophilia
88. purpura
89. C
90. thrombocytopenia
91. C
92. F
93. F
94. T
95. T
96. F
97. T
98. T
99. T
100. failure in production of red blood cells
101. lack of enough iron either in diet or absorption, which causes insufficient production of hemoglobin
102. insufficient vitamin B12, which causes abnormal red blood cell shape
103. hereditary blood disorder with insufficient hemo-globin production
104. hereditary red blood cell disorder with misshapen cells and breakdown in cell membranes that creates problems with carrying oxygen to the tissues
105. aplastic anemia, a failure of the bone marrow to pro-duce enough red blood cells
106. Yes; anemia is a complica-tion that should be dealt with first because of the probability of further blood loss during surgery.
107. No. He cannot afford to lose more blood.
108. Vitamin B12
109. coagulants; hemostatics
110. anticoagulant
111. relapse
112. remission
113. cholesterol; HDL; LDL;
114. thyroid function

CHAPTER

13

The Lymphatic and Immune Systems

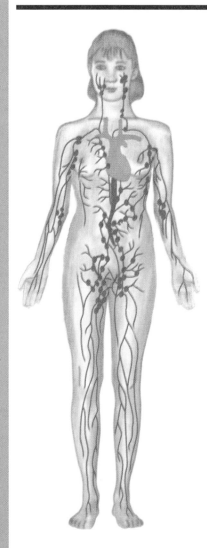

After studying this chapter, you will be able to:

- Name the parts of the lymphatic and immune systems and discuss the function of each part

- Define combining forms used in building words that relate to the lymphatic and immune system

- Identify the meaning of related abbreviations

- Name the common diagnoses, clinical procedures, and laboratory tests used in treating the lymphatic and immune systems

- List and define the major pathological conditions of the lymphatic and immune systems

- Explain the meaning of surgical terms related to the lymphatic and immune systems

- List common pharmacological agents used in treating disorders of the lymphatic and immune systems

Structure and Function

The lymphatic and immune systems share some of the same structures and functions. Both the lymphatic and immune systems contain the lymph nodes, spleen, and thymus gland, and produce some of the disease-fighting immune cells. Separately, the lymphatic system contains lymph vessels and the lymph itself, while the immune system includes all the types of immunity either inherent (or natural) in or acquired by the body. Figure 13-1a shows the lymphatic and immune systems. Figure 13-1b shows how lymph circulates throughout the body.

Lymphatic Organs and Structures

The lymphatic system is similar to both the cardiovascular and blood systems. A network of *lymphatic vessels* transports a fluid (**lymph**) to and from the

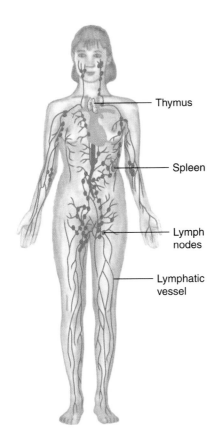

Thymus

Spleen

Lymph nodes

Lymphatic vessel

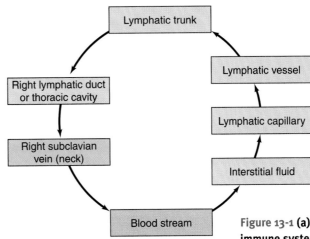

Lymphatic trunk

Right lymphatic duct or thoracic cavity

Right subclavian vein (neck)

Blood stream

Lymphatic vessel

Lymphatic capillary

Interstitial fluid

Figure 13-1 (a) The lymphatic and immune systems are the body's major defense against foreign substances; (b) Flowchart of the path of lymph through the body.

Figure 13-2 Lymphatic capillaries gather the lymph from the space between tissues.

bloodstream. Like the blood system, lymph transports various substances around the body. Unlike blood, lymph does not contain either red blood cells or platelets. It does contain white blood cells. It carries less protein than blood, but about the same amount of water, salts, sugar, and waste material.

Microscopic *lymphatic capillaries* are the smallest part of the *lymphatic pathways*, the vessels that transport the lymph around the body. The capillaries have thin walls that allow the fluid in tissues to flow between the capillaries and the tissues. Figure 13-2 illustrates the flow of lymph from the lymphatic capillaries within the lymphatic system to lymphatic vessels and nodes in the body. This fluid in the spaces between tissues is called *interstitial fluid*. When this fluid flows into the lymphatic capillaries, it is called lymph.

The capillaries merge to form larger pathways, the lymphatic vessels. These vessels bring lymph to the **lymph nodes,** specialized organs that both produce lymph cells (**lymphocytes**) and filter harmful substances from the tissues (Figure 13-3). The lymph nodes contain special cells (**macrophages**) that devour foreign substances. Lymph nodes become swollen with lymph cells and macrophages. The lymphocytes produce **antibodies,** specialized proteins that fight

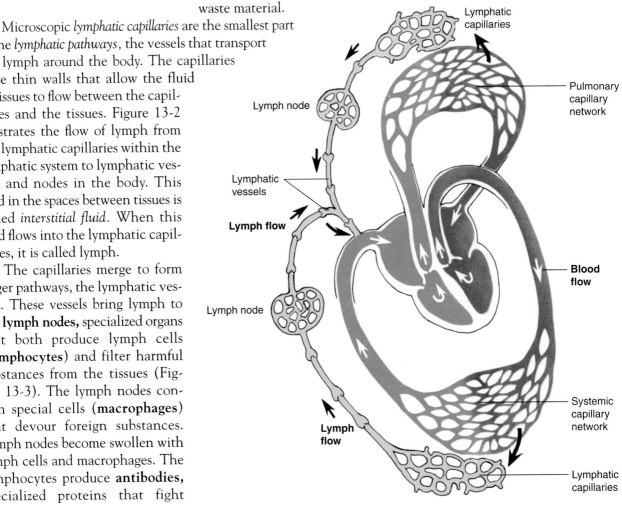

Lymphatic capillaries

Pulmonary capillary network

Lymph node

Lymphatic vessels

Lymph flow

Blood flow

Lymph node

Systemic capillary network

Lymph flow

Lymphatic capillaries

Figure 13-3 Lymph nodes contain cells (lymphocytes and macrophages) that ingest foreign substances.

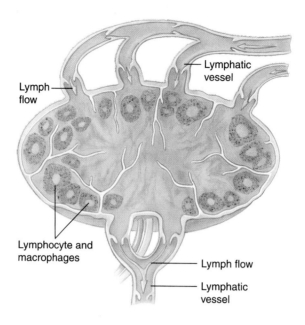

Lymphatic vessel

Lymph flow

Lymphocyte and macrophages

Lymph flow

Lymphatic vessel

disease, to help rid the body of the diseased cells. Substances called **antigens** also fight disease by provoking an immune response in other cells. The lymph vessels also gather fluid and substances that have leaked from the blood capillaries into the tissues and transport them back to the bloodstream where they are needed. In addition, they bring lipids from the small intestine to the bloodstream where parts of the lipids are used. Excess lipids can form plaque in blood vessels. Lymph travels in only one direction, toward the thoracic cavity, where it empties into the *right lymphatic duct* and the *thoracic duct*. The two ducts carry the lymph into the subclavian veins in the neck, where the lymph flows into the blood system. The blood system circulates the blood to the body's tissues, where the process of fluid and substances leaking into the lymphatic capillaries begins again (see Figure 13-1b).

Lymph nodes are located throughout the body except in the central nervous system. The major groups of lymph nodes are located in the throat (the tonsils and adenoids are actually lymph tissue), neck, armpit, mediastinum, and groin.

Two organs of the lymph system are the **spleen** and the **thymus gland.** The largest lymphatic organ, the spleen, is located in the upper left portion of the abdominal cavity, where it can easily be injured and ruptured. In such cases, it must be repaired or removed (its functions are taken over by the lymph nodes, liver, and bone marrow). The function of the spleen is to filter foreign material from the blood, to store blood, to destroy old red blood cells, and to activate lymphocytes that destroy some of the foreign substances filtered from the blood (Figure 13-4).

The thymus gland is a soft gland with two lobes (Figure 13-5). It is large during infancy and early childhood when immunity is most crucial, but gradually shrinks until it is often quite small in adulthood (when the body has acquired other types of immunities). The thymus gland contains certain important cells called **thymocytes,** some of which mature into **T cells (T lymphocytes).** T cells provide immunity after they leave the thymus. Their movement is aided by **thymosin,** a hormone secreted by the thymus.

Figure 13-4 The spleen, like the lymph nodes, contains cells that destroy foreign substances.

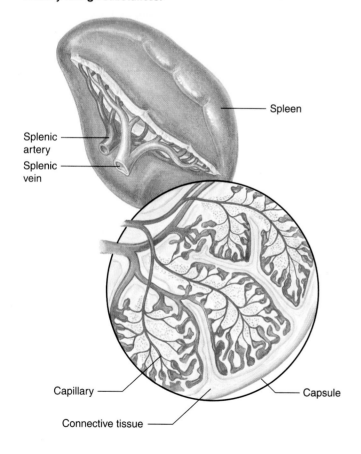

Spleen

Splenic artery

Splenic vein

Capillary

Connective tissue

Capsule

Immune System

The immune system consists of a series of defenses against intruders, such as viruses and bacteria. The immune system shares several parts with the lymphatic system (lymph nodes, spleen, and thymus gland). These parts serve as defense mechanisms protecting the body. Parts of other systems, such as the skin, also play an important role in protecting the body from disease.

The human body includes a number of mechanical, chemical, and other defenses against disease. When disease-causing agents, **pathogens,** try to enter the body, they are often stopped by the skin, the cilia in the nostrils, and by various mucous membranes—all of which are mechanical barriers to intrusion. If some pathogens get past the mechanical defenses, they may be stopped by chemical barriers, such as gastric juices in the stomach. Pathogens in the bloodstream may be destroyed by **phagocytosis,** the ingesting of foreign substances by specialized cells like macrophages. In addition, humans are resistant to some diseases that affect other animals and vice versa. This natural resistance may occur because the pathogen finds the human's internal environment harmful to its survival. On the other hand, some pathogens prefer the environment of the human body as opposed to that of other animals, so they affect humans but not animals. Some tick-borne diseases such as Lyme disease can have devastating consequences to humans but remain dormant in animals. Some bacteria are beneficial in humans because they help ward off disease.

These defenses work together with the immune system to avert or attack disease. The specific defenses of the immune system provide **immunity,** resistance to particular pathogens. There are three major types of immunity—natural immunity, acquired active immunity, and acquired passive immunity.

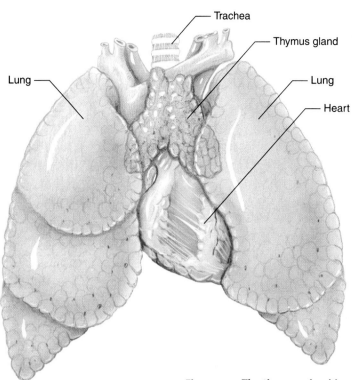

Figure 13-5 The thymus gland is located between the lungs.

Increasingly, people are trying alternative treatments designed to build the strength of their immune systems. Old-fashioned remedies are now being revived in an effort to prevent disease. Olive oil and other oils are thought to protect one from infection. Garlic is thought to prevent certain conditions.

Natural Immunity

Natural immunity is the human body's natural resistance to certain diseases. This natural resistance varies for individuals, even to the extent that persons of certain racial backgrounds tend to have more or less resistance to certain diseases. Natural resistance depends on the individual's genetic characteristics and on some of the natural chemical defenses.

Acquired Active Immunity

The body develops **acquired active immunity** either by having a disease and producing natural antibodies to it or by being *vaccinated* against the disease. A **vaccination** or **vaccine** is an antigen from a different organism that causes active immunity.

Acquired active immunity is further divided into two types. The first, **humoral immunity,** is immunity provided by **plasma cells,** which produce

When a disease has been irradicated from the population, research institutions often keep the actual virus in a safe place in order to create vaccines for future use.

antibodies called **immunoglobulins.** These are the five major types of immuno-globulins and their functions:

- *Immunoglobulin G (IgG)* is effective against bacteria, viruses, and toxins.

- *Immunoglobulin A (IgA)* is common in exocrine gland secretions, such as breast milk, tears, nasal fluid, gastric juice, and so on.

- *Immunoglobulin M (IgM)* develops in the blood plasma in response to certain antigens within the body or from foreign sources. It is the first antigen to be produced after infection.

- *Immunoglobulin D (IgD)* is important in B-cell activation, which helps immunity by transforming itself into a plasma cell in the presence of a specific type of antigen.

- *Immunoglobulin E (IgE)* appears in glandular secretions and is associated with allergic reactions.

The second type of acquired active immunity, **cell-mediated immunity,** is provided by the action of T cells. The T cells respond to antigens by multiplying rapidly and producing proteins (for example, **interferons** and **interleukins**) that have antiviral properties. Three types of other specialized T cells are:

- **Helper cells** or CD4 cells that stimulate the immune response.

- **Cytotoxic cells** or CD8 cells that help in the destruction of infected cells.

- **Suppressor cells** or T cells (mainly CD8 and some CD4) that suppress B cells and other immune cells.

Acquired Passive Immunity

Acquired passive immunity is immunity provided in the form of anti-bodies or antitoxins that have been developed in another person or another species. Acquired passive immunity is necessary in cases of snakebite and tetanus or any problem where immediate immunity is needed. In such cases, a dose of **antitoxin** (antibody directed against specific toxins) is given to provide antibodies. Passive immunity may also be administered to lessen the chance of catching a disease or to lessen the severity of the course of the disease. **Gamma globulin** is a preparation of collected antibodies given to prevent or lessen certain diseases, such as hepatitis A, varicella, and rabies.

Vocabulary Review

In the previous section, you learned terms relating to the lymphatic and immune systems. Before going on to the exercises, review the terms below and refer to the previous section if you have any questions.

Term	Word Analysis	Definition
acquired active immunity		Resistance to a disease acquired naturally or developed by previous exposure or vaccination.
acquired passive immunity		Inoculation against disease or poison, using antitoxins or antibodies from or in another person or another species.

Term	Word Analysis	Definition
antibody	[ĂN-tē-bŏd-ē] anti-, against + body	Specialized protein that fights disease.
antigen	[ĂN-tǐ-jěn] anti(body) + -gen, producing	Any substance in the bloodstream that can provoke an immune response.
antitoxin	[ăn-tē-TŎK-sǐn] anti-, against + toxin	Antibodies directed against a particular disease or poison.
cell-mediated immunity		Resistance to disease mediated by T cells.
cytotoxic cell	[sī-tō-TŎK-sǐk] cyto-, cell + toxic	T cell that helps in destruction of infected cells throughout the body.
gamma globulin	[GĂ-mă GLŎB-yū-lǐn]	Antibodies given to prevent or lessen certain diseases.
helper cell		T cell that stimulates the immune response.
humoral immunity	[HYŪ-mōr-ăl]	Resistance to disease provided by plasma cells and antibody production.
immunity	[ǐ-MYŪ-nǐ-tē] Latin *immunitas*, freedom from service	Resistance to particular pathogens.
immunoglobulin	[ĬM-yū-nō-GLŎB-yū-lǐn] immuno-, immunity + globulin	Type of antibody.
interferon	[ǐn-těr-FĒR-ŏn]	Protein produced by T cells and other cells; destroys disease-causing cells with its antiviral properties.
interleukin	[ǐn-těr-LŪ-kǐn] inter-, among + leuk(ocyte)	Protein produced by T cells; helps regulate immune system.
lymph	[lǐmf] Latin *lympha*, clear spring water	Fluid containing white blood cells and other substances that flows in the lymphatic vessels.
lymph node		Specialized organ that produces lymphocytes and filters harmful substances from the tissues.
lymphocytes	[LĬM-fō-sīts] lympho-, lymph + -cyte, cell	Lymph cells.

Term	Word Analysis	Definition
macrophage	[MĂK-rō-fāj] macro-, large + -phage, eating	Special cell that devours foreign substances.
natural immunity		Inherent resistance to disease found in a species, race, family group, or certain individuals.
pathogen	[PĂTH-ō-jĕn] patho-, disease + -gen, producing	Disease-causing agent.
phagocytosis	[FĂG-ō-sī-TŌ-sĭs] phagocyt(e) + -osis, condition	Ingestion of foreign substances by specialized cells.
plasma cell	[PLĂZ-mă]	Specialized lymphocyte that produces immunoglobulins.
spleen	[splēn] Greek splen	Organ of lymph system that filters, stores, removes blood, and activates lymphocytes.
suppressor cell	[sŭ-PRĔS-ōr]	T cell that suppresses B cells and other immune cells.
T cells		Specialized cells that develop in the thymus and are responsible for cellular immunity.
thymocyte	[THĪ-mō-sīt] thym(us) + -cyte, cell	Cell of the thymus gland that can mature into a T cell.
thymosin	[THĪ-mō-sĭn]	Hormone secreted by the thymus gland that aids in distribution of thymocytes.
thymus gland	[THĪ-mŭs] Greek thymos, sweetbread	Soft gland with two lobes that is involved in immune responses; located in mediastinum.
T lymphocytes		See T cells.
vaccination , vaccine	[VĂK-sĭ-NĀ-shŭn], [VĂK-sēn] Latin vaccinus, relating to a cow	Injection of an antigen from a different organism to cause active immunity.

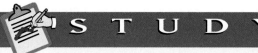

CASE STUDY

Researching a Cure

Some hospitals are part of large university complexes. These hospitals often do many kinds of research and offer *tertiary care*, medical care at a center that has a unit specializing in certain diseases. They may provide data on drug trials. They may work on improving diagnostic testing. Some research trials work on diseases that are infectious and for which there is not yet a cure. The goal of many studies is to produce a vaccine.

Critical Thinking

1. Why would researchers want to produce a vaccination?

2. What form of immunity would a vaccination provide?

Structure and Function Exercises

Find a Match

Match the correct definition in the right-hand column with the terms in the left-hand column.

3. T cell

4. pathogen

5. immunoglobulin E

6. IgD

7. helper cell

8. cytoxic cell

9. suppressor cell

10. antitoxin

11. antibody

12. gamma globulin

a. T cell that helps destroy foreign substances

b. T cell that regulates the amounts of antibody

c. T cell that stimulates antibody production

d. antibody important in B-cell activation

e. agent given to prevent or lessen disease

f. mature thymocyte

g. antigen that helps produce resistance to a disease or a poison

h. specialized cell that fights diseased cells

i. disease-causing agent

j. antibody associated with allergic reactions

Check Your Knowledge

Fill in the blanks

13. People are born with some _____ immunity.

14. Vaccinations give _____ _____ immunity.

15. Antitoxins give _____ _____ immunity.

16. The special lymph node cells that ingest foreign substances are called _____.

17. Lymph contains _____ blood cells.

18. The thymus gland produces cells that mature into _____ _____.

19. Agents of T cells that destroy disease-causing cells are _____ and _____.

20. The fluid in the space between tissues is called _____ _____.

Combining Forms and Abbreviations

The lists below include combining forms and abbreviations that relate specifically to the lymphatic and immune systems. Pronunciations are provided for the examples.

Combining Form	Meaning	Example
aden(o)	gland	adenocarcinoma [ĂD-ē-nō-kăr-sĬ-NŌ-mă], glandular cancer
immun(o)	immunity	immunosuppressor [ĬM-yū-nō-sŭ-PRĔS-ōr], agent that suppresses the immune response
lymph(o)	lymph	lymphocyte [LĬM-fō-sĬt], white blood cell formed in lymphatic tissue
lymphaden(o)	lymph nodes	lymphadenopathy [lĭm-făd-ē-NŎP-ă-thē], disease affecting the lymph nodes
lymphangi(o)	lymphatic vessels	lymphangitis [lĭm-făn-JĪ-tĭs], inflammation of the lymphatic vessels
splen(o)	spleen	splenectomy [splē-NĔK-tō-mē], removal of the spleen
thym(o)	thymus	thymectomy [thī-MĔK-tō-mē], removal of the thymus
tox(o), toxi, toxico	poison	toxicosis [tŏk-sĬ-KŌ-sĬs], systemic poisoning

Abbreviation	Meaning	Abbreviation	Meaning
AIDS	acquired immunodeficiency syndrome	CML	chronic myelogenous leukemia
ALL	acute lymphocytic leukemia	CMV	cytomegalovirus
AML	acute myelogenous leukemia	EBV	Epstein-Barr virus
AZT	Azidothymidine	EIA, ELISA	Enzyme-linked immunosorbent assay
CLL	chronic lymphocytic leukemia	HIV	human immunodeficiency virus

Abbreviation	Meaning		Abbreviation	Meaning
HSV	herpes simplex virus		IgM	immunoglobulin M
IgA	immunoglobulin A		PCP	Pneumocystis carinii pneumonia
IgD	immunoglobulin D		SLE	systemic lupus erythematosus
IgE	immunoglobulin E		ZDV	Zidovudine
IgG	immunoglobulin G			

C A S E S T U D Y

Checking for Immunity

Jill, a three-year-old girl, was playing barefoot in her back-yard when she stepped on a rusty nail. The nail punctured her skin and made her vulnerable to tetanus, a muscle disease (see Chapter 5). Jill is up to date on all her vaccinations. The most common early childhood vacinnation is DPT (diphtheria, pertussis, and tetanus). The vacinnations last for a number of years.

Critical Thinking

21. Is it likely that Jill will contract tetanus? Why or why not?

22. What type of immunity to tetanus does Jill have?

Combining Forms and Abbreviations Exercises

Build Your Medical Vocabulary

Fill in the missing word part.

23. Removal of lymph nodes: _____ectomy.

24. Hemorrhage from a spleen: _____rrhagia

25. Cell that develops in the thymus: _____cyte.

26. Lacking in some immune function_____deficient.

27. Cell of a gland: _____cyte.

28. Skin disease caused by a poison: _____derma

29. Dilation of the lymphatic vessels: _____ectasis

30. Resembling lymph: _____oid

Find a Match

Match the term on the left with the correct definition on the right.

31. toxicologist

32. splenomegaly

33. lymphangiosarcoma

34. splenomyelomalacia

35. lymphocele

36. lymphadenitis

37. toxanemia

a. anemia resulting from a poison

b. malignancy in the lymphatic vessels

c. cystic mass containing lymph

d. inflammation of a lymph node

e. spleen enlargement

f. expert in the science of poisons

g. softening of the spleen and bone marrow

Diagnostic, Procedural, and Laboratory Terms

Abnormalities of lymph organs can be checked in a CAT scan. Several blood tests that indicate the number and condition of white blood cells are used in diagnosing lymph and immune systems diseases. HIV infection is diagnosed mainly with two blood serum tests, **enzyme-linked immunosorbent assay (EIA, ELISA)** and **Western blot.** ELISA tests blood for the antibody to the HIV virus (as well as antibodies to other specific viruses, such as hepatitis B), and the Western blot is a confirming test for the presence of HIV antibodies. Other more reliable AIDS tests are being developed.

Vocabulary Review

In the previous section, you learned terms relating to diagnosis, clinical procedures, and laboratory tests. Before going on to the exercises, review the terms below and refer to the previous section if you have any questions.

Term	Word Analysis	Definition
enzyme-linked immunosorbent assay (EIA, ELISA)		Test used to screen blood for the presence of antibodies to different viruses or bacteria.
Western blot		Test primarily used to check for antibodies to HIV in serum.

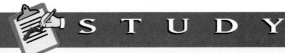

CASE STUDY

Handling the Emergency

Kyle, a seven-year-old boy, came to the emergency room at the hospital in respiratory distress. His mother says that he often has respiratory allergies. He was taken to the imaging area for chest x-rays. His lungs show some restricted areas. He is also given a thorough medical exam to make sure that nothing other than an allergic reaction is causing the breathing difficulties. If the examination is normal, Kyle will be sent to an allergist to determine the cause of his allergic reaction. The resident performing the exam marks the chart as follows:

 Critical Thinking

38. Why did Kyle need a thorough physical exam?

39. Did the physical exam show any abnormalities other than respiratory allergies?

GENERAL: He is a well-developed, well-nourished male in moderate respiratory distress.

HEENT: Tympanic membranes unremarkable. Eyes, nose, mouth, and throat normal.

NECK: No masses. Supple.

LUNGS: Breath sounds clear bilaterally with somewhat decreased air exchange and diffuse expiratory wheeze. Work of breathing is mildly to moderately increased.

CARDIAC: No murmur or gallop. Pulses 2+ and symmetrical.

ABDOMEN: Soft and nontender without organomegaly or mass.

GU: Normal male.

EXTREMITIES: Unremarkable.

NEUROLOGIC: Alert and appropriate. Cranial nerves intact. Reflexes 2+ and symmetrical.

Diagnostic, Procedural, and Laboratory Terms Exercises

Check Your Knowledge

Circle T for true or F for false.

40. The ELISA tests for HIV. T F

41. A lymphangiogram is taken after a contrast medium is injected into the bloodstream. T F

42. An analysis of white blood cells can help in diagnosing lymph and immune system diseases. T F

Pathological Terms

Diseases of the lymph and immune systems include diseases that attack lymph tissue itself; diseases that are spread through the lymphatic pathways; and diseases that flourish because of a *suppression* of the *immune response*. Disorders of the lymph and immune systems can be caused by an overly vigorous response to an immune system invader. This is the case with some diseases of other body systems, such as multiple sclerosis, in which the immune system attacks some of the nervous system's protective covering, myelin. It is also the case with **allergy,** an immune overresponse to a stimulus.

The most widespread **immunosuppressive disease** is **acquired immunodeficiency syndrome (AIDS).** AIDS is caused by the **human immunodeficiency virus (HIV),** a virus spread by sexual contact, exchange of bodily fluids, or intravenous exposure. The HIV virus is a type of **retrovirus,** a ribonucleic acid (RNA) that causes reversal of normal cell copying. The retro- (reverse) is the opposite of the ordinary method of DNA copying itself onto RNA. AIDS patients are subject to a number of **opportunistic infections,** infections that take hold because of the lowered immune response. Many of these infections are present in other body systems. Table 13-1 lists some opportunistic infections commonly present in AIDS patients and the parts of the body affected. AIDS affects the entire body with diseases such as herpes, candidiasis, and Kaposi's sarcoma appearing on the skin, and Pneumocystis carinii pneumonia (PCP) appearing in the lungs.

A disease such as AIDS brings with it many social issues. Many people with AIDS consider confidentiality a major requirement of receiving treatment. The government, on the other hand, is trying to control this infectious disease by reducing exposure.

Table 13-1 Some Opportunistic Malignancies and Infections that often Accompany AIDS

Opportunistic Infection	Type of Malignancy or Infection	Areas Affected
candidiasis	caused by fungus— Candida albicans	digestive tract, respiratory tract, skin, and some reproductive organs (particularly the vagina)
cytomegalovirus	Herpesviridae	can infect various cells or organs (like the eyes); causes swelling
Kaposi's sarcoma	malignancy arising from capillary linings	skin and lymph nodes
Mycobacterium avium-intracellulare (MAI)	caused by bacterium found in soil and water	systemic infection with fever, diarrhea, lung and blood disease, and wasting
Pneumocystis carinii pneumonia (PCP)	caused by parasite— Pneumocystis carinii	lungs—particularly dangerous type of pneumonia

Lymphoma, cancer of the lymph nodes, is a relatively common cancer with high cure rates. Some AIDS patients are especially susceptible to lymphomas because of their lowered immune systems. There are many different types of lymphomas. Two of the most common are **Hodgkin's lymphoma (Hodgkin's disease)**, a type of lymph cancer of uncertain origin that generally appears in early adulthood, and **non-Hodgkin's lymphoma,** a cancer of the lymph nodes with some cells resembling healthy cells and spreading in a diffuse pattern. It usually appears in mid-life. Depending on how far the disease has spread (**metastasis**), both types can be arrested with chemotherapy and radiation. Surgery (bone marrow transplantation) is also useful in Hodgkin's lymphoma.

Malignant tumors appear in many places in the lymph system. A **thymoma** is a malignancy of the thymus gland. Hodgkin's lymphoma is a malignancy of the lymph nodes and spleen. Enlarged lymph nodes, enlarged spleen (**splenomegaly**), and overactive spleen (**hypersplenism**) characterize this disease. Non-Hodgkin's lymphoma is a disease with malignant cells that resemble large lymphocytes (**lymphocytic lymphoma**) or large macrophages (called histiocytes, hence the name **histiocytic lymphoma**).

Non-malignant lesions on the lymph nodes, lungs, spleen, skin, and liver can indicate the presences of **sarcoidosis,** an inflammatory condition that can affect lung function. Swollen lymph nodes (**lymphadenopathy**) can also indicate the presence of **infectious mononucleosis,** an acute infectious disease caused by the *Epstein-Barr virus*. Infectious mononucleosis is often called the "kissing disease," because it is usually transmitted through mouth-to-mouth contact during kissing, sharing drinks, and sharing eating utensils. Rest is generally the only cure.

Allergies are a problem of the immune system that affect millions of people. They are due to the production of IgE antibodies against an **allergen,** an allergy-causing substance (Figure 13-6). Allergies vary for different people depending on time of year, amount of exposure to different allergens, and other immunological problems. **Hypersensitivity** increases as exposure increases, sometimes resulting in **anaphylaxis** (or *anaphylactic reaction* or *shock*), a reaction so severe that it can be life-threatening by decreasing blood pressure, affecting breathing, and causing loss of consciousness. Some people are extremely allergic to peanuts. A person with a severe peanut allergy who ingests even a tiny amount of peanuts (as in a cookie) will immediately go into

MORE ABOUT...

Contracting AIDS

When the AIDS epidemic began in the United States, many people feared that the HIV virus could be spread by casual contact. In fact, time has shown that there are very few specific ways it can be transmitted. These are the ways that AIDS is transmitted and how it is not transmitted.

How HIV Is Transmitted

Sexual contact, particularly vaginal, anal, and oral intercourse

Contaminated needles (intravenous drug use, accidental needle stick in medical setting)

During birth from an infected mother

Receiving infected blood or other tissue (rare; precautions usually prevent this)

How HIV Is NOT Transmitted

Casual contact (social kissing, hugging, handshakes)

Objects—toilet seats, deodorant sticks, doorknobs

Mosquitoes

Sneezing and coughing

Sharing food

Swimming in the same water as an infected person

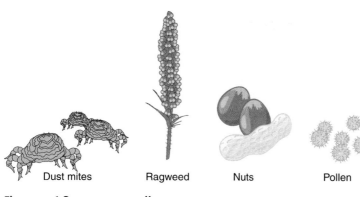

Dust mites   Ragweed   Nuts   Pollen

Figure 13-6 Some common allergens that provoke a response in many people.

an anaphylactic reaction. Some people are allergic in the same way to other foods and to bee stings. Most severely allergic people carry a dose of epinephrine to slow the reaction.

The immune system can also turn against its own healthy tissue. **Autoimmune diseases,** such as rheumatoid arthritis, lupus, and scleroderma, result from the proliferation of T cells that react as though they were fighting a virus, but are actually destroying healthy cells. An **autoimmune response** is the result of T cells that attack one's own healthy cells. Autoimmune responses often result from the body's need to fight an actual infection, during which the immune system becomes overactive.

Vocabulary Review

In the previous section, you learned terms relating to pathology. Before going on to the exercises, review the terms below and refer to the previous section if you have any questions.

Term	Word Analysis	Definition
acquired immuno-deficiency disease	[ĬM-yū-nō-dē-FĬSH-ĕn-sē]	AIDS.
AIDS		Most widespread immunosuppressive disease; caused by the HIV virus.
allergen	[ĂL-ĕr-jĕn] allerg(y) + -gen, producing	Substance to which exposure causes an allergic response.
allergy	[ĂL-ĕr-jē]	Production of IgE antibodies against an allergen.
anaphylaxis	[ĂN-ă-fĭ-LĂK-sĭs]	Life-threatening allergic reaction.
autoimmune disease	[ăw-tō-ĭ-MYŪN] auto-, self + immune	Any of a number of diseases, such as rheumatoid arthritis, lupus, and scleroderma, caused by an autoimmune response.
autoimmune response		Overactivity in the immune system against oneself causing destruction of one's own healthy cells.
histiocytic lymphoma	[HĬS-tē-ō-SĪT-ĭk]	Lymphoma with malignant cells that resemble histiocytes.
Hodgkin's lymphoma, Hodgkin's disease	After Thomas Hodgkin (1798–1866), British physician	Type of lymph cancer of uncertain origin that generally appears in early adulthood.

Term	Word Analysis	Definition
human immuno-deficiency virus (HIV)	[ĬM-yū-nō-dē-FĬSH-ĕn-sē]	Virus that causes AIDS; spread by sexual contact and exchange of body fluids.
hypersensitivity	[HĪ-pĕr-sĕn-si-TĬV-i-tē] hyper-, excessive + sensitivity	Abnormal reaction to an allergen.
hypersplenism	[hĭ-pĕr-SPLĒN-ĭzm]	Overactive spleen.
immunosuppressive disease	[ĬM-yū-nō-sŭ-PRĔS-ĭv]	Disease that flourishes because of lowered immune response.
infectious mononucleosis	[MŎN-ō-nū-klē-Ō-sĭs] mono-, one + nucle(us) + -osis, condition	Acute infectious disease caused by the Epstein-Barr virus.
lymphadenopathy	[lĭm-făd-ĕ-NŎP-ă-thē]	Swollen lymph nodes.
lymphocytic lymphoma	[lĭm-fō-SĬT-ĭk]	Lymphoma with malignant cells that resemble large lymphocytes.
lymphoma	[lĭm-FŌ-mă] lymph-, lymph + -oma, tumor	Cancer of the lymph nodes.
metastasis	[mĕ-TĂS-tă-sĭs] Greek, a removing	Spread of a cancer from a localized area.
non-Hodgkin's lymphoma		Cancer of the lymph nodes with some cells resembling healthy cells and spreading in a diffuse pattern.
opportunistic infection	[ŏp-pōr-tū-NĬS-tĭk]	Infection that takes hold because of lowered immune response.
retrovirus	[rĕ-trō-VĪ-rŭs]	Type of virus that spreads by using DNA in the body to help it replicate its RNA.
sarcoidosis	[săr-kŏy-DŌ-sĭs] sarcoid, former word for sarcoma + -osis	Inflammatory condition with lesions on the lymph nodes and other organs.
splenomegaly	[splēn-ō-MĔG-ă-lē] spleno-, spleen + -megaly, enlargement	Enlarged spleen.
thymoma	[thĭ-MŌ-mă] thym(us) + -oma, tumor	Tumor of the thymus gland.

C A S E S T U D Y

Helping to Manage a Disease

University Hospital has an extensive oncology department involved in research. Jane Bryant is a 32-year-old woman with AIDS. Recently, Kaposi's sarcoma has appeared on her arms and back. She was referred to the oncology department for chemotherapy. In addition, her doctors prescribed a new medication that increases T-cell count and the effectiveness of the immune response.

Critical Thinking

43. What might be the advantage for a chronically ill person to be treated in a research hospital?

44. Jane has AIDs, an immunosuppressive disease. Why is she being referred to the oncology department?

Pathological Terms Exercises

Spell It Correctly

Put a C after each word that is spelled correctly; if a word is incorrectly spelled, write it correctly.

45. retorvirus_____

46. immunosuppressive_____

47. imunodeficiency_____

48. sarcodosis_____

49. lumphoma_____

50. mononucleosis_____

51. anphylaxis_____

52. histocytic_____

53. metastasis_____

54. thimoma_____

Check Your Knowledge

For each of the following statements, write either **lymph** or **immune** in the blank to complete the sentence.

55. Allergies involve a(n) _____ response.

56. Splenomegaly is a symptom of _____ system disease.

57. Multiple sclerosis is a disease in which the _____ system attacks some of the body's cells.

58. Sarcoidosis is an inflammatory condition of the _____ system.

59. AIDS is a disease of the _____ system.

Surgical Terms

Cancers of the lymph system may require a **lymph-node dissection,** removal of cancerous lymph nodes for microscopic examination. A **lymphadenectomy** is the removal of a lymph node, and a **lymphadenotomy** is an incision into a lymph node. A **splenectomy** is removal of the spleen, which is usually required if it is ruptured. Other organs of the body, such as the liver, will take over the functions of the spleen if it is removed. A **thymectomy** is removal of the thymus gland, which is very important to the maturation process but not as serious once a patient reaches adulthood.

M O R E   A B O U T...
Lymph Node Surgery

A person with a malignant neoplasm in the breast must have further tests to determine if the cancer has metastasized. The usual biopsy included removal of many lymph nodes until one without cancer was found. Research trials on a procedure called *sentinel node biopsy* is showing encouraging results. A contrast medium is injected into the area around the tumor. The first node it reaches is the sentinel node. It is checked for malignancy. If that node is clean, then no further biopsy is done on the other lymph nodes, and the patient is spared painful surgical side effects.

Vocabulary Review

In the previous section, you learned terms relating to surgery. Before going on to the exercises, review the terms below and refer to the previous section if you have any questions.

Term	Word Analysis	Definition
lymphadenectomy	[lĭm-făd-ĕ-NĔK-tō-mē] lymphaden-, lymph node + -ectomy, removal	Removal of a lymph node.
lymphadenotomy	[lĭm-făd-ĕ-NŎ-Tō-mē] lymphadeno-, lymph node + -tomy, a cutting	Incision into a lymph node.
lymph node dissection		Removal of a cancerous node for microscopic examination.
splenectomy	[splē-NĔK-tō-mē] splen-, spleen + -ectomy	Removal of the spleen.
thymectomy	[thī-MĔK-tō-mē] thym(us) + -ectomy	Removal of the thymus gland.

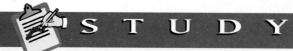

C A S E   S T U D Y

Getting an Examination

John Latella, a patient with AIDS, came to the hospital's clinic for his monthly T-cell test and to review the medications he is taking. He seems to be feeling more energetic, so John believes his T-cell test will show improvement. During the examination, however, the doctor notices an enlargement in John's lymph nodes. He sends John to the outpatient surgical unit for a biopsy.

Critical Thinking

60. If the node is malignant, what kind of surgery will most likely be performed?

61. A malignancy may have to be treated with radiation and/or chemotherapy, both of which destroy some healthy cells at the same time that they destroy malignant cells. Why would such treatment be especially risky for an AIDS patient?

Surgical Terms Exercises

Build Your Medical Vocabulary

Write and define the lymph and immune system combining forms in the following words.

62. splenectomy_____

63. lymphadenotomy_____

64. thymectomy_____

65. lymphadenectomy_____

Pharmacological Terms

Diseases of the lymph and immune systems are often treated with relatively high doses of chemotherapy and/or radiation. Advances in AIDS research have made it possible to manage this disease (i.e., to prolong patient's life) once thought fatal. A "cocktail" of *anti-HIV drugs*, a potential AIDS vaccine, and other newer drug compounds are bringing hope for long-term vitality to people with AIDS. Other drug compounds have been developed to fight opportunistic infections. Table 13-2 lists some of the important immune system medications.

Table 13-2 Medications Used to Treat Disorders of the Lymphatic and Immune System

Drug Class	Purpose	Generic	Trade Name
antiviral used in AIDS	to block virus growth	zidovudine (ZDV)	Retrovir, AZT
antimicrorganism agent used in AIDS	to prevent PCP	pentamidine	Pentam 300, Pneumopent
antihistamines	to prevent or lessen allergic reactions	loratidine diphenhydramine terfenadine	Claritin Allerdryl, Benadryl, Diahist Seldane

C A S E S T U D Y

Getting Good News

John Latella's biopsy reveals that the node is not malignant. The swelling is thought to be an infection. Further blood tests show that it is. John already takes a number of prophylactic medications aimed at preventing infection. For this infection, he is put on a course of antibiotics.

Critical Thinking

66. Why does John find it difficult to fight infections?

67. What results are the antibiotics supposed to provide?

Pharmacological Terms Exercises

Check Your Knowledge

Fill in the blanks.

68. AIDS patients often have to take many medications, including some to avoid _____ infections.

69. Lymphomas are generally treatable with _____ and _____.

70. An AIDS drug that blocks virus growth is _____.

71. One body substance manufactured and given in high doses in immune disorders is _____.

The clinic at University Hospital is treating a young woman with AIDS. She is monitored monthly at the clinic. Her latest blood test is shown here.

Laboratory Report			
University Hospital			
3 Center Drive			
Westford, NH 11114			
900-546-8000			

Patient: Amy Carr   Patient ID: 099-00-1200   Date of Birth: 12/04/81
Date Collected: 04/30/XXXX   Time Collected: 16:05   Total Volume: 2000
Date Received: 04/30/XXXX   Date Reported: 5/06/XXXX

Test	Result	Flag	Reference
Complete Blood Count			
WBC	13.2	*	3.9-11.1
RBC	4.11		3.80-5.20
HCT	39.7		34.0-47.0
MCV	96.5		80.0-98.0
MCH	32.9		27.1-34.0
MCHC	34.0		32.0-36.0
MPV	8.6		7.5-11.5
NEUTROPHILS %	45.6		38.0-80.0
NEUTROPHILS ABS.	1.82		1.70-8.50
LYMPHOCYTES %	36.1		15.0-49.0
LYMPHOCYTES ABS.	1.44		1.00-3.50
EOSINOPHILS %	4.5		0.0-8.0
EOSINOPHILS ABS.	0.18		0.03-0.55
BASOPHILS %	0.7		0.0-2.0
BASOPHILS ABS.	0.03		0.000-0.185
PLATELET COUNT	229		150-400
Automated Chemistries			
GLUCOSE	80		65-109
UREA NITROGEN	17		6-30
CREATININE (SERUM)	0.6		0.5-1.3
UREA NITROGEN/CREATININE	28		10-29
SODIUM	140		135-145
POTASSIUM	4.4		3.5-5.3
CHLORIDE	106		96-109
CO_2	28		20-31
ANION GAP	6		3-19
CALCIUM	9.8		8.6-10.4
PHOSPHORUS	3.6		2.2-4.6
AST (SGOT)	28		0-30
ALT (SGPT)	19		0-34
BILIRUBIN, TOTAL	0.5		0.2-1.2
PROTEIN, TOTAL	7.8		6.2-8.2
ALBUMIN	4.3		3.5-5.0
GLOBULIN	3.5		2.1-3.8
URIC ACID	2.4		2.0-7.5
CHOLESTEROL	172		120-199
TRIGLYCERIDES	68		40-199
IRON	85		30-150
HDL CHOLESTEROL	54		35-59
CHOLESTEROL/HDL RATIO	3.2		3.2-5.7
LDL, CALCULATED	80		70-129
T3, UPTAKE	32		24-37
T4, TOTAL	6.9		4.5-12.8

72. Is this lab test a test for AIDS?

73. Which lab test results are indicative of opportunistic infections?

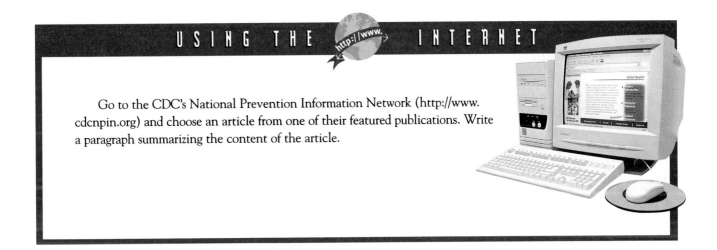

USING THE INTERNET

Go to the CDC's National Prevention Information Network (http://www.cdcnpin.org) and choose an article from one of their featured publications. Write a paragraph summarizing the content of the article.

CHAPTER REVIEW

Definitions

Write the definitions in the space provided.

Word	Definition
acquired active immunity	
acquired passive immunity	
acquired immunodeficiency [ĬM-yū-nō-dē-FĬSH-ĕn-sē] disease	
aden(o)	
AIDS	
allergen [ĂL-ĕr-jĕn]	
allergy [ĂL-ĕr-jē]	
anaphylaxis [ĂN-ă-fĭ-LĂK-sĭs]	
antibody [ĂN-tē-bŏd-ē]	
antigen [ĂN-tĭ-jĕn]	
antitoxin [ăn-tē-TŎK-sĭn]	
autoimmune [ăw-tŏ-ĭ-MYŪN] disease	
autoimmune response	
cell-mediated immunity	
cytotoxic [sī-tō-TŎK-sĭk] cell	
enzyme-linked immunosorbent assay (EIA, ELISA)	
gamma globulin [GĂ-mă GLŎB-yū-lĭn]	
helper cell	
histiocytic [HĬS-tē-ō-SĬT-ĭk] lymphoma	
Hodgkin's lymphoma, Hodgkin's disease	
human immunodeficiency [ĬM-yū-nō-dē-FĬSH-ĕn-sē] virus (HIV)	
humoral [HYŪ-mōr-ăl] immunity	
hypersensitivity [HĪ-pĕr-sĕn-sĭ-TĬV-ĭ-tē]	
hypersplenism [hī-pĕr-SPLĒN-ĭzm]	
immun(o)	

Word	Definition
immunity [ĭ-MYŪ-nĭ-tē]	
immunoglobulin [ĬM-yū-nō-GLŎB-yū-lĭn]	
immunosuppressive [ĬM-yū-nō-sŭ-PRĔS-ĭv] disease	
infectious mononucleosis [MŎN-ō-nū-klē-Ō-sĭs]	
interferon [ĭn-tĕr-FĒR-ŏn]	
interleukin [ĭn-tĕr-LŪ-kĭn]	
lymph [lĭmf]	
lymph(o)	
lymphaden(o)	
lymphadenectomy [lĭm-fă-dō-NĔK-tō-mē]	
lymphadenopathy [lĭm-făd-ĕ-NŎP-ă-thē]	
lymphadenotomy [lĭm-fă-dō-NŎ-tō-mē]	
lymphangi(o)	
lymph node	
lymph node dissection	
lymphocytes [LĬM-fō-sīts]	
lymphocytic [lĭm-fō-SĬT-ĭk] lymphoma	
lymphoma [lĭm-FŌ-mă]	
macrophage [MĂK-rō-fāj]	
metastasis [mĕ-TĂS-tă-sĭs]	
natural immunity	
non-Hodgkin's lymphoma	
opportunistic [ŏp-pōr-tū-NĬS-tĭk] infection	
pathogen [PĂTH-ō-jĕn]	
phagocytosis [FĂG-ō-sī-TŌ-sĭs]	
plasma [PLĂZ-mă] cell	
retrovirus [rĕ-trō-VĪ-rŭs]	
sarcoidosis [săr-kŏy-DŌ-sĭs]	
spleen [splēn]	
splen(o)	
splenectomy [splē-NĔK-tō-mē]	

Word	Definition
splenomegaly [splēn-ō-MĔG-ă-lē]	
suppressor [sŭ-PRĔS-ōr] cell	
T cells	
thym(o)	
thymectomy [thī-MĔK-tō-mē]	
thymocyte [THĪ-mō-sīt]	
thymoma [thī-MŌ-mă]	
thymosin [THĪ-mō-sĭn]	
thymus [THĪ-mŭs] gland	
T lymphocytes	
tox(o) , toxi, toxico	
vaccination [VĂK-sĭ-NĀ-shŭn], vaccine [VĂK-sēn]	
Western blot	

Abbreviation	Meaning
AIDS	
ALL	
AML	
AZT	
CLL	
CML	
CMV	
EBV	
EIA, ELISA	
HIV	
HSV	
IgA	
IgD	
IgE	
IgG	
IgM	
PCP	
SLE	
ZDV	

1. to lessen the progress of or to prevent disease
2. acquired active immunity
3. f
4. i
5. j
6. d
7. c
8. a
9. b
10. g
11. h
12. e
13. natural
14. acquired active
15. acquired passive
16. macrophages
17. white
18. T cells
19. interferon, interleukin
20. interstitial fluid
21. No, since she has already been vaccinated, tetanus should not develop.
22. acquired active immunity
23. lymphaden
24. spleno
25. thymo
26. immuno
27. adeno
28. toxi
29. lymphangi
30. lymph
31. f
32. e
33. b
34. g
35. c
36. d
37. a
38. to see if his breathing problems are caused by something other than allergies
39. no, just the blocked breathing caused by allergies
40. T
41. T
42. T
43. the patient might be eligible to be part of a new drug testing program
44. Jane has a type of cancer— Kaposi's sarcoma
45. retrovirus
46. C
47. immunodeficiency
48. sarcoidosis
49. lymphoma
50. C
51. anaphylaxis
52. histiocytic
53. C
54. thymoma
55. immune
56. lymph
57. immune
58. lymph
59. immune
60. lymphadenectomy
61. AIDS patients already have compromised immune systems. Any destruction of healthy cells can be devastating to their immune system and may allow other infections to take hold.
62. splen-, spleen
63. lymphadeno-, lymph node
64. thym-, thymus gland
65. lymphaden-, lymph node
66. AIDS has resulted in a compromised immune system that does not provide sufficient immune response.
67. They should resolve the lymph node infection.
68. opportunistic
69. radiation, chemotherapy
70. ZDV
71. interferon
72. No. It is a blood profile.
73. WBC

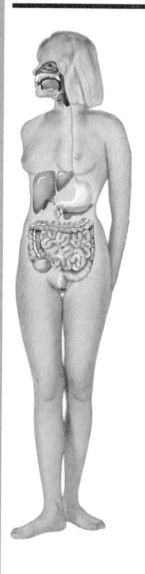

CHAPTER 14

The Digestive System

After studying this chapter, you will be able to:

- ◆ Name the parts of the digestive system and discuss the function of each part
- ◆ Define combining forms used in building words that relate to the digestive system
- ◆ Identify the meaning of related abbreviations
- ◆ Name the common diagnoses, clinical procedures, and laboratory tests used in treating the digestive system
- ◆ List and define the major pathological conditions of the digestive system
- ◆ Explain the meaning of surgical terms related to the digestive system
- ◆ Recognize common pharmacological agents used in treating disorders of the digestive system

Structure and Function

Digestion is the process of breaking down foods into nutrients that can be absorbed by cells. The digestive system consists of the **alimentary canal** (*digestive tract* or *gastrointestinal tract*) and several accessory organs. Food enters the alimentary canal through the **mouth,** passes through the **pharynx** and **esophagus** into the **stomach,** then into the **small intestine** and **large intestine** or **bowels,** and then into the **anal canal.** Figure 14-1a shows the digestive system, and Figure 14-1b diagrams the digestive process.

The alimentary canal is a tube that extends from the mouth to the **anus.** The wall of the alimentary canal has four layers that aid in the digestion of the food that passes through it. The outer covering is a serous layer of tissue that protects the canal and lubricates the outer surface so that organs within the abdominal cavity can slide freely near the canal and will not get lodged next to it. The next layer is the muscular layer, which contracts and expands in wavelike motions called **peristalsis,** to move food along the canal. The third layer is made of loose connective tissue that holds various vessels, glands, and nerves that both nourish and carry away waste from surrounding tissue. The innermost layer is a mucous membrane that secretes mucus and digestive enzymes while protecting the tissues within the canal. Digestive **enzymes** convert complex proteins into **amino acids,** compounds that can be absorbed by the body. Complex sugars are reduced to **glucose** and other simpler sugars,

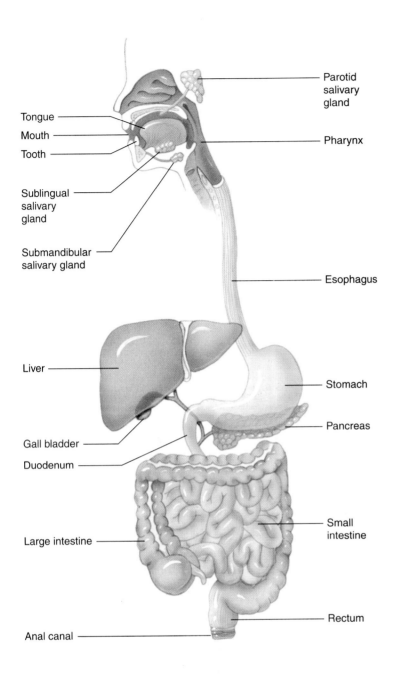

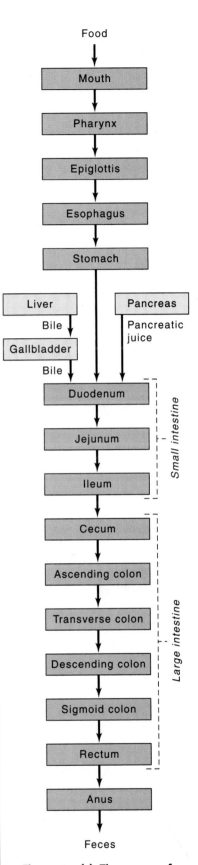

and fat molecules are reduced to **fatty acids** and other substances through the action of the digestive enzymes.

Mouth

The **lips** sense the food that is about to enter the mouth (Figure 14-2). They sense the temperature and texture of the food and serve to protect the mouth from receiving food that is too hot or too rough on the surface. Food is then taken into the oral cavity (mouth). Once inside, food is chewed with the help of the muscles of the **cheeks** (the walls of the oral cavity), and the **tongue** (which moves food during **mastication,** chewing), and **deglutition** (swallowing). The tongue has **papillae,** small raised areas that contain the taste buds (cell that provide the sensation of taste). The tongue is connected to the floor of the mouth by a mucous membrane called a **frenulum.** At the back of

Figure 14-1 **(a). The process of digestion begins in the mouth. (b). A diagram of the pathway of food through the body.**

the tongue, **lingual tonsils** form two mounds of rounded tissue that play an important role in the immune system (see Chapter 13).

The roof of the mouth is formed by the **hard palate,** the hard anterior part of the palate with irregular ridges of mucous membranes called **rugae,** and the **soft palate,** the soft posterior part of the palate. At the back of the soft palate is a downward cone-shaped projection called the **uvula.** On either side of the back of the mouth are rounded masses of lymphatic tissue called the **palatine tonsils.** The role of both kinds of tonsils in the lymphatic and immune systems is explained in Chapter 13. The mouth also contains the **gums,** the fleshy sockets that hold the *teeth.* Chapter 20 discusses the teeth.

Digestion of food begins in the mouth with mastication. In addition, the three sets of **salivary glands** surrounding the oral cavity secrete **saliva,** a fluid containing enzymes (such as **amylase,** an enzyme that begins the digestion of carbohydrates) that aid in breaking down food. Each gland has ducts through which the saliva travels to the mouth. The three pairs of salivary glands are the *parotid glands,* located inferior to the cheekbone; the *submandibular glands,* located below the mandible; and the *sublingual glands,* located in the base of the mouth below the tongue.

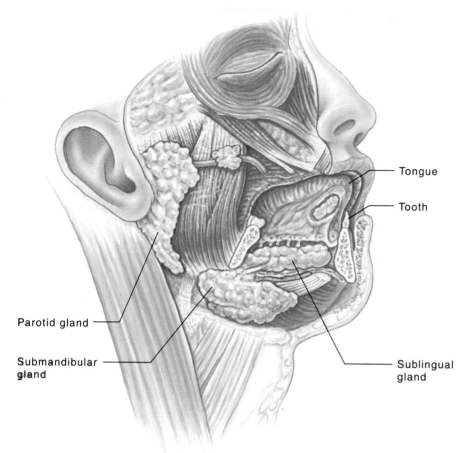

Tongue

Tooth

Sublingual gland

Parotid gland

Submandibular gland

Figure 14-2 The salivary glands release fluids that start the digestive process.

Pharynx

From the mouth, food goes through the pharynx (**throat**). Both food and air share this passageway. The pharynx is a muscular tube (about 5 inches long in adults) that moves food into the *esophagus.* Air moves through the trachea (windpipe). When we eat and swallow food, a flap of tissue (the **epiglottis**) covers the trachea until the food is moved into the esophagus. The epiglottis prevents food from entering the larynx (the voice box). Food that happens to get into the larynx when we are eating causes choking.

Esophagus

The esophagus is a muscular tube (9 to10 inches long in the average

---

M O R E   A B O U T...

Choking

People have died of choking, even when efforts were made to save them. If an object such as a chicken bone became lodged in the windpipe, it was difficult to remove it while still allowing the person to breathe. A doctor, Harry J. Heimlich, discovered that a simple series of movements can prevent choking to death in most cases. The movements involve placing arms around the abdomen just below the diaphragm, grasping fists, and thrusting upward to dislodge the item. Testimony from around the world affirms that this maneuver is put to good use every day.

adult) that contracts rhythmically (peristalsis) to push food toward the stomach. At the bottom of the esophagus, just above the stomach, is a group of thickened muscles in the esophageal wall called the *lower esophageal sphincter* (*cardiac sphincter*). This group of muscles contracts and closes the entrance to the stomach when food is present to prevent **reflux** (backflow), **emesis,** or **regurgitation** (*vomiting*). Every time more food comes through the esophagus to the stomach, the muscles relax and allow the food to pass.

Stomach

The stomach is a pouchlike organ in the left hypochondriac region of the abdominal cavity. The stomach receives food from the esophagus and mixes it with *gastric juice*. The enzyme **pepsin** in the gastric juice begins protein digestion. Table 14-1 shows the major components of gastric juice. Gastric juice is produced by the *gastric glands*, which are stimulated to produce this substance continuously but in varying amounts depending on the amount of food being absorbed.

Many people find relief from excess gastric juice by taking antacids.

Table 14-1 Major Components of Gastric Juice

Component	Function
pepsin	digests almost all types of protein
hydrochloric acid	provides acidic environment for action of pepsin
mucus	provides alkaline protective layer on the inside of the stomach wall

Figure 14-3 **The stomach has four regions and rugae in its lining.**

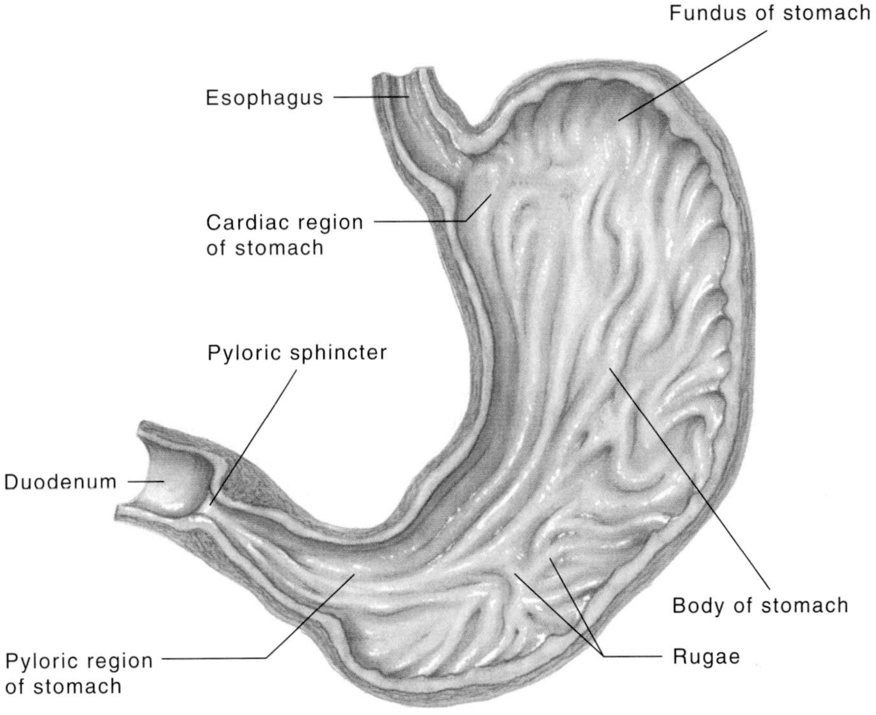

The stomach has four regions (Figure 14-3). The *cardiac region*, the region closest to the heart, is where the cardiac sphincter allows food to enter the stomach and prevents regurgitation. The **fundus** is the upper, rounded portion of the stomach. The **body** is the middle portion. The **pylorus,** the narrowed bottom part of the stomach, has a powerful, circular muscle at its base, the *pyloric sphincter*. This sphincter controls the emptying of the stomach's contents into the small intestine. The lining of the stomach is relatively thick with many folds of mucous tissue called *rugae*. As the stomach fills up, the wall distends and the folds disappear.

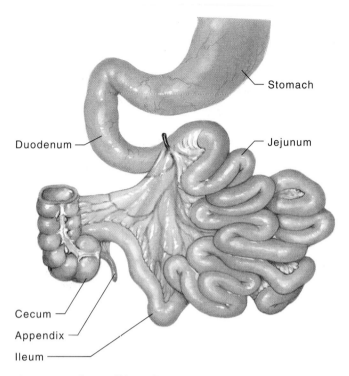

Stomach

Duodenum

Jejunum

Cecum

Appendix

Ileum

Figure 14-4 The small intestine connects the stomach to the large intestine.

After a meal, the muscular movements of the stomach and the mixing of food with gastric juice forms a semifluid mass called **chyme.** Chyme may consist of food that has been in the stomach for several hours, or it may contain food that is broken down in as little as one hour. The type of food and the amounts eaten determine how long it takes for the stomach to release the chyme. The muscles of the stomach release the chyme in small batches at regular intervals into the small intestine, where further digestion takes place.

Small Intestine

The small intestine receives chyme from the stomach, bile from the liver, and pancreatic juice from the pancreas (Figure 14-4). The small intestine has three parts—the **duodenum,** the **jejunum,** and the **ileum.** Together, these sections are about 20 feet long from the stomach to the large intestine. The small intestine lies within the abdominopelvic cavity, where it is held in place by the **mesentery,** a membranous tissue that attaches both the small and large intestines to the muscle wall at the dorsal part of the abdomen. **Absorption** (passage of material through the walls to the bloodstream) begins in the small intestines.

In the duodenum (only about 10 inches long), chyme mixes with bile to aid in fat digestion; with pancreatic juice to aid in digestion of starch, proteins, and fat; and with *intestinal juice* to aid in digesting sugars (*glucose*). Glands in the walls of the small intestine excrete intestinal juice. The juices also help change starch (**glycogen**) into glucose. The entire small intestine is lubricated by secretions from mucous glands. The small intestine is lined with **villi,** tiny, one-cell-thick fingerlike projections with capillaries through which digested nutrients are absorbed into the bloodstream and lymphatic system.

The digestive process continues through the jejunum, an eight-foot section of the small intestine. The next section of the small intestine, the ileum, connects the small intestine to the large intestine. Chyme takes from one to six hours to travel through the small intestine before it enters the large intestine. The length of time for digestion varies depending on the food being digested and the health of the digestive system.

Large Intestine

The large intestine, which is about five feet long, has four parts—the cecum, the colon, the sigmoid colon, and the rectum (Figure 14-5). The ileum is attached to the large intestine at the **cecum,** a pouch. Located at the bottom of the ileum is the ileocecal sphincter muscle that relaxes to allow undigested and unabsorbed food material into the large intestine in fairly regular waves. Other muscular contractions segment the ileum and prevent waste material from the cecum from backing up into the small intestine. The entire large intestine forms a rectangle around the tightly packed small intestine. Undigestible waste products from digestion usually remain in the large intestine from 12 to 24 hours.

The cecum has three openings: one from the ileum into the cecum; one from the cecum into the colon; and another from the cecum into a worm-like pouch on the side, the **appendix** (also called the *vermiform appendix*). The appendix is filled with lymphatic tissue, but is considered an **appendage,** an accessory part of the body that has no central function, because it has no role in the digestive process. The appendix can, however, become inflamed and may require surgical removal. Within the cecum, the process of turning waste material into semisolid waste (**feces**) begins as water and certain necessary substances are absorbed back into the bloodstream. As the water is removed, a semisolid mass is formed and moved into the colon.

The **colon** is further divided into three parts—the *ascending colon,* the *transverse colon,* and the *descending colon.* The ascending colon extends upward from the cecum to a place under the liver where it makes a right-angle bend known as the *hepatic flexure.* After the bend, the transverse colon continues across the abdomen from right to left where it makes a right-angle bend (the *splenic flexure*) toward the spleen. After the bend, the descending colon extends down to the rim of the pelvis where it connects to the sigmoid colon.

The **sigmoid colon** is an s-shaped body that goes across the pelvis to the middle of the sacrum, where it connects to the rectum. The **rectum** attaches to the *anal canal.* Feces (**stool**) then pass from the anal canal into the anus. The anus and anal canal open during the release of feces from the body (**defecation**). At other times, they are compressed by sphincter muscles.

Liver

The **liver** is an important digestive organ located in the right, upper quadrant of the abdominal cavity. Although it is not within the digestive tract, it performs many digestive functions. The liver is a relatively large organ weighing about 3 pounds in the average adult. It is divided into two lobes, the *right lobe* and the *left lobe* (Figure 14-6). The *hepatic portal system* is the group of blood vessels that transports blood and other substances to and from the liver. The liver changes food nutrients into usable substances. It secretes **bile** (yellowish-brown to greenish fluid), which is stored in the gallbladder for use in breaking down fats and other digestive functions. It stores glucose and

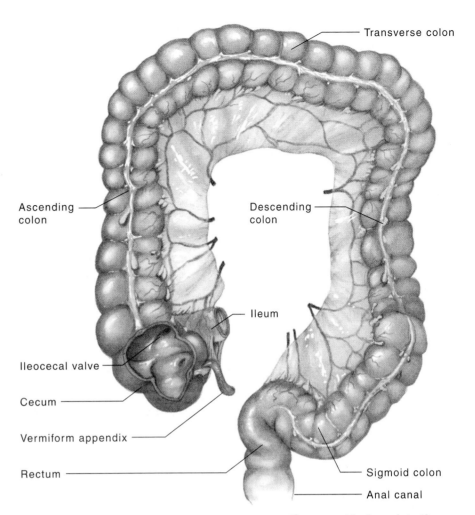

Figure 14-5 The large intestine leads from the small intestine to the anal canal.

A high-fiber diet helps to move waste through the large intestine.

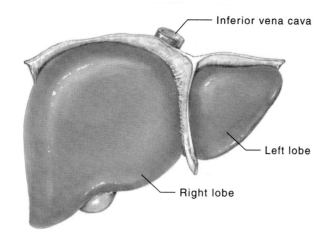

Figure 14-6 **The liver secretes bile, a fluid that is important in digestion of fats.**

certain vitamins for release when the body needs them. The liver also secretes **bilirubin,** a bile pigment, that is combined with bile and excreted into the duodenum.

Gallbladder

The bile released from the liver to the *hepatic duct* is then released into the *cystic duct*, which brings the substance into the **gallbladder.** The gallbladder stores bile until it is needed for digestion. Then it is forced out of the cystic duct into the *common bile duct*. At the entrance to the duodenum, bile mixes with pancreatic juices and enters the duodenum from the common bile duct. There the bile aids in **emulsification,** the breaking down of fats.

Pancreas

The chyme that empties into the small intestine mixes with secretions from the pancreas and liver. The **pancreas** is five to six inches long and lies across the posterior side of the stomach. The pancreas is a digestive organ in that it secretes digestive fluids into the small intestine through its system of ducts. The digestive fluid is called *pancreatic juice*, which includes various enzymes such as *amylase* and **lipase.** The pancreas is also an endocrine gland that regulates blood sugar through the release of insulin (a hormone) and, as such, is discussed in Chapter 15.

Vocabulary Review

In the previous section, you learned terms relating to the digestive system. Before going on to the exercises, review the terms below and refer to the previous section if you have any questions.

Term	Word Analysis	Meaning
absorption	[ăb-SŎRP-shŭn] Latin *absorptio*, a swallowing	Passing of nutrients into the bloodstream.
alimentary canal	[ăl-ĭ-MĔN-tĕr-ē]	Muscular tube from the mouth to the anus; digestive tract; gastrointestinal tract.
amino acid	[ă-MĒ-nō]	Chemical compound that results from digestion of complex proteins.
amylase	[ĂM-ĭl-ās]	Enzyme that is part of pancreatic juice and saliva and that begins the digestion of carbohydrates.
anal canal	[Ā-năl]	Part of the digestive tract extending from the rectum to the anus.
anus	[Ā-nŭs]	Place at which feces exit the body.

Term	Word Analysis	Meaning
appendage	[ă-PĔN-dĭj]	Any body part (inside or outside) either subordinate to a larger part or having no specific central function.
appendix	[ă-PĔN-dĭks] Latin, appendage	Wormlike appendage to the cecum.
bile	[bīl] Latin *bilis*	Yellowish-brown to greenish fluid secreted by the liver and stored in the gallbladder; aids in fat digestion.
bilirubin	[bĭl-ĭ-RŪ-bĭn] bili-, bile + Latin *ruber*, red	Pigment contained in bile.
body		Middle section of the stomach.
bowel	[bŏwl] Latin *botulus*, sausage	Intestine.
cecum	[SĒ-kŭm] Latin, blind	Pouch at the top of the large intestine connected to the bottom of the ileum.
cheeks		Walls of the oral cavity.
chyme	[kīm] Greek *chymos*, juice	Semisolid mass of partially digested food and gastric juices that passes from the stomach to the small intestine.
colon	[KŌ-lŏn] Greek *kolon*	Major portion of the large intestine.
defecation	[dĕ-fĕ-KĀ-shŭn] Laitn *defaeco*, to remove the dregs	Release of feces from the anus.
deglutition	[dē-glū-TĬSH-ŭn] Latin *deglutio*, to swallow	Swallowing.
digestion	[dī-JĔS-chŭn] Latin *digestio*	Conversion of food into nutrients for the body and into waste products for release from the body.
duodenum	[dū-ō-DĒ-nŭm] Latin *duodeni*, twelve (about equal in size to the width of twelve fingers)	Top part of the small intestine where chyme mixes with bile, pancreatic juices, and intestinal juice to continue the digestive process.
emesis	[ĕ-MĒ-sĭs]	*See* regurgitation.

Term	Word Analysis	Meaning
emulsification	[ĕ-MŬL-sĭ-fĭ-KĀ-shŭn]	Breaking down of fats.
enzyme	[ĔN-zīm]	Protein that causes chemical changes in substances in the digestive tract.
epiglottis	[ĕ-pĭ-GLŎ-tĭs]	Movable flap of tissue that covers the trachea.
esophagus	[ĕ-SŎF-ă-gŭs]	Part of alimentary canal from the pharynx to the stomach.
fatty acid		Acid derived from fat during the digestive process.
feces	[FĒ-sēz] Latin *faeces*, dregs	Semisolid waste that moves through the large intestine to the anus, where it is released from the body.
frenulum	[FRĔN-yū-lŭm] Latin, small bridle	Mucous membrane that attaches the tongue to the floor of the mouth.
fundus	[FŬN-dŭs] Latin, bottom	Upper portion of the stomach.
gallbladder	[GĂWL-blăd-ĕr]	Organ on lower surface of liver; stores bile.
glucose	[GLŪ-kōs]	Sugar found in fruits and plants and in various parts of the body.
glycogen	[GLĬ-kō-jĕn]	Starch that can be converted into glucose.
gums	[gŭmz]	Fleshy sockets that hold the teeth and aid in chewing.
hard palate	[PĂL-ăt]	Hard anterior portion of the palate at the roof of the mouth.
ileum	[ĬL-ē-ŭm]	Bottom part of the small intestine that connects to the large intestine.
jejunum	[jĕ-JŪ-nŭm] Latin *jejunus*, empty	Middle section of the small intestine.
large intestine		Passageway in intestinal tract for waste received from small intestine to be excreted through the anus; also, place where water reabsorption takes place.
lingual tonsils	[LĬNG-gwăl TŎN-sĭls]	Two mounds of lymph tissue at the back of the tongue.
lipase	[LĬP-ās]	Enzyme contained in pancreatic juice.

Term	Word Analysis	Meaning
lips	Old English *lippa*	Two muscular folds formed around the outside boundary of the mouth.
liver	[LĬV-ĕr] Old English *lifer*	Organ important in digestive and metabolic functions; secretes bile.
mastication	[măs-tĭ-KĀ-shŭn] Latin *mastico*, to chew	Chewing.
mesentery	[MĔS-ĕn-tĕr-ē] Greek *mesenterion*	Membranous tissue that attaches small and large intestines to the muscular wall at the dorsal part of the abdomen.
mouth	Old English *muth*	Cavity in the face in which food and water is ingested.
palatine tonsils	[PĂL-ă-tĭn]	Mounds of tissue on either side of the pharynx.
pancreas	[PĂN-krē-ăs] Greek *pankreas*, sweetbreads	Digestive organ that secretes digestive fluids; endocrine gland that regulates blood sugar.
papilla (pl. papillae)	[pă-PĬL-ă (-ē)] Latin, nipple	Tiny projection on the superior surface of the tongue that contains taste buds.
pepsin	[PĔP-sĭn] Greek *pepsis*, digestion	Digestive enzyme of gastric juice.
peristalsis	[pĕr-ĭ-STĂL-sĭs] peri-, around + Greek *stalsis*, constriction	Coordinated, rhythmic contractions of smooth muscle that force food through the digestive tract.
pharynx	[FĂR-ĭngks] Greek, throat	Tube through which food passes to the esophagus.
pylorus	[pī-LŌR-ŭs] Latin, gatekeeper	Narrowed bottom part of the stomach.
rectum	[RĔK-tŭm] Latin, straight	Bottom portion of large intestine; connected to anal canal.
reflux	[RĒ-flŭks] re-, back + Latin *fluxus*, a flow	*See* regurgitation.
regurgitation	[rē-GĔR-jĭ-TĀ-shŭn] re- + Latin *gurgito*, to flood	Backward flow from the normal direction.
rugae	[RŪ-gē] Latin, wrinkles	Folds in stomach lining.

Term	Word Analysis	Meaning
saliva	[să-LĪ-vă] Latin	Fluid secreted by salivary glands.
salivary glands	[SĂL-ĭ-văr-ē]	Glands in the mouth that secrete fluids that aid in breaking down food.
sigmoid colon	[SĬG-mŏyd]	S-shaped part of large intestine connecting at the bottom to the rectum.
small intestine		Twenty-foot long tube that continues the process of digestion started in the stomach; place where most absorption takes place.
soft palate	[PĂL-āt]	Soft posterior part of the palate in the mouth.
stomach	[STŬM-ŭk] Latin *stomachus*	Large sac between the esophagus and small intestine; place where food is broken down.
stool	[stūl] Old English *stol*, seat	Feces.
throat	Old English *throtu*, throat	Pharynx.
tongue	[tŭng] Old English *tunge*	Fleshy part of the mouth that moves food during mastication.
uvula	[YŪ-vyū-lă] Latin, small grape	Cone-shaped projection hanging down from soft palate.
villus (pl. villi)	[VĬL-ŭs (-ī)] Latin, shaggy animal hair	Tiny, fingerlike projection on the lining of the small intestine with capillaries through which digested nutrients are absorbed into the bloodstream and lymphatic system.

C A S E S T U D Y

Getting a Referral

Asmin Sahib reported burning chest pains to her general practitioner. Ms. Sahib feared that the pains indicated that she was having a heart attack. After a thorough examination, including an ECG, the physician found Ms. Sahib to have no cardiovascular pathology. The general practitioner referred Asmin to Mary Walker, M.D., a gastroenterologist (specialist in the digestive system).

 Critical Thinking

1. Why might Asmin feel she is having a heart attack?

2. What parts of the body will the gastroenterologist treat?

Structure and Function Exercises

Complete the Diagram

3. Label the digestive system parts in the following illustration.

a.

b.

c.

d.

e.

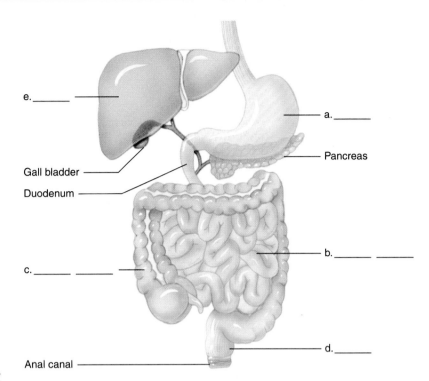

e._____

a._____

Pancreas

Gall bladder

Duodenum

c._____ _____ _____

b._____ _____

d._____

Anal canal

Check Your Knowledge

For each of the following words, write C in the space provided if the word is spelled correctly. If it is not, spell the word correctly.

4. papilae_____

5. frenelum_____

6. deglutition_____

7. chime_____

8. glycogen_____

9. villi_____

10. amylase_____

11. lypase_____

12. bilirubin_____

Fill in the blanks.

13. Food is moved along the alimentary canal by a process called _____.

14. The four regions of the stomach are _____, _____, _____, and _____.

15. The three parts of the small intestine are the _____, _____, and _____.

16. The four parts of the large intestine are the _____, _____, _____, and _____.

17. The longest intestine is the _____ intestine.

18. A group of blood vessels that transports blood and other substances to and from the liver is called the _____ _____ _____.

19. Two enzymes in pancreatic juice are _____ and _____.

20. Bile aids in the breaking down of fats, called _____.

Combining Forms and Abbreviations

The lists below include combining forms and abbreviations that relate specifically to the circulatory system. Pronunciations are provided for the examples.

Combining Form	Meaning	Example
an(o)	anus	*anoplasty* [ā-nō-PLĂS-tē], surgical repair of the anus
append(o), appendic(o)	appendix	*appendicitis* [ă-pĕn-dĭ-SĪ-tĭs], inflammation of the appendix
bil(o), bili	bile	*biliverdin* [bĭl-ĭ-VĔR-dĭn], green bile pigment
bucc(o)	cheek	*buccogingival* [bŭk-ō-JĬN-jĭ-văl], pertaining to the cheeks and gums
cec(o)	cecum	*cecopexy* [SĒ-kō-pĕk-sē], surgical repair or fixing of the cecum to correct excessive mobility
celi(o)	abdomen	*celioma* [SĒ-lē-ō-mă], tumor in the abdomen
chol(e), cholo	bile	*choleic* [kō-LĒ-ĭk], pertaining to bile
cholangi(o)	bile vessel	*cholangiogram* [kō-LĂN-jē-ō-grăm], x-ray image of the bile vessels
cholecyst(o)	gallbladder	*cholecystectomy* [kō-lē-sĭs-TĔK-tō-mē], removal of the gallbladder
choledoch(o)	common bile duct	*choledochotomy* [kō-lĕd-ō-KŎT-ō-mē], incision into the common bile duct
col(o), colon(o)	colon	*colectomy* [kō-LĔK-tō-mē], removal of all or part of the colon
duoden(o)	duodenum	*duodenitis* [dū-ŏd-ĕ-NĪ-tĭs], inflammation of the duodenum
enter(o)	intestines	*enteropathy* [ĕn-tĕr-ŎP-ă-thē], any intestinal disease

Combining Form	Meaning	Example
esophag(o)	esophagus	*esophagoscopy*, [ĕ-sŏf-ă-GŎS-kō-pē], examination of the interior of the esophagus
gastr(o)	stomach	*gastralgia* [găs-TRĂL-jē-ă], stomachache
gloss(o)	tongue	*glossopharyngeal* [GLŎS-ō-fă-RĬN-jē-ăl], of the tongue and pharynx
gluc(o)	glucose	*glucogenesis* [glū-kō-JĔN-ĕ-sĭs], formation of glucose
glyc(o)	sugar	*glycosuria* [glī-kō-SŪ-rē-ă], abnormal excretion of carbohydrates in urine
glycogen(o)	glycogen	*glycogenolysis* [GLĪ-kō-jĕ-NŎL-ĭ-sĭs], breakdown of glycogen to glucose
hepat(o)	liver	*hepatitis* [hĕp-ă-TĪ-tĭs], liver disease or inflammation
ile(o)	ileum	*ileitis* [ĭl-ē-Ī-tĭs], inflammation of the ileum
jejun(o)	jejunum	*jejunostomy* [jĕ-jū-NŎS-tō-mē], surgical opening to the outside of the body for the jejunum
labi(o)	lip	*labioplasty* [LĀ-bē-ō-plăs-tē], surgical repair of lips
lingu(o)	tongue	*linguodental* [lĭng-gwō-DĔN-tăl], pertaining to tongue and teeth
or(o)	mouth	*orofacial* [ōr-ō-FĀ-shăl], pertaining to mouth and face
pancreat(o)	pancreas	*pancreatitis* [păn-krē-ă-TĪ-tĭs], inflammation of the pancreas
periton(eo)	peritoneum	*peritonitis* [PĔR-ĭ-tō-NĪ-tĭs], inflammation of the peritoneum
pharyng(o)	pharynx	*pharyngotonsillitis* [fă-RĬN-jō-tŏn-sĭ-LĪ-tĭs], inflammation of tonsils and pharynx
proct(o)	anus, rectum	*proctologist* [prŏk-TŎL-ō-jĭst], specialist in study and treatment of diseases of the anus and rectum
pylor(o)	pylorus	*pylorospasm* [pĭ-LŎR-ō-spăzm], involuntary contraction of the pylorus
rect(o)	rectum	*rectoabdominal* [RĔK-tō-ăb-DŎM-ĭ-năl], of the rectum and abdomen
sial(o)	saliva, salivary gland	*sialism* [SĪ-ă-lĭzm], excessive secretion of saliva

Combining Form	Meaning	Example
sialaden(o)	salivary gland	*sialoadenitis* [SĪ-ă-lō-ă-dĕ-NĪ-tĭs], inflammation of the salivary glands
sigmoid(o)	sigmoid colon	*sigmoidoscopy* [SĬG-mŏy-DŎS-kō-pē], visual examination of the sigmoid colon
steat(o)	fats	*steatorrhea* [stē-ă-tō-RĒ-ă], greater than normal amounts of fat in the feces
stomat(o)	mouth	*stomatitis* [STŌ-mă-TĪ-tĭs], inflammation of the lining of the mouth

Abbreviation	Meaning	Abbreviation	Meaning
ALT, AT	alanine transaminase	IBD	inflammatory bowel disease
AST	aspartic acid transaminase	IBS	irritable bowel syndrome
BE	barium enema	NG	nasogastric
BM	bowel movement	NPO	nothing by mouth (Latin, *nul per os*)
EGD	esophagogastroduodenoscopy	SGOT	serum glutamic oxaloacetic transaminase
ERCP	endoscopic retrograde cholangiopancreatography	SGPT	serum glutamic pyruvic transaminase
GERD	gastroesophageal reflux disease	TPN	total parenteral nutrition
GI	gastrointestinal	UGI(S)	upper gastrointestinal (series)

C A S E S T U D Y

Seeing a Specialist

Dr. Walker reviewed Asmin Sahib's family history. It showed that two members of her immediate family had died from cancer of the digestive tract. Her father had stomach cancer, and her sister had liver cancer. Since Asmin has always known the risks associated with digestive cancers, she maintained a healthy diet and had regular checkups to detect any signs of the kind of cancers that has afflicted her family.

Critical Thinking

21. Why is family history important in evaluating a patient?

22. Before cancer was detected in her family members, they suffered from chronic stomach and liver inflammations. What are the medical names for these two conditions?

Combining Forms and Abbreviations Exercises

Build Your Medical Vocabulary

Use the following combining forms or roots along with suffixes you learned in Chapter 2 to give the missing term.

gastr(o) esophag(o) proct(o) chol(o) cholecyst(o) choledoch(o) hepat(o) pancreat(o) colon(o) duoden(o) rect(o)

23. Excision (removal of the stomach) *gastrectomy*

24. Inflammation of the esophagus _____

25. Prolapse of the rectum _____

26. Pertaining to the duodenum _____

27. Excision of a part of the common bile duct _____

28. Inflammation of the pancreas _____

29. Pain in the rectum_____

30. Visual examination of the colon _____

31. Enlargement of the liver _____

32. Suture of the stomach _____

33. Specialist in the study of diseases and treatment of the rectum and anus _____

34. Inflammation of the gallbladder _____

35. Liver tumor _____

Find the Combining Forms

For the following terms, write the gastrointestinal combining form(s) in the space provided and define each term.

36. pyloroduodenal: _____

37. perianal: _____

38. enterocolostomy: _____

39. ileocecal: _____

40. sublingual: _____

Diagnostic, Procedural, and Laboratory Terms

The digestive or gastrointestinal system is examined in many different ways to diagnose a number of problems. Gastroenterologists (specialists in the digestive system) perform procedures to examine the internal health of various organs. They order blood tests to look for signs of infection or disease and also use some of the extensive number of imaging procedures available for this body system.

A stool specimen may be tested to identify disease-causing organisms, such as parasites. This test is called a *stool culture*. A *stool culture and sensitivity test* is used to try out different medications on microorganisms to check for effectiveness. A chemical test of a stool specimen (*hemoccult test* or *stool guaiac*) indicates whether there is bleeding in the digestive tract. Guaiac is a substance added to the stool sample that reacts with any occult (not visible) blood.

Various types of endoscopes are used to examine the digestive system, either through the mouth, the anus, or an opening into the abdominal cavity. An **esophagoscopy** is the use of an *esophagoscope* to illuminate the esophagus as it is passed through the mouth and into the esophagus. A *gastroscope* is used to examine the stomach in **gastroscopy.** A **colonoscopy** is the use of an endoscope to examine the colon. A *proctoscope* is used to examine the rectum and anus in a **proctoscopy.** A *sigmoidoscope* is used to examine the sigmoid colon in **sigmoidoscopy.** *Endoscopic retrograde cholangiopancreatography (ERCP)* is a procedure used to examine the biliary ducts with x-ray, a contrast medium, and the use of an endoscope. **Peritoneoscopy** or *laparoscopy* is the examination of the abdominal cavity with an instrument called a *peritoneoscope* or a *laparoscope*.

X-rays and other imaging techniques are used extensively to search for abnormalities. They also show if a foreign object has been swallowed (Figure 14-7). An MRI shows the major organs of the digestive system. A CAT scan provides a visual image of the abdominal cavity and the digestive tract. To examine more specific areas, patients are usually given a contrast medium or other substance that stands out against the background of the x-ray produced. A *barium swallow* is the ingestion of a barium solution before an x-ray of the esophagus, which is generally used to locate foreign objects that have been swallowed (Figure 14-7). A *barium enema* is the administration of a barium solution through an enema before taking a series of x-rays of the colon called a *lower GI series*. An *upper GI series* provides x-rays of the esophagus, stomach, and duodenum, usually after the patient swallows a barium solution or other contrast medium. A *cholangiogram* is an image of the bile vessels taken in **cholangiography,** an x-ray of the bile ducts. A *cholecystogram* is an image of the gallbladder taken in **cholecystography,** an x-ray of the gallbladder taken after the patient swallows iodine. A *liver scan*, done after injection of radioactive material, can reveal abnormalities. Ultrasound is used to provide images of the entire abdominal area, as in *abdominal ultrasonography*.

Several serum tests indicate how the liver is functioning. A *serum glutamic oxaloacetic transaminase (SGOT)* or an *aspartate transaminase (AST)* measures the enzyme levels in serum that have leaked from damaged liver cells. Another serum test for liver function is the *serum glutamic pyruvic transaminase (SGPT)*. This test is also known as an *alanine transaminase (ALT, AT)*. A *serum bilirubin*

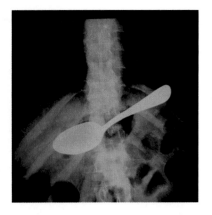

Figure 14-7 When children swallow foreign objects, they often need an x-ray.

measures bilirubin in the blood as an indicator of jaundice. An *alkaline phosphatase* reveals levels of the enzyme, alkaline phosphatase, in serum as an indicator of liver disease, especially liver cancer.

A *nasogastric (NG) tube* is passed through the nose to the stomach to relieve fluid buildup or to take stomach content samples for analysis (Figure 14-8). This process is called *nasogastric intubation*.

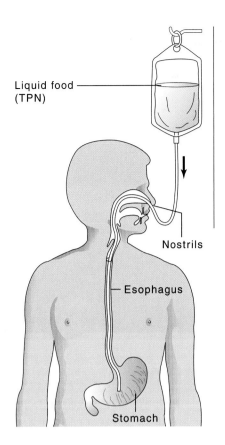

Liquid food (TPN)

Nostrils

Esophagus

Stomach

Figure 14-8 Liquid nourishment can be provided through a nasogastric (NG) tube. This type of tube may also be used to relieve fluid buildup in the stomach or to take stomach content samples.

Vocabulary Review

In the previous section, you learned terms relating to diagnosis, clinical procedures, and laboratory tests. Before going on to the exercises, review the terms below and refer to the previous section if you have any questions.

Term	Word Analysis	Meaning
cholangiography	[kō-lăn-jē-ŎG-ră-fē] cholangio-, bile vessel + -graphy, a recording	X-ray of the bile ducts.
cholecystography	[kō-lē-sĭs-TŎG-ră-fē] chole-, bile + cysto-, bladder + -graphy	X-ray of the gallbladder.
colonoscopy	[kō-lŏn-ŎS-kō-pē] colono-, colon + -scopy, a viewing	Examination of the colon using an endoscope.
esophagoscopy	[ĕ-sŏf-ă-GŎS-kō-pē] esophago-, esophagus + -scopy	Examination of the esophagus with an esophagoscope.
gastroscopy	[găs-TRŎS-kō-pē] gastro-, stomach + -scopy	Examination of the stomach using an endoscope.

Term	Word Analysis	Meaning
peritoneoscopy	[PĔR-ĭ-tō-nē-ŎS-kō-pē] peritoneo-, peritoneum + -scopy	Examination of the abdominal cavity using a peritoneoscope.
proctoscopy	[prŏk-TŎS-kō-pē] procto-, rectum + -scopy	Examination of the rectum and anus using a proctoscope.
sigmoidoscopy	[SĬG-mŏy-DŎS-kō-pē] sigmoido-, sigmoid colon + -scopy	Examination of the sigmoid colon using a sigmoidoscope.

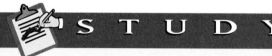

CASE STUDY

Treating the Symptoms

Dr. Walker finds Asmin to be a healthy 49-year-old except for the burning sensations in her chest. Dr. Walker has decided to have Asmin try a bland diet, sleeping with the head of the bed raised, and avoidance of spicy food, alcohol, and caffeine. He prescribes a mild antacid. Dr. Walker suggests a return visit in three weeks to see if the steps to avoid esophageal reflux are showing improvement.

After three weeks, Asmin has shown marked improvement. Dr. Walker tells her she can add some spicy foods slowly back into her diet, but to continue to avoid alcohol and caffeine. Asmin will need a checkup with Dr. Walker in six months.

Critical Thinking

41. What diagnostic test will Dr. Walker use to check Asmin's reflux condition in six months?

42. What other tests might Dr. Walker prescribe for someone with a family history of intestinal cancer?

Diagnostic, Procedural, and Laboratory Terms Exercises

Find a Match

Match the diagnostic test in the left-hand column with the definition or possible diagnosis resulting from the test in the right-hand column.

43. serum bilirubin

    a. x-ray of esophagus, stomach, and duodenum

44. alkaline phosphatase

    b. barium

45. upper GI series

    c. cholangiogram

46. image of bile vessels

    d. nasogastric tube

47. testing of waste for disease-causing organisms

    e. SGOT

48. tube to retrieve stomach contents for examination   f. stool guaiac

49. element in a solution used in x-rays   g. jaundice

50. test for liver function   h. liver cancer

51. x-rays of the intestines and anal canal   i. stool culture

52. hemoccult test   j. lower GI series

Pathological Terms

The digestive system is both the site and the source of many diseases and disorders. What we take into our mouths determines the type of nutrition our body receives. Eating disorders can be the catalyst for disease processes to start. **Anorexia** is a morbid refusal to eat because the person wishes to be dangerously thin. **Bulimia** is a disease wherein binging on food and then purposely purging or vomiting is also a quest for abnormal weight loss. Both anorexia and bulimia can produce many health problems and symptoms, such as hair loss, amenorrhea, and heart damage. **Obesity** is often the result of overeating, although recent gene studies indicate a possible hereditary defect in many obese people. Obesity can be one of the factors in many health problems, such as heart disease and diabetes. Many eating disorders can be treated with psychological counseling, but others, such as anorexia, often result in death, particularly of adolescents.

Areas in the mouth can become inflamed from an infection, an allergy, an injury, or an internal disorder. **Cheilitis** occurs on the lips; **glossitis** occurs on the tongue; **sialoadenitis** occurs in the salivary glands; and **parotitis** or **parotiditis** occurs in the parotid glands. Various other dental disorders may similarly cause inflammation (see Chapter 20). **Halitosis** is unusually foul mouth odor, which may be caused by poor dental hygiene, gum disease, certain foods, or by an internal disorder such as a sinus infection. **Ankyloglossia** is a condition in which the tongue is partially or completely attached to the floor of the mouth, thereby preventing normal movement. Normal swallowing is an important part of maintaining good nutrition. People with swallowing disorders usually have to have their diet supplemented via a tube. **Aphagia** is an inability to swallow; **dysphagia** is difficulty in swallowing.

Diseases of the pharynx are discussed in Chapter 7 as part of the respiratory system. Food travels into the mouth, through the pharynx, and into the esophagus. *Esophageal varices* are twisted veins in the esophagus that are prone to hemorrhage and ulcers. **Esophagitis** is any inflammation of the esophagus. *Gastroesophageal reflux disease* (GERD) or *esophageal reflux* involves malfunctioning of the sphincter muscle at the bottom of the esophagus. It opens at the wrong time to allow backflow of stomach contents into the esophagus, causing irritation of the esophageal lining. **Achalasia** is the failure of the same esophageal sphincter to relax during swallowing and allow food to pass easily from the esophagus into the stomach to continue the digestive process. This disorder interferes with the intake of normal amounts of nutrients.

The stomach is also the site of many disorders. Some people are sensitive to various foods (such as very spicy dishes) or have allergies to others (as milk products). **Achlorhydria** is the lack of hydrochloric acid in the stomach, a chemical necessary for digestion. **Dyspepsia** is difficulty in digesting food, particularly in the stomach. **Gastritis** is any stomach inflammation. **Gastroenteritis** is an inflammation of both the stomach and small intestine. **Flatulence** is an accumulation of gas in the stomach or intestines. **Eructation** (belching) may release some of this gas. **Nausea** is a sick feeling in the stomach caused by illness or the ingestion of spoiled food. Nausea may also be felt in certain situations such as early pregnancy or when repetitive motion causes discomfort as in car sickness, sea sickness, and so on. **Hematemesis** is the vomiting of blood from the stomach, usually a sign of a severe disorder. *Stomach ulcers* or *gastric ulcers* are a type of **peptic ulcer,** a sore on the mucous membrane of any part of the gastrointestinal system. A **hiatal hernia** is a protrusion of the stomach through an opening in the diaphragm called the hiatal opening. The pyloric sphincter can become abnormally narrow and cause the condition known as *pyloric stenosis*.

Ulcers can become so severe that they bleed. Bleeding ulcers are dangerous and require aggressive treatment.

Secretions of the liver, pancreas, and gallbladder mix with the stomach contents that move into the duodenum. The liver can be the site of **jaundice** or **icterus,** excessive bilirubin in the blood (**hyperbilirubinemia**) causing a yellow discoloration of the skin. Newborn jaundice may be a result of liver disease or many other factors. It is sometimes treated with exposure to artificial lights or sunlight. **Hepatomegaly** is an enlarged liver. **Hepatopathy** is a general term for liver disease, and **hepatitis** is a term for several types of contagious diseases, some of which are sexually transmitted (see Chapter 10). **Cirrhosis** is a chronic liver disease usually caused by poor nutrition and excessive alcohol consumption. **Pancreatitis** is an inflammation of the pancreas. (Other pancreatic diseases are discussed in Chapter 15.)

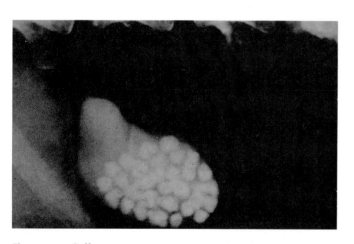

Figure 14-9 Gallstones can cause severe pain.

The gallbladder can be the site of calculi (**gallstones** or **cholelithiasis**) that block the bile from leaving the gallbladder (Figure 14-9). The presence of gallstones in the common bile duct is called *choledocholithiasis*. **Cholangitis** is any inflammation of the bile ducts. **Cholecystitis** is any inflammation of the gallbladder, either acute or chronic. The duodenum can be the site of **duodenal ulcers** or hernias. Duodenal ulcers are a type of peptic ulcer and are thought to be bacterial (H. pylori) in origin. This discovery has lead to the widespread use of antibiotics to treat many types of ulcers. On the side of the duodenum lies the appendix, which can become inflamed if gastric substances leak into it from the duodenum. This condition is called **appendicitis,** which usually requires surgery to prevent it from bursting.

The small and large intestines can have ulcers, obstructions, irritations, inflammations, abnormalities, and cancer. An **ileus** is an intestinal blockage, which may be caused by lack of sufficient moisture to move waste material through the system or by an internal disorder. **Enteritis** and **colitis** are general terms for inflammations in the small intestine. **Ulcerative colitis** is a chronic type of *irritable bowel disease* (IBD) or *inflammatory bowel disease* with recurring ulcers and inflammations. Other symptoms may include cramping, abdominal pain, and diarrhea. IBDs are often associated with stress. **Crohn's disease** is another type of IBD with symptoms similar to ulcerative colitis and sometimes with the production of **fistulas,** abnormal passages or openings in tissue walls.

Colic is a condition (usually in infants) of gastrointestinal distress due to allergies, an underdeveloped digestive tract, or other conditions that prevent easy digestion of food. In infants, colic usually resolves itself within a few months as the infant matures. **Diverticulosis** is a condition in which **diverticula**, small pouches in the intestinal wall, trap food or bacteria. **Diverticulitis** is an inflammation of the diverticula. **Ileitis** is an inflammation of the ileum. **Dysentery** is a general term for irritation of the intestinal tract with loose stools and other symptoms, such as abdominal pain and weakness. It is often caused by bacteria such as those found in many underdeveloped countries. **Polyposis** is a general term for a condition in which polyps develop in the intestinal tract. Polyps can become cancerous so they are often checked or removed to detect any abnormalities at an early stage. *Colonic polyposis* is polyps in the colon, which have a high likelihood of changing to *colorectal cancer*.

The intestines can become twisted or herniated. An *inguinal hernia* is a protrusion of the intestine through a weakness in the abdomen (Figure 14-10). A **volvulus,** an intestinal blockage caused by twisting of the intestine on itself, requires emergency surgery (Figure 14-11). An **intussusception** is the prolapse of an intestinal part into a neighboring part (Figure 14-12). The abdominal and peritoneal regions surrounding the intestinal tract can become filled with fluid (**ascites**) or inflamed (**peritonitis**).

The rectum, anus, and stool may play a role in some disorders. **Proctitis** is an inflammation of the rectum and anus. **Constipation** is a condition with infrequent or difficult release of bowel movements, sometimes the result of insufficient moisture to soften and move stools. **Diarrhea** is loose, watery stools that may be the result of insufficient roughage or of an internal disorder. **Flatus** is the release of gas through the anus. The analysis of stool for blood, bacteria, and other elements can provide a clue to various ailments. **Melena** is a condition in which blood that is not fresh appears in the stool as a black, tarry mass. **Hematochezia** is bright red blood in the stool. **Steatorrhea** is fat in the stool.

A small opening in the anal canal is called an **anal fistula.** Waste material can enter the abdominal cavity through a fistula. The anus may be the site of **hemorrhoids,** swollen, twisted veins that can cause great discomfort.

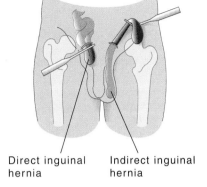
Figure 14-10 An inguinal hernia usually requires surgery.

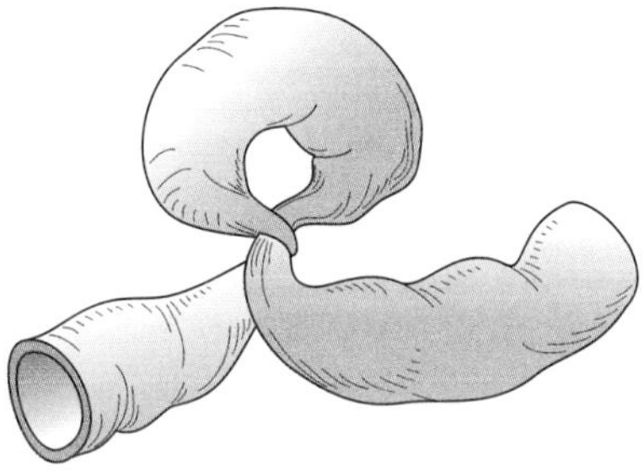

Direct inguinal hernia   Indirect inguinal hernia

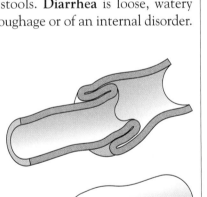

Figure 14-11 A volvulus is a twisting of the intestine that causes a blockage and requires surgery.

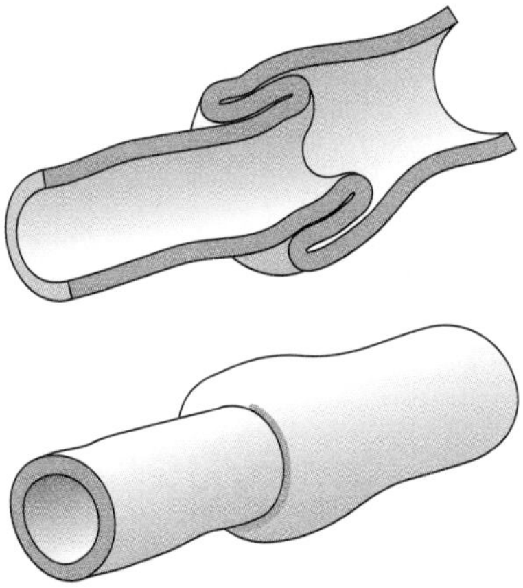

Figure 14-12 An intussusception occurs most often in children and requires surgical correction.

Vocabulary Review

In the previous section, you learned terms relating to pathology. Before going on to the exercises, review the terms below and refer to the previous section if you have any questions.

Term	Word Analysis	Definition
achalasia	[ăk-ă-LĀ-zē-ă] a-, without + Greek *chalasis*, a relaxing	Inability of a muscle, particularly the cardiac sphincter, to relax.
achlorhydria	[ā-klōr-HĬ-drē-ă]	Lack of hydrochloric acid in the stomach.
anal fistula	[FĬS-tyū-lă]	Small opening in the anal canal through which waste matter can leak.
ankyloglossia	[ĂNG-kĭ-lō-GLŎS-ē-ă] Greek *ankylos*, bent + *glossus*, tongue	Condition of the tongue being partially or completely attached to the bottom of the mouth.
anorexia	[ăn-ō-RĔK-sē-ă] an-, without + Greek *orexis*, appetite	Eating disorder with extreme weight loss.
aphagia	[ă-FĀ-jē-ă] a-, without + -phagia, eating	Inability to swallow.
appendicitis	[ă-pĕn-dĭ-SĬ-tĭs] appendic-, appendix + -itis, inflammation	Inflammation of the appendix.
ascites	[ă-SĬ-tēs] Latin, bags	Fluid buildup in the abdominal and peritoneal cavities.
bulimia	[bū-LĒM-ē-ă] Greek *boux*, ox + *limos*, hunger	Eating disorder with binging and purging.
cheilitis	[kĭ-LĬ-tĭs] Greek *cheilos*, lip + -itis	Inflammation of the lips.
cholangitis	[kō-lăn-JĬ-tĭs] cholangi-, bile vessel + -itis	Inflammation of the bile ducts.
cholecystitis	[KŌ-lē-sĭs-TĬ-tĭs] chole-, bile + cyst-, bladder +-itis	Inflammation of the gallbladder.
cholelithiasis	[KŌ-lē-lĭ-THĬ-ă-sĭs] chole- + Greek *lithos*, stone + -iasis, condition	Gallstones in the gallbladder.
cirrhosis	[sĭr-RŌ-sĭs] Greek *kirrhos*, yellow + -osis, condition	Liver disease, usually caused by alcoholism.

Term	Word Analysis	Definition
colic	[KŎL-ĭk] Greek *kolikos*, of the colon	Gastrointestinal distress, especially of infants.
colitis	[kō-LĪ-tĭs] col-, colon + -itis	Inflammation of the colon.
constipation	[kŏn-stĭ-PĀ-shŭn] Latin *constipo*, to press together	Difficult or infrequent defecation.
Crohn's disease	[krōnz] After Burrill Crohn (1884–1983), U. S. gastroenterologist	Type of irritable bowel disease with no ulcers.
diarrhea	[dī-ă-RĒ-ă] Greek *diarrhoia*, a flowing through	Loose, watery stool.
diverticula	[dī-vĕr-TĬK-yū-lă] Latin *diverticulum*, a side road	Small pouches in the intestinal walls.
diverticulitis	[DĪ-vĕr-tĭk-yū-LĪ-tĭs] diverticul(a) + -itis	Inflammation of the diverticula.
diverticulosis	[DĪ-vĕr-tĭk-yū-LŌ-sĭs] diverticul(a) + -osis	Condition in which diverticula trap food or bacteria.
duodenal ulcer	[DŪ-ō-DĒ-năl]	Ulcer in the duodenum.
dysentery	[DĬS-ĕn-tăr-ē] Greek *dysenteria*, bad bowels	Irritation of the intestinal tract with loose stools.
dyspepsia	[dĭs-PĔP-sē-ă] dys-, bad + -pepsia, digestion	Indigestion.
dysphagia	[dĭs-FĀ-jē-ă] dys- + -phagia, eating	Difficulty in swallowing.
enteritis	[ĕn-tĕr-Ī-tĭs] enter-, intestine + -itis	Inflammation of the small intestine.
eructation	[ē-rŭk-TĀ-shŭn] Latin *eructo*, to belch	Belching.
esophagitis	[ĕ-sŏf-ă-JĪ-tĭs] esophag-, esophagus + -itis	Inflammation of the esophagus.

Term	Word Analysis	Definition
fistula	[FĬS-tyū-lă] Latin, a pipe	Abnormal opening in tissue.
flatulence	[FLĂT-yū-lĕns]	Gas in the stomach or intestines.
flatus	[FLĂ-tŭs] Latin, a blowing	Gas in the lower intestinal tract that can be released through the anus.
gallstones		Calculi in the gallbladder.
gastritis	[găs-TRĬ-tĭs] gastr-, stomach + -itis	Inflammation of the stomach.
gastroenteritis	[GĂS-trō-ĕn-tĕr-Ĭ-tĭs] gastro- + enter- + -itis	Inflammation of the stomach and small intestine.
glossitis	[glŏ-SĪ-tĭs] gloss-, tongue + -itis	Inflammation of the tongue.
halitosis	[hăl-ĭ-TŌ-sĭs] Latin *halitus*, breath + -osis	Foul mouth odor.
hematemesis	[hē-mă-TĔM-ē-sĭs] hemat-, blood + emesis	Blood in vomit.
hematochezia	[HĒ-mă-tō-KĒ-zē-ă] hemato-, blood + Greek *chezo*, to go to stool	Red blood in stool.
hemorrhoids	[HĔM-ō-rŏydz]	Swollen, twisted veins in the anus.
hepatitis	[hĕp-ă-TĪ-tĭs] hepat-, liver + -itis	Inflammation or disease of the liver.
hepatomegaly	[HĔP-ă-tō-MĔG-ă-lē] hepato-, liver + -megaly, enlargement	Enlarged liver.
hepatopathy	[hĕp-ă-TŎP-ă-thē] hepato- + -pathy, disease	Liver disease
hiatal hernia	[hī-Ā-tăl]	Protrusion of the stomach through an opening in the diaphragm.
hyperbilirubinemia	[HĪ-pĕr-BĬL-ĭ-rū-bĭ-NĒ-mē-ă] hyper-, excessive + bilirubin + -emia, blood	Excessive bilirubin in the blood.

Term	Word Analysis	Definition
icterus	[ĬK-tĕr-ŭs] Greek *ikteros*	Jaundice.
ileitis	[ĭl-ē-Ĭ-tĭs] ile-, ileum + -itis	Inflammation of the ileum.
ileus	[ĬL-ē-ŭs] Latin, a twisting	Intestinal blockage.
intussusception	[ĬN-tŭs-sŭ-SĔP-shŭn] Latin *intus*, within + *suscipio*, to take up	Prolapse of an intestinal part into a neighboring part.
jaundice	[JĂWN-dĭs]	Excessive bilirubin in the blood causing yellowing of the skin.
melena	[mĕ-LĒ-nă] Greek *melaina*, black	Old blood in the stool.
nausea	[NĂW-zē-ă] Latin, seasickness	Sick feeling in the stomach.
obesity	[ō-BĒS-ĭ-tē] Latin *obesus*, fat	Abnormal accumulation of fat in the body.
pancreatitis	[PĂN-krē-ă-TĪ-tĭs] pancreat-, pancreas + -itis	Inflammation of the pancreas.
parotitis, parotiditis	[păr-ō-TĪ-tĭs, pă-rŏt-ĭ-DĪ-tĭs] parot(id gland) + -itis	Inflammation of the parotid gland.
peptic ulcer		Sore on the mucous membrane of the digestive system; stomach ulcer or gastric ulcer.
peritonitis	[PĔR-ĭ-tō-NĪ-tĭs] periton-, peritoneum + -itis	Inflammation of the peritoneum.
polyposis	[PŎL-ĭ-PŌ-sĭs] polyp + -osis	Condition with polyps, as in the intestines.
proctitis	[prŏk-TĪ-tĭs] proct-, rectum + -itis	Inflammation of the rectum and anus.
sialoadenitis	[SĪ-ă-lō-ăd-ĕ-NĪ-tĭs] sialoaden-, salivary gland + -itis	Inflammation of the salivary glands.

Term	Word Analysis	Definition
steatorrhea	[STĒ-ă-tō-RĒ-ă] steato-, fat + -rrhea, a flowing	Fat in the blood.
ulcerative colitis	[kō-LĪ-tĭs]	Inflammation of the colon with ulcers.
volvulus	[VŎL-vyū-lŭs] Latin *volvo*, to roll	Intestinal blockage caused by the intestine twisting on itself.

C A S E   S T U D Y

Testing and Diagnosing

Dr. Walker has morning hours at a local hospital several days a week. Today, Jim Santarelli is scheduled for a colonoscopy. His chart reads as follows:

 Critical Thinking

53. What might Dr. Walker be looking for in this procedure?

54. If the examination shows a clear colon, what lifestyle changes might Dr. Walker recommend?

PROCEDURE: colonoscopy

SURGEON: Dr. Walker

INDICATION: This man has a two-year history of increasing, intermittent, sudden bouts of diarrhea without mucus or blood. Antispasmodic treatment with Bentyl has failed. He had a negative barium enema 3½ months ago. Stools have been hemoccult negative. There are no systemic symptoms. The frequency of the diarrhea is once every other day to twice a week.

With the patient turned onto his left side, he was monitored using continuous SAO2 pulse monitoring and intermittent blood pressure monitoring. An IV was started in the left forearm. Mr. Santarelli was given 50 mg of Demerol and 10 mg of Valium by slow intravenous injection. After adequate sedation was achieved, the colonoscopy was performed.

Pathological Terms Exercises

Find a Match

Match the terms in the left-hand column with the correct definition in the right-hand column.

55. bulimia	a. intestinal blockage caused by the intestine twisting on itself
56. colitis	b. red blood in the stool
57. diverticula	c. prolapse of an intestinal part into a neighboring part
58. eructation	d. eating disorder with binging and purging
59. hematochezia	e. inflammation of the colon
60. intussusception	f. inflammation of the peritoneum
61. jaundice	g. fat in the stool
62. peritonitis	h. small pouches in the intestinal wall
63. steatorrhea	i. icterus
64. volvulus	j. belching

Check Your Knowledge

Circle the correct term that completes the sentence.

65. Jane's parents have brought her to see an internist. Jane is 5'10" and weighs 105 pounds. Jane thinks she is fat. The doctor suspects Jane's problem is _____. (obesity, anorexia, aphasia)

66. John was seen in the emergency room. He complained of abdominal pain with cramping and diarrhea. He was concerned that he might have _____.(constipation, irritable bowel disease, hemorrhoids)

67. Jean has been complaining of severe pain in the RUQ following the ingestion of food, especially foods like nuts and ice cream. She believes she might have _____. (pancreatitis, appendicitis, cholecystitis)

68. Dora is feeling sluggish and unwell. She complains to her doctor that she has been unable to have a bowel movement for the past 5 days. She is diagnosed with _____. (diarrhea, hematochezia, constipation)

69. Many people cannot lie flat after eating because of a burning sensation in the chest and throat. The pain makes the person feel that he or she is having a heart attack. This condition, seen frequently in the emergency room, is called _____. (inguinal hernia, dysentery, gastroesophageal reflux)

Spell It Correctly

For each of the following words, write C if the spelling is correct. If it is not, write the correct spelling.

70. dypepsia_____

71. hyperbilirubinemia_____

72. diverticuli_____

73. hematochazia_____

74. inginal hernia_____

75. iliitis_____

76. polyposis_____

77. cirrosis_____

78. hietal hernia_____

79. achlorhydria_____

80. flatusence_____

Surgical Terms

Treating the digestive tract often includes biopsies, surgeries, and observation using endoscopes. **Abdominocentesis** or **paracentesis** is an incision into the intestinal tract to relieve fluid pressure, as in ascites. **Cholelithotomy** is an incision for the removal of stones. **Choledocholithotomy** is an incision for removal of stones in the common bile duct. **Cholelithotripsy** is the crushing of gallstones using sound waves or other techniques. Surgical repair of the digestive tract includes **cheiloplasty** (lip repair); **glossorrhaphy** (tongue suturing); **esophagoplasty** (esophagus repair); and **proctoplasty** (repair of the rectum and anus). Some parts of the digestive tract may require removal because of malignancies or chronic inflammation. A **glossectomy** is removal of the tongue. A **polypectomy** is the removal of polyps, particularly in areas such as the colon, which are susceptible to cancer. An **appendectomy** is the removal of a diseased appendix that is in danger of rupturing. A **cholecystectomy** is the removal of the gallbladder, particularly one that is constantly inflamed and susceptible to painful bouts of gallstones. A **gastrectomy** is removal of some or all of the stomach. It may be followed by a **gastric resection,** to repair the remaining part of the stomach. A **colectomy** is the removal of some or all of the colon. This may be a temporary operation that is followed by a surgical reconnection of parts of the colon or it may require the use of a colostomy bag. An **anastomosis,** a surgical union of two hollow tubes, is sometimes used to bypass parts of the intestines as in the case of removal of a section of the intestines. A **pancreatectomy** is removal of the pancreas usually only in cases with malignancy. A **hemorrhoidectomy** is the removal of hemorrhoids. A **hepatic lobectomy** is removal of one or more lobes of the liver. It is usually preceded by a **liver biopsy** to determine the type and extent of disease. People can live with only part of a liver. However, if a person with a completely diseased liver does not receive an organ transplant, he or she will usually die. An anal fistula is removed in an **anal fistulectomy. Billroth's I** and **Billroth's II** are two types of operations. The first is the excision of the pylorus, and the second is the resectioning of the pylorus with the stomach.

Openings may have to be made in the gastrointestinal tract. Sometimes they are temporary to allow evacuation of waste material. In some cases, they are permanent as when intestinal parts cannot be reconnected. An **ileostomy** is the creation of an opening in the abdomen, which is attached to the ileum to allow fecal matter to discharge into a bag outside the body. A **colostomy** is an opening in the colon to the abdominal wall to create a place for waste to exit the body other than through the anus. A colostomy is sometimes required in the case of diseases such as cancer and ulcerative colitis. Figure 14-13 shows an ileostomy or colostomy appliance.

Some patients with colostomies have reconstructive surgery to create a new passageway to the anus.

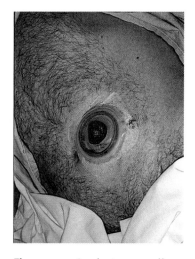

Figure 14-13 A colostomy appliance is attached to the opening after a colectomy.

Vocabulary Review

In the previous section, you learned terms relating to surgery. Before going on to the exercises, review the terms below and refer to the previous section if you have any questions.

Term	Word Analysis	Definition
abdominocentesis	[ăb-DŎM-ĭ-nō-sĕn-TĒ-sĭs] Latin *abdominis*, abdomen + -centesis, puncture	Incision into the abdomen to remove fluid.
anal fistulectomy	[Ā-năl fĭs-tyū-LĔK-tō-mē]	Removal of an anal fistula.
anastomosis	[ă-NĂS-tō-MŌ-sĭs] Greek *anastomoo*, to furnish with a mouth	Surgical union of two hollow structures.
appendectomy	[ăp-pĕn-DĔK-tō-mē] append-, appendix + -ectomy, removal	Removal of the appendix.
Billroth's I	[BĬLL-rŏthz] After C. A. Billroth (1829–1894), Austrian surgeon	Excision of the pylorus.
Billroth's II		Resection of the pylorus with the stomach.
cheiloplasty	[KĪ-lō-plăs-tē] Greek *cheilos*, lip + -plasty, repair	Repair of the lips.
cholecystectomy	[KŌ-lē-sĭs-TĔK-tō-mē] cholecyst-, gallbladder + -ectomy	Removal of the gallbladder.
choledocholithotomy	[kō-LĔD-ō-kō-lĭ-THŎT-ō-mē] choledocho-, common bile duct + Greek *lithos*, stone + -tomy, a cutting	Removal of stones from the common bile duct.
cholelithotomy	[KŌ-lē-lĭ-THŎT-ō-mē] chole-, bile + Greek *lithos*, stone + -tomy	Removal of gallstones.
cholelithotripsy	[kō-lē-LĬTH-ō-trĭp-sē] chole- + Greek *lithos*, stone + *tripsis*, a rubbing	Breaking up or crushing of stones in the body, especially gallstones.

Term	Word Analysis	Definition
colectomy	[kō-LĔK-tō-mē] col-, colon + -ectomy	Removal of the colon.
colostomy	[kō-LŎS-tō-mē] colo-, colon + -stomy, mouth, opening	Creation of an opening from the colon into the abdominal wall.
esophagoplasty	[ĕ-SŎF-ă-gō-plăs-tē] esophago-, esophagus + -plasty	Repair of the esophagus.
gastrectomy	[găs-TRĔK-tō-mē] gastr-, stomach + -ectomy	Removal of part or all of the stomach.
gastric resection		Removal of part of the stomach and repair of the remaining part.
glossectomy	[glŏ-SĔK-tō-mē] gloss-, tongue + -ectomy	Removal of the tongue.
glossorrhaphy	[glŏ-SŌR-ă-fē] glosso-, tongue + -rrhapy, suturing	Suture of the tongue.
hemorrhoidectomy	[HĔM-ō-rŏy-DĔK- tō-mē] hemorrhoid(s) + -ectomy	Removal of hemorrhoids.
hepatic lobectomy	[hĕ-PĂT-ĭk lō-BĔK- tō-mē]	Removal of one or more lobes of the liver.
ileostomy	[ĬL-ē-ŎS-tō-mē] ileo-, ileum + -stomy	Creation of an opening into the ileum.
liver biopsy		Removal of a small amount of liver tissue to examine for disease.
pancreatectomy	[PĂN-krē-ă-TĔK-tō-mē] pancreat-, pancreas + -tomy	Removal of the pancreas.
paracentesis	[PĂR-ă-sĕn-TĒ-sĭs] Greek *parakentesis*, a tapping for edema	Incision into the intestinal tract.
polypectomy	[pŏl-ĭ-PĔK-tō-mē] polyp + -ectomy	Removal of polyps.
proctoplasty	[PRŎK-tō-plăs-tē] procto-, rectum + -plasty	Repair of the rectum and anus.

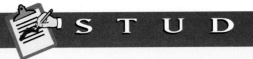

C A S E S T U D Y

Performing Surgery

Dr. Walker has another patient scheduled for a colonoscopy. Laura Martinez had an earlier colonoscopy, which was negative. Since then, she has experienced some rectal bleeding. This time her colonoscopy shows several suspicious-looking polyps near the rectum. Dr. Walker biopsies several of them. The result is positive for cancer, but the area of malignancy that needs removal is limited.

Critical Thinking

81. What operation will likely be performed?

82. Why might the operation include a colostomy?

Surgical Terms Exercises

Fill in the blanks.

83. Removal of a liver lobe is a(n) _____ _____.

84. Repair of a part of the stomach is a(n) _____ _____.

85. Two openings that allow waste to exit the body other than through the anus are a(n) _____ and a(n) _____.

86. The crushing of gallstones is called _____.

87. Incision into the intestinal tract is _____.

Pharmacological Terms

Aside from treatments for cancer, medications for the digestive tract counteract situations that occur in various parts of the tract. **Antacids** neutralize stomach acid. Many antacids are taken before meals to prevent the building up of excess stomach acids. Others are taken after symptoms appear. **Antiemetics** prevent vomiting. **Antispasmodics** relieve spasms in the gastrointestinal tract. A **laxative** or **cathartic** stimulates movement of bowels. An **antidiarrheal** helps to control loose, watery stools. Table 14-2 lists some common medications used to treat the intestinal tract.

Many antacids are a good source of calcium.

Table 14-2 Medications Used to Treat Digestive Disorders

Drug Class	Purpose	Generic	Trade Name
antacid	to neutralize stomach acid	magaldrate magnesium hydroxide cimetidine famotodine sodium bicarbonate	Riopan Phillip's Milk of Magnesia Tagamet Pepcid Arm and Hammer baking soda
antidiarrheal	to control loose stools	attapulgite loperamide bismuth subsalicylate	Kaopectate, Diasorb Imodium A-D Pepto-Bismol
antiemetic	to prevent regurgitation	dimenhydrinate trimethobenzamide	Dramamine, Nauseatol Tigan, Trimazide
antispasmodic	to calm spasms in the intestinal tract	glycopyrrolate propantheline	Robinul Pro-Banthine
cathartic	to cause vomiting (after ingestion of poison); to relieve constipation; to empty bowels for medical procedures	ipecac syrup psyllium	none Metamucil
laxative	to relieve constipation	psyllium glycerine bisacodyl lactulose magnesium salts phenolphthalein senna	Metamucil Glycerol, Fleet Dulcolax Emulose, Lactulax Phillip's Milk of Magnesia Ex-Lax Senokot

Vocabulary Review

In the previous section, you learned terms relating to pharmacology. Before going on to the exercises, review the terms below and refer to the previous section if you have any questions.

Term	Word Analysis	Definition
antacid	[ănt-ĂS-ĭd] ant-, against + acid	Agent that neutralizes stomach acid.
antidiarrheal	[ăn-tē-dī-ă-RĔ-ăl] anti-, against + diarrhea	Agent that controls loose, watery stools.
antiemetic	[ĂN-tē-ĕ-MĔT-ĭk] anti- + emetic, related to vomiting	Agent that prevents vomiting.

Term	Word Analysis	Definition
antispasmodic	[ăn-tē-spăz-MŎD-ĭk] anti- + spasmodic	Agent that controls intestinal tract spasms.
cathartic	[kă-THĂR-tĭk] Greek *katharsis*, purification	Laxative.
laxative	[LĂX-ă-tĭv] Latin *laxativus*	Agent that softens stool to relieve constipation.

C A S E   S T U D Y

Resolving a Complaint

Dora, a patient complaining of constipation, was given a laxative to regulate her bowel movements. Doctors found that Dora avoided high roughage foods because of an acid condition in her stomach.

💡 **Critical Thinking**

88. Why is it important that Dora eat foods with high roughage content?

89. What other medication might the doctor prescribe to make it easier for her to digest such foods?

Pharmacological Terms Exercises

Find a Match

Match the pharmacological agent in the left-hand column with its use in the right-hand column.

90. antacid

91. antidiarrheal

92. antiemetic

93. antispasmodic

94. cathartic

95. laxative

a. relieves constipation

b. calms spasms

c. prevents regurgitation

d. relieves constipation

e. controls loose, watery stools

f. relieves burning sensation in digestive disorder

CHALLENGE SECTION

The chart for Dr. Walker's patient, Holly Berger, shows a history of gastrointestinal problems. Dr. Walker performed a procedure that allowed a full examination and biopsies of certain sections of Holly's intestinal tract. The procedure was performed in the hospital, and the patient was able to leave after a few hours in the recovery room.

Challenge Section Exercises

96. Why did Dr. Walker take biopsies of various intestinal tract areas?

97. From his examination of the stomach and duodenum, what most likely made Dr. Walker able to rule out Crohn's disease?

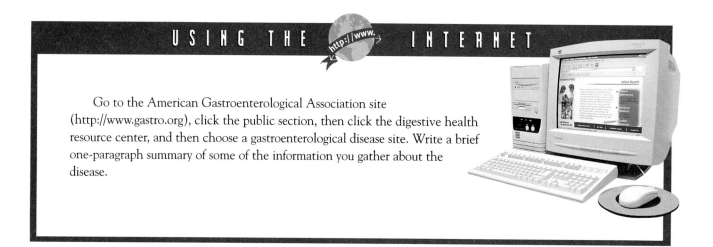

USING THE INTERNET

Go to the American Gastroenterological Association site (http://www.gastro.org), click the public section, then click the digestive health resource center, and then choose a gastroenterological disease site. Write a brief one-paragraph summary of some of the information you gather about the disease.

CHAPTER REVIEW

Definitions

Define the following terms and combining forms. Review the chapter before starting. Make sure you know how to pronounce each term as you define it.

Word	Definition
abdominocentesis [ăb-DŎM-ĭ-nō-sĕn-TĒ-sĭs]	
absorption [ăb-SŎRP-shŭn]	
achalasia [ăk-ă-LĀ-zē-ă]	
achlorhydria [ā-klōr-HĪ-drē-ă]	
alimentary [ăl-ĭ-MĔN-tĕr-ē] canal	
amino [ă-MĒ-nō] acid	
amylase [ĂM-ĭl-ās]	
anal [Ā-năl] canal	
anal fistula [FĬS-tyū-lă]	
anal fistulectomy [Ā-năl fĭs-tyū-LĔK-tō-mē]	
anastomosis [ă-NĂS-tō-MŌ-sĭs]	
ankyloglossia [ĂNG-kĭ-lō-GLŎS-ē-ă]	
an(o)	
anorexia [ăn-ō-RĔK-sē-ă]	
antacid [ănt-ĂS-ĭd]	
antidiarrheal [ăn-tē-dī-ă-RĒ-ăl]	
antiemetic [ĂN-tē-ĕ-MĔT-ĭk]	
antispasmodic [ăn-tē-spăz-MŎD-ĭk]	
anus [Ā-nŭs]	
aphagia [ā-FĀ-jē-ă]	
append(o), appendic(o)	
appendage [ă-PĔN-dĭj]	
appendectomy [ăp-pĕn-DĔK-tō-mē]	
appendicitis [ă-pĕn-dĭ-SĪ-tĭs]	
appendix [ă-PĔN-dĭks]	

Word	Definition
ascites [ă-SĪ-tēs]	
bil(o), bili	
bile [bīl]	
bilirubin [bĭl-ĭ-RŪ-bĭn]	
Billroth's [BĬLL-rŏthz] I	
Billroth's II	
body	
bowel [bŏwl]	
bucc(o)	
bulimia [bū-LĒM-ē-ă]	
cathartic [kă-THĂR-tĭk]	
cec(o)	
cecum [SĒ-kŭm]	
celi(o)	
cheeks	
cheilitis [kī-LĪ-tĭs]	
cheiloplasty [KĪ-lō-plăs-tē]	
chol(e), cholo	
cholangi(o)	
cholangiography [kō-lăn-jē-ŎG-ră-fē]	
cholangitis [kō-lăn-JĪ-tĭs]	
cholecyst(o)	
cholecystectomy [KŌ-lē-sĭs-TĔK-tō-mē]	
cholecystitis [KŌ-lē-sĭs-TĪ-tĭs]	
cholecystography [kō-lē-sĭs-TŎG-ră-fē]	
choledoch(o)	
choledocholithotomy [kō-LĔD-ō-kō-lĭ-THŎT-ō-mē]	
cholelithiasis [KŌ-lē-lĭ-THĪ-ă-sĭs]	
cholelithotomy [KŌ-lē-lĭ-THŎT-ō-mē]	
cholelithotripsy [kō-lē-LĪTH-ō-trĭp-sē]	
chyme [kīm]	
cirrhosis [sĭr-RŌ-sĭs]	
col(o), colon(o)	

Word	Definition
colectomy [kō-LĔK-tō-mē]	
colic [KŎL-ĭk]	
colitis [kō-LĪ-tĭs]	
colon [KŌ-lŏn]	
colonoscopy [kō-lŏn-ŎS-kō-pē]	
colostomy [kō-LŎS-tō-mē]	
constipation [kŏn-stĭ-PĀ-shŭn]	
Crohn's [krōnz] disease	
defecation [dĕ-fĕ-KĀ-shŭn]	
deglutition [dē-glū-TĬSH-ŭn]	
diarrhea [dī-ă-RĒ-ă]	
digestion [dī-JĔS-chŭn]	
diverticula [dī-vĕr-TĬK-yū-lă]	
diverticulitis [DĪ-vĕr-tĭk-yū-LĪ-tĭs]	
diverticulosis [DĪ-vĕr-tĭk-yū-LŌ-sĭs]	
duoden(o)	
duodenal [DŪ-ō-DĒ-năl] ulcer	
duodenum [dū-ō-DĒ-nŭm]	
dysentery [dĭs-ĕn-tăr-ē]	
dyspepsia [dĭs-PĔP-sē-ă]	
dysphagia [dĭs-FĀ-jē-ă]	
emesis [ĕ-MĒ-sĭs]	
emulsification [ĕ-MŬL-sĭ-fĭ-KĀ-shŭn]	
enter(o)	
enteritis [ĕn-tĕr-Ī-tĭs]	
enzyme [ĔN-zīm]	
epiglottis [ĕp-ĭ-GLŎ-tĭs]	
eructation [ē-rŭk-TĀ-shŭn]	
esophag(o)	
esophagitis [ĕ-sŏf-ă-JĪ-tĭs]	
esophagoplasty [ĕ-SŎF-ă-gō-plăs-tē]	
esophagoscopy [ĕ-sŏf-ă-GŎS-kō-pē]	
esophagus [ĕ-SŎF-ă-gŭs]	
fatty acid	

Word	Definition
feces [FĒ-sēz]	
fistula [FĬS-tyū-lă]	
flatulence [FLĂT-yū-lĕns]	
flatus [FLĂ-tŭs]	
frenulum [FRĔN-yū-lŭm]	
fundus [FŬN-dŭs]	
gallbladder [GĂWL-blăd-ĕr]	
gallstones	
gastrectomy [găs-TRĔK-tō-mē]	
gastric resection	
gastritis [găs-TRĪ-tĭs]	
gastr(o)	
gastroenteritis [GĂS-trō-ĕn-tĕr-Ī-tĭs]	
gastroscopy [găs-TRŎS-kō-pē]	
gloss(o)	
glossectomy [glŏ-SĔK-tō-mē]	
glossitis [glŏ-SĪ-tĭs]	
glossorrhaphy [glō-SŌR-ă-fē]	
gluc(o)	
glucose [GLŪ-kōs]	
glyc(o)	
glycogen(o)	
glycogen [GLĪ-kō-jĕn]	
gums [gŭmz]	
halitosis [hăl-ĭ-TŌ-sĭs]	
hard palate [PĂL-ăt]	
hematemesis [hē-mă-TĔM-ē-sĭs]	
hematochezia [HĒ-mă-tō-KĒ-zē-ă]	
hemorrhoidectomy [HĔM-ō-rŏy-DĔK-tō-mē]	
hemorrhoids [HĔM-ō-rŏydz]	
hepat(o)	
hepatic lobectomy [hĕ-PĂT-ĭk lō-BĔK-tō-mē]	
hepatitis [hĕp-ă-TĪ-tĭs]	

Word	Definition
hepatomegaly [HĔP-ă-tō-MĔG-ă-lē]	
hepatopathy [hĕp-ă-TŎP-ă-thē]	
hiatal [hī-Ā-tăl] hernia	
hyperbilirubinemia [HĪ-pĕr-BĬL-ĭ-rū-bĭ-NĒ-mē-ă]	
icterus [ĬK-tĕr-ŭs]	
ile(o)	
ileitis [ĭl-ē-Ī-tĭs]	
ileostomy [ĬL-ē-ŎS-tō-mē]	
ileum [ĬL-ē-ŭm]	
ileus [ĬL-ē-ŭs]	
intussusception [ĬN-tŭs-sŭ-SĔP-shŭn]	
jaundice [JĂWN-dĭs]	
jejun(o)	
jejunum [jĕ-JŪ-nŭm]	
labi(o)	
large intestine	
laxative [LĂX-ă-tĭv]	
lingu(o)	
lingual tonsils [LĬNG-gwăl TŎN-sĭls]	
lipase [LĬP-ās]	
lips	
liver [LĬV-ĕr]	
liver biopsy	
mastication [măs-tĭ-KĀ-shŭn]	
melena [mĕ-LĒ-nă]	
mesentery [MĔS-ĕn-tĕr-ē]	
mouth	
nausea [NĂW-zē-ă]	
obesity [ō-BĒS-ĭ-tē]	
or(o)	
palatine [PĂL-ă-tīn] tonsils	
pancreas [PĂN-krē-ăs]	
pancreat(o)	

Word	Definition
pancreatectomy [PĂN-krē-ă-TĔK-tō-mē]	
pancreatitis [PĂN-krē-ă-TĪ-tĭs]	
papilla (pl. papillae) [pă-PĬL-ă (-ī)]	
paracentesis [PĂR-ă-sĕn-TĒ-sĭs]	
parotitis, parotiditis [păr-ō-TĪ-tĭs, pă-rŏt-ĭ-DĪ-tĭs]	
pepsin [PĔP-sĭn]	
peptic ulcer	
peristalsis [pĕr-ĭ-STĂL-sĭs]	
periton(eo)	
peritoneoscopy [PĔR-ĭ-tō-nē-ŎS-kō-pē]	
peritonitis [PĔR-ĭ-tō-NĪ-tĭs]	
pharyng(o)	
pharynx [FĂR-ĭngks]	
polypectomy [pŏl-ĭ-PĔK-tō-mē]	
polyposis [PŎL-ĭ-PŌ-sĭs]	
proct(o)	
proctitis [prŏk-TĪ-tĭs]	
proctoplasty [PRŎK-tō-plăs-tē]	
proctoscopy [prŏk-TŎS-kō-pē]	
pylor(o)	
pylorus [pī-LŌR-ŭs]	
rect(o)	
rectum [RĔK-tŭm]	
reflux [RĒ-flŭxs]	
regurgitation [rē-GĔR-jĭ-TĀ-shŭn]	
rugae [RŪ-gē]	
saliva [să-LĪ-vă]	
salivary [SĂL-ĭ-vār-ē] glands	
sial(o)	
sialaden(o)	
sialoadenitis [SĪ-ă-lō-ăd-ē-NĪ-tĭs]	
sigmoid(o)	
sigmoid [SĬG-mŏyd] colon	

Word	Definition
sigmoidoscopy [SĬG-mŏy-DŎS-kō-pē]	
small intestine	
soft palate [PĂL-āt]	
steat(o)	
steatorrhea [STĒ-ă-tō-RĒ-ă]	
stomat(o)	
stomach [STŬM-ŭk]	
stool [stūl]	
throat	
tongue [tŭng]	
ulcerative colitis [kō-LĪ-tĭs]	
uvula [YŪ-vyū-lă]	
villus (pl. villi) [VĬL-ŭs (-ī)]	
volvulus [VŎL-vyū-lŭs]	

Abbreviations

Write the full meaning for each abbreviation.

Abbreviation	Meaning
ALT, AT	
AST	
BE	
BM	
EGD	
ERCP	
GERD	
GI	
IBD	
IBS	
NG	
NPO	
SGOT	
SGPT	
TPN	
UGI(S)	

Answers to Chapter Exercises

1. Burning chest pains may also be a sign of a heart attack.
2. Esophagus and stomach, because the burning sensation is probably related to backflow from the stomach to the esophagus.
3. a. stomach; b. small intestine; c. large intestine; d. rectum; e. liver
4. papillae
5. frenulum
6. C
7. chyme
8. C
9. C
10. C
11. lipase
12. C
13. peristalsis
14. cardiac region, fundus, body, pylorus
15. duodenum, jejunum, ileum
16. cecum, colon, sigmoid colon, rectum
17. small
18. hepatic portal system
19. amylase, lipase
20. emulsification
21. Many diseases are either directly hereditary or may be the result of a hereditary tendency. Early detection may enable better treatment.
22. gastritis and hepatitis
23. gastrectomy
24. esophagitis
25. rectocele
26. duodenal
27. choledochectomy
28. pancreatitis
29. rectodynia, rectalgia
30. colonoscopy
31. hepatomegaly
32. gastrorrhaphy
33. proctologist
34. cholecystitis
35. hepatoma
36. pyloro, duoden, of the pylorus and duodenum
37. an-, around the anus
38. entero, colo-, opening between the small intestine and colon
39. ileo-, cec-, of the ileum and cecum
40. lingu-, under the tongue
41. gastroscopy
42. biopsies for cancer, blood tests for liver function
43. g
44. h
45. a
46. c
47. i
48. d
49. b
50. e
51. j
52. f
53. colitis, colon cancer, or other colon disorders
54. bland diet, avoiding alcohol and caffeine
55. d
56. e
57. h
58. j
59. b
60. c
61. i
62. f
63. g
64. a
65. anorexia
66. irritable bowel disease
67. cholecystitis
68. constipation
69. gastroesophageal reflux
70. dyspepsia
71. C
72. diverticula
73. hematochezia
74. inguinal hernia
75. ileitis
76. C
77. cirrhosis
78. hiatal hernia
79. C
80. flatulence
81. colectomy
82. At least until reconstructive surgery is done, an alternative waste excretion site will be needed.
83. hepatic lobectomy
84. gastric resection
85. ileostomy, colostomy
86. cholelithotripsy
87. abdominocentesis or paracentesis
88. A diet high in roughage, may eliminate constipation.
89. antacid
90. f
91. e
92. c
93. b
94. a or d
95. d or a
96. to check for cancer
97. There were ulcerations.

15
The Endocrine System

After studying this chapter, you will be able to

◆ Name the parts of the endocrine system and discuss the function of each part

◆ Define combining forms used in building words that relate to the endocrine system

◆ Identify the meaning of related abbreviations

◆ Name the common diagnoses, clinical procedures, and laboratory tests used in treating disorders of the endocrine system

◆ List and define the major pathological conditions of the endocrine system

◆ Define surgical terms related to the endocrine system

◆ Recognize common pharmacological agents used in treating disorders of the endocrine system

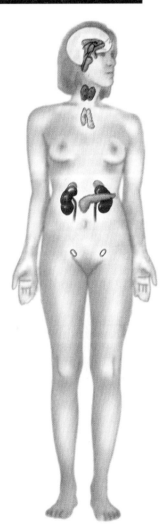

Structure And Function

The endocrine system is a group of glands that act as the body's master regulator (Figure 15-1a). It regulates many bodily functions as diagrammed in Figure 15-1b. It helps to maintain homeostasis by regulating the production of chemicals that affect most functions of the body. It secretes substances that aid the nervous system in reacting to stress, and it is an important regulator of growth and development. The endocrine system is made up of various **glands** and other tissue that secrete **hormones,** specialized chemicals, into the bloodstream. The hormones are effective only in specific **target cells,** cells that have **receptors** that recognize a compatible hormone. A group of such cells forms *target tissue*. Minute amounts of hormones can initiate a strong reaction in some target cells.

Unlike **exocrine glands,** which secrete substances into ducts directed toward a specific location, **endocrine glands** or tissue secrete hormones into the bloodstream. They are also known as **ductless glands.** Some endocrine glands are also exocrine glands. For example, as an endocrine gland, the pancreas secretes insulin, and as an exocrine gland, it releases digestive juices through ducts to the small intestine.

Hormones are various substances manufactured from raw materials in cells and secreted into the capillaries between cells to enter the bloodstream. Aside from the specific target cells and functions, hormones are differentiated by their properties. Some hormones are fat-soluble steroids, others are water-

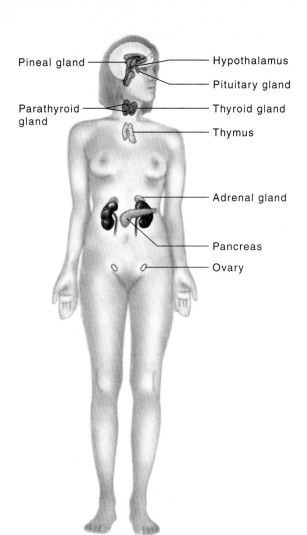

Pineal gland — Hypothalamus
— Pituitary gland
Parathyroid — — Thyroid gland
gland
— Thymus

— Adrenal gland

— Pancreas
— Ovary

soluble proteins, and still others are derived from amino acids. Each type of hormone is transported differently throughout the body because of its chemical properties.

Hypothalamus

The **hypothalamus** is a part of the nervous system that serves as an endocrine gland because it releases hormones that regulate pituitary hormones. The hormones released by the hypothalamus have either a **releasing** (allowing the secretion of other hormones to take place) or an **inhibiting** (preventing the secretion of other hormones) factor. The hypothalamus is located in the brain superior to the pituitary gland.

Pineal Gland

The **pineal gland** is located superior and posterior to the pituitary gland. It releases **melatonin,** a hormone that is believed to affect sleep and the functioning of the gonads.

Pituitary Gland

The **pituitary gland,** also called the **hypophysis,** is located at the base of the brain in an area called the sella turcica. The pituitary is the body's master gland regulating or aiding in the secretion of essential hormones. Table 15-1 describes the functions of all parts of the endocrine system.

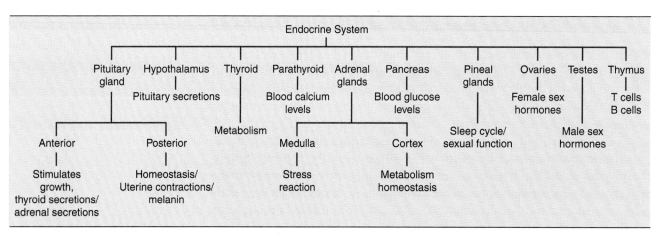

Figure 15-1 (a) The endocrine system secretes hormones that affect all parts of the body. (b) The bodily functions affected by the endocrine hormones.

Pineal comes from Latin *pineus,* pine cone, referring to the shape of the gland.

The pituitary consists of an *anterior lobe* (**adenohypophysis**) and a *posterior lobe* (**neurohypophysis**).

Thyroid Gland

The **thyroid gland** consists of a left lobe and a right lobe. The lobes sit on either side of the trachea. The two lobes are connected by the **isthmus,** a narrow strip of tissue on the ventral surface of the trachea. Above the thyroid gland sits the *thyroid cartilage,* a large piece of cartilage that covers the larynx and produces the protrusion on the neck known as the **Adam's apple.** Thyroid secretions control metabolism and blood calcium concentrations. Two of the hormones secreted, **thyroxine** or *tetraiodothyronine* **(T_4)** and **triiodothyronine (T_3)** are produced in the thyroid gland using iodine from blood that circulates through the gland. T_3 and T_4 differ in the number of iodine atoms in each cell, with T_3 having three atoms and T_4 having four. These compounds circulate throughout the bloodstream helping to stimulate and control various bodily functions, such as regulating the metabolizing of carbohydrates, lipids, and proteins. **Calcitonin** is secreted from the outside surface of thyroid cells. It is a hormone that helps lower blood calcium concentration.

Parathyroid Glands

The **parathyroid glands** are four oval-shaped glands located on the dorsal side of the thyroid. The parathyroids helps regulate calcium and phosphate levels, two elements necessary to maintain homeostasis.

Thymus Gland

The **thymus gland** is considered an endocrine gland because it secretes a hormone and is ductless; however, it is also part of the immune system. The hormone stimulates the production of T and B cells, important to the development of an immune response. (Chapter 13 discusses the immune system.)

Adrenal Glands

The **adrenal glands** (or **suprarenal glands**) are a pair of glands. Each of the glands sits atop a kidney. Each gland consists of two parts—the **adrenal cortex** (the outer portion) and the **adrenal medulla** (the inner portion). The adrenal glands regulate **electrolytes** (substances that conduct electricity and are decomposed by it) or essential mineral salts in the body. The mineral salts affect metabolism and blood pressure. They are also **sympathomimetic,** imitative of the sympathetic nervous system, as in response to stress. The adrenal medulla secretes a class of hormones, **catecholamines** (epinephrine and norepinephrine), in response to stress.

Pancreas

The **pancreas** helps in maintaining a proper level of blood glucose. Within the pancreas, the **islets of Langerhans,** specialized hormone-producing cells, secrete **insulin** when blood sugar levels are high and **glucagon** when it is low.

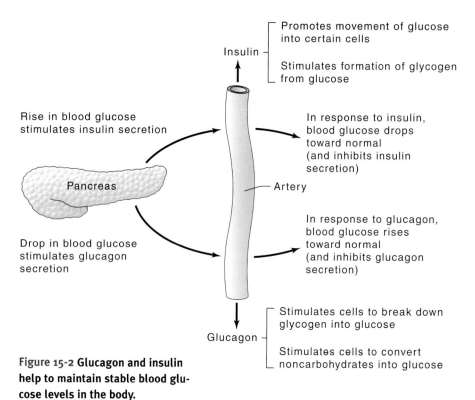

Insulin
- Promotes movement of glucose into certain cells
- Stimulates formation of glycogen from glucose

Rise in blood glucose stimulates insulin secretion

Pancreas

Drop in blood glucose stimulates glucagon secretion

In response to insulin, blood glucose drops toward normal (and inhibits insulin secretion)

Artery

In response to glucagon, blood glucose rises toward normal (and inhibits glucagon secretion)

Glucagon
- Stimulates cells to break down glycogen into glucose
- Stimulates cells to convert noncarbohydrates into glucose

Figure 15-2 Glucagon and insulin help to maintain stable blood glucose levels in the body.

Insulin is produced by **beta cells** in the islets of Langerhans, and glucagon is produced by **alpha cells** in the islets. When insulin is released in response to high blood sugar levels, it stimulates the glucose to be sent to the body's cells for energy as needed and to be converted to a starchy substance, **glycogen,** that is stored for later use in the liver. When glucagon is released in response to low blood sugar levels, it stimulates stored glycogen to be transformed into glucose again. Figure 15-2 shows the glucagon/glucose production process.

The pancreas is both an exocrine and an endocrine gland. The islets of Langerhans serve its endocrine functions, and the remaining cells its exocrine ones (as discussed in the digestive system in Chapter 14).

Ovaries

The **ovaries** are in the female pelvic region, one at the top of each fallopian tube. (Chapter 10 describes the female reproductive system.) The ovaries produce the immature ovum, which, when fertilized, becomes the fetus. The ovaries also produce the female sex hormones—estrogen and progesterone.

Testes

The two **testes** (or **testicles**) are located in the scrotum, a sac on the outside of the male body. The testes produce spermatozoa, which fertilize ova. The testes also produce male sex hormones called **androgens.** The major androgen is *testosterone.* (Chapter 11 describes the male reproductive system.)

Table 15-1 Endocrine Glands, Their Secretions and Their Functions

Endocrine Gland or Tissue	Hormone	Function
hypothalamus	pituitary-regulating hormones	either stimulate or inhibit pituitary secretions
neurohypophysis (pituitary gland—posterior)	antidiuretic hormone (ADH), vasopressin	increase water reabsorption
	oxytocin	stimulates uterine contractions and lactation
	melanocyte-stimulating hormone	stimulates production of melanin

Table 15-1 (continued)

Endocrine Gland or Tissue	Hormone	Function
adenohypophysis (pituitary gland—anterior)	growth hormone (GH), somatotropic hormone (STH)	stimulate bone and muscle growth; regulate some metabolic functions, such as the rate that cells utilize carbohydrates and fats
	thyroid-stimulating hormone (TSH)	stimulates thyroid gland to secrete hormones
	adrenocorticotropic hormone (ACTH)	stimulates secretion of adrenal cortex hormones
	follicle-stimulating hormone (FSH), luteinizing hormone (LH)	stimulate development of ova and production of female hormones
	prolactin	stimulates breast development and milk production
thyroid	thyroxine (T_4); triiodothyronine (T_3)	regulates metabolism; stimulates growth
	calcitonin	lowers blood calcium as necessary to maintain homeostasis
parathyroid	parathormone, parathyroid hormone (PTH)	increase blood calcium as necessary to maintain homeostasis
adrenal medulla	epinephrine (adrenaline), norepinephrine (*noradrenaline*)	work with the sympathetic nervous system to react to stress
adrenal cortex	glucocorticoids (cortisol, corticosteroids, *corticosterone*), mineralocorticoids (aldosterone), gonadocorticoids (androgens)	affect metabolism, growth, and aid in electrolyte and fluid balances
pancreas (in islets of Langerhans)	insulin, glucagon	maintain homeostasis in blood glucose concentration
pineal gland	melatonin	affects sexual functions and wake-sleep cycles
ovaries	estrogen (estradiol, the most powerful estrogen), progesterone	promote development of female sex characteristics, menstrual cycle, reproductive functions
testes	androgen, testosterone	promote development of male sex characteristics, sperm production
thymus gland	thymosin, thymic humoral factor (THF), factor thymic serum (FTS)	aid in development of T cells and some B cells; function not well understood

Vocabulary Review

In the previous section you learned terms related to the endocrine system. Before going on to the exercises, review the terms below and refer to the previous section if you have any questions.

Term	Word Analysis	Meaning
Adam's apple		Protrusion in the neck caused by a fold of thyroid cartilage.
adenohypophysis	[ĂD-ē-nō-hī-PŎF-ĭ-sĭs] adeno-, gland + hypophysis	Anterior lobe of the pituitary gland.
adrenal cortex	[ă-DRĒ-năl KŌR-tĕks]	Outer portion of the adrenal gland; helps control metabolism, inflammations, sodium and potassium retention, and effects of stress.
adrenal gland		One of two glands, each of which is situated on top of each kidney.
adrenaline	[ă-DRĔ-nă-lĭn]	Epinephrine; secreted by adrenal medulla.
adrenal medulla	[mĕ-DŪL-lă]	Inner portion of adrenal glands; releases large quantities of hormones during stress.
adrenocorticotropic hormone (ACTH)	[ă-DRĒ-nō-KŌR-tĭ-kō-TRŌ-pĭk] adreno-, adrenal glands + cortico(steroid) + -tropic, turning	Hormone secreted by anterior pituitary; involved in the control of the adrenal cortex.
aldosterone	[ăl-DŎS-tēr-ōn]	Hormone secreted by adrenal cortex; mineralocorticoid.
alpha cells		Specialized cells that produce glucagon in the pancreas.
androgen	[ĂN-drō-jĕn] andro-, man + -gen, producing	Any male hormone, such as testosterone.
antidiuretic hormone (ADH)	[ĂN-tē-dī-yū-RĔT-ĭk] anti-, against + diuretic	Posterior pituitary hormone that increases water reabsorption.
beta cells		Specialized cells that produce insulin in the pancreas.
calcitonin	[kăl-sĭ-TŌ-nĭn] calci-, calcium + Greek *tonos*, a stretching	Hormone secreted by the thyroid gland and other endocrine glands; helps control blood calcium levels.
catecholamines	[kăt-ĕ-KŌL-ă-mēnz]	Hormones, such as epinephrine, released in response to stress.
corticosteroids	[KŌR-tĭ-kō-STĒR-ŏydz]	Steroids produced by the adrenal cortex.

Term	Word Analysis	Meaning
cortisol	[KŌR-tĭ-sōl]	Hydrocortisone.
ductless gland		Endocrine gland.
electrolyte	[ē-LĔK-trō-līt]	Any substance that conducts electricity and is decomposed by it.
endocrine gland	[ĔN-dō-krĭn] endo-, within + -crine, secreting	Gland that secretes substances into the bloodstream instead of into ducts.
epinephrine	[ĔP-ĭ-NĔF-rĭn] epi-, upon + nephr-, kidney + -ine, chemical compound	Hormone released by the adrenal medulla in response to stress; adrenaline.
exocrine gland	[ĔK-sō-krĭn] exo-, external + -crine	Any gland that releases substances through ducts to a specific location.
follicle-stimulating hormone (FSH)		Hormone released by the anterior pituitary to aid in production of ova and sperm.
gland	Latin *glans*, acorn	Any organized mass of tissue secreting or excreting substances.
glucagon	[GLŪ-kă-gŏn] gluc-, glucose + -gen	Hormone released by the pancreas to increase blood sugar.
glucocorticoid	[glū-kō-KŌR-tĭ-kŏyd] gluco- + corticoid	Hormone released by the adrenal cortex.
glycogen	[GLĬ-kō-jĕn] glyco-, glycogen + -gen	Converted glucose stored in the liver for future use.
growth hormone (GH)		Hormone released by the anterior pituitary.
hormone	[HŌR-mōn] Greek *hormon*, rousing	Substance secreted by glands and carried in the bloodstream to various parts of the body.
hypophysis	[hī-PŎF-ĭ-sĭs] Greek, undergrowth	Pituitary gland.
hypothalamus	[HĪ-pō-THĂL-ă-mŭs] hypo-, beneath + thalamus	Gland in the nervous system that releases hormones to aid in regulating pituitary hormones.
inhibiting		Preventing the secretion of other hormones.
insulin	[ĬN-sū-lĭn] Latin *insula*, island	Substance released by the pancreas to lower blood sugar.

Term	Word Analysis	Meaning
islets of Langerhans	[LĂN-gĕr-hănz] After Paul Langerhans (1847-1888), German anatomist	Specialized cells in the pancreas that release insulin and glucagon.
isthmus	[ĬS-mŭs] Greek *isthmos*, narrow band	Narrow band of tissue connecting the two lobes of the thyroid gland.
luteinizing hormone (LH)	[LŪ-tē-ĭn-ĪZ-ĭng]	Hormone released to aid in maturation of ova and ovulation.
melanocyte-stimulating hormone (MSH)		Hormone released by the pituitary gland.
melatonin	[mĕl-ă-TŌN-ĭn] Greek *melas*, dark + *tonos*, a stretching	Hormone released by the pineal gland; affects sexual function and sleep patterns.
mineralocorticoid	[MĬN-ĕr-ăl-ō-KŌR-tĭ-kŏyd] mineral + corticoid, steroid secretion	Steroid secreted by adrenal cortex.
neurohypophysis	[NŪR-ō-hī-PŎF-ĭ-sĭs] neuro-, nerve + hypophysis	Posterior lobe of pituitary gland.
norepinephrine	[NŌR-ĕp-ĭ-NĔF-rĭn]	Hormone secreted by adrenal medulla.
ovary	[Ō-vār-ē] Latin *ovum*, egg	One of two female reproductive glands that secrete hormones in the endocrine system.
oxytocin	[ŏk-sĭ-TŌ-sĭn] Greek *oxytokos*, swift birth	Hormone released by the posterior pituitary gland to aid in uterine contractions and lactation.
pancreas	[PĂN-krē-ăs] Greek *pankreas*, sweetbread	Gland of both the endocrine system (blood sugar control) and the digestive system (as an exocrine gland).
parathormone (PTH)	[păr-ă-THŌR-mōn] parath(yroid) + (h)ormone	Parathyroid hormone.
parathyroid gland	[păr-ă-THĪ-rŏyd] para-, adjacent + thyroid	One of four glands located adjacent to the thyroid gland on its dorsal surface that help maintain levels of blood calcium.
parathyroid hormone		Hormone released by parathyroid glands to help raise blood calcium levels.

Term	Word Analysis	Meaning
pineal gland	[PĬN-ē-ăl] Latin *pineus*, relating to pine	Gland located above pituitary gland; secretes melatonin.
pituitary gland	[pĭ-TŪ-ĭ-tār-ē] Latin *pituita*	Major endocrine gland; secretes hormones essential to metabolic functions.
receptor	[rē-SĔP-tōr] Latin, receiver	Part of a target cell with properties compatible with a particular substance (hormone).
releasing		Allowing secretion of other hormones.
somatotrophic hormone (STH)	[SŌ-mă-tō-TRŌF-ĭk] somato-, sleep + -trophic, nutritional	Hormone secreted by anterior pituitary glands; important in growth and development.
suprarenal gland	[SŪ-pră-RĒ-năl] supra-, above + renal	Adrenal gland.
sympathomimetic	[SĬM-pă-thō-mĭ-MĔT-ĭk] sympath(etic) + Greek *mimikos*, imitating	Mimicking functions of the sympathetic nervous system.
target cell		Cell with receptors that are compatible with specific hormones.
testis, testicle	[TĔS-tĭs], [TĔS-tĭ-kl] Latin	One of two male organs that secrete hormones in the endocrine system.
thymus gland	[THĪ-mŭs] Greek *thymos*, sweetbread	Gland that is part of the immune system as well as part of the endocrine system; aids in the maturation of T and B cells.
thyroid gland	[THĪ-rŏyd] Greek *thyreos*, oblong shield	Gland with two lobes located on either side of the trachea; helps control blood calcium levels and metabolic functions.
thyroid-stimulating hormone (TSH)		Hormone secreted by anterior pituitary gland; stimulates release of thyroid hormones.
thyroxine (T$_4$)	[thĭ-RŎK-sēn, -sĭn]	Compound found in or manufactured for thyroid gland; helps regulate metabolism.
triiodothyronine (T$_3$)	[trĭ-Ī-ō-dō-THĪ-rō-nēn]	Thyroid hormone that stimulates growth.
vasopressin	[vā-sō PRĔS-ĭn]	Hormone secreted by pituitary gland; raises blood pressure.

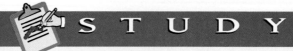

Checking the Symptoms

Gail Woods is a 45-year-old woman who has noticed some disturbing symptoms, such as unusual fatigue, since her last checkup. She called her physician, Dr. Tyler, for an appointment. Dr. Tyler examined her and sent her to a lab for several tests.

 Critical Thinking

1. Dr. Tyler ordered a urinalysis and blood tests. Why?

2. If Dr. Tyler is able to limit the symptoms to one body system, will he probably send Gail to a specialist?

Structure and Function Exercises

Find a Match

Match each hormone with its function by writing the name of the hormone on the appropriate line.

ADH prolactin insulin aldosterone oxytocin thyroxine testosterone thymosin melatonin epinephrine

3. may affect sleep habits _____

4. reacts to stress_____

5. decreases urine output _____

6. stimulates uterine contractions and lactation_____

7. helps transport glucose to cells and decreases blood sugar _____

8. stimulates breast development and lactation _____

9. affects electrolyte and fluid balances_____

10. regulates rate of cellular metabolism _____

11. promotes growth and maintenance of male sex characteristics and sperm production_____

12. aids in development of the immune system_____

Check Your Knowledge

For each of the following words, write C if the spelling is correct. If it is not, write the correct spelling.

13. adenohypophysis _____

14. adenal _____

15. hypophisis _____

16. suparenal _____

17. sympathomimetic _____

18. pituatary _____

19. lutinizing _____

20. triiodothyronine _____

Combining Forms and Abbreviations

The lists below include combining forms and abbrevations that relate specifically to the endocrine system. Pronunciations are provided for the examples.

Combining Form	Meaning	Example
aden(o)	gland	*adenopathy* [ă-dĕ-NŎP-ă-thē], glandular or lymph node disease
adren(o), adrenal(o)	adrenal glands	*adrenomegaly* [ă-drē-nō-MĔG-ă-lē], enlargement of the adrenal glands
gluc(o)	glucose	*glucogenesis* [glū-kō-JĔN-ĕ-sĭs], production of glucose
glyc(o)	glycogen	*glycolysis* [glī-KŎL-ĭ-sĭs], conversion of glycogen to glucose
gonad(o)	sex glands	*gonadotropin* [gō-NĂD-ō-trō-pĭn], hormone that aids in growth of gonads
pancreat(o)	pancreas	*pancreatitis* [păn-krē-ă-TĪ-tĭs], inflammation of the pancreas
parathyroid(o)	parathyroid	*parathyroidectomy* [pă-ră-thī-rŏy-DĔK-tō-mē], excision of the parathyroid glands
thyr(o), thyroid(o)	thyroid gland	*thyrotoxic* [thī-rō-TŎK-sĭk], having excessive amounts of thyroid hormones

Abbreviation	Meaning	Abbreviation	Meaning
ACTH	adrenocorticotropic hormone	IDDM	insulin-dependent diabetes mellitus
ADH	antidiuretic hormone	LH	luteinizing hormone
CRH	corticotropin-releasing hormone	MSH	melanocyte-stimulating hormone
DM	diabetes mellitus	NIDDM	noninsulin-dependent diabetes mellitus
FSH	follicle-stimulating hormone	PRL	prolactin
GH	growth hormone	PTH	parathyroid hormone, parathormone
GTT	glucose tolerance test	STH	somatotropin hormone
HCG	human chorionic gonadotropin	TSH	thyroid-stimulating hormone

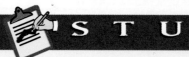
Getting the Results

Gail's tests came back with abnormally high blood sugar. Her lab results are shown here:

 Critical Thinking

21. Were any other tests abnormal?

22. What body system is the likely origin of Gail's abnormal tests?

John Colter, M.D. 3 Windsor Street Nome, AK 66660 777-546-7890	Laboratory Report Grandview Diagnostics 12 Settlers Drive Nome, AK 66661 777-546-7000	
Patient: Gail Woods Date Collected: 04/27/XXXX Date Received: 04/27/XXXX	Patient ID: 099-00-1200 Time Collected: 16:05 Date Reported: 10/06/XXXX	Date of Birth: 06/10/59 Total Volume: 2000

Test	Result	Flag	Reference
Complete Blood Count			
WBC	4.0		3.9-11.1
RBC	4.11		3.80-5.20
HCT	39.7		34.0-47.0
MCV	96.5		80.0-98.0
MCH	32.9		27.1-34.0
MCHC	34.0		32.0-36.0
MPV	8.6		7.5-11.5
NEUTROPHILS %	45.6		38.0-80.0
NEUTROPHILS ABS.	1.82		1.70-8.50
LYMPHOCYTES %	36.1		15.0-49.0
LYMPHOCYTES ABS.	1.44		1.00-3.50
EOSINOPHILS %	4.5		0.0-8.0
EOSINOPHILS ABS.	0.18		0.03-0.55
BASOPHILS %	0.7		0.0-2.0
BASOPHILS ABS.	0.03		0.000-0.185
PLATELET COUNT	229		150-400
Automated Chemistries			
GLUCOSE	275	*	65-109
UREA NITROGEN	17		6-30
CREATININE (SERUM)	0.6		0.5-1.3
UREA NITROGEN/CREATININE	28		10-29
SODIUM	152	*	135-145
POTASSIUM	4.4		3.5-5.3
CHLORIDE	106		96-109
CO_2	28		20-31
ANION GAP	6		3-19
CALCIUM	9.8		8.6-10.4
PHOSPHORUS	3.6		2.2-4.6
AST (SGOT)	28		0-30
ALT (SGPT)	19		0-34
BILIRUBIN, TOTAL	0.5		0.2-1.2
PROTEIN, TOTAL	7.8		6.2-8.2
ALBUMIN	4.3		3.5-5.0
GLOBULIN	3.5		2.1-3.8
URIC ACID	2.4		2.0-7.5
CHOLESTEROL	195		120-199
TRIGLYCERIDES	68		40-199
IRON	85		30-150
HDL CHOLESTEROL	73		35-59
CHOLESTEROL/HDL RATIO	3.2		3.2-5.7
LDL, CALCULATED	126		70-129
T3, UPTAKE	32		24-37
T4, TOTAL	6.9		4.5-12.8

Combining Forms and Abbreviations Exercises

Build Your Medical Vocabulary

Using the combining forms learned in this chapter, construct five words about the endocrine system that fit the definitions provided.

23. inflammation of a gland _____

24. disease of the pancreas _____

25. producing glycogen _____

26. enlargement of the thyroid gland _____

27. beneficial thyroid function _____

Know the Meaning

Write the definitions for the following terms.

28. adrenalectomy _____

29. pancreatectomy _____

30. adenoma _____

31. gonadotropin _____

32. thyromegaly _____

Diagnostic, Procedural, and Laboratory Terms

Endocrine functions affect homeostasis, the maintenance of fluid balance in the body. Levels of hormones, minerals, glucose, and other substances affect overall health. Blood and urine test results can often confirm a suspected diagnosis (usually based on symptoms such as sudden weight loss, fatigue, and abnormal thirst as in the case of diabetes). Blood sugar levels vary depending on when the last meal was eaten. A **fasting blood sugar** test and a **glucose tolerance test** are both taken after a 12-hour fast. However, the glucose tolerance test is repeated every hour for 5 or 6 hours after the patient ingests a glucose solution. Patients can check **blood sugar** or **blood glucose** levels themselves to track fluctuations in blood sugar. A **postprandial blood sugar** is a test for blood sugar usually taken about 2 hours after a meal. A **urine sugar** is a test for ketones and/or sugar in urine, both of which may indicate diabetes.

Overall endocrine functioning is tested in a serum test. Many hormones and electrolytes are present in serum. Endocrine function can be tested in the plasma by using a **radioactive immunoassay,** a test using radioactive iodine to locate various substances in the plasma. Thyroid functioning can be tested in a **thyroid function test,** which is a blood test for various hormones secreted by the thyroid. A **radioactive iodine uptake** is a measure of how quickly ingested iodine is taken into the thyroid gland. A **thyroid scan** is a test for cancer or other abnormality using radionuclide imaging.

Vocabulary Review

In the previous section you learned terms related to diagnosis, clinical procedures, and laboratory tests. Before going on to the exercises, review the terms below and refer to the previous section if you have any questions.

Term	Word Analysis	Meaning
blood sugar, blood glucose		Test for glucose in blood.
fasting blood sugar		Test for glucose in blood following a fast of 12 hours.
glucose tolerance test (GTT)		Blood test for body's ability to metabolize carbohydrates; taken after a 12-hour fast, then repeated every hour for 4 to 6 hours after ingestion of a sugar solution.
postprandial blood sugar		Test for glucose in blood, usually about two hours after a meal.
radioactive immunoassay (RIA)		Test for measuring hormone levels in plasma; taken after radioactive solution is ingested.
radioactive iodine uptake		Test for how quickly the thyroid gland pulls in ingested iodine.
thyroid function test or study		Test for levels of TSH, T_3, and T_4 in blood plasma to determine thyroid function.
thyroid scan		Imaging test for thyroid abnormalities.
urine sugar		Test for diabetes; determined by presence of ketones or sugar in urine.

C A S E S T U D Y

Referring to a Specialist

Dr. Tyler reviewed Gail's symptoms and test results with her. She has lost 12 pounds rapidly over the last couple of months, is feeling abnormally tired, and is unusually thirsty. Dr. Tyler referred her to an endocrinologist.

Critical Thinking

33. What disease does Dr. Tyler think Gail has?

34. What test for blood glucose is taken after a meal

Diagnostic, Procedural, and Laboratory Terms Exercises

Match the Test

Match the test with the possible diagnosis. Write D if it is a test for diabetes or T if it is a test for thyroid function.

35. fasting blood sugar _____

36. radioactive iodine uptake _____

37. radioactive immunoassay _____

38. urine sugar _____

39. glucose tolerance test _____

Pathological Terms

Diseases of the endocrine system commonly involve *lack* of homeostasis. In other words, either too much or too little of a hormone or substance in the body creates an imbalance and, often, a disorder or disease. The remarkable work and importance of hormones is seen in their pathology. Sometimes a minute difference in the amount of hormone can make a huge difference in the seriousness of an illness. Most endocrine illnesses are the result of **hypersecretion** (oversecretion) or **hyposecretion** (undersecretion) of one or more hormones.

Pituitary abnormalities include **acromegaly** (hypersecretion of growth hormone after puberty), which causes abnormal enlargement of features after childhood. Hypersecretion of growth hormone from the pituitary gland may result in **gigantism,** which causes abnormal growth, even to over 8 feet tall. Hyposecretion of the same growth hormone may result in **dwarfism,** which is stunted growth. Dwarfism caused by hyposecretion of growth hormone results in an extremely small person, but one with normally proportioned features. Dwarfism with disproportionate features is usually caused by the congenital absence of the thyroid gland or by another genetic defect.

In addition to growth problems, hyposecretion of vasopressin or antidiuretic hormone causes **diabetes insipidus,** a disease with **polyuria** (excessive amount of water secreted in the urine) and **polydipsia** (excessive and constant thirst). It can be treated with an antidiuretic medication. Hypersecretion of antidiuretic hormone causes **syndrome of inappropriate ADH (SIADH),** which results in excessive water retention. **Cushing's syndrome** results from an oversecretion of ACTH.

The thyroid gland may become overactive, causing **hyperthyroidism,** also known as **Graves' disease** or **thyrotoxicosis.** Hyperthyroidism is characterized by **exophthalmos,** bulging of the eyes. A **goiter** can also be caused by hypersecretion, a tumor, or lack of iodine in the diet, causing the gland to expand and create a massive growth in the neck. **Hypothyroidism,** underactivity of

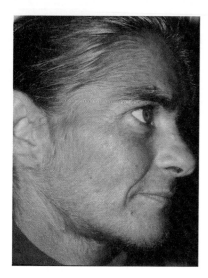

Figure 15-3 Excess androgen can cause hirsutism.

the thyroid gland, causes sluggishness and slow pulse, often resulting in obesity. **Myxedema** is a specific type of hypothyroidism in adults with a range of symptoms, including puffiness in the extremities, slow muscular response, and excessively dry skin. As with other types of hypothyroidism, myxedema can be treated with synthetic hormones. Fetal hypothyroidism may result in a form of dwarfism (once called *cretinism;* now referred to as *congenital hypothyroidism*) which results in small physical stature as well as slow mental development. If caught early enough, it can be treated with a synthetic form of thyroxine.

The parathyroid glands help control blood calcium levels, which contribute to bone growth and muscular health. **Hyperparathyroidism** (overactivity of the parathyroid glands) is usually caused by a tumor in the parathyroid gland. It often results in many clinical symptoms, from bone loss to severe cases of kidney failure. **Hypoparathyroidism** (underactivity of the parathyroid glands) results in low blood calcium levels, causing many symptoms such as bone loss and some muscle paralysis (**tetany**). Medications and supplements that increase calcium absorption are available treatments that may be prescribed.

The adrenal glands may be overactive (**hyperadrenalism**) or underactive (**hypoadrenalism**). Hyperadrenalism is usually caused by an adrenal tumor. It is usually cured by removal of the tumor. *Adrenogenital syndrome* results in symptoms of excessive androgens both in men and women, which, in turn, can result in **hirsutism,** abnormal hair growth (Figure 15-3). **Virilism** is also a condition with excessive androgen secretion. Virilism results in mature masculine features in children. Administration of steroids can keep the overactivity in balance. Hypoadrenalism is also known as **Addison's disease.** It may result in anemia, abnormal skin pigment, and general malaise. It can be controlled with cortisone.

Sometimes, the pancreas may become inflamed, as in **pancreatitis.** Hypersecretion of insulin may cause **hypoglycemia,** a lowering of blood sugar levels that deprives the body of needed glucose. It can be controlled with dietary changes. Hyposecretion of insulin can cause **diabetes mellitus,** a widespread disease that affects about 4 percent of the U.S. population. Diabetes occurs either as **Type I (insulin-dependent) diabetes** or as **Type II (noninsulin-dependent) diabetes.** Type I occurs in childhood and is the result of underproduction of insulin by the beta cells. Glucose accumulates and overflows into the urine (**glucosuria, glycosuria**). Type I diabetes can be treated with con-

MORE ABOUT...

Diabetes and Diet

For many years, doctors prescribed a high-protein, low-carbohydrate diet for diabetics. In recent years, increased understanding of how food is metabolized by the body has led to changes in diets prescribed for diabetics. Most newly diagnosed diabetics are given a varied diet by a physician or a dietitian tailored to their specific needs—current weight, level of diabetes (mild, moderate, severe), and lifestyle. The American Dietetic Association and the American Diabetes Association provide dietary information on which most diets for diabetics are based. A diabetic's personalized daily diet might include four fruit exchanges, three protein exchanges, three bread exchanges, and 7 vegetable exchanges. Many suppliers of processed food, particularly those foods aimed at the health-conscious consumer, now list exchanges as part of their nutrition labels as shown here.

Nutrition Facts	
Serving Size 1 cup (246g)	
Servings Per Container about 2	
Amount Per Serving	
Calories 100	Calories from Fat 5
	% Daily Value*
Total Fat 0.5g	1%
Saturated Fat 0g	0%
Cholesterol 0mg	0%
Sodium 430mg	18%
Total Carbohydrate 23g	8%
Dietary Fiber 2g	8%
Sugars 1g	
Protein	4g
Vitamin A 30% • Vitamin C 15%	
Calcium 4% • Iron 6%	
* Percent Daily Values are based on a 2,000 calorie diet	

DIETARY EXCHANGES PER SERVING:
1 Bread
1 Vegetable

Diet exchanges are based on Exchange Lists for Meal Planning, © 1989, the American Diabetes Assoc., Inc. and the American Dietetic Assoc.

trolled doses of insulin. Type II diabetes occurs in adulthood, usually in over-weight people whose responsiveness to insulin is abnormally low. This response is called *insulin resistance*. The complications of this type of diabetes cover a wide range of ailments from circulatory problems to infections to organ failure. **Diabetic nephropathy** is a kidney disease resulting from serious diabetes. **Diabetic neuropathy** is loss of sensation in the extremities. **Diabetic retinopathy** is gradual visual loss leading to blindness. The body uses stored fat to replace glucose, thereby causing **acidosis, ketoacidosis,** and **ketosis,** the abnormal presence of ketone bodies in the blood and urine. Mild Type II diabetes is controllable by exercise and diet. More severe cases need medication to control sensitivity to insulin or to add insulin to the body.

Cancers occur commonly in the endocrine system. Many, such as thyroid cancer, can be treated with removal of the affected gland and supplementation with a synthetic version of the necessary hormones that are then missing from the body. Some cancers, such as pancreatic cancer, are almost always fatal since no good treatments are available.

Researchers are now looking at how chromium, a mineral found in the body, affects blood sugar. Regulation of chromium may be a key to controlling blood sugar.

Before the discovery of insulin as a compound that affects blood sugar levels, people with diabetes usually died of some of the many complications of the disease. Diabetes is still not curable, just controllable.

Vocabulary Review

In the previous section you learned terms related to pathology. Before going on to the exercises, review the terms below and refer to the previous section if you have any questions.

Term	Word Analysis	Meaning
acidosis	[ăs-ĭ-DŌ-sĭs] acid + -osis, condition	Abnormal release of ketones in the body.
acromegaly	[ăk-rō-MĔG-ă-lē] acro-, extreme + -megaly, enlargement	Abnormally enlarged features resulting from a pituitary tumor and hypersecretion of growth hormone.
Addison's disease	[ĂD-ĭ-sŏnz] After Thomas Addison (1793–1860), English physician	Underactivity of the adrenal glands.
Cushing's syndrome	[KŬSH-ĭngs] After Harvey Cushing (1869–1939), U. S. neurosurgeon	Group of symptoms caused by overactivity of the adrenal glands.
diabetes	[dī-ă-BĒ-tēz] Greek, a siphon	*See* Type I diabetes, Type II diabetes.
diabetes insipidus	[ĬN-sĭp-ĭ-dŭs]	Condition caused by hyposecretion of antidiuretic hormone.
diabetes mellitus	[MĔL-ĭ-tŭs, mĕ-LĪ-tŭs]	*See* Type I diabetes, Type II diabetes.
diabetic nephropathy	[dī-ă-BĔT-ĭk nĕ-FRŎP-ă-thē]	Kidney disease due to diabetes.

Term	Word Analysis	Meaning
diabetic neuropathy	[nū-RŎP-ă-thē]	Loss of sensation in the extremities due to diabetes.
diabetic retinopathy	[rĕt-ĭ-NŎP-ă-thē]	Gradual loss of vision due to diabetes.
dwarfism	[DWŌRF-ĭzm] dwarf + -ism, state	Abnormally stunted growth caused by hyposecretion of growth hormone, congenital lack of a thyroid gland, or a genetic defect.
exophthalmos	[ĕk-sŏf-THĂL-mŏs] ex-, out of + Greek *ophthalmos*, eye	Abnormal protrusion of the eyes typical of Graves' disease.
gigantism	[JĪ-găn-tĭzm] Greek *gigas*, giant + -ism	Abnormally fast and large growth caused by hypersecretion of growth hormone.
glucosuria	[glū-kō-SŪ-rē-ă] gluco-, glucose + -uria, urine	Glucose in the urine.
glycosuria	[glī-kō-SŬ-rē-ă] glyco-, glycogen + -uria, urine	Glucose in the urine
goiter	[GŎY-tĕr] Latin *guttur*, throat	Abnormal enlargement of the thyroid gland as a result of its overactivity or lack of iodine in the diet.
Graves' disease	[grāvz] After Robert Graves (1796–1853), Irish physician	Overactivity of the thyroid gland.
hirsutism	[HĔR-sū-tĭzm] hirsut(e), hairy + -ism	Abnormal hair growth due to an excess of androgens.
hyperadrenalism	[HĪ-pĕr-ă-DRĔN-ă-lĭzm] hyper-, excessive + adrenal + -ism	Overactivity of the adrenal glands.
hyperparathyroidism	[HĪ-pĕr-pă-ră-THĪ-rŏyd-ĭzm] hyper- + parathyroid + -ism	Overactivity of the parathyroid glands.
hypersecretion	[HĪ-pĕr-sē-KRĒ-shŭn] hyper- + secretion	Abnormally high secretion, as from a gland.
hyperthyroidism	[hī-pĕr-THĪ-rŏyd-ĭzm] hyper- + thyroid + -ism	Overactivity of the thyroid gland.

Term	Word Analysis	Meaning
hypoadrenalism	[HĪ-pō-ă-DRĔN-ă-lĭzm] hypo-, below normal + adrenal + -ism	Underactivity of the adrenal glands.
hypoglycemia	[HĪ-pō-glī-SĒ-mē-ă] hypo- + glyc- + -emia	Abnormally low level of glucose in the blood.
hypoparathyroidism	[HĪ-pō-pă-ră-THĪ-rŏyd-ĭzm] hypo- + parathyroid + -ism	Underactivity of the parathyroid glands.
hyposecretion	[HĪ-pō-sē-KRĒ-shŭn] hypo- + secretion	Abnormally low secretion, as from a gland.
hypothyroidism	[HĪ-pō-THĪ-rŏyd-ĭzm] hypo- + thyroid + -ism	Underactivity of the thyroid gland.
insulin-dependent diabetes mellitus (IDDM)		*See* Type I diabetes.
ketoacidosis	[KĒ-tō-ă-sĭ-DŌ-sĭs] keto(ne) + acidosis	Condition of high acid levels caused by the abnormal release of ketones in the body.
ketosis	[kē-TŌ-sĭs] ket(one) + -osis, condition	Condition caused by the abnormal release of ketones in the body.
myxedema	[mĭk-sě-DĒ-mă] Greek *myxa*, mucus + edema	Advanced adult hypothyroidism.
noninsulin-dependent diabetes mellitus (NIDDM)		*See* Type II diabetes.
pancreatitis	[PĂN-krē-ă-TĪ-tĭs] pancreat-, pancreas + -itis, inflammation	Inflammation of the pancreas.
polydipsia	[pŏl-ē-DĬP-sē-ă] poly-, much + Greek *dipsa*, thirst	Excessive thirst.
polyuria	[pŏl-ē-YŪ-rē-ă] poly- + -uria	Excessive amount of water in the urine.
syndrome of inappropriate ADH (SIADH)		Excessive secretion of antidiuretic hormone.

Term	Word Analysis	Meaning
tetany	[TĔT-ă-nē] Greek *tetanos*, convulsive tension	Muscle paralysis, usually due to decreased levels of ionized calcium in the blood.
thyrotoxicosis	[THĪ-rō-tŏk-sĭ-KŌ-sĭs] thyro-, thyroid + toxic + -osis	Overactivity of the thyroid gland.
Type I diabetes		Endocrine disorder with abnormally low levels of insulin; also known as insulin-dependent diabetes mellitus (IDDM).
Type II diabetes		Disease caused by failure of the body to recognize insulin that is present or by an abnormally low level of insulin; also known as noninsulin-dependent diabetes mellitus (NIDDM); usually adult onset.
virilism	[VĬR-ĭ-lĭzm] Latin *virilis*, masculine	Condition with excessive androgen production, often resulting in the appearance of mature male characteristics in young children.

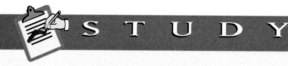

Getting a Diagnosis

Gail went for an appointment with an endocrinologist to work out a treatment plan for her diabetes. The specialist, Dr. Malpas, encouraged her to think that most patients in her condition can control diabetes with diet and exercise once the blood sugar is under control. Because Gail is overweight, Dr. Malpas suspects her body is not sensitive to insulin. He prescribes a medication to make her body more sensitive. He tells her to test her blood sugar with a prescribed measuring device. He also gives her a special diet.

 Critical Thinking

40. What type of diabetes does Gail appear to have?

41. What is special about Gail's diet?

Pathological Terms Exercises

Write A for adrenal, PA for pancreas, PI for pituitary, and T for thyroid to indicate the gland from which each of the following diseases arises.

42. acromegaly_____

43. diabetes mellitus_____

44. exophthalmos_____

45. gigantism_____

46. goiter_____

47. myxedema_____

48. Cushing's syndrome_____

49. Graves' disease_____

50. Addison's disease_____

51. dwarfism_____

52. cretinism_____

Surgical Terms

Certain endocrine glands that become diseased can be surgically removed. Synthetic versions of the hormones they produce are given to the patients to help their bodies perform the necessary endocrine functions once the glands are removed.

An **adenectomy** is the removal of any gland. An **adrenalectomy** is the removal of an adrenal gland. Removal of the pituitary gland is a **hypophysectomy.** The pancreas is removed in a **pancreatectomy.** Removal of the parathyroid gland is performed in a **parathyroidectomy,** and removal of the thymus gland is performed in a **thymectomy.** A **thyroidectomy** is the removal of the thyroid. Some of these operations may remove only the diseased part of a gland, leaving the remaining part to take over the endocrine function.

Vocabulary Review

In the previous section you learned terms related to surgery. Before going on to the exercises, review the terms below and refer to the previous section if you have any questions.

Term	Word Analysis	Meaning
adenectomy	[ă-dĕ-NĔK-tō-mĕ] aden-, gland + -ectomy, removal	Removal of a gland.
adrenalectomy	[ă-drē-năl-ĔK-tō-mē] adrenal + -ectomy	Removal of an adrenal gland.
hypophysectomy	[hī-pŏf-ĭ-SĔK-tō-mē] hypophys(is) + -ectomy	Removal of the pituitary gland.

Term	Word Analysis	Meaning
pancreatectomy	[PĂN-krē-ă-TĔK-tō-mē] pancreat-, pancreas + -ectomy	Removal of the pancreas.
parathyroidectomy	[PĂ-ră-thī-rŏy-DĔK-tō-mē] parathyroid + -ectomy	Removal of one or more of the parathyroid glands.
thymectomy	[thī-MĔK-tō-mē] thym(us) + -ectomy	Removal of the thymus gland.
thyroidectomy	[thī-rŏy-DĔK-tō-mē] thyroid + -ectomy	Removal of the thyroid.

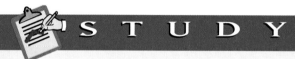

Controlling the Disease

Dr. Malpas is pleased that Gail is controlling her diabetes, losing weight slowly, and exercising regularly. Her outlook is favorable. Dr. Malpas has another patient, Will Burns, who has had an overactive thyroid since he was a child. Lately, Will's hyperthyroidism has increased. Dr. Malpas biopsies Will's thyroid and tells Will it would be best to remove the thyroid.

 Critical Thinking

53. What did Dr. Malpas probably find that necessitated thyroid removal?

54. What medications should Will be given after the operation?

Surgical Terms Exercises

Build Your Medical Vocabulary

Supply the missing part of the term:

55. removal of a gland: _____ectomy

56. removal of the pituitary gland: _____ectomy

57. removal of an adrenal gland: _____ectomy

58. removal of the thymus gland_____ectomy

59. removal of part of the pancreas: _____ectomy

60. removal of the thyroid gland: _____ectomy

61. removal of one or more of the parathyroid glands: _____ectomy

After completing the terms in items 55 through 61, use them to define the following treatments:

62. Treatment for Graves' disease: _____

63. Treatment for severe virilism:_____

64. Treatment for a cancerous gland: _____

65. Treatment for hyperparathyroidism: _____

66. Treatment for acromegaly: _____

Pharmacological Terms

Hormonal deficiencies are sometimes treated by **hormone replacement therapy (HRT).** Common types of hormone therapy include synthetic thyroid, estrogen, and testosterone. Other medications include those that regulate levels of substances in the body, such as glucose levels in diabetics. An **antihypoglycemic** raises blood sugar. An **antihyperglycemic** or **hypoglycemic** lowers blood sugar. Instead of or in addition to using drugs to regulate blood sugar, many diabetics are now treated with medications that increase their sensitivity to their own insulin. **Human growth hormone** occurs naturally in the body. In some cases of dwarfism, it is given to promote growth. **Steroids** are used in controlling symptoms and treating many diseases within and outside the endocrine system. Table 15-2 lists common pharmacological agents used in treating the endocrine system.

Many cancers of the endocrine system require removal and/or chemotherapy or radiation. A thyroid tumor may also be treated with **radioactive iodine therapy** to eradicate the tumor.

Women who are in perimenopause or menopause itself must weigh the risks of HRT (increased risk of cancer and clots in some studies) with the benefits (alleviation of symptoms, prevention of heart disease and osteoporosis).

Table 15-2 Agents Used in Treating the Endocrine System

Agent	Purpose	Generic	Trade Name
antihyperglycemic	to lower blood sugar	insulin chlorpropamide	Humulin, Novolin Diabinese
antihypoglycemic	to prevent or relieve severe hypoglycemia or insulin reaction	dextrose	Insta-Glucose, Glutose
human growth hormone	to increase height in cases of abnormal lack of growth	somatotropin	Humatrope, Protropin
steroid	to increase growth; to relieve symptoms of various diseases	methylprednisolone prednisone cortisone hydrocortisone	Medrol, Duralone Prednisolone, Predcor Cortone CaldeCort, Cortaid, Hydrocortone

Vocabulary Review

In the previous section you learned terms related to pharmacology. Before going on to the exercises, review the terms below and refer to the previous section if you have any questions.

Term	Word Analysis	Meaning
antihyperglycemic	[ĂN-tē-HĪ-pĕr-glĭ-SĒ-mĭk] anti-, against + hyperglycem(ia) + -ic, pertaining to	Agent that lowers blood glucose.
antihypoglycemic	[ĂN-tē-HĪ-pō-glĭ-SĒ-mĭk] anti- + hyperglycem(is) + -ic	Agent that raises blood glucose.
hormone replacement therapy (HRT)		Ingestion of hormones to replace missing or low levels of needed hormones.
human growth hormone		Naturally occurring substance in the body that promotes growth; synthesized substance that serves the same function.
hypoglycemic	[HĪ-pō-glĭ-SĒ-mĭk] hypoglycem(ia) + -ic	Agent that lowers blood glucose.
radioactive iodine therapy		Use of radioactive iodine to eliminate thyroid tumors.
steroid	[STĔR-ŏyd, STĒR-ŏyd] ster(ol), alcohol compound + -oid, like	A hormone or chemical substance released by several endocrine glands or manufactured in various medications.

C A S E S T U D Y

Learning the Outcome

Gail is beginning to feel symptoms of menopause, at the same time as her diabetes is diagnosed. Women in the late forties and throughout their fifties represent a large con- centration of newly diagnosed diabetics. Will has had his thyroid removed. Both Gail and Will need hormone replacement therapy.

 Critical Thinking

67. What hormones are likely to be prescribed for Gail?

68. What hormones are likely to be prescribed for Will?

Pharmacological Terms Exercises

Build Your Medical Vocabulary

In the space provided, write the name of the gland from which a hormone is needed to relieve symptoms of the disease.

69. Addison's disease _____

70. hyperglycemia _____

71. diabetes insipidus _____

72. myxedema _____

73. panhypopituitarism _____

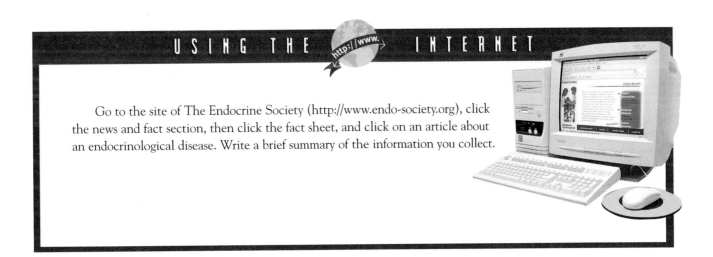

USING THE http://www. INTERNET

Go to the site of The Endocrine Society (http://www.endo-society.org), click the news and fact section, then click the fact sheet, and click on an article about an endocrinological disease. Write a brief summary of the information you collect.

The laboratory report shown here is for a woman on hormone replacement therapy who also takes thyroid medications.

Pathologist's Laboratory
West Lake Road
West Lake, CT 00008
555-678-8900

Patient Name: Sally Benedict	**Age/Sex:** 50/F	**Patient Number:** 41983
Requesting Physician: Jane Merdin, MD	**D.O.B.:** 10/28/50	
Source: 09/30/XXXX	**Collected:** 03-27-XXXX 0826	**Reported:** 03-28-XXXX 1649
Comments: Fasting 12 hrs. Thyroid & Hormone Meds.		**Operator:** _____ **Reviewed by:** _____

Test	Results	Normal Range	
		FEMALE (Adjusted For Age)	
CPK	66	24-170	IU/L
LDH	122	122-220	IU/L
SGOT (AST)	21	0-31	IU/L
SGPT (ALT)	28	0-31	IU/L
ALK PHOSPHATASE	54	39-117	IU/L
GGTP	21	7-33	IU/L
TOTAL BILIRUBIN	0.3	.0-1.0	MG/DL
URIC ACID	3.5	2.4-5.7	MG/DL
TRIGLYCERIDE	105	0-200	MG/DL
CHOLESTEROL	229	0-240	MG/DL
TRIG/CHOL RATIO	0.5		
GLUCOSE	103	70-105	MG/DL
BUN	14	5-23	MG/DL
CREATININE	1.0	.6-1.1	MG/DL
BUN/CREAT RATIO	14.0		
PHOSPHORUS	3.2	2.7-4.5	MG/DL
CALCIUM	8.1	8.7-10.4	MG/DL
TOTAL PROTEIN	6.7	6.5-8.0	GM/DL
ALBUMIN	4.2	3.5-5.5	GM/DL
GLOBULIN	2.5	2.2-4.2	GM/DL
A/G RATIO	1.7	1.2-2.2	
SODIUM	140	135-148	MEQ/L
POTASSIUM	4.0	3.5-5.3	MEQ/L
CHLORIDE	106	100-112	MEQ/L
IRON	79	40-145	UG/DL
**THYROID			
T UPTAKE	29.5	27.8-40.8	%
THYROXINE	7.5	4.5-13.0	UG/DL
F.T.I. (T7)	2.2	1.8-4.4	

74. From the results of the lab report, do you think the patient's thyroid medication is sufficient?

CHAPTER REVIEW

Definitions

Define the following terms and combining forms. Review the chapter before starting. Make sure you know how to pronounce each term as you define it.

Word	Definition
acidosis [ăs-ĭ-DŌ-sĭs]	
acromegaly [ăk-rō-MĔG-ă-lē]	
Adam's apple	
Addison's [ĂD-ĭ-sŏnz] disease	
aden(o)	
adenectomy [ă-dĕ-NĔK-tō-mĕ]	
adenohypophysis [ĂD-ē-nō-hī-PŎF-ĭ-sĭs]	
adren(o), adrenal(o)	
adrenal cortex [ă-DRĒ-năl KŌR-tĕks]	
adrenalectomy [ă-drē-năl-ĔK-tō-mē]	
adrenal gland	
adrenaline [ă-DRĔN-ă-lĭn]	
adrenal medulla [mĕ-DŪL-lă]	
adrenocorticotropic [ă-DRĒ-nō-KŌR-tĭ-kō-TRŌP-ĭk] hormone (ACTH)	
aldosterone [ăl-DŎS-tēr-ōn]	
alpha cells	
androgen [ĂN-drō-jĕn]	
antidiuretic [ĂN-tē-dī-yū-RĔT-ĭk] hormone (ADH)	
antihyperglycemic [ĂN-tē-HĪ-pĕr-glī-SĒ-mĭk]	
antihypoglycemic [ĂN-tē-HĪ-pō-glī-SĒ-mĭk]	
beta cells	
blood sugar, blood glucose	
calcitonin [kăl-sĭ-TŌ-nĭn]	

Word	Definition
catecholamines [kăt-ĕ-KŌL-ă-mēnz]	
corticosteroids [KŌR-tĭ-kō-STĒR-ŏydz]	
cortisol [KŌR-tĭ-sōl]	
Cushing's [KŬSH-ĭngs] syndrome	
diabetes [dī-ă-BĒ-tēz]	
diabetes insipidus [ĬN-sĭp-ĭ-dŭs]	
diabetes mellitus [MĔL-ĭ-tŭs, mĕ-LĪ-tŭs]	
diabetic nephropathy [dī-ă-BĔT-ĭk nĕ-FRŎP-ă-thē]	
diabetic neuropathy [nū-RŎP-ă-thē]	
diabetic retinopathy [rĕt-ĭ-NŎP-ă-thē]	
ductless gland	
dwarfism [DWŎRF-ĭzm]	
electrolyte [ē-LĔK-trō-līt]	
endocrine [ĔN-dō-krĭn] gland	
epinephrine [ĔP-ĭ-NĔF-rĭn]	
exocrine [ĔK-sō-krĭn] gland	
exophthalmos [ĕk-sŏf-THĂL-mŏs]	
fasting blood sugar	
follicle-stimulating hormone (FSH)	
gigantism [JĪ-găn-tĭzm]	
gland	
gluc(o)	
glucagon [GLŪ-kă-gŏn]	
glucocorticoid [glū-kō-KŌR-tĭ-kŏyd]	
glucose tolerance test (GTT)	
glucosuria [glū-kō-SŪ-rē-ă]	
glyc(o)	
glycogen [GLĪ-kō-jĕn]	
glycosuria [glī-kō-SŪ-rē-ă]	
goiter [GŎY-tĕr]	
gonad(o)	
Graves' [grāvz] disease	
growth hormone (GH)	
hirsutism [HĬR-sū-tĭzm]	

Word	Definition
hormone [HŌR-mōn]	
hormone replacement therapy (HRT)	
human growth hormone (HCG)	
hyperadrenalism [HĪ-pĕr-ă-DRĔN-ă-lĭzm]	
hyperparathyroidism [HĪ-pĕr-pă-ră-THĪ-rŏyd-ĭzm]	
hypersecretion [HĪ-pĕr-sē-KRĒ-shŭn]	
hyperthyroidism [hī-pĕr-THĪ-rŏyd-ĭzm]	
hypoadrenalism HĪ-pō-ă-DRĔN-ă-lĭzm]	
hypoglycemia [HĪ-pō-glī-SĒ-mē-ă]	
hypoglycemic [HĪ-pō-glī-SĒ-mĭk]	
hypoparathyroidism [hī-pō-pă-ră-THĪ-rŏyd-ĭzm]	
hypophysectomy [HĪ-pŏf-ĭ-SĔK-tō-mē]	
hypophysis [hī-PŎF-ĭ-sĭs]	
hyposecretion [HĪ-pō-sē-KRĒ-shŭn]	
hypothalamus [HĪ-pō-THĂL-ă-mŭs]	
hypothyroidism [HĪ-pō-THĪ-rŏyd-ĭzm]	
inhibiting	
insulin [ĬN-sū-lĭn]	
insulin-dependent diabetes mellitus (IDDM)	
islets of Langerhans [LĂN-gĕr-hănz]	
isthmus [ĬS-mŭs]	
ketoacidosis [KĒ-tō-ă-sĭ-DŌ-sĭs]	
ketosis [kē-TŌ-sĭs]	
luteinizing [LŬ-tē-ĭn-ĪZ-ĭng] hormone (LH)	
melanocyte-stimulating hormone (MSH)	
melatonin [mĕl-ă-TŌN-ĭn]	
mineralocorticoid [MĬN-ĕr-ăl-ō-KŌR-tĭ-kŏyd]	
myxedema [mĭk-sĕ-DĒ-mă]	
neurohypophysis [NŪR-ō-hī-PŎF-ĭ-sĭs]	

Word	Definition
noninsulin-dependent diabetes mellitus (NIDDM)	
norepinephrine [NŌR-ĕp-ĭ-NĔF-rĭn]	
ovary [Ō-vār-ē]	
oxytocin [ŏk-sĭ-TŌ-sĭn]	
pancreas [PĂN-krē-ăs]	
pancreat(o)	
pancreatectomy [PĂN-krē-ă-TĔK-tō-mē]	
pancreatitis [PĂN-krē-ă-TĪ-tĭs]	
parathormone [păr-ă-THŌR-mōn] (PTH)	
parathyroid(o)	
parathyroidectomy [PĂ-ră-thī-rŏy-DĔK-tō-mē]	
parathyroid [păr-ă-THĪ-rŏyd] gland	
parathyroid hormone	
pineal [PĬN-ē-ăl] gland	
pituitary [pĭ-TŪ-ĭ-tār-ē] gland	
polydipsia [pŏl-ē-DĬP-sē-ă]	
polyuria [pŏl-ē-YŪ-rē-ă]	
postprandial blood sugar	
radioactive immunoassay (RIA)	
radioactive iodine therapy	
radioactive iodine uptake	
receptor [rē-SĔP-tōr]	
releasing	
somatotrophic [SŌ-mă-tō-TRŌF-ĭk] hormone (STH)	
steroid [STĔR-ŏyd, STĒR-ŏyd]	
suprarenal [SŪ-pră-RĒ-năl] gland	
sympathomimetic [SĬM-pă-thō-mĭ-MĔT-ĭk]	
syndrome of inappropriate ADH (SIADH)	
target cell	
testis [TĔS-tĭs], testicle [TĔS-tĭ-kl]	

Word	Definition
tetany [TĔT-ă-nē]	_____
thymectomy [thĭ-MĔK-tō-mē]	_____
thymus [THĬ-mŭs] gland	_____
thyr(o), thyroid(o)	_____
thyroidectomy [thĭ-rŏy-DĔK-tō-mē]	_____
thyroid function test or study	_____
thyroid [THĬ-rŏyd] gland	_____
thyroid scan	_____
thyroid-stimulating hormone (TSH)	_____
thyrotoxicosis [THĬ-rō-tŏk-sĭ-KŌ-sĭs]	_____
thyroxine [thĭ-TRŎK-sēn, -sĭn] (T_4)	_____
triiodothyronine [trī-Ī-ō-dō-THĬ-rō-nēn] (T_3)	_____
Type I diabetes	_____
Type II diabetes	_____
urine sugar	_____
vasopressin [vā-sō-PRĔS-ĭn]	_____
virilism [VĬR-ĭ-lĭzm]	_____

Abbreviations

Write the full meaning of each abbreviation.

Abbreviation	Meaning
ACTH	_____
ADH	_____
CRH	_____
DM	_____
FSH	_____
GH	_____
GTT	_____
HCG	_____
IDDM	_____
LH	_____
MSH	_____
NIDDM	_____

Abbreviation	Meaning
PRL	
PTH	
STH	
TSH	

1. to eliminate various diseases and to test for others
2. possibly yes, if her symptoms are serious enough
3. melatonin
4. epinephrine
5. ADH
6. oxytocin
7. insulin
8. prolactin
9. aldosterone
10. thyroxine
11. testosterone
12. thymosin
13. C
14. adrenal
15. hypophysis
16. suprarenal
17. C
18. pituitary
19. luteinizing
20. C
21. yes, sodium
22. endocrine
23. adenitis
24. pancreatopathy
25. glycogenesis
26. thyromegaly
27. euthyroid
28. removal of an adrenal gland
29. removal of part of the pancreas
30. glandular tumor
31. aid in sex cell development
32. abnormally large thyroid
33. diabetes
34. postparandial blood sugar
35. D
36. T
37. T
38. D
39. D
40. Type II
41. food exchanges and exact quantities
42. PI
43. PA
44. T
45. PI
46. T
47. T
48. A
49. T
50. A
51. PI
52. T
53. cancer
54. thyroid hormones
55. adenectomy
56. hypophysectomy
57. adrenalectomy
58. thymectomy
59. pancreatectomy
60. thyroidectomy
61. parathyroidectomy
62. thyroidectomy
63. adrenalectomy
64. adenectomy
65. parathyroidectomy
66. hypophysectomy
67. estrogen, progesterone
68. thyroxine, triiodothyronine
69. adrenal
70. pancreas
71. pituitary
72. thyroid
73. pituitary
74. Yes, thyroxine and thyroid uptake are normal.

CHAPTER 16

The Sensory System

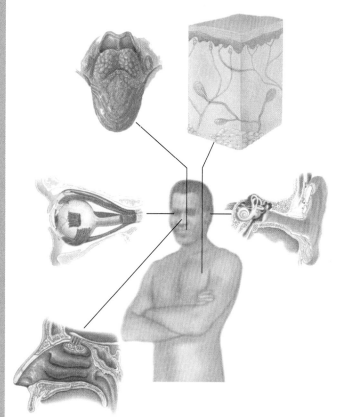

After studying this chapter, you will be able to:

- Name the parts of the sensory system and discuss the function of each part

- Define combining forms used in building words that relate to the sensory system

- Identify the meaning of related abbreviations

- Name the common diagnoses, clinical procedures, and laboratory tests used in treating disorders of the sensory system

- List and define the major pathological conditions of the sensory system

- Explain the meaning of surgical terms related to the sensory system

- Recognize common pharmacological agents used in treating disorders of the sensory system

Structure and Function

The **sensory system** includes any organ or part involved in the perceiving and receiving of stimuli from the outside world and from within our bodies. Aristotle, a Greek philosopher who lived more than 2000 years ago, identified the five senses—**sight, touch, hearing, smell,** and **taste.** These senses are popularly thought of as the sensory system even though most of the senses are based on stimulation of nerves in the nervous system. While all five are the basic senses of the body and the main structures for reacting to environmental stimuli, there are other ways in which our bodies "sense" and react to stimuli. For example, the islets of Langherhans sense high blood sugar and are stimulated to release insulin. This is but one example of a type of sense response in the body; however, the major parts of the sensory system relate specifically to the organs of the five senses and related senses felt by those organs. Figure 16-1a shows the major organs of the sensory system. Figure 16-1b charts the location in the body where stimuli are sensed.

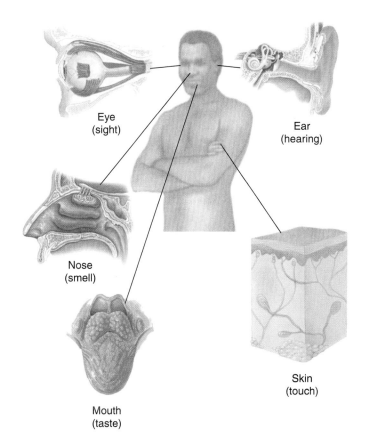

Sense		Sensory Organ
Sight	⟶	Eyes
Touch	⟶	Skin
Hearing	⟶	Ears
Smell	⟶	Nose
Taste	⟶	Mouth

Figure 16-1b The locations where stimuli are sensed.

Eye (sight)

Ear (hearing)

Nose (smell)

Skin (touch)

Mouth (taste)

Figure 16-1a The sensory system includes organs of the five senses.

Sensory organs are also known as **sensory receptors.** All sensory receptors contain specialized receptor cells that are able to receive stimuli. They are designed to receive only certain stimuli (such as sound in the ear and light waves in the eye). Sensory receptor cells send impulses to the afferent (conductive) nerves in the central nervous system to interpret the stimuli.

Sight—the Eye

The **eyes,** organs of sight, contain about 70 percent of all the receptors in the human body. Each eye is a sphere with an outer layer, a middle layer, and an inner layer. The outer layer is covered by the **eyelid.** The anterior surface of the eye and the posterior surface of the eyelid are lined with a mucous membrane (the **conjunctiva**).

The smooth, firm, white posterior section called the **sclera** is made of a thick, tough membrane. The sclera supports the eyeball. The **cornea** is the transparent, anterior section which is the first place where light is bent or refracted as it enters the eye. The sclera is white and has blood vessels that nourish the cornea (which has no blood supply). The cornea is transparent, has no blood vessels, and bends (or refracts) light rays in a process called **refraction.**

The middle layer is the vascular layer of blood vessels, consisting of a thin posterior membrane, the **choroid.** Anteriorly, this is continuous with the **ciliary body,** which contains the ciliary muscles, used for focusing the eyes. Vision is the process that begins when light is refracted as it hits the cornea and again when it hits the *retina.* Light passes through the **pupil,** the black circular center of the eye, then passes through the **lens,** a colorless, flexible transparent body behind the **iris,** the colored part of the eye that expands and contracts in response to light, thereby opening and closing the pupil. From there it goes to the lens, which is suspended by ligaments that extend to the ciliary body. The ciliary body contracts to change the shape of the lens in a process called *accommodation.* Accommodation allows the eye to focus on objects at varying distances. This region of the eye which includes the iris, ciliary body, and choroid is known as the **uvea.**

The interior layer of the eye is called the *retinal layer.* It contains a light sensitive membrane, the **retina,** that can decode the light waves and send the information on to the brain, which interprets what we see. The retina itself has many layers. The thick layer of nervous tissue is called the **neuroretina.** The neuroretina consists of specialized nerve receptor cells called **rods,** sensors of black and white shades, and **cones,** sensors of color and the brightest light. There are three types of cones, one each for red, green, and blue. There are approximately 125 million rods and 7 million cones in each eye, along with other nerve cells, that convert the light images received to nerve impulses that are then transmitted through the **optic nerve** to the appropriate lobes of the brain. The region where the retina connects to the optic nerve is called the *optic disk,* an area where there are no rods or cones to receive images, which is called the *blind spot.* Light causes a chemical change in the rods and cones that allows them to convert the images to nerve impulses. The thin layer of the retina is made of pigmented epithelial tissue, which, along with the choroid, absorbs stray light that is not absorbed by the neuroretina and prevents reflections from the back of the retina. The center of the retina directly behind the lens has a small yellowish area called the **macula lutea,** which has a depression in the center called the **fovea centralis,** the area of sharpest vision.

The eyeball is divided into three cavities called *chambers.* The *anterior chamber* lies between the cornea and iris. The *posterior chamber* lies between the iris and the lens. Both the anterior and posterior chambers are filled with *aqueous humor,* a thin, watery liquid that provides nourishment to the lens and cornea and maintains a constant pressure within the eyeball. The tissue that holds the aqueous humor in until it exits the eye is made up of *trabeculae,* bundles of supportive fiber. The *vitreous chamber,* located posterior to the lens, occupies about 80 percent of the space in the eyeball. It is filled with *vitreous humor,* a gelatinous substance that nourishes parts of the eyes and maintains a supportive structure to keep the eye from collapsing.

Several other structures are important to the eye. The eyelids close to protect the eyes or to allow rest and sleep. The **eyebrows** and **eyelashes** help keep foreign particles from entering the eye. The **lacrimal glands** secrete moisture into the *lacrimal ducts*

MORE ABOUT...

Eye Color

Newborns with light skin are almost always born with blue eyes, even though their eyes may later turn brown or green. Eye color is determined by heredity. It takes several months for the melanocytes to be distributed to the anterior portion of the eye. Babies with darker skin normally have a higher concentration of melanocytes to begin with, and their eyes at birth are almost always dark. Albinos are born with no melanocytes in their body and they are, therefore, much more sensitive to light and have no pigment in the iris of their eyes.

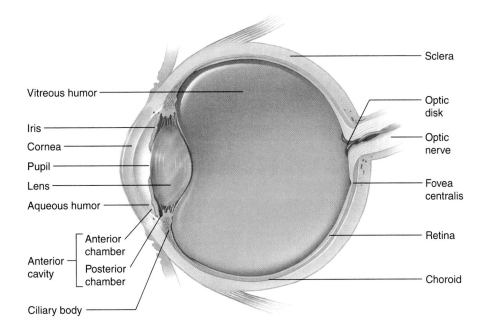

Vitreous humor	Sclera
Iris	Optic disk
Cornea	Optic nerve
Pupil	
Lens	Fovea centralis
Aqueous humor	
Anterior chamber	Retina
Anterior cavity — Posterior chamber	Choroid
Ciliary body	

Figure 16-2 The eye is the organ of sight.

or *tear ducts*. The resulting **tears** moisten the eyes, wash foreign particles off the eye, and distribute water and nutrients to parts of the eye. Tears may be secreted more heavily than necessary as a reaction to allergies, infections, or emotional upset. Figure 16-2 shows the eye.

Hearing and Equilibrium—the Ear

The **ear** is an organ of hearing and **equilibrium** (balance). The three major divisions of the ear are the *external ear*, the *middle ear*, and the *inner ear*. The external ear begins on the outside of the head with a funnel-like structure called the **auricle** or **pinna.** This structure leads through part of the skull known as the *temporal bone* (which itself has a bony projection called the *mastoid process*) to an s-shaped tube called the *external auditory meatus*. The external auditory meatus contains glands that secrete *cerumen* or ear wax, a brownish yellow, waxy substance.

Next, the middle ear includes the *tympanic cavity*, in which sits the **eardrum (tympanic membrane)** and the **auditory ossicles,** three small, specially shaped bones. The eardrum is an oval, semitransparent membrane with skin on its outer surface and a mucous membrane on the inside. Sound waves change the pressure on the eardrum, which moves back and forth, thereby producing vibrations. The three ossicles are the **malleus** (hammer), **incus** (anvil), and **stapes** (stirrup). They are all attached to the tympanic cavity by tiny ligaments. The malleus is attached to the eardrum to help it maintain its oval and conic shape. Vibrations are carried from the eardrum through the malleus to the incus. The incus passes the movement onto the stapes, which is connected to the wall near the *oval window,* an opening leading to the inner ear. The middle ear is connected to the pharynx through the **eustachian tube** (*auditory tube*). This

MORE ABOUT...

Ears

Driving down a mountain sometimes causes you to feel and hear a popping sound. The eustachian tubes react quickly to equalize the pressure caused by exposure to a high altitude when the eardrum membrane is stretched. The eardrum "pops" back into place when pressure is equalized.

tube helps equalize air pressure on both sides of the eardrum, which is essential to hearing.

The inner ear is a system of two tubes—the **osseus labyrinth** and the **membranous labyrinth.** The osseus labyrinth is a bony canal in the temporal bone. The membranous labyrinth is a tube within the osseus labyrinth and separated from it by **perilymph,** a liquid secreted by the walls of the osseus labyrinth. Inside the membranous labyrinth is another fluid, **endolymph.** The labyrinths include three **semicircular canals,** structures important to equilibrium, and a **cochlea,** a snail-shaped structure important to hearing. The cochlea is further divided into the *scala vestibuli*, which leads from the oval window to the apex of the cochlea, and the *scala tympani*, which leads from the apex of the cochlea to a covered opening in the inner ear called the *round window*. The cochlea has a membrane called the *basilar membrane* that has hairlike receptor cells located in the **organ of Corti** on the membrane's surface. The hairs move back and forth in response to sound waves and eventually send messages via neurotransmitters through the eighth cranial nerve and to the brain for interpretation. Table 16-1 shows various **decibel** (intensity of sound) levels that can be heard by a normal human ear. The scale of decibels gives the intensity of sound in progressions multiplied by 10. So 10dB is 10 times greater than the lowest perceptible decibel, 20dB is 100 times as great as 10dB, and so on. The easy availability of electronic equipment and the sound generated by modern machines have raised the decibel levels to which each successive generation is exposed.

Table 16-1 Decibel Levels

Decibel Level	Intensity of Sound	Effect on Hearing
40dB	10,000 times as great as 10dB	A whisper—perceptible to most people with normal hearing
60dB	1 million times as great as 10dB	Regular conversational speech
80dB	100 million times as great as 10dB	High noise such as in a crowded room or heavy traffic
130dB	10 trillion times as great as 10dB	Extremely loud rock concert; can cause ear damage.
140dB	100 trillion times as great as 10dB	Sound of a jet engine on takeoff. Hearing can be damaged.

MORE ABOUT...

Equilibrium

Motion sickness in a vehicle or airplane is the result of many sudden changes in body motion that occur when the organs of equilibrium are disrupted. People experience motion sickness at different rates. Some medications relieve the feelings of dizziness and nausea that accompany motion sickness.

The sense of equilibrium is the ability to maintain steady balance either when still, *static equilibrium*, or when moving, *dynamic equilibrium*. The bony chamber between the semicircular canal and the cochlea is called the **vestibule.** The vestibule contains a membranous labyrinth divided into two chambers, the *utricle* and *saccule*. Both of these chambers contain a

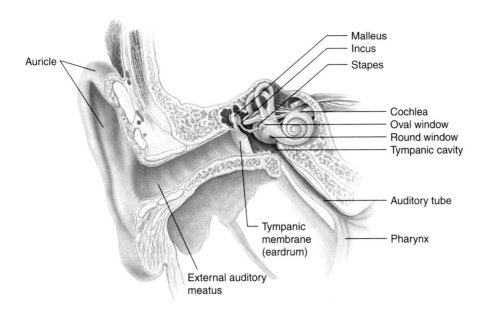

Auricle

Malleus
Incus
Stapes

Cochlea
Oval window
Round window
Tympanic cavity

Auditory tube

Pharynx

Tympanic membrane (eardrum)

External auditory meatus

Figure 16-3 The ear is the organ of hearing.

macula, a structure with many hairlike sensory receptors that move forward, backward, or upward to move the gelatinous mass inside the inner ear. This mass contains **otoliths,** small calcifications that move to maintain gravitational balance. The semicircular canals also respond to movement and aid in maintaining balance. Figure 16-3 illustrates the structures of the ear.

Touch, Pain, and Temperature—the Skin

The skin's layers sense different intensities of touch. Light touch is felt in the top layer of skin, whereas touch with harder pressure is felt in the middle or bottom layer. The skin's receptors can sense touch, pressure, pain, and hot and cold temperatures. The skin also has pain receptors that sense any injury to skin tissue.

Smell—the Nose

The sense of smell or *olfactory stimulation* is activated by *olfactory receptors* located at the top of the nasal cavity. The olfactory receptors are neurons covered with cilia that send smell messages to the brain. The receptors are located within the **olfactory organs,** yellowish-brown masses along the top of the nasal cavity. For the sense of smell to sense an object, the object must be dissolved in a liquid in the olfactory organs. The sense of smell is closely related to the sense of taste.

Taste—the Tongue and Oral Cavity

Taste buds are organs that sense the taste of food. Most taste buds are on the surface of the tongue in small raised structures called **papillae,** but some also line the roof of the mouth and the walls of the pharynx. Each taste bud contains receptor cells,

MORE ABOUT...

Skin

One of the remarkable advances in genetic engineering is the ability to grow replacement skin. The new skin is grown from cells of skin from various parts of the body and can be used to replace burned or injured areas. If the skin is working once it is put in place, it will continue to grow and function like normal skin—helping to regulate body temperature, preventing foreign material from entering the body, and protecting inner organs from bruises.

The ability to taste is affected by conditions, such as colds or inflammations of the mouth. Smoking lessens the ability to taste.

called **taste cells.** Nerve fibers wrapped around the taste cells transmit impulses to the brain. The taste buds are activated when the item being tasted dissolves in the watery fluid surrounding the taste buds. The salivary glands secrete this fluid. There are at least four types of taste buds to match the primary taste sensations—sweet, sour, salty, and bitter. Different sections of the tongue contain concentrations of receptors for each of the taste sensations. There are also receptors that sense the texture, odor, and temperature of food. In the case of food that is too hot, too spicy, or too cold, some pain receptors are activated.

Vocabulary Review

In the previous section, you learned terms relating to the sensory system. Before going on to the exercises, review the terms below and refer to the previous section if you have any questions.

Term	Word Analysis	Meaning
auditory ossicles	[ĂW-dĭ-tōr-ē ŎS-ĭ-klz]	Three specially shaped bones in the middle ear that anchor the eardrum to the tympanic cavity and that transmit vibrations to the inner ear.
auricle	[ĂW-rĭ-kl] From Latin *auris*, ear	Funnel-like structure leading from the external ear to the external auditory meatus; also called pinna.
choroid	[KŌ-rŏyd] Greek *chorioeides*, like a membrane	Thin posterior membrane in the middle layer of the eye.
ciliary body	[SĬL-ē-ăr-ē]	Thick anterior membrane in the middle layer of the eye.
cochlea	[KŌK-lē-ă] Latin, snail shell	Snail-shaped structure in the inner ear that contains the organ of Corti.
cones	[kōnz]	Specialized receptor cells in the retina that perceive color and bright light.
conjunctiva (pl. conjunctivae)	[kŏn-JŬNK-tĭ-vă (-vē)] From Latin *conjungo*, to join together	Mucous membrane lining the eyelid.
cornea	[KŌR-nē-ă] Latin, like a horn	Transparent anterior section of the eyeball that bends light in a process called refraction.
decibel	[DĔS-ĭ-bĕl] Latin *decimus*, tenth + bel, sound	Measure of the intensity of sound.
ear	[ēr] Old English eare	Organ of hearing.

Term	Word Analysis	Meaning
eardrum	[ĔR-drŭm] ear + drum	Oval, semitransparent membrane that moves in response to sound waves and produces vibrations.
endolymph	[ĔN-dō-lĭmf] endo-, within + lymph	Fluid inside the membranous labyrinth important to hearing and equilibrium.
equilibrium	[ē-kwĭ-LĬB-rē-ŭm] Latin *aequilibrium*, horizontal position	Sense of balance.
eustachian tube	[yū-STĀ-shŭn, yū-STĀ-kē-ăn] After Bartolommeo Eustachio (1524–1574), Italian anatomist	Tube that connects the middle ear to the pharynx.
eye	[ī] Old English eage	Organ of sight.
eyebrow	[Ī-brŏw] eye + brow	Clump of hair, usually about ½-inch above the eye, that helps to keep foreign particles from entering the eye.
eyelashes	[Ī-lăsh-ĕz] eye + lashes	Group of hairs protruding from the end of the eyelid; helps to keep foreign particles from entering the eye.
eyelid	[Ī-lĭd] eye + lid	Moveable covering over the eye.
fovea centralis	[FŌ-vē-ă sĕn-TRĂL-ĭs]	Depression in the center of the macula lutea; perceives sharpest images.
hearing		Ability to perceive sound.
incus	[ĬN-kŭs] Latin, anvil	One of the three auditory ossicles; the anvil.
iris	[Ī-rĭs] Greek, iris, rainbow	Colored part of the eye that contains muscles that expand and contract in response to light.
lacrimal glands	[LĂK-rĭ-măl]	Glands that secrete liquid to moisten the eyes and produce tears.
lens	[lĕnz] Latin, lentil	Colorless, flexible transparent body behind the iris.
macula	[MĂK-yū-lă] Latin, spot	Inner ear structure containing hairlike sensors that move to maintain equilibrium.

Term	Word Analysis	Meaning
macula lutea	[lū-TĒ-ă]	Small, yellowish area located in the center of the retina, which has a depression called the fovea centralis.
malleus	[MĂL-ē-ŭs] Latin, hammer	One of the three auditory ossicles; the hammer.
membranous labyrinth		One of the two tubes that make up the semicircular canals.
neuroretina	[nūr-ō-RĔT-ĭ-nă] neuro-, nerve + retina	Thick layer of nervous tissue in the retina.
olfactory organs	[ōl-FĂK-tō-rē]	Organs at the top of the nasal cavity containing olfactory receptors.
optic nerve		Nerve that transmits nerve impulses from the eye to the brain.
organ of Corti	[KŌR-tī]	Structure on the basilar membrane with hairlike receptors that receive and transmit sound waves.
osseus labyrinth	[ŎS-sē-ŭs]	One of the two tubes that make up the semicircular canals.
otoliths	[Ō-tō-lĭthz] oto-, ear + -lith, stone	Small calcifications in the inner ear that help to maintain balance.
papillae	[pă-PĬL-ē] Latin papilla, small pimple	Small, raised structures that contain the taste buds.
perilymph	[PĔR-ĭ-lĭmf] peri-, around + lymph	Liquid secreted by the walls of the osseus labyrinth.
pinna	[PĬN-ă] Latin, feather	Auricle.
pupil	[PYŪ-pĭl] Latin pupilla	Black circular center of the eye; opens and closes when muscles in the iris expand and contract in response to light.
refraction	[rē-FRĂK-shŭn] From Latin refractus, broken up	Process of bending light rays.
retina	[RĔT-ĭ-nă]	Oval, light-sensitive membrane in the interior layer of the eye; decodes light waves and transmits information to the brain.
rods	[rŏdz]	Specialized receptor cells in the retina that perceive black to white shades.

Term	Word Analysis	Meaning
sclera (pl. sclerae)	[SKLĒR-ă (-ē)] Greek *skleros*, hard	Thick, tough membrane in the outer eye layer; supports eyeball structure.
semicircular canals		Structures in the inner ear important to equilibrium.
sensory receptors		Specialized tissue containing cells that can receive stimuli.
sensory system		Organs or tissue that perceive and receive stimuli from outside or within the body.
sight		Ability to see.
smell		Ability to perceive odors.
stapes (pl. stapes, stapedes)	[STĀ-pēz (STĀ-pĕ-dēz)]	One of the three auditory ossicles; the stirrup.
taste		Ability to perceive the qualities of ingested matter.
taste buds		Organs that sense the taste of food.
taste cells		Specialized receptor cells within the taste buds.
tears		Moisture secreted from the lacrimal glands.
touch		Ability to perceive pressure on the skin.
tympanic membrane	[tĭm-PĂN-ĭk]	Eardrum.
uvea	[YŪ-vē-ă] Latin *uva*, grape	Region of the eye containing the iris, choroid membrane, and ciliary bodies.
vestibule	[VĔS-tĭ-būl] Latin *vestibulum*, space	Bony chamber between the semicircular canal and the cochlea.

C A S E   S T U D Y

Checking Symptoms

John James, a 67-year-old male, presented at his family doctor's office very nervous and upset. His general health is excellent and, although he was widowed one year ago, he is proud of the way he has maintained his independence. His only complaint is diminished vision. He says his night vision is so bad that he has given up night driving. His family doctor gives him a general physical including laboratory tests. All of the test results prove normal. Mr. James is then referred to an ophthalmologist (eye specialist).

 Critical Thinking

1. In addition to the general physical, why did the family doctor refer Mr. James to an ophthalmologist?

2. Why is a general physical necessary?

Structure and Function Exercises

Find a Match

Match the terms in the left-hand column with the definitions in the right-hand column.

3. iris

a. tough, white, outer coating of eyeball

4. sclera

b. dark opening of the eye, surrounded by the iris

5. pupil

c. ear wax

6. optic disc

d. hammer

7. eustachian

e. eardrum

8. incus

f. anvil

9. malleus

g. stirrup

10. stapes

h. auditory tube

11. tympanic membrane

i. pinna

12. auricle

j. blind spot of the eye

13. cerumen

k. colored portion of the eye

Check Your Knowledge

Circle T for true or F for false.

14. The aqueous humor is a thick, gelatinous substance. T F

15. The sharpest images are perceived in the optic disk. T F

16. Rods and cones are receptor cells that sense light and color. T F

17. Olfactory receptors perceive light rays. T F

18. Semicircular canals in the ears are important to equilibrium. T F

19. Refraction is the focusing on distant objects. T F

20. The papillae house the taste buds. T F

Combining Forms and Abbreviations

The lists below include combining forms and abbreviations that relate specifically to the sensory system. Pronunciations are provided for the examples.

Combining Form	Meaning	Example
audi(o), audit(o)	hearing	*audiometer* [ăw-dē-ŎM-ĕ-tĕr], instrument for measuring hearing
aur(o), auricul(o)	hearing	*auriculocranial* [ăw-RĬK-yū-lō-KRĀ-nē-ăl], pertaining to the auricle of the ear and the cranium
blephar(o)	eyelid	*blepharitis* [blĕf-ă-RĪ-tĭs], inflammation of the eyelid
cerumin(o)	wax	*ceruminolytic* [sĕ-rū-mĭ-nō-LĬT-ĭk], agent for softening ear wax
cochle(o)	cochlea	*cochleovestibular* [kōk-lē-ō-vĕs-TĬB-yū-lăr], pertaining to the cochlea and the vestibule of the ear
conjunctiv(o)	conjunctiva	*conjunctivoplasty* [kŏn-JŬNK-tĭ-vō-plăs-tē], plastic surgery on the conjunctiva
cor(o), core(o)	pupil	*coreoplasty* [KŌR-ē-ō-plăs-tē], surgical correction of the size and shape of a pupil
corne(o)	cornea	*corneoscleral* [kōr-nē-ō-SKLĔR-ăl], pertaining to the cornea and sclera
cycl(o)	ciliary body	*cyclodialysis* [sī-klō-dī-ĂL-ĭ-sĭs], method of relieving introcular pressure in glaucoma
dacry(o)	tears	*dacryolith* [DĂK-rē-ō-lĭth], calculus in the tear duct
ir(o), irid(o)	iris	*iridoptosis* [ĭr-ĭ-dŏp-TŌ-sĭs], prolapse of the iris
kerat(o)	cornea	*keratoconus* [kĕr-ă-tō-KŌ-nŭs], abnormal protrusion of the cornea
lacrim(o)	tears	*lacrimotomy* [LĂK-rĭ-mă-tō-mē], incision into the lacrimal duct
mastoid(o)	mastoid process	*mastoiditis* [măs-tŏy-DĪ-tĭs], inflammation of the mastoid process
myring(o)	eardrum, middle ear	*myringitis* [mĭr-ĭn-JĪ-tĭs], inflammation of the tympanic membrane
nas(o)	nose	*nasosinusitis* [nās-zō-sĭ-nŭ-SĪ-tĭs], inflammation of the nasal and sinus cavities
ocul(o)	eye	*oculodynia* [ŏk-yū-lō-DĬN-ē-ă], pain in the eyeball
ophthalm(o)	eye	*ophthalmoscope* [ŏf-THĂL-mō-skōp], instrument for studying the interior of the eyeball

Combining Form	Meaning	Example
opt(o), optic(o)	eye	*optometer* [ŏp-TŎM-ĕ-tĕr], instrument for determining eye refraction
ossicul(o)	ossicle	*ossiculectomy* [ŎS-ĭ-kyū-LĔK-tō-mē], removal of one of the ossicles of the middle ear
phac(o), phak(o)	lens	*phacoma* [fā-KŌ-mă], tumor of the lens
pupill(o)	pupil	*pupillometer* [pyū-pĭ-LŎM-ĕ-tĕr], instrument for measuring the diameter of the pupil
retin(o)	retina	*retinitis* [rĕt-ĭ-NĪ-tĭs], inflammation of the retina
scler(o)	white of the eye	*sclerectasia* [sklĕr-ĕk-TĀ-zē-ă], bulging of the sclera
scot(o)	darkness	*scotometer* [skō-TŎM-ĕ-tĕr], instrument for evaluating a scotoma or blind spot
tympan(o)	eardrum, middle ear	*tympanoplasty* [tĭm-pă-nō-PLĂS-tē], repair of a damaged middle ear
uve(o)	uvea	*uveitis* [yū-vē-Ī-tĭs], inflammation of the uvea

Abbreviation	Meaning
acc.	accommodation
AD	right ear
ARMD	age-related macular degeneration
AS	left ear
AU	both ears
D	diopter
dB	decibel
DVA	distance visual acuity
ECCE	extracapsular cataract extraction
EENT	eye, ear, nose, and throat
ENT	ear, nose, and throat
ICCE	intracapsular cataract cryoextraction
IOL	intraocular lens
IOP	intraocular pressure
NVA	near visual acuity
OD	right eye

Abbreviation	Meaning
OM	otitis media
OS	left eye
OU	each eye
PERRLA	pupils equal, round, reactive to light and accommodation
PE tube	polyethylene ventilating tube (placed in the eardrum)
SOM	serious otitis media
VA	visual acuity
VF	visual field
+	plus/convex
−	minus/concave

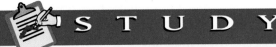
Seeing a Specialist

Mr. James was next referred to an ophthalmologist who discovered that Mr. James had a cataract in his right eye that should be removed. He also had one in the left eye that did not need treatment at this time. During surgery an IOL implant was placed in the right eye. After surgery, the ophthalmologist prescribed eyeglasses. The prescription form is used to instruct the optometrist or optician as to what corrective powers are necessary.

 Critical Thinking

21. Through which eye can Mr. James see distant objects more clearly?

22. Did Mr. James need a corrective lens for his left eye?

Dr. Janet Maitland
3000 Blue Willow Lane
Forest Park, IL 99999
999-000-5555

NAME *John James* DATE *2/3/XXXX*

Rx

	SPH.	CYL.	AXIS	PRISM
R	-.75	+.75	180	20/20
L	-2.00	+.75	005	20/50

Remarks
1st Rx after cataract Sx OD

ADD	
R	+2.50
L	+2.50

P.D.		
DIST 64	60	NEAR

☒ Janet Maitland, M.D.

EXPIRES *2/XXXX*

Janet Maitland, M.D.
IL. LIC. NO. 7yytt8

Combining Forms and Abbreviations Exercises

Find the Roots

From the following list of combining forms and from the list of suffixes in Chapter 2, write the word that matches the definition.

audi(o)   kerat(o)
blephar(o)   opt(o)
core(o)   ot(o)
dacryocyst(o)   retin(o)
irid(o)   scler(o)

23. _____ inflammation of the ear

24. _____ instrument for determining eye refraction

25. _____ study of the ear

26. _____ inflammation of the cornea

27. _____ instrument to examine the cornea

28. _____ disease of the iris

29. _____ pain in the tear sac

30. _____ repair of the pupil

31. _____ softening of the sclera

32. _____ inflammation of the sclera and cornea

33. _____ swelling in the eyelid

34. _____ pertaining to the retina

35. _____ paralysis of the iris

36. _____ earache

37. _____ study of hearing (disorders)

38. _____ inflammation of the eyelid

39. _____ hemorrhage from the ear

40. _____ instrument to measure hearing

Diagnostic, Procedural, and Laboratory Terms

Diagnosis of the sensory system usually includes testing of the sense in question and examination of the sensory structures. Loss of a sense can cause serious problems for an individual. In some cases, senses can be partially or totally restored through the use of prosthetic devices, transplants, or medication. In other cases, patients must adapt to the loss of a sense.

Diagnosing the Eye

An **ophthalmologist** (medical doctor who specializes in treatment and surgeries of the eye) and an **optometrist** (a trained nonmedical specialist who can examine patients for vision problems and prescribe lenses) both perform routine eye examinations. The most common diagnostic test of the eye is the *visual acuity test*, which measures the ability to see objects clearly at measured distances. The most common chart is the *Snellen Chart* (Figure 16-4). Perfect vision measures 20/20 on such a test. The first number, 20, is the distance (typically 20 feet) from which the person being tested reads a chart with black letters of different size. The second number is the distance from which the person being tested can read the size of the letters in relation to someone

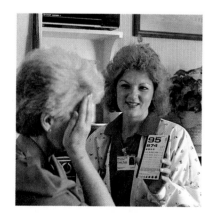

Figure 16-4 A Snellen Chart is used in an eye examination.

with normal vision. If the test shows that the subject can read only the letters on the 400 line, then the vision would be measured as 20/400. The 400 line means that someone with normal vision would be able to see from 400 feet away what the person being tested can see without corrective lenses at only twenty feet. A reading that shows less than 20/20 (for example 20/13) means that a person can read something at 20 feet that most people with 20/20 vision would only be able to read at 13 feet.

The next step in a routine eye examination is to examine *peripheral vision,* the area one is able to see to the side with the eyes looking straight ahead. This is usually done by telling a patient to follow a finger placed in front of their eyes while facing straight ahead. (In diagnosing some diseases, peripheral vision is tested in an examination called *visual field examination.*) Depending on the patient's age, most routine eye examinations also include **tonometry,** a measurement of pressure within the eye (a test for glaucoma) and **ophthalmoscopy** (visual examination of the interior of the eye). If the patient needs corrective lenses, an **optician** (trained technician who makes and fits corrective lenses) can fill the prescription written by an ophthalmologist or an optometrist. Most optometrists and some ophthalmologists also fill prescriptions for lenses. A prescription includes the **diopter,** the unit of refracting power needed in a lens.

For further diagnosis of the eye, a *slit lamp ocular* device is used to view the interior of the eye magnified through a microscope (Figure 16-5). *Fluorescein angiography* is the injection of a contrast medium into the blood vessels to observe the movement of blood throughout the eye. This test is for people with diabetes and other diseases that show lesions on various parts of the eye.

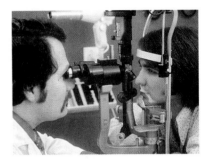

Figure 16-5 **A split lamp ocular device is a viewing device that magnifies the interior of the eye.**

Tuning forks are also used by musicians to establish a definite pitch for their instruments. Concert A is a note with a specific number of vibrations per second.

Diagnosing the Ear

Hearing tests are given to young children to see if they have any hearing deficit. Later, hearing is checked when a person notices hearing loss or when that person's friends and family suspect it. An **otologist** is an ear specialist, and an **audiologist** is a nonmedical hearing specialist. They both perform thorough examinations that include **otoscopy,** visual examination of the ear using an *otoscope,* a lighted viewing device (Figure 16-6). Such an examination might also include **audiometry,** the measurement of various acoustic frequencies to determine what frequencies the patient can or cannot hear. The device used is an *audiometer,* and the results of the test are plotted on a graph, an **audiogram.** The inside of the ear may be tested using a *pneumatic otoscope,* an otoscope that allows air to be blown into the ear to view the movement of the eardrum. A *tuning fork* compares the conduction of sound in one ear or between the two ears. The *Rinne test* and the *Weber test* are two tuning fork tests.

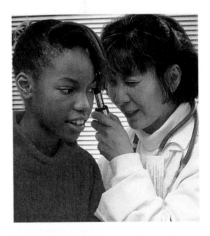

Figure 16-6 **An otoscope is used to perform a visual examination of the ear.**

Diagnosing Other Senses

The nose is usually observed as part of a general examination or, more specifically, a respiratory examination. Loss of the sense of smell is often the result of a disease process or of aging. The tongue and other parts of the mouth and the skin are also observed during a general examination. Loss of taste or touch may also be part of a disease process or of aging.

Vocabulary Review

In the previous section, you learned diagnostic, procedural, and laboratory terms. Before going on to the exercises, review the terms below and refer to the previous section if you have any questions.

Term	Word Analysis	Meaning
audiogram	[ăw-dē-Ō-grăm] audio- + -gram, a recording	Graph that plots the acoustic frequencies being tested.
audiologist	[ăw-dē-ŎL-ō-jĭst] audio- + -logist, one who specializes	Specialist in evaluating hearing function.
audiometry	[ăw-dē-ŎM-ĕ-trē] audio- + -metry, measurement	Measurement of acoustic frequencies using an audiometer.
diopter	[dī-ŎP-tĕr] Greek *dioptra*, leveling instrument	Unit of refracting power of a lens.
ophthalmologist	[ŏf-thăl-MŎL-ō-jĭst] ophthalmo-, eye + -logist	Medical specialist who diagnoses and treats eye disorders.
ophthalmoscopy	[ŏf-thăl-MŎS-kō-pē] ophthalmo- + -scopy, viewing	Visual examination of the interior of the eye.
optician	[ŏp-TĬSH-ăn]	Technician who makes and fits corrective lenses.
optometrist	[ŏp-TŎM-ĕ-trĭst] opto-, eye + Greek *metron*, measure	Nonmedical specialist who examines the eyes and prescribes lenses.
otologist	[ō-TŎL-ō-jĭst] oto-, ear + -logist	Medical specialist in ear disorders.
otoscopy	[ō-TŎS-kō-pē] oto- + -scope	Inspection of the ear using an otoscope.
tonometry	[tō-NŎM-ĕ-trē] tono-, tension + -metry	Measurement of tension or pressure within the eye.

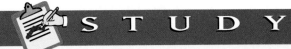

Another Problem Arises

Mr. James returned to the ophthalmologist in four months complaining of cloudy vision in his left eye. The ophthalmologist determined that it was time to remove the cataract in the left eye and replace it with an artificial lens or IOL. After a few weeks, Mr. James had regained night vision, even proclaiming that he could see better now than he had years before. His eyeglass prescription was changed. He only really needed his glasses for reading. The ophthalmologist also recommended sunglasses for most outdoor daytime activities, because ultraviolet rays can harm the eyes.

Critical Thinking

41. An artificial lens replaces what part of the eye?

42. Does a lens implant change eye color?

Diagnostic, Procedural, and Laboratory Terms Exercises

Know Your Senses

For each of the following diagnostic tests or devices, write A for eye, B for ear, or C for both eye and ear.

43. audiogram _____

44. otoscope _____

45. Rinne test _____

46. visual acuity _____

47. tuning fork _____

48. Snellen chart _____

49. tonometer _____

50. ophthalmoscope _____

Pathological Terms

Lost or damaged senses are illnesses in themselves. The disruption of losing or damaging a sense organ can lead to related illnesses. Much of the pathology of the sensory system results from age-related disorders or just age-related wear and tear on the senses.

Eye Disorders

The most common eye disorders involve defects in the curvature of the cornea and/or lens or defects in the refractive ability of the eye due to an abnormally short or long eyeball. Such disorders are usually managed with corrective lenses. Corrective lenses may be placed in frames to be worn on the face or may be in the form of **contact lenses,** which are placed directly over the cornea of the eye centered on the pupil. Contact lenses come in a variety of types, including disposable, hard, soft, and long-term wear. The degree of correction of the lenses depends on the results of a visual acuity examination.

An eye examination may reveal an **astigmatism,** distortion of sight because light rays do not come to a single focus on the retina (Figure 16-7). It may also reveal **hyperopia (farsightedness)** or **myopia (nearsightedness).** All three are errors of refraction, the bending of light that causes light rays to fall at one point on the retina. Hyperopia is the focusing of light rays behind the retina, and myopia is the focusing of light rays in front of the retina. Figure 16-8 shows hyperopia and myopia. **Strabismus** is eye misalignment (sometimes called "cross-eyed"). Two types of strabismus are **esotropia,** deviation of one eye inward, and **exotropia,** deviation of one eye outward. **Presbyopia** is loss of close reading vision due to lessened ability to focus and accommodate, a common disorder after age 40. **Asthenopia** or **eyestrain** is a condition in which the eyes tire easily because of weakness of the ocular or ciliary muscles. Symptoms may include pain in or around the eyes, headache, dimness of vision, dizziness, and light nausea. **Diplopia** is double vision. **Photophobia** is extreme sensitivity to light, sometimes as a result of a disease. **Cataracts** are cloudiness of the lens of the eye. They are usually a result of the aging process, but can be congenital or the result of a disease process or injury. Also, some types of medication may hasten the clouding of the lens. Removal of a cataract results in **aphakia,** absence of a lens. A **pseudophakia** is an implanted lens used to replace one that has been removed. A **scotoma** is a blind spot in vision. **Glaucoma** is any disease caused by abnormally high pressure within the eye. It can be treated in most cases by the use of special eye medications or surgical procedures to relieve the pressure. If not treatable, it can lead to **blindness,** loss of vision. There are many other causes of blindness, such as congenital defects, trauma to the eyes, and **macular degeneration.** Macular degeneration is the breakdown of macular tissue, which leads to loss of central vision, the vision we use for reading, driving, and watching television. Some specific conditions within the eye may affect vision. One such is *papilledema* or edema of the optic disk. Diseases of other body systems can affect

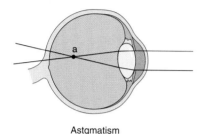

Astgmatism

Figure 16-7 An astigmatism distorts light rays.

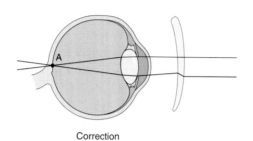

Correction

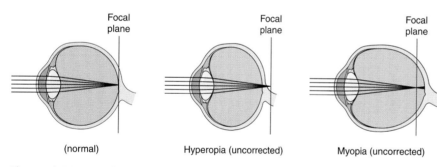

Focal plane   Focal plane   Focal plane

(normal)   Hyperopia (uncorrected)   Myopia (uncorrected)

Figure 16-8 Hyperopia and myopia are errors of refraction.

the senses. *Diabetic retinopathy* is a complication of diabetes mellitus that can result in vision loss. **Retinitis pigmentosa** is a progressive, inherited disorder, usually accompanied by scarring on the retina and **nyctalopia,** night blindness. The retina can tear or become detached and need surgical repair. Many of these conditions and other situations can lead to a form of partial blindness known as *legal blindness.* Legal blindness is a range of sight set by states. For example, someone whose vision can only be corrected to 20/400 may be considered legally blind.

The eyeball can protrude abnormally, as in **exophthalmus** or **exophthalmos,** usually caused by hyperthyroidism (Figure 16-9). **Lacrimation** or **epiphora** is excessive tearing, and **nystagmus** is excessive eyeball movement.

Inflammations and conditions of the eyelid include **blepharospasm,** involuntary eyelid movement causing excessive blinking; **blepharitis,** inflammation of the eyelid; **conjunctivitis** or **pinkeye,** a highly infectious inflammation of the conjunctiva; **blepharochalasis** or **dermatochalasis,** loss of elasticity of the eyelid; and **blepharoptosis,** paralysis of the eyelid causing drooping. A **chalazion** is a nodular inflammation that usually forms on the eyelid. **Trichiasis** is abnormal growth of eyelashes in a direction that causes them to rub on the eye. A **hordeolum** or **sty** is an infection of a sebaceous gland in the eyelid.

Inflammations of other parts of the eye include **dacryoadenitis,** inflammation of a lacrimal gland; **dacryocystitis,** inflammation of a tear duct; **iritis,** inflammation of the iris; **keratitis,** inflammation of the cornea; **retinitis,** inflammation of the retina; and **scleritis,** inflammation of the sclera.

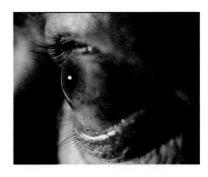

Figure 16-9 Exophthalmos is usually caused by hyperthyroidism.

Ear Disorders

The sense of hearing can be diminished or lost in a number of situations. **Anacusis** is total loss of hearing. **Paracusis** is impaired hearing. **Deafness** is either partial or total hearing loss. **Presbyacusis** or *presbycusis* is age-related hearing loss. *Conductive hearing loss* is caused by lessening of vibrations of the ear. *Sensorineural hearing loss* (also known as *nerve deafness*) is caused by lesions or dysfunction of those parts of the ear necessary to hearing. *Cerumen impaction,* abnormal wax buildup, can diminish hearing. **Otosclerosis** is the hardening of bone within the ear. **Tinnitus** is a constant ringing or buzzing in the ear. **Otalgia** or *earache* can interfere with hearing. **Otorrhagia,** bleeding in the ear, and **otorrhea,** purulent matter draining from the ear, can also impair hearing, usually temporarily. The sense of equilibrium is disturbed in **vertigo,** dizziness.

Various ear inflammations can diminish hearing or cause pain. **Otitis media** is inflammation of the middle ear and is often found in children. It may result in *eustachian obstruction,* blockage of the eustachian tube with fluid. **Otitis externa** is an inflammation of the external ear canal. **Labyrinthitis** is inflammation of the labyrinth. **Myringitis** or **tympanitis** is inflammation of the eardrum. **Mastoiditis** is inflammation of the mastoid process. Changes in atmospheric pressure, as in air travel, can result in **aerotitis media,** inflammation of the middle ear.

An *acoustic neuroma* is a benign tumor of the eighth cranial nerve that can affect hearing. A **cholesteatoma** is a fatty cyst within the middle ear. **Meniere's disease** is elevated fluid pressure within the cochlea, causing disturbances of the equilibrium and vertigo.

People without the ability to hear often learn to communicate in other ways, such as by using a sign language. American Sign Language is a widely used form of deaf communication.

Vocabulary Review

In the previous section, you learned terms relating to pathology. Before going on to the exercises, review the terms below and refer to the previous section if you have any questions.

Term	Word Analysis	Meaning
aerotitis media	[ār-ō-TĪ-tĭs MĒ-dē-ă]	Inflammation of the middle ear caused by air pressure changes, as in air travel.
anacusis	[ăn-ă-KŪ-sĭs] an-, without + Greek *akousis*, hearing	Loss of hearing.
aphakia	[ă-FĀ-kē-ă] a-, without + Greek *phakos*, lentil-shaped	Absence of a lens.
asthenopia	[ăs-thĕ-NŌ-pē-ă] Greek *astheneia*, weakness + *ops*, eye	Weakness of the ocular or ciliary muscles that causes the eyes to tire easily.
astigmatism	[ă-STĬG-mă-tĭzm] a-, without + Greek *stigma*, point + -ism, state	Distortion of sight because of lack of focus of light rays at one point on the retina.
blepharitis	[blĕf-ă-RĪ-tĭs] blephar-, eyelid + -itis, inflammation	Inflammation of the eyelid.
blepharochalasis	[blĕf-ă-rō-KĂL-ă-sĭs] blepharo-, eyelid + Greek *chalasis*, a slackening	Loss of elasticity of the eyelid.
blepharoptosis	[blĕf-ă-RŎP-tō-sĭs] blepharo- + Greek *ptosis*, a falling	Drooping of the eyelid.
blepharospasm	[BLĔF-ă-rō-spăzm] blepharo- + spasm	Involuntary eyelid movement; excessive blinking.
blindness		Loss or absence of vision.
cataract	[CĂT-ă-răkt] Latin *cataracta*	Cloudiness of the lens of the eye.
chalazion	[kă-LĀ-zē-ŏn] Greek, little sty	Nodular inflammation that usually forms on the eyelid.

Term	Word Analysis	Meaning
cholesteatoma	[kō-lĕs-tē-ă-TŌ-mă] chole(sterol) + Greek *stear*, fat + -oma, tumor	Fatty cyst within the middle ear.
conjunctivitis	[kŏn-jŭnk-tĭ-VĪ-tĭs] conjunctiv-, conjunctiva + -itis	Inflammation of the conjunctiva of the eyelid.
contact lenses		Corrective lenses worn on the surface of the eye.
dacryoadenitis	[DĂK-rē-ō-ăd-ĕ-NĪ-tĭs] dacryo-, lacrimal gland + aden, gland + -itis	Inflammation of the lacrimal glands.
dacryocystitis	[DĂK-rē-ō-sĭs-TĪ-tĭs] dacryo- + cyst + -itis	Inflammation of a tear duct.
deafness		Loss or absence of hearing.
dermatochalasis	[DĔR-mă-tō-kă-LĀ-sĭs] dermato-, skin + Greek *chalasis*, a slackening	Loss of elasticity of the eyelid.
diplopia	[dĭ-PLŌ-pē-ă] diplo-, double + -opia, vision	Double vision.
epiphora	[ĕ-PĬF-ō-ră] Greek, a sudden flow	Excessive tearing.
esotropia	[ĕs-ō-TRŌ-pē-ă] Greek *eso*, inward + -tropia, a turning	Deviation of one eye inward.
exophthalmos, exophthalmus	[ĕk-sŏf-THĂL-mōs] ex-, out of + Greek *ophthalmos*, eye	Abnormal protrusion of the eyeballs.
exotropia	[ĕk-sō-TRŌ-pē-ă] exo-, outward + -tropia	Deviation of one eye outward.
eyestrain	eye + strain	Asthenopia.
farsightedness		Hyperopia.
glaucoma	[glăw-KŌ-mă] Greek *glaukoma*, opacity	Any of various diseases caused by abnormally high eye pressure.
hordeolum	[hōr-DĒ-ō-lŭm	Infection of a sebaceous gland of the eyelid; sty.

Term	Word Analysis	Meaning
hyperopia	[hī-pĕr-Ō-pē-ă] hyper-, excessive + -opia, vision	Focusing behind the retina causing vision distortion; farsightedness.
iritis	[ī-RĪ-tĭs] ir-, iris + -itis	Inflammation of the iris.
keratitis	[kĕr-ă-TĪ-tĭs] kerat-, cornea + -itis	Inflammation of the cornea.
labyrinthitis	[LĂB-ĭ-rĭn-THĪ-tĭs] labyrinth + -itis	Inflammation of the labyrinth.
lacrimation	[lăk-rĭ-MĀ-shŭn]	Secretion of tears, usually excessively.
macular degeneration	[MĂK-yū-lăr]	Gradual loss of vision caused by degeneration of tissue in the macula.
mastoiditis	[măs-tŏy-DĪ-tĭs] mastoid + -itis	Inflammation of the mastoid process.
Meniere's disease	[mĕn-YĒRZ] After Prosper Meniere (1799–1862), French physician	Elevated pressure within the cochlea.
myopia	[mī-Ō-pē-ă] Greek, from my-, muscle + -opia, vision	Focusing in front of the retina causing vision distortion; nearsightedness.
myringitis	[mĭr-ĭn-JĪ-tĭs] myring-, eardrum + -itis	Inflammation of the eardrum.
nearsightedness		Myopia.
nyctalopia	[nĭk-tă-LŌ-pē-ă] nyct-, night + Greek *alaos*, obscure + -opia, vision	Night blindness.
nystagmus	[nĭs-STĂG-mŭs] Greek *nystagmos*, a nodding	Excessive involuntary eyeball movement.
otalgia	[ō-TĂL-jē-ă] ot-, ear + -algia, pain	Pain in the ear.
otitis externa	[ō-TĪ-tĭs ĕks-TĔR-nă]	Inflammation of the external ear canal.
otitis media	[MĒ-dē-ă]	Inflammation of the middle ear.

Term	Word Analysis	Meaning
otorrhagia	[ō-tō-RĀ-jē-ă] oto-, ear + -rrhagia, hemorrhage	Bleeding from the ear.
otorrhea	[ō-tō-RĒ-ă] oto- + -rrhea, flow	Purulent discharge from the ear.
otosclerosis	[ō-tō-sklĕ-RŌ-sĭs] oto- + sclerosis	Hardening of bones of the ear.
paracusis	[PĂR-ă-KŪ-sĭs] para-, beyond + Greek *akousis*, hearing	Impaired hearing.
photophobia	[fō-tō-PHŌ-bē-ă] photo-, light + -phobia, fear	Extreme sensitivity to light.
pinkeye		Conjunctivitis.
presbyacusis	[prĕz-bē-ă-KŪ-sĭs] presby-, old age + Greek *akousis*, hearing	Age-related hearing loss.
presbyopia	[prĕz-bē-Ō-pē-ă] presby- + -opia	Age-related diminished ability to focus or accommodate.
pseudophakia	[sū-dō-FĀ-kē-ă] pseudo-, fake + Greek *phakos*, lentil	Eye with an implanted lens after cataract surgery.
retinitis	[rĕt-ĭ-NĪ-tĭs] retin-, retina + -itis	Inflammation of the retina.
retinitis pigmentosa	[pĭg-mĕn-TŌ-să]	Progressive, inherited disease with a pigmented spot on the retina and poor night vision.
scleritis	[sklĕ-RĪ-tĭs]	Inflammation of the sclera.
scotoma	[skō-TŌ-mă] Greek *skotoma*, vertigo	Blind spot in vision.
strabismus	[stră-BĬZ-mŭs] Greek *strabismos*, a squinting	Eye misalignment.
sty, stye	[stī] Old English *stigan*, to rise	Hordeolum.

Term	Word Analysis	Meaning
tinnitus	[tĭ-NĪ-tŭs, TĬ-nĭ-tŭs] Latin, a jingling	Constant ringing or buzzing in the ear.
trichiasis	[trĭ-KĪ-ă-sĭs] trich-, hair + -iasis, condition	Abnormal growth of eyelashes in a direction that causes them to rub on the eye.
tympanitis	[tĭm-pă-NĪ-tĭs] tympan-, eardrum + -itis	Inflammation of the eardrum.
vertigo	[VĔR-tĭ-gō, vĕr-TĬ-gō] Latin	Dizziness.

C A S E S T U D Y

Getting Treatment

After his 69th birthday, Mr. James noticed that his hearing had seriously diminished in the last year. His physician referred him to a specialist. It was found that Mr. James had a buildup of wax in his ear. After treatment, his hearing improved slightly, but not enough for Mr. James to feel comfortable.

Critical Thinking

51. What other condition might explain this patient's hearing loss?

52. What type of specialist should Mr. James be referred to?

Pathological Terms Exercises

Sense the Diseases

For each of the diseases listed below, write A for eye, B for ear, or C for nose to indicate the organ associated with that disease.

53. conjunctivitis _____

54. cataract _____

55. nyctalopia _____

56. aerotitis media _____

57. presbyopia _____

58. allergic rhinitis _____

59. scotoma _____

60. nasosinusitis _____

61. Meniere's disease _____

Check Your Knowledge

Circle T for true or F for false.

62. A hordeolum is a sty. T   F

63. The focusing of light rays behind the retina is myopia. T   F

64. Myringitis is an inflammation of the tympanic membrane. T   F

65. A chalazion is a nodular inflammation typically occurring in the nose. T   F

66. Labyrinthitis occurs in the labyrinth of the eye. T   F

Surgical Terms

Some of the sense organs require surgery at various times. *Corneal transplants* or **keratoplasty** may give or restore sight. Implantation of new sound wave devices may give or restore hearing. The eye, ear, and the nose are also the site of plastic surgery to correct congenital defects or the signs of aging. Microscopic laser surgery or microsurgery is often used to operate on the small, delicate sensory organs.

Plastic surgery is used in **blepharoplasty,** eyelid repair; **otoplasty,** surgical repair of the outer ear; and **tympanoplasty,** eardrum repair. In some cases, removal of part of a sensory organ becomes necessary to treat a disorder or because a part has become damaged or cancerous.

Cataract extraction is the removal of a cloudy lens from the eye. It is usually followed by an *intraocular lens (IOL) implant,* during which an artificial lens is implanted to replace the natural lens of the eye that was removed (Figure 16-10). It is unusual for patients to be unable to tolerate the implant. In such cases, special glasses are prescribed that allow the patient some, usually limited, sight. Ultrasound can be used to break up and remove cataracts in **phacoemulsification.** A **dacryocystectomy** is the removal of a lacrimal sac. **Enucleation** is the removal of an eyeball. **Iridectomy** is removal of part of the iris. A **trabeculectomy** is an incision into and removal of part of the trabeculae to allow aqueous humor to flow freely around the eye. An **iridotomy** is an incision into the iris to allow aqueous humor to flow from the posterior to the anterior chambers. Correction of nearsightedness is also available with a laser procedure that changes the curvature of the cornea by making spokelike incisions around it. A retina can tear or become detached due to a trauma. **Cryoretinopexy** or *cryopexy* is the use of extreme cold to repair the damage to the retina, which can also be repaired using laser surgery.

In the ear, hearing can sometimes be aided by a **stapedectomy,** removal of the stapes to correct otosclerosis and insertion of tissue to substitute for a damaged stapes. A **myringotomy** is the insertion of a small, *polyethylene (PE) tube* to help drain fluid, thereby relieving some of the symptoms of otitis media. This operation is done frequently on infants and children with recurring ear infections.

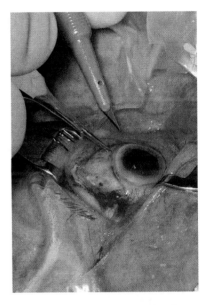

Figure 16-10 Cataract extraction is the removal of a cloudy lens from the eye (and often, its replacement with an artificial lens).

Nearsightedness correction is advancing rapidly. New, more advanced lasers are used widely to perform this common surgery.

Vocabulary Review

In the previous section, you learned terms relating to surgery. Before going on to the exercises, review the terms below and refer to the previous section if you have any questions.

Term	Word Analysis	Meaning
blepharoplasty	[BLĔF-ă-rō-plăst-ē] blepharo-, eyelid + -plasty, repair	Surgical repair of the eyelid.
cryoretinopexy	[krī-ō-rĕ-tĭn-nō-PĔKS-ē] cryo-, cold + retino-, retina + -pexy, a fixing	Fixing of a torn retina using extreme cold.
dacryocystectomy	[dăk-rē-ō-sĭs-TĔK-tō-mē] dacryo-, lacrimal gland + cyst + -ectomy, removal	Removal of a lacrimal sac.
enucleation	[ē-nū-klē-Ā-shŭn] From Latin *enucleo*, to remove the kernel	Removal of an eyeball.
iridectomy	[ĭr-ĭ-DĔK-tō-mē] irid-, iris + -ectomy	Removal of part of the iris.
iridotomy	[ĭr-ĭ-DŎT-ō-mē] irido-, iris + -tomy, a cutting	Incision into the iris to relieve pressure.
keratoplasty	[KĔR-ă-tō-plăs-tē] kerato-, cornea + -plasty	Corneal transplant.
myringotomy	[mĭr-ĭng-GŎT-ō-mē] myringo-, middle ear + -tomy	Insertion of a small tube to help drain fluid from the ears (particularly of children).
otoplasty	[Ō-tō-plăs-tē] oto-, ear + -plasty	Surgical repair of the outer ear.
phacoemulsification	[PHĀ-kō-ē-mŭls-ĭ-fĭ-KĀ-shŭn] phaco-, lens + emulsification	Use of ultrasound to break up and remove cataracts.
stapedectomy	[stā-pĕ-DĔK-tō-mē] stapes + -ectomy	Removal of the stapes to cure otosclerosis.
trabeculectomy	[tră-BĔK-yū-LĔK-tō-mē] trabecul(um) + -ectomy	Removal of part of the trabeculum to allow aqueous humor to flow freely around the eye.
tympanoplasty	[TĬM-pă-nō-plăs-tē] tympano- + -plasty	Repair of an eardrum.

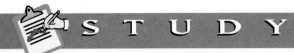

CASE STUDY

Getting Help

Mr. James's great grandson came for a few days' visit with his mother. The two-year-old had had fairly frequent ear infections, but they seemed to have subsided for a month or two, so his mother decided to risk the overnight stay. The boy woke up screaming and clutching his ear. A local 24-hour clinic diagnosed severe otitis media and prescribed medication. When the boy returned

home, his pediatrician wrote the following notes on his chart.

 Critical Thinking

67. Is the child's otitis media infectious for Mr. James?

68. Why did the doctor suggest a myringotomy?

Patient name	*Everett James*	Age _2_	Current Diagnosis _____
DATE/TIME 3/3/XXXX	Notes: *Frequent otitis media (7 times in the last 11 months). Suggest*		
	myringotomy. (Note: schedule during mother's work vacation 5/4–5/11.)		
	J. Redpine, M.D.		

Surgical Terms Exercises

Check Your Knowledge

69. A patient sustaining a third-degree burn to the pinna would likely require _____.

70. A stapedectomy would be performed to correct _____.

71. Cryoretinopexy would be performed to correct a _____ retina.

72. A corneal _____ may restore sight.

73. A child with chronic otitis media may need a _____.

Pharmacological Terms

Eyes and ears can both be treated with the *instillation* of drops. *Antibiotic ophthalmic solution* is an antibacterial agent used to treat eye infections, such as conjunctivitis. A **mydriatic** solution dilates the pupil during an eye examination. A **miotic** solution causes the pupil to contract. The eye and the ear can both be *irrigated,* flushed with water or solution to remove foreign objects. *Ear irrigation (lavage)* is the irrigation of the ear canal to remove excessive cerumen buildup. Antibiotics, antihistamines, anti-inflammatories, and decongestants are used to relieve ear infections, allergies, inflammations, and congestion. Table 16-2 (on page 576) lists various medications used for disorders of the senses.

Table 16-2 Medications used to treat disorders of the senses.

Drug Class	Purpose	Generic	Trade Name
antiseptic ear drops	to cleanse ears by dispelling earwax	alcohol carbamide peroxide	EarSol Murine Ear Drops
anti-inflammatory ear drops	to reduce ear inflammation	hydrocortisone	Ear-Eze, EarSol-HC
eye drops	to reduce eye congestion	tetrahydrozoline HCL	Murine Plus, Visine
eye moisturizer	to moisten eyes	methylcellulose	Murocel
miotic	contraction of the pupil	carbachol	Isoptocarbachol, Miostat
mydriatic	dilation of the pupil	atropine	Atropisol
nasal decongestant	to reduce nasal congestion	tetrahydrozoline	Tyzine

Vocabulary Review

In the previous section, you learned terms relating to pharmacology. Before going on to the exercises, review the terms below and refer to the previous section if you have any questions.

Term	Word Analysis	Meaning
miotic	[mī-ŎT-ĭk] From Greek *meion*, less	Agent that causes the pupil to contract.
mydriatic	[mĭ-drē-ĂT-ĭk] Greek *mydriasis*, excessive pupil dilation	Agent that causes the pupil to dilate.

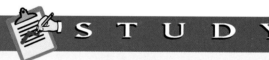

C A S E   S T U D Y

Feeling Better

When his great grandson came to visit the following year, Mr. James was hearing better with the help of a hearing aid. His eyesight was nearly perfect, and at age 70, he was happy to remain independent. His great-grandson's operation had proved effective. The boy had gone for about 10 months without any ear inflam-

mations. On the second day of the visit, however, the boy started rubbing his eyes and complained of itching. His mother noticed a reddish area around the edge of his eyelid.

 Critical Thinking

74. What was the likely cause of the child's itchy eyelids?

75. Is it surprising that Mr. James, who played with his great grandson frequently, developed the same condition five days later?

Check Your Knowledge

Fill in the blanks.

76. What medication might be prescribed for conjunctivitis? _____

77. During an eye exam, what agent helps to open a part of the eye for better viewing? _____

_____

78. What medication might be prescribed for otitis media? _____

CHALLENGE SECTION

A letter from an opthalmologist to a family practitioner is shown below.

Dr. Janet Maitland
3000 Blue Willow Lane
Forest Park, IL 99999
999-000-5555

5/6/XXXX

William Gonzalez, M.D.
7 Steele Drive
Forest Park, IL 99999
999-000-5444

Dear Dr. Gonzalez:

I was happy to evaluate our mutual patient, Joseph Consalvo, with regards to his recent Plaquenil prescription.

IMPRESSION: I do not see any evidence of Plaquenil toxicity on his examination, although there is a fair amount of macular disease due to previous diabetic retinopathy and subsequent laser therapy. He has recovered well from his cataract surgery, and his vision has returned to the expected level.

RECOMMENDATION: I think that I would continue to monitor him for problems every four to six months, both in regard to Plaquenil and with regard to his history of relatively severe nonproliferative diabetic retinopathy. We made an appointment for an examination after this period of time and he is to report any sudden changes in his vision to me directly.

I hope this information is helpful. Please let me know if I can be of any further help.

Sincerely,

Janet Maitland, M.D.

Janet Maitland, M.D.

JM/lrc

Challenge Section Exercises

79. What eye conditions does this diabetic patient have?

80. What condition does he have that is probably not caused by diabetes?

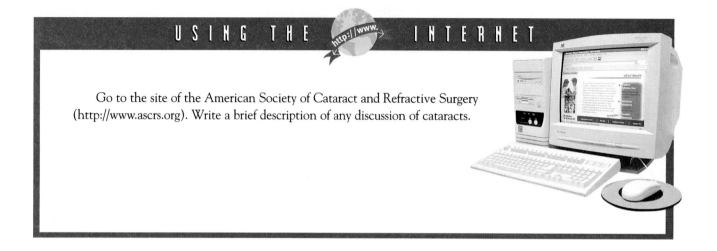

USING THE http://www. INTERNET

Go to the site of the American Society of Cataract and Refractive Surgery (http://www.ascrs.org). Write a brief description of any discussion of cataracts.

CHAPTER REVIEW

Definitions

Define the following terms and combining forms. Review the chapter before starting. Make sure you know how to pronounce each term as you define it.

Word	Definition
aerotitis media [ār-ō-TĪ-tĭs MĒ-dē-ă]	
anacusis [ăn-ă-KŪ-sĭs]	
aphakia [ā-FĀ-kē-ă]	
asthenopia [ăs-thĕ-NŌ-pē-ă]	
astigmatism [ă-STĬG-mă-tĭzm]	
audi(o)	
audiogram [ăw-dē-Ō-grăm]	
audiologist [ăw-dē-ŎL-ō-jĭst]	
audiometry [ăw-dē-ŎM-ĕ-trē]	
audit(o)	
auditory ossicles [ĂW-dĭ-tōr-ē ŎS-ĭ-klz]	
aur(o), auricul(o)	
auricle [ĂW-rĭ-kl]	
blephar(o)	
blepharitis [blĕf-ă-RĪ-tĭs]	
blepharochalasis [blĕf-ă-rō-KĂL-ă-sĭs]	
blepharoplasty [BLĔF-ă-rō-plăst-ē]	
blepharoptosis [blĕf-ă-RŎP-tō-sĭs]	
blepharospasm [BLĔF-ă-rō-spăzm]	
blindness	
cataract [CĂT-ă-răkt]	
cerumin(o)	
chalazion [kă-LĀ-zē-ŏn]	
cholesteatoma [kō-lĕs-tē-ă-TŌ-mă]	
choroid [KŌ-rŏyd]	
ciliary [SĬL-ē-ăr-ē] body	

Word	Definition
cochle(o)	
cochlea [KŌK-lē-ǎ]	
cones [kōnz]	
conjunctiv(o)	
conjunctiva (pl. conjunctivae) [kŏn-JŬNK-tǐ-vǎ (-vē)]	
conjunctivitis [kŏn-jŭnk-tǐ-VĪ-tǐs]	
contact lenses	
cor(o), core(o)	
corne(o)	
cornea [KŌR-nē-ǎ]	
cryoretinopexy [krī-ō-rě-tǐn-nō-PĚKS-ē]	
cycl(o)	
dacry(o)	
dacryoadenitis [DĂK-rē-ō-ǎd-ě-NĪ-tǐs]	
dacryocystectomy [dǎk-rē-ō-sǐs-TĚK-tō-mē]	
dacryocystitis [DĂK-rē-ō-sǐs-TĪ-tǐs]	
deafness	
decibel [DĚS-ǐ-běl]	
dermatochalasis [DĚR-mǎ-tō-kǎ-LĀ-sǐs]	
diopter [dī-ŎP-těr]	
diplopia [dǐ-PLŌ-pē-ǎ]	
ear [ēr]	
eardrum [ĒR-drŭm]	
endolymph [ĚN-dō-lǐmf]	
enucleation [ē-nū-klē-Ā-shŭn]	
epiphora [ě-PĬF-ō-rǎ]	
equilibrium [ē-kwǐ-LĬB-rē-ŭm]	
esotropia [ěs-ō-TRŌ-pē-ǎ]	
eustachian [yū-STĀ-shŭn, yū-STĀ-kē-ǎn] tube	
exophthalmos, exophthalmus [ěk-sǒf-THĂL-mōs]	
exotropia [ěk-sō-TRŌ-pē-ǎ]	

Word	Definition
eye [ī]	
eyebrow [Ī-brŏw]	
eyelashes [Ī-lăsh-ĕz]	
eyelid [Ī-lĭd]	
eyestrain	
farsightedness	
fovea centralis [FŌ-vē-ă sĕn-TRĂL-ĭs]	
glaucoma [glăw-KŌ-mă]	
hearing	
hordeolum [hōr-DĒ-ō-lŭm]	
hyperopia [hī-pĕr-Ō-pē-ă]	
incus [ĬN-kŭs]	
ir(o), irid(o)	
iridectomy [ĭr-ĭ-DĔK-tō-mē]	
iridotomy [ĭr-ĭ-DŎT-ō-mē]	
iris [Ī-rĭs]	
iritis [ĭ-RĪ-tĭs]	
kerat(o)	
keratitis [kĕr-ă-TĪ-tĭs]	
keratoplasty [KĔR-ă-tō-plăs-tē]	
labyrinthitis [LĂB-ĭ-rĭn-THĪ-tĭs]	
lacrim(o)	
lacrimal [LĂK-rĭ-măl] glands	
lacrimation [lăk-rĭ-MĀ-shŭn]	
lens [lĕnz]	
macula [MĂK-yū-lă]	
macula lutea [lū-TĒ-ă]	
macular [MĂK-yū-lăr] degeneration	
malleus [MĂL-ē-ŭs]	
mastoid(o)	
mastoiditis [măs-tŏy-DĪ-tĭs]	
membranous labyrinth	
Meniere's [mĕn-YĒRZ] disease	
miotic [mī-ŎT-ĭk]	

Word	Definition
mydriatic [mĭ-drē-ĂT-ĭk]	
myopia [mī-Ō-pē-ă]	
myring(o)	
myringitis [mĭr-ĭn-JĪ-tĭs]	
myringotomy [mĭr-ĭng-GŎT-ŏ-mē]	
nas(o)	
nearsightedness	
neuroretina [nūr-ō-RĔT-ĭ-nă]	
nyctalopia [nĭk-tă-LŌ-pē-ă]	
nystagmus [nĭs-STĂG-mŭs]	
ocul(o)	
olfactory [ōl-FĂK-tō-rē] organs	
ophthalm(o)	
ophthalmologist [ŏf-thăl-MŎL-ō-jĭst]	
ophthalmoscopy [ŏf-thăl-MŎS-kō-pē]	
opt(o), optic(o)	
optician [ŏp-TĬSH-ăn]	
optic nerve	
optometrist [ŏp-TŎM-ĕ-trĭst]	
organ of Corti [KŌR-tĭ]	
osseus [ŎS-sē-ŭs] labyrinth	
ossicul(o)	
otalgia [ō-TĂL-jē-ă]	
otitis externa [ō-TĪ-tĭs ĕks-TĔR-nă]	
otitis media [MĒ-dē-ă]	
otoliths [Ō-tō-lĭthz]	
otologist [ō-TŎL-ō-jĭst]	
otoplasty [Ō-tō-plăs-tē]	
otorrhagia [ō-tō-RĀ-jē-ă]	
otorrhea [ō-tō-RĒ-ă]	
otosclerosis [ō-tō-sklĕ-RŌ-sĭs]	
otoscopy [ō-TŎS-kō-pē]	
papillae [pă-PĬL-ē]	
paracusis [PĂR-ă-KŪ-sĭs]	

Word	Definition
perilymph [PĔR-ĭ-lĭmf]	
phac(o), phak(o)	
phacoemulsification [PHĀ-kō-ē-mŭls-ĭ-fĭ-KĀ-shŭn]	
photophobia [fō-tō-PHŌ-bē-ă]	
pinkeye	
pinna [PĬN-ă]	
presbyacusis [prĕz-bē-ă-KŪ-sĭs]	
presbyopia [prēz-bē-Ō-pē-ă]	
pseudophakia [sū-dō-FĀ-kē-ă]	
pupil [PYŪ-pĭl]	
pupill(o)	
refraction [rē-FRĂK-shŭn]	
retin(o)	
retina [RĔT-ĭ-nă]	
retinitis [rĕt-ĭ-NĪ-tĭs]	
retinitis pigmentosa [pĭg-mĕn-TŌ-să]	
rods [rŏdz]	
scler(o)	
sclera (pl. sclerae) [SKLĒR-ă (-ē)]	
scleritis [sklĕ-RĪ-tĭs]	
scot(o)	
scotoma [skō-TŌ-mă]	
semicircular canals	
sensory receptors	
sensory system	
sight	
smell	
stapedectomy [stā-pĕ-DĔK-tō-mē]	
stapes (pl. stapes, stapedes) [STĀ-pēz (STĀ-pĕ-dēz)]	
strabismus [stră-BĬZ-mŭs]	
sty, stye [stī]	
taste	

Word	Definition
taste buds	
taste cells	
tears	
tinnitus [tǐ-NĪ-tŭs, TĬ-nǐ-tŭs]	
tonometry [tō-NŎM-ě-trē]	
touch	
trabulectomy [trǎ-BĚK-yū-LĚK-tō-mē]	
trichiasis [trǐ-KĪ-ǎ-sǐs]	
tympan(o)	
tympanic [tǐm-PĂN-ǐk] membrane	
tympanitis [tǐm-pǎ-NĪ-tǐs]	
tympanoplasty [TĬM-pǎ-nō-plǎs-tē]	
uve(o)	
uvea [YŪ-vē-ǎ]	
vertigo [VĚR-tǐ-gō, věr-TĪ-gō]	
vestibule [VĚS-tǐ-bŭl]	

Abbreviations

Write the full meaning of each abbreviation.

Abbreviation	Meaning
acc.	
AD	
ARMD	
AS	
AU	
D	
dB	
DVA	
ECCE	
EENT	
ENT	
ICCE	
IOL	
IOP	

NVA _____

OD _____

OM _____

OS _____

OU _____

PERRLA _____

PE tube _____

SOM _____

VA _____

VF _____

+ _____

− _____

Answers to Chapter Exercises

1. None of the general tests showed abnormal results so Mr. James's problem needs further investigation.
2. Eye disease can be part of a systemic problem.
3. k
4. a
5. b
6. j
7. h
8. f
9. d
10. g
11. e
12. i
13. c
14. F
15. F
16. T
17. F
18. T
19. F
20. T
21. right eye
22. yes
23. otitis
24. optometer
25. otology
26. keratitis
27. keratometer

28. iridopathy
29. dacryocystalgia
30. coreoplasty
31. scleromalacia
32. sclerokeratitis
33. blepharedema
34. retinal
35. iridoplegia
36. otalgia
37. otology/audiology
38. blepharitis
39. otorrhagia
40. otometer/ audiometer
41. lens
42. No, the lens is inside the eye; the iris determines eye color.
43. B
44. B
45. B
46. A
47. B
48. A
49. A
50. A
51. nerve deafness of old age or other systemic condition such as an infection
52. otologist
53. A
54. A

55. A
56. B
57. A
58. C
59. A
60. C
61. B
62. T
63. F
64. T
65. F
66. F
67. No—it is an inflammation of the middle ear.
68. to relieve the recurring ear infections
69. otoplasty
70. otosclerosis
71. detached
72. transplant
73. myringotomy
74. conjunctivitis
75. No, it is highly infectious.
76. antibiotic ophthalmic solution
77. mydriatic
78. antibiotic
79. diabetic retinopathy, cataracts
80. cataracts

CHAPTER 17

Human Development

After reading this chapter, you will be able to

• Describe each stage of human development

• Name medical specialists that treat the disorders in each stage of the lifespan

• List the diseases and disorders common to each stage of the lifespan

Stages of Development

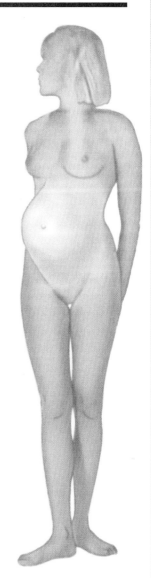

The time between conception and death is the period of an individual's development. The average *lifespan* (length of life) varies from country to country. Each stage (see Table 17-1) is described in this chapter, along with specialists who typically treat patients in a particular time in the lifespan. Pathology of the lifespan is also discussed.

Table 17-1 Stages of Human Development

Lifespan Period	Average Time	Developmental Characteristics
fetus	period from eight weeks gestation to birth	development of all body systems that are present at birth
neonate	first 4 weeks of infancy	adjustment to life outside the uterus
infancy	first year of life	many physical and emotional developmental strides
toddler	age 1 to 3	walking, talking, and becoming somewhat independent from caretakers
childhood	age 3 to puberty	cognitive and physical development, usually including schooling
puberty	about 8 to 12	development of secondary sex characteristics

(continued on next page)

Table 17-1 (continued)

Lifespan Period	Average Time	Developmental Characteristics
adolescence	period from puberty to full physical maturity	physical maturation and often psychological separation from the family, leading to independence
young adulthood	ages 20-39	period of establishment of adult work and lifestyle situations
middle adulthood	ages 40-59	often stressful period of continued career and family development
old age	ages 60 on	period of diminishing of physical and, sometimes, mental faculties
oldest old	ages 90 on	period of late life, often with many physical and emotional difficulties
death	end of life	cessation of cardiovascular, respiratory, and nervous system functions

Freezing of sperm or eggs has allowed people to have a child at a later time (as after treatment for cancer) with the help of laboratories specializing in fertility.

Fertilization, Pregnancy, and Birth

Fertilization can occur as the result of sexual intercourse between a male and a female. It may also occur in a laboratory in cases of infertility. However it occurs, fertilization is the union of an egg cell (ovum) with a spermatozoon. (In rare cases, more eggs are fertilized by several sperm or one egg divides into identical twins, triplets, and so on.) After traveling through the fallopian tube, the fertilized ovum (also called an **embryo**) is **implanted** or attached to the wall of the uterus. Once attached, the ovum remains *in utero,* or within the uterus, until development and birth. It takes an average of 40 weeks from the time that the ovum is fertilized until birth. This period of development is known as **gestation.** The ovum begins to change during the first 8 weeks of gestation. After that, the ovum becomes a **fetus,** the developing product of conception prior to birth. For the mother, this is the period known as *pregnancy.* Chapters 10 and 11 cover the female and male reproductive systems.

The birth process usually includes a period of **labor,** the process of expelling the fetus and the placenta from the uterus. Labor may end in a vaginal birth. If not, a **cesarean section,** removal of the fetus surgically through the abdomen, is performed. The reasons for performing a cesarean section vary widely, but may include fetal or maternal distress, complications (as in multiple births or premature birth), or extended labor without dilation of the cervix. The fetus, in the majority of circumstances, is in a *cephalic* position or head down in the birth canal. A fetus may be positioned in a **breech** position (infant in birth canal with feet first) or may be *transverse*, sideways. *Obstetricians*, specialists in **obstetrics,** which includes fertility, pregnancy, and birth, assist in the vaginal birth of a breech baby, or turn a transverse baby so that it can be born vaginally. A breech or tranverse baby cannot exit the vagina without being harmed unless it is maneuvered into a position to allow it to come through the birth canal. Often, infants in such positions are at risk during the birth process and are much more likely to be born by cesarean section. Figure 17-1 shows cephalic and breech birth positions.

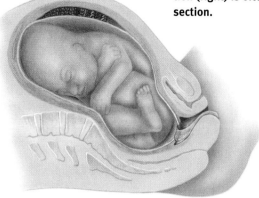

Figure 17-1. Birth position can determine whether a birth is vaginal or by caesarean section. Cephalic presentation (left) is usually vaginal. Breech presentation (right) is often by caesarean section.

(a) Cephalic presentation   (b) Breech presentation

Infancy

A baby, also referred to as a newborn or *infant*, is born. For the first four weeks of life, the infant is referred to as a **neonate** (Figure 17-2). **Neonatology** is the medical specialty concerned with the care and treatment of neonates with severe health problems or who may have been born prematurely. *Neonatologists* are specialists in neonatology. The remainder of the infancy period lasts the first year. During the next period, the child is often referred to as a *toddler*. The toddler is a young child who becomes competent at walking, begins to speak, and begins to handle some of the activities of daily living by himself or herself. This occurs in the period between the end of the first year and age three. **Pediatrics** is the specialty that treats children from the neonate stage through adolescence. *Pediatricians* are the practitioners of this specialty.

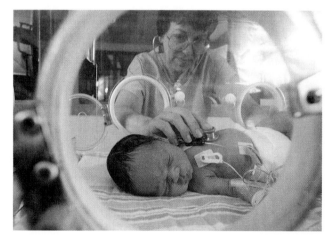

Childhood

Childhood is the period of life from infancy to puberty. *Puberty* is a sequence of development of secondary sex characteristics beginning around ages 8 to 12. Childhood years vary because puberty may start very early or very late. Also, the onset of puberty is generally earlier in girls than in boys.

Figure 17-2. A neonate is an infant under 4 weeks old.

Adolescence

Adolescence is the period of physical maturation, usually between ages 13 and 19. During this time, the secondary sex characteristics fully develop (girls develop breasts, underarm hair, pubic hair; boys develop facial hair, pubic hair, underarm hair, voice change). It is the period when most people start to take the emotional steps that will lead them to be independent of their parents. Adolescents often experience the conflict of being more physically mature than emotionally ready to handle such things as pregnancy and parenthood.

Adulthood

Young adulthood comprises the period from ages 20 to 40. This is usually the period in which adults set up their first homes, become parents, and build their careers. Middle adulthood or *middle age* is the period from ages 40 to 60. Young adults may choose an *internist* or *family practitioner* as their primary physician. During middle adulthood, many physical changes (i.e., menopause, diminution of strength, reduction in hearing ability) occur. Middle adulthood is often the time that disorders are discovered and treatments are begun.

Old Age

Old age begins around age 60 and encompasses the years until death. The quality of life in old age usually reflects your family's genetic history, general health, and emotional attitudes. Some people live well into their 90s or early 100s independently and in good health. People who have such *longevity*, length of life beyond the average, are often referred to as the *oldest old* (Figure 17-3). Others may have heart attacks or other illnesses during middle age that lead to an old age that includes many periods of illness and may even include early death. **Gerontology** is the medical specialty that diagnoses and treats disorders present in old age. *Gerontologists* are specialists in treating ailments of the aging.

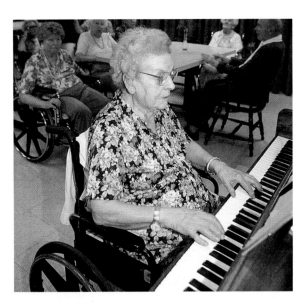

Preventive medicine now encompasses many alternatives, such as vitamin and herbal supplements and mediation.

Figure 17-3. A 101-year-old woman playing piano in a nursing home.

Death

Death, the end of life, occurs when the heart, respiratory system, and central nervous system cease functioning. This definition of death is being changed by life-support machines that are able to keep someone with respiratory or other body failure alive indefinitely. Because of the controversies surrounding the use of life-support machines near the end of life, several legal changes have been made in recent years. The practice of **euthanasia** or *assisted suicide* is allowed in certain countries in the world. In the United States, most states forbid this method of helping very sick people die comfortably. The field of *bioethics*, study of ethical medical treatment and research, has grown in the last part of the twentieth century.

A *living will* is considered a legal document signed by a patient who prefers to be allowed to die rather than be kept alive by artificial means if there is no reasonable expectation of recovery. Some people appoint a *health care proxy* to make decisions for them in case of their own disability. Such legal statements are called *advance directives*, something that provides instructions for the future in the event of certain circumstances. The movement toward *hospice*, a program of supportive care for dying patients in a nonhospital setting, has spread to all parts of the country. Hospice provides end-of-life pain relief (called *palliation*) and care, but does not try to artificially prolong life or resuscitate a patient who has stopped breathing.

Vocabulary Review

In the previous section, you learned terms about stages of development. Before going on to the exercises, review the terms below and refer to the previous section if you have any questions.

Term	Word Analysis	Definition
breech	[brēch]	Birth canal position with feet first.
cesarean section	[sĕ-ZĀ-rē-ăn] From Latin *lex caesaria*, Roman law	Surgical removal of the fetus through the abdomen.
embryo	[ĔM-brē-ō] Greek *embryon*	Fertilized ovum until about 8 weeks of gestation.
euthanasia	[yū-thă-NĀ-zē-ă] eu-, good + Greek *thanatos*, death	Assisting in the suicide of or putting a person with an incurable or painful disease to death.
fertilization	[FĔR-tĭl-ĭ-ZĀ-shŭn]	Union of an egg cell(s) with sperm.
fetus	[FĒ-tŭs]	Developing product of conception from 8 weeks to birth.
gerontology	[JĔR-ŏn-TŎL-ō-jē] geronto-, old age + -logy, study of	Medical specialty that diagnoses and treats disorders of old age.
gestation	[jĕs-TĀ-shŭn] Latin *gestatio*	Period of fetal development from fertilization until delivery.
implant	[ĭm-PLĂNT]	To attach to the lining of the uterus in the first stage of pregnancy.
labor	[LĀ-bōr]	Process of expelling the fetus and placenta from the uterus.
neonate	[NĒ-ō-nāt] neo-, new + Latin *natus*, born	Infant under four weeks old.
neonatology	[NĒ-ō-nā-TŎL-ō-jē] neonat(e) + -logy	Medical specialty that diagnoses and treats disorders of neonates.
obstetrics	[ŏb-STĔT-rĭks] Latin *obstetrix*, midwife	Medical specialty that guides women and treats disorders throughout fertilization, pregnancy, and birth.
pediatrics	[PĒ-dē-ĂT-rĭks] From Greek *pais*, child + *iatrikos*, of medicine	Medical specialty that diagnoses and treats disorders in children from infancy through adolescence.

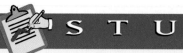

C A S E S T U D Y

Spanning the Generations

Maria and Paul Adams were overjoyed upon discovering Maria's pregnancy at age 36. Maria's mother had her children later in life. She was now turning 77, living alone since her husband died. Maria and Paul are part of what is called the *"sandwich" genera-tion*—those people caring for their young children and their older parents at the same time. Maria's mother had a myocardial infarction a few years ago. She lives in the same town as Maria, who does her grocery shopping, takes her to doctors, and visits with her about four times a week. Maria also works as a systems analyst. Her paycheck is impor-tant to the couple, and Maria plans to go back to work after several months of pregnancy leave.

Critical Thinking

1. What stages of life will Maria and her child be going through simultaneously?

2. Will Paul and Maria need a neonatologist for their child?

Stages of Development Exercises

Know the Lifespan

Write the lifespan period(s) that best fits each description or profession.

3. In utero_____

4. Neonatologist_____

5. Secondary sex characteristics_____

6. First walking_____

7. Early schooling_____

8. Cessation of body functions_____

9. Establishment of adult work_____

10. Physical maturation_____

11. Two weeks old_____

12. Obstetrician_____

13. Gerontologist_____

Pathology of the Lifespan

The majority of diseases occur at the beginning (infancy) and at the end (old age) of life. Diseases or disorders may be determined or caused by **genetics,** the science of biological inheritance, environmental causes (as exposure to a virus or bacteria), or trauma (sudden, massive injury). A *geneticist* is a specialist in genetics who can counsel people with genetic abnor-malities who wish to have children. Some congenital diseases (severe spina bifida, anencephaly) are devastating. In some cases, geneticists can predict the odds of the newborn inheriting a gene. It is also possible to observe (via ultra-sound) the fetus during its development. Fetuses are treated **in utero,** while in the uterus, either with medication or surgically, for a number of conditions. In addition, blood tests reveal genetic clues to disorders carried by the parents (Figure 17-4).

Neonates born **prematurely,** after less than 37 weeks of gestation, often have underdeveloped lungs and other problems. Advances in neonatology save many premature infants. Birth after 40 weeks of gestation may also cause or indicate fetal problems that can include high fetal weight. Infants may die suddenly in an unknown manner (**sudden infant death syndrome** or **SIDS**), usually while sleeping. Safety measures that can prevent some suffocation deaths and/or respiratory problems are to place the infant on its back to sleep, avoid pillows or stuffed animals in the crib, and to avoid smoking in the house. Infants may also experience trauma (as in falls) or may contract infections (such as streptococcus or strep throat).

As children grow, they experience many of the diseases of the body systems covered in each of the body system chapters in this book. Some childhood diseases help to strengthen the immune system for later life. For example, a childhood bout with chicken pox usually offers lifelong immunity against a disease that can have much more devastating effects in older people.

Middle age is often the period during which the stress and wear and tear of daily life begin to take their toll. In this period, particularly, an unhealthy lifestyle can bring on major diseases. A high-fat diet can raise cholesterol, a major risk factor for coronary artery disease. Smoking increases the risk of heart disease and lung cancer. Lack of exercise can be a major factor in cardiovascular disease. Many diseases in this period can be prevented with systematic attention to lifestyle issues and to early warning tests, such as mammograms and PSA tests. The diseases of middle age usually worsen in the next stage of life.

Most of the pathology in life takes place in old age, with the wearing down of bone, the weakening of the musculoskeletal structure, and the diminishing of the central nervous system. Many doctors and patients focus on **preventive medicine,** a medical specialty concerned with preventing disease. Prevention may include lifestyle changes, medications (as Tamoxifen for women with a family history of breast cancer), or frequent checkups (as for people with previous cancers). Table 17-2 lists some diseases common to the various stages of the lifespan. Some of these diseases appear at all stages of the lifespan, but occur most frequently in a particular stage.

At the end of life, death is declared by a medical person. The exact definition of death varies but most states use the standards set forth in the federal Uniform Determination of Death Act that was proposed by a presidential commission. Most states have adopted the two criteria for brain death—cessation of circulatory and respiratory functions, and the entire brain, including the brain stem, has irreversibly ceased to function. A physician checks for reflexes and responses before declaring brain death.

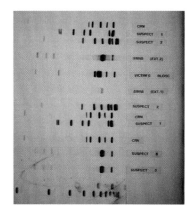

Figure 17-4. A genetic screen can reveal the presence of genetic disorders.

Table 17-2 Pathology in Human Development

Lifespan Period	Average Time	Some Diseases Most Prevalent at Each Stage — (See body systems chapters for further discussion of pathology.)
fetus	during 40 weeks of gestation	hydrocephaly, spina bifida, Rh incompatibility (erythroblastosis fetalis)
neonate	first 4 weeks of infancy	jaundice, diarrhea, allergies, SIDS, hydrocephaly, spina bifida, premature birth, hyaline membrane disease, Down syndrome, Tay-Sach's disease, sickle cell anemia, pyloric stenosis

(continued on next page)

Table 17-2 (continued)

Lifespan Period	Average Time	Some Diseases Most Prevalent at Each Stage — (See body systems chapters for further discussion of pathology.)
infancy	first year of life	Down syndrome, SIDS, otitis media, strep throat, allergies, diarrhea
toddler	ages 1 to 3	otitis media, strep throat, roseola, allergies, diarrhea
childhood	ages 3 to puberty	strep throat, otitis media, and if not vaccinated, measles, mumps, chicken pox, polio
puberty	about ages 8 to 12	same as during childhood
adolescence	period from puberty to full physical maturity	some childhood diseases, plus emotional problems (such as depression and anxiety)
young adulthood	ages 20-39	schizophrenia, multiple sclerosis, early cancers (prostate, cervical, uterine, and breast)
middle adulthood	ages 40-59	heart disease, stroke, cancer, Parkinson's disease, Alzheimer's disease, osteoporosis
old age	ages 60 on	same as middle adulthood plus senile dementia, depression
oldest old	ages 90 on	same as old age
death	end of life	cessation of cardiovascular, respiratory, and nervous system functions

Vocabulary Review

In the previous section, you learned terms relating to the pathology of the lifespan. Before going on to the exercises, review the terms below and refer to the previous section if you have any questions.

Term	Word Analysis	Definition
genetics	[jĕ-NĔT-ĭks] From Greek *genesis*, origin	Science of biological inheritance.
in utero	[ĭn YŪ-tĕr-ō] Latin	Within the uterus; unborn.
premature	[PRĒ-mă-chūr] Latin *praematurus*, too early	Born before 37 weeks gestation.
preventive medicine		Medical specialty concerned with preventing disease.
sudden infant death syndrome (SIDS)		Death of an infant, usually while sleeping, of unknown cause.

C A S E   S T U D Y

Dealing with Complications

Maria's age prompted a question from her obstetrician about a test for fetal abnormalities. Maria decided to have amniocentesis, a test for fetal abnormalities. It came back normal. Meanwhile, Maria's mother had another heart attack. Maria and her mother decided to look for a living situation that would provide independence for her mother while providing care as necessary. They settled on an assisted living complex in the next town. This seemed to be ideal—Maria would

have fewer tasks, and her mother would be around people all the time.

Around the beginning of Maria's seventh month of pregnancy, a routine visit to the doctor showed that her blood pressure had spiked to dangerous levels. Maria had a kidney infection and was dealing with a very stressful situation. She also had noticed some vague cramps. The kidney infection was treated, but, in addition, Maria was told to cut her work hours and spend more time resting in bed in prepara-

tion for the final stage of pregnancy. The cramps were a sign of possible early labor.

 Critical Thinking

14. What is the danger to the fetus if Maria's obstetrician is not able to prevent early labor?

15. What are some of the abnormalities that might be seen on an ultrasound as opposed to those tested for in amniotic fluid?

Pathology of the Lifespan Exercises

Following the Stages of Life

Write the lifespan stage(s) during which each disease is most likely to occur. You may want to review Table 17-2 before proceeding with this exercise.

16. Senile dementia_____

17. Chicken pox_____

18. SIDS_____

19. Alzheimer's disease_____

20. Erythroblastosis fetalis_____

U S I N G   T H E   I N T E R N E T

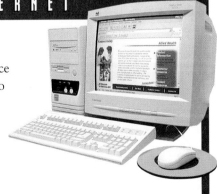

Go to the Hospice Foundation of America's web site (http://www.hospice foundation.org) and write a short paragraph on the goals of hospice. Also, go to http://www.mediacareinfo.com and write a brief paragraph on "advanced directives."

CHAPTER REVIEW

Definitions

Define the following terms. Review the chapter before starting. Make sure you know how to pronounce each term as you define it.

Word	Definition
breech [brēch]	
cesarean [sĕ-ZĀ-rē-ăn] section	
embryo [ĔM-brē-ō]	
euthanasia [yū-thă-NĀ-zē-ă]	
fertilization [FĔR-tĭl-ĭ-ZĀ-shŭn]	
fetus [FĒ-tŭs]	
genetics [jĕ-NĔT-ĭks]	
gerontology [JĔR-ŏn-TŎL-ō-jē]	
gestation [jĕs-TĀ-shŭn]	
implant [ĭm-PLĂNT]	
in utero [ĭn YŪ-tĕr-ō]	
labor [LĀ-bōr]	
neonate [NĒ-ō-nāt]	
neonatology [NĒ-ō-nā-TŎL-ō-jē]	
obstetrics [ŏb-STĔT-rĭks]	
pediatrics [PĒ-dē-ĂT-rĭks]	
premature [PRĒ-mă-chūr]	
preventive medicine	
sudden infant death syndrome (SIDS)	

1. Maria will be in the young adulthood stage up to the time her child will finish the toddler stage. Then middle adulthood will coincide with the child's development through to young adulthood.

2. Not necessarily. Although Maria's age puts the fetus at higher risk for certain abnormalities, such as Down syndrome, only testing can determine if a fetus needs a specialist in neonatology.

3. fetus
4. neonate
5. puberty
6. toddler
7. childhood
8. death
9. young adulthood
10. adolescence
11. neonate
12. pregnancy
13. old age, oldest old
14. Maria's baby might be born prematurely with physical problems due to underdevelopment.
15. limb abnormalities, spina bifida, hydrocephaly, and others that show up externally on the fetus
16. old age and oldest old
17. childhood, puberty
18. infancy
19. middle adulthood, old age, oldest old
20. fetus

CHAPTER 18

Terms in Oncology
Cancer and Its Causes

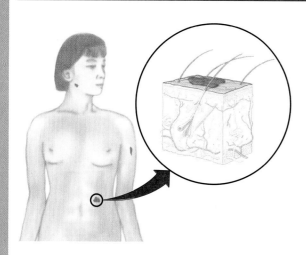

After studying this chapter, you will be able to

♦ Name the types of cancers, discuss the major pathological conditions, and list some of their possible causes

♦ Define the combining forms used in building words that relate to oncology

♦ Identify the meaning of related abbreviations

♦ Name the laboratory tests and clinical procedures used in testing and treating cancer

♦ Describe pathological terms related to cancer

♦ Define surgical terms related to cancer

♦ List common pharmacological agents used in treating cancer

Tumors: Types and Causes

Tumors

Oncology is the study, diagnosis, and treatment of tumors. **Tumors** or **neoplasms** are growths made up of cells that reproduce abnormally. Cells in the body normally reproduce only at a rate to replace cells that have died. Cells also have a mechanism that signals them to die when they have passed a certain point of usefulness. Tumors are made up of cells that seem to be missing the mechanism that tells them either to stop reproducing or to die. The death of normal cells in a normal time cycle is called **apoptosis.**

Tumors can be **benign** (usually retained safely within a capsule of thick, connective tissue or *encapsulated*) or **malignant** (not held within a capsule; reproducing rapidly in an uncontrollable pattern). Lumps in the breast can be either benign or malignant. Malignant neoplasms are categorized by the types of tissue from which they develop.

A *carcinoma*, the most common type of cancer, originates from epithelial tissue. Also called **solid tumors,** carcinomas make up about 90 percent of all tumors. Common sites are in the skin, lungs, breasts, colon, stomach, mouth, and uterus. Carcinomas spread by way of the lymphatic system. A **sarcoma,**

Survival rates for various malignant cancers have improved, but the incidence of cancer has increased dramatically. Some of this is due to improved detection rates.

which is fairly rare, originates in muscle or connective tissue and lymph. A *mixed-tissue tumor* derives from tissue that is capable of separating into either epithelial or connective tissue because it is composed of several types of cells. Such a tumor can be found in the kidneys, ovaries, or testes. Mixed-tissue tumors can be **teratomas,** growths containing bone, muscle, skin, and glandular tissue as well as other types of cells. There is also a class of cancers that arise from blood, lymph, or nervous system cells. Cancers such as leukemia fall into this category. As mentioned in Chapter 12, some leukemias are also sarcomas.

Benign tumors are **encapsulated,** held within a capsule, and are not life-threatening (Figure 18-1a). They are made up of **differentiated** cells that reproduce abnormally but in an orderly fashion. Some benign tumors can cause pain from pressure exerted on an organ or tissue. Often, removal cures the problem. Malignant tumors are **invasive,** extending beyond the tissue to infiltrate other organs (Figure 18-1b). Malignant tumors can be life-threatening. These tumors are made up of **dedifferentiated** cells, which lack the normal orderly arrangement of the cells from which they arise. *Undifferentiated* cells lack a defined mature cell structure. This loss of cell differentiation is called **anaplasia.** Any abnormal tissue development is known as **dysplasia** or **heteroplasia.** The first stages of cancer development may be classified as dysplasia because they represent the beginning of abnormal tissue development. Detection of cancers at this early stage plays a vital role in treatment. The next stage may be a *carcinoma in situ*, a tumor in one place that affects all layers of tissue. Finally, a *malignancy* occurs when the cells break loose and become invasive to surrounding tissue. The spread of a malignancy to other areas of the body is called **metastasis.** In earlier chapters, you learned about *homeostasis*, the maintaining of balance throughout the body. Metastasis is a state of imbalance, with cells spreading uncontrollably.

Causes of Cancer

Tumors appear under a number of different circumstances or combination of circumstances. One such is the exposure to *carcinogens*, cancer-causing agents. Carcinogens include environmental agents, such as chemicals, radiation, and viruses. Many chemicals, environmental factors, and viruses may be carcinogens, but they have not been tested thoroughly, and may not be for years. The process of proving a link between an agent and a resulting cancer is a long and tedious process. In some localities, cancer clusters (an unusually high number of cancers in a limited area) have led researchers to classify certain chemicals as carcinogens. Exposure to certain agents, such as tobacco smoke, asbestos, insecticides, some dyes, and certain hormones, are known to increase the risk of cancer.

Another cause of cancer is from an inherited defect transmitted from parent(s) to child in the genetic material of the cell, *DNA (deoxyribonucleic acid)*. Figure 18-2 shows DNA in the nucleus of a cell. DNA contains coded material called genes that direct the growth of cells and the production of new proteins. When a cell divides into two cells in normal cell growth, exactly the same DNA appears in both cells. This process is called **mitosis.** Some genes in DNA may become

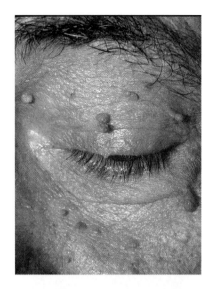
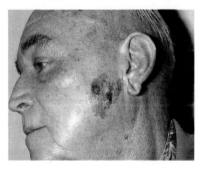

Figure 18-1. **(a) Benign tumors are not cancerous. In many cases, they do not have to be removed. (b) Malignancies have to be treated or they will spread.**

Many people are concerned about cancer and do their best to engage in prevention. Some methods that are helpful in prevention are: healthy diets, exercise, avoidance of tobacco, avoidance of sun exposure, and avoidance of carcinogens.

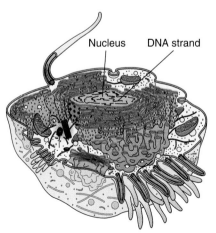

Nucleus   DNA strand

Figure 18-2. **DNA strands contain genetic information in the cell.**

defective in a process of change, called **mutation,** that often results from exposure to carcinogens. Mutations are then replicated over and over again and can lead to malignancies. Mutated DNA can predispose someone to cancer through heredity. Breast cancer and ovarian cancer are examples of largely inherited cancers. People with a family history of cancers are more likely to develop cancer. That does not mean, however, that people with no family history of a certain cancer (such as breast cancer) should ignore regular checkups. The other function of DNA is to copy its code onto another molecule called *RNA (ribonucleic acid)*. RNA carries coded messages from the nucleus to the outer material of the cell, the **cytoplasm.** The messages signal what proteins are needed.

Viruses heighten cancer risk (such as Kaposi's sarcoma from HIV). A virus that causes cancer is known as an *oncogenic* agent. An **oncogene** is a DNA fragment that converts normal cells into malignancies.

Vocabulary Review

In the previous section, you learned terms relating to oncology. Before going on to the exercises, review the terms below and refer to the previous section if you have questions.

Term	Word Analysis	Meaning
anaplasia	[ăn-ă-PLĀ-zē-ă] ana-, up + -plasia, formation	Loss of cell differentiation.
apoptosis	[ăp-ō-TŌ-sĭs] Greek, a dropping off	Normal death of cells.
benign	[bĕ-NĪN] From Latin *benignus*, kind	Encapsulated; not malignant.
cytoplasm	[SĪ-tō-plăzm] cyto-, cell + -plasm, formation	Outer portion of a cell surrounding the nucleus.
dedifferentiated	[dē-DĬF-ĕr-ĕn-shē-Ā-tĕd] de-, away from + differentiated	Lacking in normal orderly cell arrangement.
differentiated	[dĭf-ĕr-ĔN-shē-ā-tĕd]	Growing in an orderly fashion.
dysplasia	[dĭs-PLĀ-zē-ă] dys-, abnormal + -plasia	Abnormal tissue growth.
encapsulated	[ĕn-KĂP-sū-lā-tĕd]	Held within a capsule; benign.
heteroplasia	[HĔT-ĕr-ō-PLĀ-zē-ă] hetero-, different + -plasia	Dysplasia.
invasive	[ĭn-VĀ-sĭv]	Infiltrating other organs; spreading.
malignant	[mă-LĬG-nănt] From Latin *maligno*, to do in a malicious manner	Growing uncontrollably.

Term	Word Analysis	Meaning
metastasis	[mĕ-TĂS-tă-sĭs] Greek: *meta-*, beyond + *stasis*, a standing still	Spread of malignant cells to other parts of the body.
mitosis	[mī-TŌ-sĭs] From Greek *mitos*, thread	Cell division.
mutation	[myū-TĀ-shŭn]	Alteration in DNA to produce defective cells.
neoplasm	[NĒ-ō-plăzm] neo-, new + -plasm	Tumor; new growth.
oncogene	[ŎNG-kō-jēn] onco-, tumor + gene	DNA fragment that causes malignancies.
sarcoma	[săr-KŌ-mă] Greek *sarkoma*, fleshy growth	Relatively rare tumor that originates in muscle, connective tissue, and lymph.
solid tumor		Carcinoma; most common type of tumor.
teratoma	[tĕr-ă-TŌ-mă] Greek *teras*, monster + -oma, tumor	Growth containing several types of tissue and various types of cells.
tumor	[TŪ-mŏr] Latin, a swelling	Growth made up of cells that reproduce abnormally.

C A S E   S T U D Y

Finding a Symptom

Alicia Alvarez is fifty years old, has no family history of cancer, and is having her annual gynecological examination. Dr. Josiah Williams is a gynecologist specializing in the care of menopausal women. He notices a grayish area on the left side of Alicia's vulva. He recommends an immediate biopsy be taken in his office. Alicia expresses surprise and mentions that there is no cancer history in her family. Dr. Williams explains to Alicia that family history is just one factor in cancer of the female reproductive system. He also points out that a biopsy does not necessarily mean the tissue is cancerous; the discoloration may also be the result of an infection or irritation. Alicia agrees to have the biopsy.

 Critical Thinking

1. The discoloration on Alicia's vulva is possibly a type of skin cancer appearing on a part of the female reproductive system. Skin discolorations are usually *not* cancer. If you have a biopsy and the results are negative, should you still examine the skin area every few months? Why?

2. Name two cancers of the female reproductive system.

Tumors: Types and Causes Exercises

Find a Match

Write the word from this list that matches each statement.

benign   deoxyribonucleic acid   anaplasia   teratoma
carcinogen   metastasis   differentiated   malignant
dedifferentiated invasive   sarcoma   oncogene

3. Lacking in normal orderly cell growth_____

4. Encapsulated, not malignant _____

5. Infiltrating other organs; spreading _____

6. Growing uncontrollably _____

7. Genetic material of a cell _____

8. DNA fragment that causes malignancies _____

9. Growth containing several types of tissue and various types of cells _____

10. Tumor that originates in muscle, connective tissue, and lymph; fairly rare _____

11. Spread of malignant cells _____

12. Cancer-causing agent _____

Spell It Correctly

For each of the following words, write C if the spelling is correct. If it is not correct, write the correct spelling.

13. mestastasis _____

14. apoptosis _____

15. carsinoma_____

16. dedifferentiated_____

17. deoxirebonuclaic_____

18. citoplasm_____

Combining Forms and Abbreviations

The lists below include combining forms, suffixes, and abbreviations that relate specifically to oncology. Pronunciations are provided for the examples.

Combining Form	Meaning	Example
blast(o)	immature cell	*blastoma* [blăs-TŌ-mă], tumor arising from an immature cell
carcin(o)	cancer	*carcinogen* [kăr-SĬN-ō-jĕn], cancer-causing agent
muta	genetic change	*mutation* [mū-TĀ-shŭn], process of genetic change
mutagen(o)	genetic change	*mutagenic* [mū-tă-JĔN-ĭk], causing genetic change
onc(o)	tumor	*oncology* [ŏn-KŎL-ō-jē], treatment and study of tumors
radi(o)	radiation, X rays	*radiation* [rā-dē-Ā-shŭn], process of exposure to or treatment with above-normal levels of radiation

Suffix	Meaning	Example
-blast	immature cell	*leukoblast* [LŪ-kō-blăst], immature white blood cell
-oma (plural -omata)	tumor	*fibroma* [fī-BRŌ-mă], benign tumor arising from connective tissue
-plasia	formation (as of cells)	*dysplasia* [dĭs-PLĀ-zē-ă], abnormal tissue development
-plasm	formation (as of cells)	*neoplasm* [NĒ-ō-plăzm], abnormal tissue formed by abnormal cell growth
-plastic	formative	*neoplastic* [nē-ō-PLĂS-tĭk], growing abnormally (as a neoplasm)

Abbreviation	Meaning	Abbreviation	Meaning
ALL	acute lymphocytic leukemia	ER	estrogen receptor
AML	acute myelogenous leukemia	METS, mets	metastases
bx	biopsy	NHL	non-Hodgkin's lymphoma
CA	carcinoma	PSA	prostate-specific antigen
CEA	carcinogenic embyronic antigen	rad	radiation absorbed dose
chemo	chemotherapy	RNA	ribonucleic acid
CLL	chronic lymphocytic leukemia	RT	radiation therapy
CML	chronic myelogenous leukemia	TNM	tumor, nodes, metastasis
DES	diethylstilbestrol	Tx	treatment
DNA	deoxyribonucleic acid	XRT	x-ray or radiation therapy
DRE	digital rectal exam		

Being Careful

Frightened by Alicia's news of possible cancer, Peter Alvarez, her husband, went to Dr. John Chin, an internist, for a physical. He had not had a physical in the last five years, but felt now that he should. Peter is 50 years old and has no history of cancer. Dr. Chin had the nurse draw blood for various tests.

Dr. Chin explained that one of the tests that should be done on a yearly basis for males over the age of 45 is the PSA.

Critical Thinking

19. What part of the body does the PSA test evaluate?

20. Peter had not had a physical in five years. Why is it important to be checked on a yearly basis for certain types of cancer when you reach certain ages?

Combining Forms and Abbreviations Exercises

Build Your Medical Vocabulary

Using the combining forms and suffixes in this chapter and in Chapter 3, write a term for each definition.

21. therapy using radiation _____

22. bone tumor_____

23. immature red blood cell_____

24. fluid-filled glandular carcinoma_____

25. tumor of the meninges _____

26. cancer of the lymph system_____

Check Your Knowledge

For each of the following cancers, name the body part involved. Refer to Chapter 3 if you need to review combining forms for body parts.

27. adenoma _____

28. neuroblastoma _____

29. myoma _____

30. retinoblastoma _____

31. lymphocytoma _____

Find the Terms

Use the combining forms above to complete the following words.

32. tumor consisting of immature cells: _____oma

33. treatment of tumors: _____therapy

34. agent that promotes a genetic change: _____gen

35. impenetrable by radiation: _____opaque

36. destructive to cancer cells: _____lytic

Diagnostic, Procedural, and Laboratory Terms

Cancer is a general term referring to any of various diseases with uncontrolled cell growth. Researchers have developed tests to detect many cancers and, in some cases, to detect cancer at its earliest stages. Survival rates have improved because of diagnostic techniques. The sooner cell growth can be normalized, the greater the possibility of survival.

Routine medical checkups often include tests for cancer. Adult females usually have a *pap smear*, a test for cervical and uterine cancer, along with a breast examination, including palpation of the breasts for lumps. Adult males usually have a blood test called a *PSA (prostate-specific antigen)* that can detect prostate cancer. A *digital rectal exam (DRE)* is also a prostate cancer screening method. Doctors also check male testicles for any signs of tumors. Testicular cancer occurs fairly commonly. Normal adult checkups usually include auscultation of the lungs, palpation of the abdomen, inspection of the rectum and an occult stool test (particularly if the patient has a family history of colon cancer or has some possible symptoms), and a discussion of any symptoms that may need further investigation. Some blood tests indicate a particular type of cancer. For example, patients with gastrointestinal tumors usually have *carcinoembryonic antigens (CEA)* in their bloodstream. An *alphafetoprotein test (AFP)* is given to detect the presence of liver or testicular cancer. HCG or *human chorionic gonadotropin* is usually present in the blood of patients with testicular cancer. CA-125 *(cancer antigen 125)* is a protein produced by ovarian cancer cells. Colorectal cancers can be detected by a *colonoscopy.*

Imaging techniques now provide a detailed picture of various parts of the body. MRIs, CAT scans, mammograms, and the insertion of lighted instruments to view various body parts have advanced diagnostic techniques. Any tumors that are found are categorized by **grade,** the maturity of the tumor, and **stage,** the degree of spread or metastasis of the tumor. A common method for grading is the **TNM** (tumor, node, metastasis) **system,** which numbers the extent of the tumor, the extent of lymph nodes affected, and the degree of metastasis. Table 18-1 describes the grading used in the TNM system. Tumors are also characterized by appearance under the microscope, and by observations made on visual examination.

Table 18-1 The TNM system of grading

Classification	Size Indicator	Meaning
T (tumor)	0-4	0 means no tumor; 1-4 mean progressively larger tumors.
N (node)	0-4	0 means no lymph node involvement; 1-4 indicates extent to which cancer affects nodes.
M (metastasis)	0-3	0 means no metastasis. 1-3 are the stages of metastasis.

Microscopic examination can determine if a tumor is **alveolar,** forming small sacs shaped like alveoli; **anaplastic,** reverting to a more immature form; *carcinoma in situ,* contained at a site without spreading; **diffuse,** spreading evenly; **dysplastic,** abnormal in cell appearance; **epidermoid,** resembling epithelial cells; **follicular,** containing glandlike sacs; **hyperchromatic,** intensely colored; **hyperplastic,** excessive in development (of cells); **hypoplastic,** under-developed as tissue; **nodular,** formed in tight cell clusters; **papillary,** having small papillae projecting from cells; **pleomorphic,** having many types of cells; **scirrhous,** made up of hard, densely packed cells; and **undifferentiated,** lacking a defined cell structure. Figure 18-3 shows microscopic views of benign and malignant growths.

Tumors are also described by their appearance during visual examination. Tumors can be described as *cystic,* filled with fluid; **fungating,** projecting from a surface in a mushroomlike pattern; *inflammatory,* having an inflamed appearance (swollen and red); **medullary,** large and fleshy; **necrotic,** containing dead tissue; **polypoid,** containing polyps; **ulcerating,** having open wounds; and **verrucous,** having wartlike, irregular growths.

Once a tumor is confirmed as malignant, doctor and patient discuss and agree on a **protocol,** a course of treatment. One of the possible treatments is **radiation,** the bombarding of the tumor with rays that damage the DNA of the tumor cells. Most radiation treatment is carefully pinpointed, but some surrounding cells usually suffer damage as well. Radiation can cause many unpleasant side effects, such as hair loss, nausea, and skin damage.

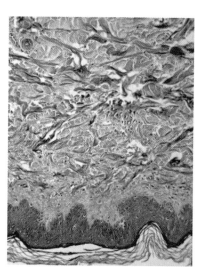 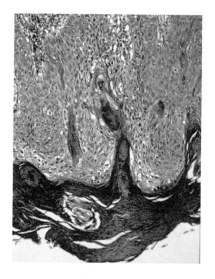

Figure 18-3. (a) Microscopic view of normal cell growth. (b) Malignancies show up under a microscope as abnormal cell growth in a particular area or areas.

Vocabulary Review

In the previous section, you learned terms relating to oncological diagnosis, clinical procedures, and laboratory tests. Before going on to the exercises, review the terms below and refer to the previous section if you have questions.

Term	Word Analysis	Meaning
alveolar	[ăl-VĒ-ō-lăr]	Forming small sacs.
anaplastic	[ăn-ă-PLĂS-tĭk] ana-, up + -plastic, forming	Reverting to a more immature form.
diffuse	[dĭ-FYŪS]	Spreading evenly.
dysplastic	[dĭs-PLĂS-tĭk] dys-, abnormal + -plastic	Abnormal in cell appearance.
epidermoid	[ĕp-ĭ-DĔR-mŏyd] epiderm(us) + -oid, like	Resembling epithelial cells.
follicular	[fŏl-LĬK-yū-lăr]	Containing glandular sacs.
fungating	[FŬNG-āt-ĭng]	Growing in a mushroomlike pattern.
grade		Maturity of a tumor.
hyperchromatic	[HĪ-pĕr-krō-MĂT-ĭk] hyper-, excessively + chromatic	Intensely colored.
hyperplastic	[hī-pĕr-PLĂS-tĭk] hyper- + -plastic	Excessive in development (of cells).
hypoplastic	[HĪ-pō-PLĂS-tĭk] hypo-, abnormally low + -plastic	Underdeveloped, as tissue.
medullary	[MĔD-ū-lăr-ē]	Large and fleshy.
necrotic	[nĕ-KRŎT-ĭk] Greek *nekrosis*, death	Containing dead tissue.
nodular	[NŌD-yū-lăr]	Formed in tight clusters.
papillary	[PĂP-ĭ-lăr-ē]	Having papillae projecting from cells.
pleomorphic	[plē-ō-MŌR-fĭk] pleo-, more + Greek *morphe*, form	Having many types of cells.

Term	Word Analysis	Meaning
polypoid	[PŎL-ĭ-pŏyd] poly(p) + -oid	Containing polyps.
protocol	[PRŌ-tō-kŏl]	Course of treatment.
radiation	[RĀ-dē-Ā-shŭn]	Bombarding of tumors with rays that damage the DNA of cells.
scirrhous	[SKĬR-ŭs] Greek *skirrhos*, hard	Hard, densely packed.
stage		Degree of tumor spread.
TNM system		Tumor, node, metastasis system of categorizing tumors.
ulcerating	[ŬL-sĕr-ā-tĭng]	Having open wounds.
undifferentiated	[ŬN-dĭf-ĕr-ĔN-shē-ā-tĕd] un-, not + differentiated	Lacking a defined cell structure.
verrucous	[vĕ-RŪ-kōs] Latin *verrucosus*	Wartlike in appearance.

C A S E S T U D Y

Getting a Diagnosis

Dr. Williams sent Alicia's biopsy to Medical Center Pathologists. He received the following report.

Critical Thinking

37. Does the report cite any unusual growth of cells?

38. Have any of the cells invaded neighboring tissue?

> MICROSCOPIC: A single slide containing sections through the submitted material is reviewed. This biopsy of skin is centrally ulcerated. The area of ulceration is surrounded by keratinizing squamous epithelium, which exhibits a full-thickness dysplasia. This dysplastic change is characterized by cells that have a vertical growth pattern, somewhat hyperchromatic nuclei, and an increased mitotic rate. Mitoses do extend to the surface. The lesion does not appear to invade the underlying and associated stroma. Mild-to-moderate dysplastic changes are seen peripherally and do extend to the surgical margins.

Find the Part

Write the body part(s) being tested for cancer by each of the following procedures:

39. mammogram: _____

40. DRE: _____

41. PSA: _____

42. pap smear: _____

Check Your Knowledge

Fill in the blanks.

43. A tumor filled with liquid is referred to as _____.

44. Some melanomas are _____, or intensely colored.

45. Chemotherapy is one _____ for treatment of cancer.

46. Tissue that is dead is referred to as _____.

47. Some cancers are _____, or wartlike in appearance.

Pathological Terms

Cancer is a pathological term. It can affect people from the fetal stage until old age. Many advances have been made in cancer prevention and treatment, but some cancers have had no increase in cure rates for many years, and others have increased within the population, some of which may be due to an increase in detection. Table 18-2 lists some common cancers.

Table 18-2 Common cancers

Type of Cancer	Where Cancer Starts	Common Sites in the Body	Specific Risk Groups (Most cancers can affect anyone.)	Prevention and Early Diagnosis
adenocarcinoma	gland	colon, stomach		high fiber diet; colonoscopy
adenoma	glandular epithelium			
astrocytoma	neuroglia	brain		

(continued on next page)

Table 18-2 (continued)

Type of Cancer	Where Cancer Starts	Common Sites in the Body	Specific Risk Groups (Most cancers can affect anyone.)	Prevention and Early Diagnosis
basal cell carcinoma	skin	skin		avoiding sun exposure; examination of skin
Burkitt's lymphoma	lymph			
carcinoma	epithelial tissue	glands, lungs, kidney, breast		avoidance of carcinogens such as tobacco, asbestos; early checkups
carcinoma in situ	encapsulated tumor	breast, cervix		self-examination; mammography
chondrosarcoma	cartilage			
Ewing's sarcoma	connective tissue			
fibrosarcoma	connective tissue			
glioblastoma	neurological tissue			
glioma	neurological	brain		
Hodgkin's disease	lymph system			
hypernephroma	kidneys			
Kaposi's sarcoma	first seen in skin of AIDS patient, then other organs		patients with HIV	preventative measures (such as safe sex)
leiomyosarcoma	smooth muscle			
leukemia	stem cells			
leukoplakia	tongue or cheeks			
liposarcoma	fat			
lymphoma	lymph system			
medulloblastoma	brain			
melanoma	skin			avoidance of sun; skin examination
multiple myeloma	bone marrow and bone			
nephrosarcoma	kidney			
neuroblastoma	adrenal glands	adrenal glands of infants and children		

(continued on next page)

Table 18-2 (continued)

Type of Cancer	Where Cancer Starts	Common Sites in the Body	Specific Risk Groups (Most cancers can affect anyone.)	Prevention and Early Diagnosis
non-Hodgkin's lymphoma	lymph tissue			
osteosarcoma	bone			
retinoblastoma	retina	eye		
rhabdomyo-sarcoma	striated muscle			
sarcoma	connective tissue			

C A S E S T U D Y

Seeing a Specialist

Alicia's cancer is a carcinoma in situ. Dr. Williams refers Alicia to a surgical oncologist who performs the surgery to remove the tumor. The surgeon, Dr. Wilma Grant, examines surrounding tissue during the surgery and decides that Alicia does not need further treatment. The surgeon cautioned Alicia to make sure she has regular six-month checkups.

Critical Thinking

48. Why did the doctor recommend six-month checkups?

49. Dr. Grant did not recommend radiation or chemotherapy. Does that mean that Alicia's cancer has metastasized?

Pathological Terms Exercises

Find the Disease

Using Table 18-2, write at least one type of cancer for each location.

50. breast_____

51. colon_____

52. bone marrow____•_____

53. skin_____

54. brain_____

55. stem cells_____

56. lymph system_____

57. bone_____

58. fat_____

59. neurological tissue_____

60. neuroglia_____

Preventing and Detecting

Answer the following questions.

61. Using Table 18-2 as a guide, write a brief paragraph about how you can minimize the risk of contracting certain cancers. _____

62. What two types of cancer are detectable by self-examination at an early stage?

_____

Spell It Correctly

For each of the following words, write C if the spelling is correct. If it is not, write the correct spelling.

63. aveolar_____

64. follicular_____

65. displastic_____

66. medulary_____

67. pleomorphic_____

Surgical Terms

Many cancers can be diagnosed and treated with surgery. First, an **incisional biopsy,** removal of a part of a tumor for examination that establishes whether the tumor is malignant, is performed. Next, a plan of treatment is established. If surgery is needed, the tumor is removed and surrounding tissue is examined for spread of the tumor in a procedure called **excisional biopsy.** The tumor is removed to an established *surgical margin* or to the point where it abuts normal tissue. Some surgeries involve **resectioning,** removal of the tumor and a large amount of the surrounding tissue, including lymph nodes, or **exenteration,** removal of an organ, tumor, and surrounding tissue. Other surgeries may involve **cryosurgery,** destruction by freezing; **electrocauterization,** destruction by burning; or **fulguration,** destruction by high-frequency current.

Vocabulary Review

In the previous section, you learned terms relating to surgery. Before going on to the exercises, review the terms below and refer to the previous section if you have questions.

Term	Word Analysis	Meaning
cryosurgery	[krī-ō-SĔR-jĕr-ē] cryo-, cold + surgery	Destruction by freezing.
electrocauterization	[ē-LĔK-trō-CĂW-tĕr-ĭ-ZĀ-shŭn] electro-, electrical + cauterization	Destruction by burning tissue.
excisional biopsy	[ĕk-SĬZH-shŭn-l BĪ-ŏp-sē]	Removal of tumor and surrounding tissue for examination.
exenteration	[ĕks-ĕn-tĕr-Ā-shŭn] ex-, out of + Greek *enteron*, bowel	Removal of an organ, tumor, and surrounding tissue.
fulguration	[fŭl-gū-RĀ-shŭn]	Destruction by high-frequency current.
incisional biopsy	[ĭn-SĬZH-shŭn-l]	Removal of a part of a tumor for examination.
resectioning	[rē-SĔK-shŭn-ĭng]	Removal of a tumor and a large amount of surrounding tissue.

CASE STUDY

Getting Information

Alicia was concerned about the possibility of a recurrence of cancer. She asked Dr. Williams for a copy of the pathologist's report. Alicia did not understand some of the language in it, so she asked Dr. Williams for an explanation.

Critical Thinking

68. How might Dr. Williams explain "The lesion does not appear to invade the underlying and associated . . .?

69. The dysplastic changes extend to the surgical margin, which is the outline out to which the removal of the cancer will take place. What determines the surgical margin?

Surgical Terms Exercises

Find a Match

Match the correct term in the right-hand column with its definition in the left-hand column

70. removal of part of a tumor   a. fulguration

71. removal of a tumor and surrounding tissue for examination   b. cryosurgery

72. form of surgery using freezing   c. electrocauterization

73. form of surgery using burning   d. incisional biopsy

74. form of surgery using high-frequency current   e. excisional biopsy

Pharmacological Terms

Aside from surgery and radiation, cancer treatment includes two other **modalities** (methods)—**chemotherapy,** use of drugs to treat cancer, and **biological therapy,** use of agents that enhance the body's own immune response in fighting tumor growth. Both chemotherapy and biological therapy have side effects, such as hair loss, nausea, and so on. All four cancer treatments may be used together or separately during the course of a protocol, a treatment plan for a particular cancer.

Radiation and chemotherapy must be specifically directed so as not to harm healthy cells while destroying unhealthy ones. Biological therapy targets cells that are receptive to the substances being injected.

Vocabulary Review

Term	Word Analysis	Meaning
biological therapy		Treatment of cancer with agents from the body that increase immune response.
chemotherapy	[KĔM-ō-thār-ă-pē, KĒ-mō-thār-ă-pē] chemo-, chemical + therapy	Treatment of cancer using drugs.
modality	[mō-DĂL-ĭ-tē]	Method of treatment.

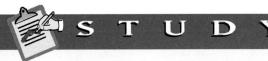

Finding Another Cancer

Alicia went for a six-month gynecological checkup. Her pap smear was normal. She encouraged her sister, Margo, to see Dr. Williams. Margo is 15 years younger than Alicia. Margo goes to the gynecologist only when she has a problem. She has never had a mammogram. Dr. Williams shows Margo how to do breast self-examination and tells her that he feels a small lump on the side of her breast. This is confirmed with a mammogram and a biopsy. After a lumpectomy, Margo is told that the cancer has spread to one lymph node which is also removed. Chemotherapy is recommended, along with biological therapy in the form of a weekly injection.

💡 Critical Thinking

75. Why did the surgeon recommend chemotherapy?

76. How might the biological therapy help Margo?

Go to the American Cancer Society's web site (http://www.cancer.org) and write a paragraph about cancer prevention.

CHAPTER REVIEW

Definitions

Define the following terms and combining forms. Review the chapter before starting. Make sure you know how to pronounce each term as you define it.

Term	Definition
alveolar [ăl-VĒ-ō-lăr]	
anaplasia [ăn-ă-PLĀ-zē-ă]	
anaplastic [ăn-ă-PLĂS-tĭk]	
apoptosis [ăp-ō-TŌ-sĭs]	
benign [bě-NĪN]	
biological therapy	
blast(o)	
-blast	
carcin(o)	
chemotherapy [KĔM-ō-thār-ă-pē, KĒ-mō-thār-ă-pē]	
cryosurgery [krī-ō-SĔR-jĕr-ē]	
cytoplasm [SĪ-tō-plăzm]	
dedifferentiated [dē-DĬF-ĕr-ĕn-shē-Ā-tĕd]	
differentiated [dĭf-ĕr-ĔN-shē-ā-tĕd]	
diffuse [dĭ-fyūs]	
dysplasia [dĭs-PLĀ-zē-Ă]	
dysplastic [dĭs-PLĂS-tĭk]	
electrocauterization [ē-LĔK-trō-CĂW-tĕr-ĭ-ZĀ-shŭn]	
encapsulated [ĕn-KĂP-sū-lā-tĕd]	
epidermoid [ĕp-ĭ-DĔR-mŏyd]	
excisional biopsy [ĕk-SĬZH-shŭn-l BĪ-ŏp-sē]	
exenteration [ĕks-ĕn-tĕr-Ā-shŭn]	
follicular [fŏl-LĬK-yū-lăr]	

Term	Definition
fulguration [fŭl-gū-RĀ-shŭn]	_____
fungating [FŬNG-āt-ĭng]	_____
grade	_____
heteroplasia [HĔT-ĕr-ō-PLĀ-zē-ă]	_____
hyperchromatic [HĪ-pĕr-krō-MĂT-ĭk]	_____
hyperplastic [hī-pĕr-PLĂS-tĭk]	_____
hypoplastic [HĪ-pō-PLĂS-tĭk]	_____
incisional [ĭn-SĬZH-shŭn-l] biopsy	_____
invasive [ĭn-VĀ-sĭv]	_____
malignant [mă-LĬG-nănt]	_____
medullary [MĔD-ū-lăr-ē]	_____
metastasis [mĕ-TĂS-tă-sĭs]	_____
mitosis [mī-TŌ-sĭs]	_____
modality [mō-DĂL-ĭ-tē]	_____
muta	_____
mutagen(o)	_____
mutation [myū-TĂ-shŭn]	_____
necrotic [nĕ-KRŎT-ĭk]	_____
neoplasm [NĒ-ō-plăzm]	_____
nodular [NŌD-yū-lăr]	_____
-oma (plural -omata)	_____
onc(o)	_____
oncogene [ŎNG-kō-jēn]	_____
papillary [PĂP-ĭ-lār-ē]	_____
-plasia	_____
-plasm	_____
-plastic	_____
pleomorphic [plē-ō-MŌR-fĭk]	_____
polypoid [PŎL-ĭ-pŏyd]	_____
protocol [PRŌ-tō-kŏl]	_____
radi(o)	_____
radiation [RĀ-dē-Ā-shŭn]	_____

Term	Definition
resectioning [rē-SĔK-shŭn-ĭng]	_____
sarcoma [săr-KŌ-mă]	_____
scirrhous [SKĬR-ŭs]	_____
solid tumor	_____
stage	_____
teratoma [tĕr-ă-TŌ-mă]	_____
TNM system	_____
tumor [TŪ-mŏr]	_____
ulcerating [ŬL-sĕr-ā-tĭng]	_____
undiffferentiated [ŬN-dĭf-ĕr-ĔN-shē-ā-tĕd]	_____
verrucous [vĕ-RŪ-kōs]	_____

Abbreviations

Write the full meaning of each abbreviation.

Abbreviation	Meaning	Abbreviation	Meaning
ALL	_____	RNA	_____
AML	_____	RT	_____
bx	_____	TNM	_____
CA	_____	Tx	_____
CEA	_____	XRT	_____
chemo	_____		
CLL	_____		
CML	_____		
DES	_____		
DNA	_____		
DRE	_____		
ER	_____		
METS, mets	_____		
NHL	_____		
PSA	_____		
rad	_____		

1. Yes. Early detection is important; and skin changes can occur fairly rapidly.
2. breast and uterine or ovarian
3. dedifferentiated
4. benign
5. invasive
6. malignant
7. deoxyribonucleic acid
8. oncogene
9. teratoma
10. sarcoma
11. metastasis
12. carcinogen
13. metastasis
14. C
15. carcinoma
16. C
17. deoxyribonucleic
18. cytoplasm
19. prostate
20. Early detection improves survival.
21. radiotherapy
22. osteoma
23. erythroblast
24. cystoadenocarcinoma
25. meningioma
26. lymphoma
27. gland
28. immature nerve cell
29. muscle tissue
30. eye
31. lymph cells
32. blast
33. onco
34. muta
35. radi(o)
36. carcino
37. yes, dysplasia
38. no, carcinoma in situ
39. breast
40. prostate
41. prostate
42. uterus and cervix
43. cystic
44. hyperchromatic
45. protocol
46. necrotic
47. verrucous
48. to find further cancer early
49. no, because metastasized cancer needs aggressive treatment
50. carcinoma in situ, carcinoma
51. adenocarcinoma
52. multiple myeloma
53. basal cell carcinoma or melanoma
54. medulloblastoma
55. leukemia
56. lymphoma
57. osteosarcoma
58. liposarcoma
59. glioblastoma
60. astrocytoma
61. Self-examination, regular checkups, colonoscopy, mammogram, and avoidance of carcinogens should be in each student's paragraph.
62. breast, skin
63. alveolar
64. C
65. dysplastic
66. medullary
67. C
68. This means the cancer has not spread.
69. how far the cancer extends out to healthy tissue
70. d
71. e
72. b
73. c
74. a
75. Margo's cancer had metastasized. There was no guarantee that all the cancer was removed.
76. Increased immune responses might attack cancer cells.
77. dysplastic, hyperchromatic
78. Yes, the margin will be just beyond the point at which dysplasia appears.

CHAPTER 19

Diagnostic Imaging and Surgery

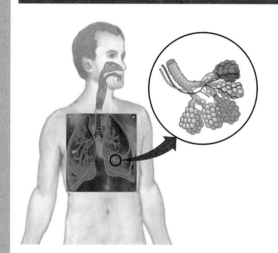

After studying this chapter, you will be able to:

◆ List the types of diagnostic imaging

◆ List the types of surgery and some important surgical tools

◆ Define the combining forms and suffixes used in building words that relate to diagnostic imaging and surgery

◆ Identify the meaning of related abbreviations

Diagnostic Imaging and Radiation Therapy

Historically, if a doctor tried to diagnose an internal ailment, surgery was the only way to actually see the tissue and organs of a person. With the advent of imaging, it is now possible to view the interior of the human body without invasive procedures. **Imaging** is the production of visual output using x-rays, sound waves, or magnetic fields. **Diagnostic imaging** is the use of imaging to diagnose problems in the interior of a part of the body without surgery. The three major types of imaging are x-rays, ultrasonography, and magnetic resonance imaging (MRI). X-ray technology was the earliest form of imaging. It now ranges from black and white images produced by electromagnetic radiation to computer-enhanced images on a computerized axial tomography (CAT) scan. X-ray technology is widely used in dentistry and for numerous diagnostic situations such as bone fractures, tumor locations, and many other conditions. Ultrasonography uses sound waves to produce a visual image of an area of the body's interior. Ultrasonography is routinely used to view the womb of a pregnant women. Magnetic resonance imaging uses a magnet to obtain images of an area of the body.

X-Ray Technology

In the early twentieth century, **x-rays** were discovered and the first images of the inside of a living person were made. X-rays are high-energy electromagnetic **radiation,** energy from the interior of a substance carried by a stream of electrically charged particles. There are three types of radioactive particles: **gamma rays** have the most penetrating ability of the three types, **alpha rays** have the least, and **beta rays** fall somewhere in the middle in penetrating ability. The use of x-rays increased dramatically until it was discovered that extensive exposure to radiation could cause health problems (cancer, birth defects, and so on). Later, lower doses of x-rays that are considered safe dramatically altered the way disease is diagnosed. Now, x-rays are commonly used to detect pathology throughout the body and to treat certain diseases.

X-rays show images in black, white, and gray (Figure 19-1). They are useful for showing abnormalities such as broken bones, internal anomalies, or dental abnormalities, as well as for use in treating certain diseases. X-rays reveal internal images by exposure of a picture on a photographic plate. The x-rays are directed toward the patient and when they travel through the patient, they come to the plate placed directly behind. Patients are positioned so that the best image may be obtained. Substances of the body may be **radiolucent,** allowing x-rays to pass through quickly (air is radiolucent) or **radiopaque,** blocking or absorbing x-rays (bone is radiopaque). In between radiolucent and radiopaque, there are many degrees of absorbability or resistance to the passage of x-rays. For example, fat is fairly absorbent; blood, lymph, and water are more so. Radiolucent substances appear black on x-ray images and radiopaque substances appear white. Substances in-between radiolucent and radiopaque appear in various shades of gray.

X-rays can be dangerous, particularly to people who administer them in a clinical setting. X-rays cannot be seen, heard, touched, or smelled. They cannot travel through lead, a very dense substance, so that the use of lead vests or aprons is very common for radiologic technologists. Also, lead vests are often used to cover parts of the patient's body not being x-rayed. X-rays **ionize,** change neutral particles to positively charged **ions,** and, in doing so, destroy cancer cells and slow the growth of tumors (Figure 19-2). Control of the x-rays has become more sophisticated; however, damage to surrounding tissue almost invariably occurs during *radiation therapy,* the use of x-rays to destroy cancer cells. Long-term, unprotected exposure to x-rays can cause cancer.

The use of computers has enhanced radiologic techniques. Not only is the detail of x-rays increased, but computer-guided x-rays can photograph at various angles and can photograph certain body parts (such as the heart) while they are working. **Tomography,** the production of three-dimensional images, provides much anatomical and diagnostic information. **CT (computed tomography)** or **CAT (computerized axial tomography) scans** show a series of images conveyed to the computer as detailed pictures of slices of an organ or body part. **Positron emission tomography** or **PET scans** are imaging tests that show the distribution of substances in tissue. They are often used to diagnose brain disorders. This is accomplished by bombarding the area being x-rayed with x-rays at many different angles. The computer interprets the normal density of various parts of the body and the density of a solution ingested. The result is a clear image of minute sections able to show abnormalities in detail. **Fluoroscopy** is another imaging technique using x-rays. Instead of a photographic plate, the image is projected onto a fluorescent screen that shows visual images as light rays that are emitted when the x-rays pass through a

In Latin, *radius* meant ray (as of light). Now, words like radiation, radiology, and radiography refer specifically to x-rays.

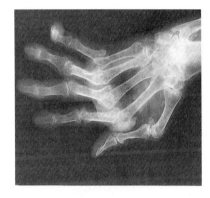

Figure 19-1 X-ray images are black, white, and gray.

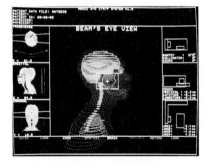

Figure 19-2 Ionizing of cells is one method of slowing or stopping tumor growth.

Diagnosing Breast Cancer

Mammograms are the most commonly used diagnostic tool for diagnosing breast tumors or lesions. They have increased early diagnosis tremendously. However, mammograms do not distinguish between benign and malignant growths, and they miss 10 percent of cancers. Researchers are working on using other imaging techniques to alleviate these two problems. PET scans are more effective at identifying benign growths. MRIs can detect 100 percent of tumors, but do not distinguish them from benign growths. The goal of the research is 100-percent detection of cancers with no unnecessary biopsies for benign growths.

In addition, radiologists are using new tools to make breast cancer treatment easier and more effective. In cases where a biopsy is necessary, a *stereotactic breast biopsy* is used to focus in on the area that needs to be examined. This technique allows radiologists and surgeons to perform the biopsy quickly and accurately.

patient. Fluoroscopy allows for observation of a body part in motion.

X-ray equipment varies depending on the intended use. For example, dental x-rays are taken with a machine that points the radiation to an area of the mouth. Chest x-rays are generally taken on a large plate that covers the front of the chest. CAT scans and PET scans also aim x-rays at particular body areas. The equipment for these scans is attached to a computer on which the image is shown.

The clarity of x-rays can be enhanced if a *contrast medium*, a dense substance that shows up as white on the x-ray film, is used for a particular area of the body. **Barium** and **iodine** substances are ingested to provide a dense substance in a particular area. A *barium swallow* (also called a *barium cookie*) is used for an upper GI series showing the esophagus, stomach, and duodenum. The barium can then be followed as it travels through the small intestine. A *barium enema* is the insertion of barium into the rectum and colon for a lower GI series.

Iodine is used in many imaging tests to highlight the interior of a cavity, tube, or vessel. *Angiography* is imaging of the blood vessels and chambers of the heart after an iodine substance is inserted through a catheter to the heart. *Digital subtraction angiography (DSA)* is a two-step imaging process described in Chapter 6. *Magnetic resonance angiography* is the imaging of the flow of blood through vessels. *Arteriography* is the imaging of arteries usually in the brain (usually to detect blockages). *Arthrography* is the imaging of joints after injection of an iodine substance. *Cholangiography* is an examination of the gallbladder and bile ducts. *Cholecystography* is an image taken after an iodine substance is swallowed and it reaches the gallbladder and bile ducts. *Hysterosalpingography* is imaging of the fallopian tubes after injection of a contrast medium containing iodine. *Lymphangiography* is imaging of the lymphatic vessels. *Myelography* is imaging of the spinal cord to examine disks and check for anomalies. *Pyelography* is the imaging of the renal pelvis and urinary tract. *Venography* is the imaging of any vein after injection of a contrast medium.

Ultrasonography

Ultrasonography or *sonography* is the use of sound waves to produce images showing the interior of the body. An **ultrasound** image or a **sonogram** results when high-frequency sound waves are reflected off the body part being observed. The waves are received by a detector that converts them to electrical impulses that can then be seen on a video monitor. The images produced are not very clear. Ultrasonography is a noninvasive method of observation. The equipment used for ultrasonography usually consists of a wand that is moved back and forth over the area being observed, which is attached to a monitor on which the image is seen. It is used most frequently in monitoring fetal development during pregnancy (Figure 19-3). It is also commonly used for diagnosis, as in *echocardiography*, a test used in cardiovascular diagnosis, and can be helpful in diagnosing disorders of many other organs (kidney, breast, uterus, gallbladder). A special type of ultrasound unit called a *doppler* is used on blood vessels.

Magnetic Resonance Imaging (MRI)

Magnetic Resonance Imaging (MRI) creates images by tracking the magnetic properties within the nuclei of various cells. As the cells move, some atoms respond to magnetic fields and emit radio waves that produce an image. MRIs are commonly used to diagnose various tumors, defects in the cardiovascular system, and brain anomalies. MRIs do not use x-rays and, therefore, are considered safe and effective. Most MRIs do not require a contrast medium, but one may be used to enhance a scan in certain cases such as in viewing blood vessels. MRI equipment generally consists of a tube into which the patient is placed. While the patient is lying absolutely still, the magnet in the equipment obtains the scan.

Nuclear Medicine

Nuclear medicine uses radioactivity to test and treat disease. Radioactive chemicals, combined with blood or urine specimens *in vitro* (in a test tube), can reveal the presence of various hormones and drugs. Such information is used to monitor the use of medications with potentially harmful side effects. One test in particular, a **radioimmunoassay (RIA)**, is a common "drug test," often given to participants in sports events, applicants for a job, or others who require regular drug testing. A radioimmunoassay is also used to determine the amount of a medication left in the body after a certain period of time. This information is useful in determining the correct dosage of certain medications.

Other studies in nuclear medicine are done *in vivo* (in the body). The basic goal of an in vivo test is to trace **radionuclides** (radioactive substances) ingested by the patient as they travel through the body. **Tracer studies** trace a specific **radiopharmaceutical** (combination of a chemical and a radionuclide designed to travel to a specific organ) while it makes its way through the organ. In this way, the function of an organ is imaged for observation and treatment. Similarly, a *scanner* (machine capable of creating **scans** or images) tracks the movement of radiopharmaceuticals within an organ to show how the organ functions. Common scans are: a *blood and heart scan*, a tracing of blood flow through the heart for diagnosing heart disease; a *bone scan* for bone cancer; a *brain scan*, for detecting anomalies in the brain that would allow a radiopharmaceutical to pass the BBB (blood-brain barrier); a *gallium scan*, using a specific radionuclide (gallium-67) to locate tumors and cysts; and a *thyroid scan*, scanning the thyroid gland for thyroid cancer and function.

An **uptake** test in nuclear medicine is used to determine how quickly a radiopharmaceutical is absorbed by a particular organ or body part, as in a radioactive iodine uptake of the thyroid gland. A *perfusion study* in nuclear medicine tracks the passage of radiopharmaceuticals throughout the capillaries of the lungs, revealing any clots. A perfusion study may be used in combination with a *ventilation study*, which tracks an inhaled gas as it fills the air sacs of the lungs.

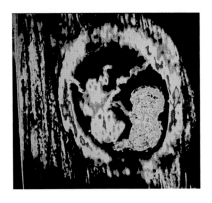

Figure 19-3 An ultrasound can detect multiple fetuses. Shown here are twins.

Radiation Therapy

X-rays and radionuclides are potentially dangerous in high doses. They can cause damage and death to cells at which they are aimed. *Radiation therapy* or *radiation oncology* is the specialty of those who treat abnormal body tissue with doses of x-rays or radionuclides (particularly those containing **cobalt**). Cells that are treated with high-dose radiation are **irradiated.** Irradiation of cells is used in treating diseases with abnormal tissue growth, such as cancer. Radiation is given in doses necessary to penetrate and destroy the malignant cells. The radiation is measured in **rads** (radiation absorbed dose), which in turn is measured in **grays (gy)**, each gray equaling 100 rads. Tissue to be irradiated is either **radiosensitive** (as are most lymphomas), needing fewer grays to kill cells, or **radioresistant** (as are most sarcomas), needing more grays to kill cells.

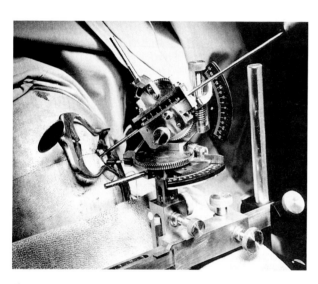

Figure 19-4 A stereotactic frame directs a radiation beam to a specific spot.

Radiation is transmitted to cells using various techniques and machines depending on the type of location of the cancerous cells needing treatment. A *linear accelerator* is an *external beam* machine used to emit radioactive particles in a straight line directed at a malignancy. A *betatron* is a circular machine for delivery of radioactive material. A **stereotactic frame** is a device placed around the patient to direct a radiation beam to a specific spot in the brain (Figure 19-4).

In addition to equipment, radiotherapy may be delivered directly in **brachytherapy,** the implanting of radioactive elements directly into a tumor (**interstitial therapy**) or into an adjacent cavity (**intracavitary therapy**). Another type of radiotherapy is the introduction of radioactive materials that have a specific use (as radioactive iodine in thyroid therapy) when placed in the bloodstream. In the case of the thyroid, it is the only body organ to use iodine, so the treatment affects only the thyroid even though the material travels through the bloodstream.

Radiation therapy may be beneficial and even lifesaving, but it does have potential side effects. Some temporary effects are *alopecia,* loss of hair; nausea, vomiting, or diarrhea; *radiation anemia,* suppression of red blood cell production after treatment with radioactive material; inflammations of the skin, mucous membranes or epithelial tissue due to breakdown of tissue exposed to the radiation; and **malaise,** general ill feeling.

Radiology or **roentgenology** is the medical specialty that analyzes the results of imaging tests. The medical specialty that uses radioactive substances to view or to treat diseases is known as **nuclear medicine.** Either a *radiologist* or a *nuclear medicine physician* is a specialist in radiology. Generally, physicians do not administer the tests or treatment. *Radiologic technologists* are trained to protect the patient and themselves while producing the clearest, most accurate image or treating a disease. Radiologic technologists may specialize as *radiographers* in **radiography,** the production of diagnostic images; *nuclear medicine technologists,* technicians who assist doctors in imaging and treatment; or *radiation therapy technologists,* technicians who give radiation therapy as ordered by a radiologist. Radiologic technologists may also become registered specifically in CT, MRI, and ultrasound technology. **Cineradiography** allows a radiologist to view a sequence of images showing how tissues or organs work in an individual.

Radiologists always need to have the clearest possible images for analysis. Correct positioning of the patient to provide the best views is the technologist's job. An image may be taken *anterior-posterior (A/P)*, from front to back. It may be taken with the patient prone, supine, or in any body position. (Chapter 3 discusses directional terms and body planes.)

Vocabulary Review

In the previous section, you learned terms relating to diagnostic imaging. Before going on to the exercises, review the terms below and refer to the previous section if you have any questions.

Term	Word Analysis	Meaning
alpha rays		Type of radioactive particle that has a low ability to penetrate the body.
barium	[BĂ-rē-ŭm] Greek *barys*, heavy	Contrast medium that shows up as white on an x-ray.
beta rays		Type of radioactive particle that has a medium ability to penetrate the body.
brachytherapy	[brăk-ē-THĀR-ă-pē] brachy-, short + therapy	Implanting of radioactive elements directly into a tumor or tissue.
CAT (computerized axial tomography) scan		Scan that shows images as detailed slices of a body part or organ.
cineradiography	[SĬN-ē-rā-dē-ŎG-ră-fē] cine-, movement + radiography	Radiography of tissues or organs in motion.
cobalt	[KŌ-băwlt]	Radioactive substance used in radiation therapy.
CT (computed tomography) scan		CAT scan.
diagnostic imaging		Use of imaging techniques in diagnosing illness.
fluoroscopy	[flūr-ŎS-kō-pē] fluoro-, light + -scopy, observing	X-ray in which the image is projected onto a fluorescent screen.
gamma rays		Commonly used radioactive particles with high penetrating ability.
gray (gy)		Unit of measure equal to 100 rads.
imaging	[ĬM-ă-jǐng]	Production of a visual output using x-rays, sound waves, or magnetic fields.

Term	Word Analysis	Meaning
interstitial therapy	[ĭn-tĕr-STĬSH-ăl]	Brachytherapy in which the radioactive substance is placed within the tissue or tumor.
intracavitary therapy	[ĬN-tră-CĂV-ĭ-tăr-ē] intra-, within + cavit(y)	Brachytherapy in which the radioactive substance is placed in a cavity near a cancerous lesion.
iodine	[Ī-ō-dīn]	Substance used in radiopharmaceuticals for contrast medium and radiation therapy.
ion	[Ī-ŏn]	Positively charged particle used to ionize tissue.
ionize	[Ī-ŏn-īz]	To destroy cells by changing neutral particles to ions using x-rays.
irradiated	[ĭ-RĀ-dē-āt-ĕd]	Treated with radiation.
magnetic resonance imaging (MRI)		Imaging produced by tracking the magnetic properties in the nuclei of various cells.
malaise	[mă-LĀZ]	General feeling of illness.
nuclear medicine		Medical specialty for treating diseases with radioactive substances.
PET (positron emission tomography) scan		A series of images that shows the distribution of substances through tissue.
rad (radiation absorbed dose)	[răd]	Unit of radioactive substance that can be absorbed in a particular period of time.
radiation	[RĀ-dē-Ā-shŭn] From Latin radius, beam	Energy carried by a stream of particles from a substance.
radiography	[RĀ-dē-ŎG-ră-fē] radio-, radiation + -graphy	Production of diagnostic images.
radioimmunoassay (RIA)	[RĀ-dē-ō-ĬM-ū-nō-ĂS-sā] radio- + immuno-, immunity + assay	In vitro test to determine the amount of drugs or medication left in the body.
radiology	[RĀ-dē-ŎL-ō-jē] radio- + -logy, study of	Medical specialty in diagnostic imaging and radiation treatment.
radiolucent	[RĀ-dē-ō-LŪ-sĕnt] radio- + Latin lucens, shining	Able to be easily penetrated by x-rays.

Term	Word Analysis	Meaning
radionuclide	[RĀ-dē-ō-NŪ-klĭd] radio- + nucl(ear)	Radioactive substance.
radiopaque	[RĀ-dē-ō-PĀK] radi-, radiation + -opaque	Not able to be easily penetrated by x-rays.
radiopharmaceutical	[RĀ-dē-ō-făr-mă-SŪ-tĭ-kăl] radio- + pharmaceutical	Chemical substance containing radioactive material.
radioresistant	[RĀ-dē-ō-rē-ZĬS-tănt] radio- + resistant	Not greatly affected by radiation.
radiosensitive	[RĀ-dē-ō-SĔN-sĭ-tĭv] radio- + sensitive	Easily affected by radiation.
roentgenology	[RĔNT-gĕn-ŎL-ō-jē] roentgeno-, roentgen + -logy	Radiology.
scan		Image obtained from the interior of the body.
sonogram	[SŎN-ō-grăm] sono-, sound + -gram, a recording	Ultrasound image.
stereotactic frame	[STĒR-ē-ō-TĂK-tĭk] stereo-, three-dimensional + Greek *taxis*, frame	Headgear worn by patients needing pinpoint accuracy in the treatment of brain anomalies.
tomography	[tō-MŎG-ră-fē] Greek *tomos*, cutting + -graphy	Type of imaging that produces three-dimensional images.
tracer study		Image that traces the passage of a radiopharmaceutical through an organ or tissue.
ultrasonography	[ŬL-tră-sō-NŎG-ră-fē] ultra-, beyond + sono- + -graphy	Use of sound waves to produce images of the interior of a body.
ultrasound	[ŬL-tră-sŏwnd] ultra- + sound	Image resulting from ultrasonography; produced by sound waves.
uptake	[ŭp-TĂK]	Speed of absorption of a radiopharmaceutical by a particular organ or body part.
x-ray	[ĕks-rā]	High-energy particles of radiation from the interior of a substance.

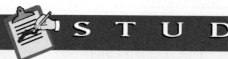
Diagnosing a Disease

Nina Thorman made an appointment with her internist to discuss some weakness on her left side. After testing her reflexes and discussing her symptoms, her doctor referred her to a neurologist. Two weeks later while talking to the neurologist, Nina discovered that a series of tests might be necessary because some diseases (particularly neurological ones) are diagnosed by a process of elimi-nation. (For example, multiple sclerosis does not show up in blood or urine tests, but does have several indicators that allow a neurologist to arrive at a diagnosis.) Nina was given an MRI to determine if a brain tumor or other brain anomaly was affecting her on one side. The MRI showed some plaque on her brain. After a series of other tests, including a spinal tap to obtain CSF (cerebral spinal fluid) for analysis, the neurologist told Nina that she has multiple sclerosis. They discussed plans for management of the disease.

 Critical Thinking

1. Why did the internist refer Nina to a neurologist for testing, rather than ordering an MRI himself?

2. Why was an MRI ordered as opposed to an x-ray?

Diagnostic Imaging Terms Exercises

Match the correct definition on the right with the term on the left.

3. ultrasound   a. blood-brain barrier

4. radiography   b. drug test

5. PET scan   c. in a test tube

6. CAT scan   d. imaging of a joint

7. cineradiography   e. loss of hair

8. arthrography   f. imaging showing slices of tissue

9. radioimmunoassay   g. imaging showing movement of substances

10. in vitro   h. device for delivering radiation

11. BBB   i. imaging of tissues or organs in motion

12. betatron   j. image using sound waves

13. alopecia   k. the production of diagnostic images

Surgical Terms

Types of Surgery

Surgery is the removal of tissue, manipulation of tissue, or insertion of a device or transplanted body part or tissue. Surgery is **preventative,** designed to prevent further disease (as in removal of a cancerous lesion likely to spread); **manipulative** or **closed,** changed without incision (as in the alignment of a fracture); **diagnostic,** helping to finalize a diagnosis (as in the removal of sample tissue for microscopic diagnosis or biopsy); **minimally invasive,** with the smallest possible incision (as in surgeries that use laparoscopes); and **reconstructive** or **cosmetic,** designed to improve on or return a part of the body to its original functioning and/or appearance. Surgery can be **cryogenic,** involving the use of freezing to destroy tissue, or **cauterizing,** involving the use of heat to destroy tissue.

Surgery and **operations,** the removal, transplant, or manipulation of tissue performed in surgery, can be described according to location on the body, obstruction being removed, machine or techniques being used, or where it is performed. Abdominal surgery is performed on the abdomen; craniofacial surgery is performed on the cranium and facial bones; hip surgery usually means repair or replacement of a hip; transplant surgery is the removal of and insertion of a body part or tissue; and dental surgery is performed on the mouth and gums. Cataract surgery is the removal of a lens of the eye, and **Mohs' surgery** is the removal of a carcinoma after mapping with a chemical to establish the narrowest possible margin of affected tissue. *Endoscopic* and *laparoscopic surgeries* are performed with the use of a camera attached to a lighted probe. *Inpatient surgery* takes place in the hospital with the patient admitted for one or more nights. *Ambulatory* or *outpatient surgery* takes place in a hospital, clinic, or office without admission to a hospital.

Surgical Implements

In the centuries before anesthesia and x-rays, surgery was basically performed using a knife and a lot of guesswork. Later, **aseptic** (germ-free) environments and instruments contributed to a gradually increasing surgical survival rate. Surgical implements include cutting and dissecting instruments, clamping devices, retracting, dilating, and probing instruments, injecting and suturing implements, and personal equipment for the surgical staff.

Cutting and dissecting instruments include various types of **scalpels** (knives), **surgical scissors,** and **curette** (also *curet*), sharp-edged instruments for scraping tissue. Surgical **clamps** or **forceps** are used to grasp and hold or remove something during surgery. Forceps may be placed around something (such as a baby's temple) to aid in pulling the baby out through the birth canal. Clamps are used to grab and hold tissue in place or to apply pressure to a blood vessel to control bleeding. **Retractors** are used to hold a surgical wound open, **dilators** are used to enlarge an opening, and **probes** are used to explore body cavities or to clear blockages. Hollow needles are used in surgery to inject or extract material. **Suture needles** and **needle holders** allow the surgeon to bind the surgical wound after surgery by sewing suturing material through the wound. **Staples** are another suturing implement. New glues and other materials can be used to suture without needles or staples.

Reconstructive surgery after burns may include the use of "manufactured skin," skin that is grown in laboratories.

Individuals participating in the surgical procedure must wear personal surgical protective clothing that includes scrub gowns or outfits (pants and top), protective headgear, face shields, protective glasses, and masks. Those people who will be performing or assisting in the surgery must also wear sterile gowns and latex or vinyl gloves. All must follow hospital and government rules (set by OSHA, Occupational Safety and Health Administration) and guidelines for **standard precautions** (set by the CDC, Centers for Disease Control and Prevention) with regard to blood and body fluids to prevent the spread of disease. Standard precautions are slightly more detailed than the previous *universal precautions* set by the government.

Vocabulary Review

In the previous section, you learned terms relating to surgery. Before going on to the exercises, review the terms below and refer to the previous section if you have any questions.

Term	Word Analysis	Meaning
aseptic	[ā-SĔP-tĭk] a-, without + sepsis, presence of pathogens	Germ-free.
cauterizing	[KĂW-tĕr-īz-ĭng] From Greek *kauterion*, branding iron	Destroying tissue by burning.
clamps	[klămps]	Implement used to grasp a body part during surgery.
closed		Performed without an incision.
cosmetic		Designed to improve the appearance of an exterior body part.
cryogenic	[krī-ō-JĔN-ĭk] cryo-, cold + -genic, producing	Destroying tissue by freezing.
curette	[kyū-RĔT]	Sharp instrument for scraping tissue.
diagnostic	[dī-ăg-NŎS-tĭk]	Helping to finalize a diagnosis.
dilator	[DĪ-lā-tĕr]	Implement used to enlarge an opening.
forceps	[FŌR-sĕps] Latin, tongs	Surgical implement used to grasp and remove something.
manipulative	[mă-NĬP-ū-lā-tĭv]	Done without an incision, as in the reduction of a fracture.
minimally invasive		Done with the smallest incision possible, such as the clearing of arterial blockages with tiny probes that use lasers.

Term	Word Analysis	Meaning
Mohs' surgery	[mōhs] After Frederic Mohs (1910–), U.S. surgeon	Removal of a carcinoma after mapping with a chemical to establish the narrowest possible margin of affected tissue.
needle holder		Surgical forceps used to hold and pass a suturing needle through tissue.
operation		Any surgical procedure, such as the removal, transplant, or manipulation of tissue.
preventative	[prē-VĔN-tă-tǐv]	Designed to stop or prevent disease.
probe		Sharp device for exploring body cavities or clearing blockages.
reconstructive	[rē-cǒn-STRŬC-tǐv]	Designed to restore a body part to its original state or appearance.
retractor	[rē-TRĂK-těr]	An instrument used to hold back edges of tissue and organs to expose other tissues or body parts; especially used in surgery.
scalpel	[SKĂL-pl] Latin *scalpellum*, small knife	Knife used in surgery or dissection.
standard precautions		Guidelines issued by the Centers for Disease Control for preventing the spread of disease.
staples		Metal devices used to suture surgical incisions.
surgery	[SĚR-jěr-ē]	Removal, transplant, or manipulation of tissue.
surgical scissors		Scissors used for cutting and dissecting tissue during surgery.
suture needles	[SŪ-chūr]	Needles used in closing surgical wounds by sewing.

C A S E   S T U D Y

Outpatient Surgery

James Wilson, an 80-year-old, scheduled his yearly appointment with his ophthalmolo- gist. James has had cataracts but they were not yet ready to be removed. However, at this visit, the ophthalmologist suggested that removal of the right cataract and insertion of an intraocular

CASE STUDY (continued)

lens would be a fast and comfortable solution to Mr. Wilson's ever-diminishing sight. The medical assistant scheduled Mr. Wilson for surgery at the Eye and Ear Center, a local outpatient clinic.

The day of the surgery, Mr. Wilson was greeted by a patient care technician who escorted him into the surgical area. There he was given a surgical gown and covers for his shoes and head. The doctor, anesthesiologist, and nurse all were in the operating room scrubbed and ready for surgery. Later that day, after several hours of rest and observation, Mr. Wilson's son picked him up to take him home.

 Critical Thinking

14. Is Mr. Wilson's surgery an example of preventative, diagnostic, or cosmetic surgery?

15. Cataract operations are simple and localized in one eye. Why is it necessary for the doctors and assistants to be surgically aseptic?

Surgical Terms Exercises

Know the Equipment

Write the name of the instrument that is being defined in each statement below.

forceps	clamps	probe	surgical scissors	curette
dilator	needle holder	retractor	staples	surgical needles

16. Sharp instrument for scraping tissue: _____

17. Needles used in closing surgical wounds by sewing: _____

18. Blunt device for exploring body cavities or clearing blockages: _____

19. Surgical forceps used to pass a suturing needle through tissue: _____

20. Instrument used to hold back edges of tissue and body organs to expose other tissues or body parts:

_____

21. Instrument used to grasp a body part especially during surgery: _____

22. Implement used to enlarge an opening: _____

23. Surgical implement used to grasp and remove: _____

24. Metal devices used to suture surgical openings: _____

25. Scissors used for cutting and dissecting tissue during surgery: _____

Combining Forms and Abbreviations

The lists below include combining forms, suffixes, and abbreviations that relate specifically to diagnostic imaging and surgery. Pronunciations are provided for the examples.

Combining Form	Meaning	Example
cine	movement	*cineradiography* [SĬN-ĕ-rā-dē-ŎG-ră-fē], radiography of an organ in motion
electr(o)	electric; electricity	*electrocardiogram* [ē-lĕk-trō-KĂR-dē-ō-grăm], graphic record of heart's electrical currents
fluor(o)	light; luminous	*fluoroscopy* [flūr-ŎS-kō-pē], deep tissue examination by x-ray
micr(o)	small; microscopic	*microsurgery* [mī-krō-SĔR-jĕr-ē], surgery performed using magnification by a microscope
radi(o)	radiation	*radiopaque* [RĀ-dē-ō-PĀK], impenetrable to radiation
son(o)	sound	*sonogram* [SŎN-ō-grăm], ultrasound image
ultra	beyond	*ultrasound* [ŬL-tră-sŏwnd], imaging using sound frequencies beyond a certain measurement

Suffix	Meaning	Example
-centesis	puncture	*amniocentesis* [ăm-nē-ō-sĕn-TĒ-sĭs], retrieval of amniotic fluid through a needle inserted into the amnion
-clasis	breaking	*osteoclasis* [ŎS-tē-ō-klă-sĭs], intentional breaking of a bone
-clast	breaking	*osteoclast* [ŎS-tē-ō-klăst], instrument for breaking a bone (also, a large bone cell)
-ectomy	removal of	*appendectomy* [ăp-pĕn-DĔK-tō-mē], removal of the appendix
-gram	a recording	*sonogram* [SŎN-ō-grăm], ultrasound image
-graph	recording instrument	*electroencephalograph* [ē-LĔK-trō-ĕn-SĔF-ă-lō-grăf], system for recording the brain's electrical activity
-graphy	process of recording	*ultrasonography* [ŬL-tră-sō-NŎG-ră-fē], imaging by the use of sound waves

Suffix	Meaning	Example
-opsy	a viewing	*biopsy* [BĪ-ŏp-sē], removal of tissue from a living patient for examination
-ostomy	opening	*colostomy* [kō-LŎS-tō-mē], surgical opening in the colon
-pexy	fixation done surgically	*nephropexy* [NĔF-rō-pĕk-sē], surgical fixation of a floating kidney
-plasty	surgical repair	*rhinoplasty* [RĪ-nō-plăs-tē], plastic surgery of the nose
-rrhaphy	surgical suturing	*herniorrhaphy* [hĕr-nē-ŎR-ă-fē], surgical repair of a hernia
-scope	instrument for observing	*microscope* [MĪ-krō-skōp], instrument for viewing small objects
-scopy	a viewing	*microscopy* [mĭ-KRŎS-kō-pē], use of microscopes
-stomy	opening	*nephrostomy* [nĕ-FRŎS-tō-mē], surgical opening between the kidney and the exterior of the body
-tome	cutting segment	*osteotome* [ŎS-tē-ō-tōm], instrument for cutting bone
-tomy	cutting operation	*laparotomy* [LĂP-ă-RŎT-ō-mē], incision in the abdomen

Abbreviation	Meaning
Ba	barium
BaE	barium enema
CAT	computerized axial tomography
C-spine	cervical spine (film)
CT	computed tomography
CXR	chest x-ray
DSA	digital subtraction angiography
ERCP	endoscopic retrograde cholangiopancreatography
Fx	fracture
Gy	unit of radiation equal to 100 rads
IVC	intravenous cholangiography
IVP	intravenous pyelogram
IVU	intravenous urography
MRA	magnetic resonance angiography

Abbreviation	Meaning
MRI	magnetic resonance imaging
MUGA	multigated acquisition scan
NMR	nuclear magnetic resonance (imaging)
PET	positron emission tomography
r	roentgen
Ra	radium
rad	radiation absorbed dose
RAI	radioactive iodine
RIA	radioimmunoassay
SPECT	single photon emission computed tomography
U/S	ultrasound
V/Q	ventilation perfusion scan
XRT	radiation therapy

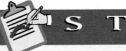
Receiving Treatment

Molly Pearl is 80 years old and is having frequent bouts of dizziness, has fallen five times, and is losing some feeling in her limbs. Her gerontologist has referred her to a clinic for neurological disorders where she is given a number of tests including an MRI and a CAT scan. The results of the tests show abnormalities that contribute to her symptoms.

 Critical Thinking

26. Why do some imaging tests require the use of a contrast medium?

27. In what part of Molly Pearl's body did the MRI likely show abnormalities?

Combining Forms, Suffixes, and Abbreviations Exercises

Build Your Medical Vocabulary

Complete the terms below by adding a suffix from the list in this section.

28. Kidney removal: nephr_____

29. Recording of the heart: cardio_____

30. Imaging of an artery: arterio_____

31. Suture of a vein: phlebo_____

32. Surgical fixing of the bladder: cysto_____

33. Instrument for viewing the uterus: hystero_____

34. Creation of an opening into the bladder: cysto_____

35. Cutting of a nerve: neuro_____

U S I N G   T H E   http://www   I N T E R N E T

The governmental Agency for Health Care Policy and Research (http://www.ahcpr.gov/consumer/surgery.htm) maintains a website containing information about surgery. Go to the site and find at least five questions to ask your doctor before you have surgery.

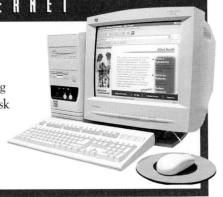

CHAPTER REVIEW

Definitions

Define the following terms, combining forms, and suffixes. Review the chapter before starting. Make sure you know how to pronounce each term as you define it.

Term	Definition
alpha rays	
aseptic [ā-SĔP-tĭk]	
barium [BĂ-rē-ŭm]	
beta rays	
brachytherapy [brăk-ē-THĂR-ă-pē]	
CAT (computerized axial tomography) scan	
cauterizing [KĂW-tĕr-īz-ĭng]	
-centesis	
cine	
cineradiography [SĬN-ē-rā-dē-ŎG-ră-fē]	
clamps [klămps]	
-clasis	
-clast	
closed	
cobalt [KŌ-băwlt]	
cosmetic	
cryogenic [krī-ō-JĔN-ĭk]	
CT (computed tomography) scan	
curette [kyū-RĔT]	
diagnostic [dī-ăg-NŎS-tĭk]	
diagnostic imaging	
dilator [DĪ-lā-tĕr]	
-ectomy	
electr(o)	
fluor(o)	

Term	Definition
fluoroscopy [flūr-ŎS-kō-pē]	_____
forceps [FŌR-sĕps]	_____
gamma rays	_____
-gram	_____
-graph	_____
-graphy	_____
gray (gy)	_____
imaging [ĬM-ă-jĭng]	_____
interstitial [ĭn-tĕr-STĬSH-ăl] therapy	_____
intracavitary [ĬN-tră-CĂV-ĭ-tăr-ē] therapy	_____
iodine [Ī-ō-dĭn]	_____
ion [Ī-ŏn]	_____
ionize [Ī-ŏn-īz]	_____
irradiated [ĭ-RĀ-dē-āt-ĕd]	_____
magnetic resonance imaging (MRI)	_____
malaise [mă-LĀZ]	_____
manipulative [mă-NĬP-ū-lā-tĭv]	_____
micr(o)	_____
minimally invasive	_____
Mohs' [mōhs] surgery	_____
needle holder	_____
nuclear medicine	_____
operation	_____
-opsy	_____
-ostomy	_____
PET (positron emission tomography) scan	_____
-pexy	_____
-plasty	_____
preventative [prē-VĔN-tă-tĭve]	_____
probe	_____
rad [răd] (radiation absorbed dose)	_____
radiation [RĀ-dē-Ā-shŭn]	_____
radi(o)	_____

Term	Definition
radiography [RĀ-dē-ŎG-ră-fē]	
radioimmunoassay (RIA) [RĀ-dē-ō-ĬM-ū-nō-ĂS-sā]	
radiology [RĀ-dē-ŎL-ō-jē]	
radiolucent [RĀ-dē-ō-LŪ-sĕnt]	
radionuclide [RĀ-dē-ō-NŪ-klĭd]	
radiopaque [RĀ-dē-ō-PĀK]	
radiopharmaceutical [RĀ-dē-ō-făr-mă-SŪ-tĭ-kăl]	
radioresistant [RĀ-dē-ō-rē-ZĬS-tănt]	
radiosensitive [RĀ-dē-ō-SĔN-sĭ-tĭv]	
reconstructive [rē-cŏn-STRŬC-tĭv]	
retractor [rē-TRĂK-tĕr]	
roentgenology [RĔNT-gĕn-ŎL-ō-jē]	
-rrhaphy	
scalpel [SKĂL-pl]	
scan	
-scope	
-scopy	
son(o)	
sonogram [SŎN-ō-grăm]	
standard precautions	
staples	
stereotactic [STĒR-ē-ō-TĂK-tĭk] frame	
-stomy	
surgery [SĔR-jĕr-ē]	
surgical scissors	
suture [SŪ-chūr] needles	
-tome	
tomography [tō-MŎG-ră-fē]	
-tomy	
tracer study	
ultra	
ultrasonography [ŬL-tră-sō-NŎG-ră-fē]	

ultrasound [ŬL-tră-sŏwnd]

uptake [ŭp-TĂK]

x-ray [ĕks-rā]

Abbreviations

Write the full meaning of each abbreviation.

Abbreviation	Meaning
Ba	
BaE	
CAT	
C-spine	
CT	
CXR	
DSA	
ERCP	
Fx	
Gy	
IVC	
IVP	
IVU	
MRA	
MRI	
MUGA	
NMR	
PET	
r	
Ra	
rad	
RAI	
RIA	
SPECT	
U/S	
V/Q	
XRT	

Answers to Chapter Exercises

1. Neurologists specialize in diagnosing central nervous system disorders, partially through imaging.
2. to check for brain anomalies not viewable on an x-ray
3. j
4. k
5. g
6. f
7. i
8. d
9. b
10. c
11. a
12. h
13. e
14. diagnostic
15. Any surgery requires aseptic conditions.
16. curette
17. surgical needles
18. probe
19. needle holder
20. retractor
21. clamps
22. dilator
23. forceps
24. staples
25. surgical scissors
26. to highlight certain areas of the body or to follow motion within the body
27. brain
28. nephrectomy
29. cardiogram
30. arteriography
31. phleborrhaphy
32. cystopexy
33. hysteroscope
34. cystostomy
35. neurotomy

CHAPTER 20

Terms in Psychiatry

After studying this chapter, you will be able to

- Describe common mental disorders
- Define combining forms used in building words that relate to mental disorders
- Identify the meaning of related abbreviations
- Name the common tests, procedures, and treatments used in treating mental disorders
- Recognize common pharmacological agents used in treating psychiatric ailments

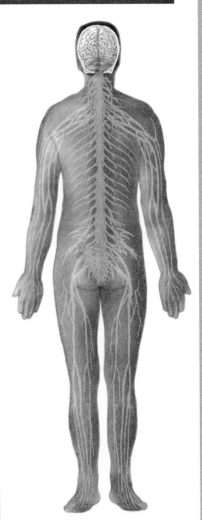

Psychiatric Disorders Terms

Psychiatric or mental disorders (disorders of the mind) can have many causes. Heredity often plays a role. Environmental stresses may also contribute to mental illness, or medication taken for other ailments may be the underlying cause of symptoms. With the advent of sophisticated diagnostic imaging, some mental disorders that result from damage to the brain can be assessed by imaging or by physical testing (as of neurological responses). Most mental disorders, however, must be assessed by a specialist trained in understanding how a group of symptoms equals a mental disorder and how to treat that disorder. Treatment usually involves either medication or psychotherapy (talk therapy) or a combination of both. It may also involve surgery or electroconvulsive therapy (ECT).

Psychiatry is the medical specialty that diagnoses and treats mental disorders, usually ones that require medication. A *psychiatrist* is a medical doctor specializing in psychiatry. Psychiatrists sometimes provide talk therapy, often in combination with medication. Nonmedical practitioners who treat mental disorders using psychotherapy alone are called *psychologists, psychotherapists,* **therapists,** or **social workers.** These people may have a master's degree or a doctorate. They usually have had extensive training in **psychology,** the profession that studies human behavior and nonmedical treatments of mental disorders. Such training gives them the ability to practice **psychotherapy,** treatment of mental disorders with verbal and nonverbal communication as opposed to treatment with medication alone. Psychotherapy is also known as *talk therapy.*

Most mental illnesses can be controlled with medication. Often, when a problem arises during treatment, it is because the patient was not sufficiently monitored, and he or she stopped taking medication because of delusions about the state of the illness.

Symptoms

Mental disorders often include many types of emotional symptoms. They may arise from an existing physical ailment, or they may lead to a physical ailment. Symptoms of emotional illnesses may include:

+ **Aggressiveness,** attacking forcefulness

+ **Agitation,** abnormal restlessness

+ **Ambivalence,** feeling of conflicting emotions about the same person or issue, as love–hate, pleasure–pain, and tenderness–cruelty

+ **Anxiety,** abnormal worry

+ **Catalepsy,** trancelike state with holding of one pose for a long time

+ *Defensiveness*, psychological process that enables an individual to deny, displace, or repress something that causes anxiety

+ **Deliriousness,** mental confusion, often with hallucinations that last for a brief period, as during a high fever

+ **Delusional,** having false beliefs resulting from disordered thinking

+ **Dementia,** disorder, particularly in older adulthood, with multiple cognitive defects

+ **Depression,** condition with feelings of despair, loneliness, and low self-esteem

+ **Paranoia,** abnormal distrust of others

+ **Phobia,** obsessive fear of something

+ **Psychosis,** extreme disordered thinking

These terms all relate to some sort of mental or personality disorder. Some of the symptoms, such as depression and anxiety, are also the name of a disorder.

MORE ABOUT...

Phobias

Many people have very specific phobias. Descriptive terms for those phobias are formed by adding the suffix phobia to a combining form that indicates the item about which the patient is phobic. For example, extreme fear of bees (api-) is apiphobia; extreme fear of darkness (nycto-) is nyctophobia; fear of heights (acro-) is acrophobia; and fear of the number thirteen (triskaideka-) is triskaidekaphobia.

Although phobias are symptoms of many mental disorders, having a phobia does not necessarily indicate disease. Rather, it may be as a result of a traumatic experience or the influence of someone else's phobia.

Mental Disorders

The American Psychiatric Association publishes the *Diagnostic and Statistical Manual of Mental Disorders,* currently in its fourth edition (1994). Known informally as DSM-IV, it lists the criteria on which mental disorders are diagnosed and categorized (Figure 20-1). The major mental disorders are as follows:

+ *Anxiety disorder* and *panic disorder*— Anxiety disorder is a condition with chronic unrealistic fear over a period of time, usually affecting concentration and sleep, and causing fatigue. Panic disorder is a condition with recurring *panic attacks,* short periods of intense and immobilizing fear. While having an attack, patients may feel they are suffering from shortness of breath and/or chest pain. Such attacks can mimic the symptoms of a heart attack, adding to the extreme fright experienced by the patient.

- *Alcohol/substance abuse*—Alcohol or substance abuse is a condition in which the patient uses alcohol or drugs recurrently and its use has affected the patient's ability to function at school or work

and at home. Such patients are **addicts,** people who have difficulty avoiding alcohol or drugs.

- **Obsessive-compulsive disorder**—Obsessive-compulsive disorder is a condition with persistent thoughts, ideas, and actions that lead to tendencies to perform acts that are recurrent, time-consuming, repetitive, and ritualistic. This disorder usually involves a patient who is a perfectionist and inflexible. If severe, this can interfere with the patient's ability to function normally in daily life.

- **Dissociative disorders**—Dissociative disorders include a gradual or sudden loss of the ability to integrate memory, identity, and other mental abilities with the environment. Patients may have more than one identity or may become depersonalized to an extreme degree.

- **Post-traumatic stress disorder (PTSD)**— PTSD is a condition of extreme traumatic stress that may occur and last for years after a traumatic incident or a period of time in an extremely stressful environment. Prisoners of war, victims of torture, combat veterans, child abuse victims, and crime victims are just some of the people who are vulnerable to PTSD. PTSD does not necessarily show up immediately. It may take years before it develops.

- *Eating disorders*—Eating disorders include conditions with grossly disturbed eating habits. In **anorexia nervosa,** patients refuse to eat enough to maintain a normal body weight, usually accompanied by a distorted body image and an obsessive need to lose weight even, in some cases, to the point of starvation and death. No matter how thin the individual is, they perceive themselves as physically fat. **Bulimia nervosa** is a condition in which the patient binges (eats uncontrollably) and then purges (forces regurgitation). **Pica** is a condition in which the patient (usually a young child) eats non-nutritive substances, such as paint, clay, or sand, for a long period of time.

- **Mental retardation**—Usually a condition of birth, such as Down syndrome, mental retardation includes far below average intellectual functioning to the point of inability to care for oneself thoroughly and inability to function within a certain range of academic skills.

- *Mood disorders*—Mood disorders include conditions in which the patient has abnormal moods or mood swings. Depression, when it is diagnosed as

---

■ **Diagnostic criteria for 298.8 Brief Psychotic Disorder**

A. Presence of one (or more) of the following symptoms:
(1) delusions
(2) hallucinations
(3) disorganized speech (e.g., frequent derailment or incoherence)
(4) grossly disorganized or catatonic behavior

Note: Do not include a symptom if it is a culturally sanctioned response pattern.

B. Duration of an episode of the disturbance is at least 1 day but less than 1 month, with eventual full return to premorbid level of functioning.

C. The disturbance is not better accounted for by a Mood Disorder With Psychotic Features, Schizoaffective Disorder, or Schizophrenia and is not due to the direct physiological effects of a substance (e.g., a drug of abuse, a medication) or a general medical condition.

Figure 20-1. The criteria for diagnosing a brief psychotic disorder is shown in this excerpt from DSM-IV.

clinical depression, is a disabling disorder with a loss of interest and pleasure in almost all activities. Clinically depressed people can become *suicidal*, in danger of killing oneself. **Manic** patients have moods that become dangerously elevated to the point of inability to work, sleep, concentrate, and maintain normal relationships. **Bipolar disorders** or **manic-depressive** or **mixed-episode** disorders include drastic swings between manic and depressive moods.

+ *Personality disorders*—Personality disorders are conditions in which a destructive pattern of behavior is part of a maladjusted person's everyday life. Included in personality disorders are *obsessive-compulsive* behavior, the characteristics of which are perfectionism and inflexibility; paranoia, extreme, unfounded mistrust of others; *dependency*, abnormal submissiveness, particularly in adulthood; and **sociopathy** or *antisocial* behavior, having an unusually callous disregard for others.

+ **Schizophrenia**—Schizophrenia has many degrees of severity. Most schizophrenics experience some hallucinations such as imagined inner voices directing their lives. New medications have made it possible for many schizophrenics to function in society. The most prominent symptom of schizophrenia is psychosis that interferes with the activities of daily living. A childhood mental disorder with morbid self-absorption, **autism,** is sometimes thought to have some of the same symptoms as schizophrenia.

+ **Somatoform disorders**—Somatoform disorders include physical symptoms having a psychological basis. **Hypochondria** is the preoccupation with imagined illnesses in the patient's body. Somatoform disorders also include intense preoccupation with imagined physical defects in one's body.

Some mental difficulties do not rise to the level of a mental disorder and usually do not require medication for an extended period of time. For example, depression may be situational, as in the death of a loved one. In that case, it would not be classified as clinical depression. Patients with anxiety disorder have levels of anxiety that interfere with their overall functioning. Many people have anxieties that do not prevent them from functioning. Such people are said to have **neuroses,** behavioral conditions that the person has learned to cope with and that do not overwhelmingly affect daily functioning.

Vocabulary Review

In the previous section, you learned terms relating to psychiatric disorders. Before going on to the exercises, review the terms below and refer to the previous section if you have any questions.

Term	Word Analysis	Definition
addict	[ĂD-ĭkt]	One who is dependent on a substance (usually illegal, as narcotics) on a recurring basis.
aggressiveness	[ă-GRĔS-ĭv-nĕs]	Abnormal forcefulness toward others.
agitation	[ă-jĭ-TĀ-shŭn]	Abnormal restlessness.

Term	Word Analysis	Definition
ambivalence	[ăm-BĬV-ă-lĕns]	Feeling of conflicting emotions about a person or an issue.
anorexia nervosa	[ăn-ō-RĔK-sē-ă nĕr-VŌ-să]	Eating disorder in which the patient refuses to eat enough to sustain a minimum weight.
anxiety	[ănks-ZĪ-ĕ-tē]	Abnormal worry.
autism	[ĂW-tĭzm]	Mental disorder usually beginning in early childhood with morbid self-absorption and difficulty in perceiving reality.
bipolar disorder	[bī-PŌ-lĕr]	Condition with drastic mood swings over a period of time.
bulimia nervosa	[BŪ-lēm-ē-ă, BŪ-lĭm-ē-ă nĕr-VŌ-să]	Eating disorder with extreme overeating followed by purging.
catalepsy	[KĂT-ă-lĕp-sē]	Trancelike state with holding of one pose for a long period of time.
deliriousness	[dē-LĬR-ē-ŭs-nĕs]	Mental confusion, often with hallucinations, usually having a physical cause such as a high fever.
delusional	[dē-LŪ-zhŭn-ăl]	Having false beliefs resulting from disordered thinking.
dementia	[dē-MĔN-shē-ă]	Disorder, particularly in older adulthood, with multiple cognitive defects.
depression	[dē-PRĔSH-ŭn]	Disabling condition with a loss of interest and pleasure in almost all activities.
dissociative disorder	[dĭ-SŌ-sē-Ă-tĭv]	Condition with a gradual or sudden loss of the ability to integrate memory, identity, and other mental abilities with the environment.
hypochondria	[hī-pō-KŎN-drē-ă]	Condition of preoccupation with imagined illnesses in the patient's body.
manic	[MĂN-ĭk]	Having a dangerously elevated mood.
manic-depressive disorder	[MĂN-ĭk dē-PRĔ-sĭv]	See *bipolar disorder*.
mental retardation		Condition with below average intellectual functioning.
mixed-episode disorder		See *bipolar disorder*.

Term	Word Analysis	Definition
neurosis	[nū-RŌ-sĭs]	Behavior condition usually involving anxiety that a patient can cope with that does not rise to the level of psychosis.
obsessive-compulsive disorder		Condition with obsessive-compulsive feelings.
paranoia	[păr-ă-NŎY-ă]	Extreme unfounded mistrust of others.
phobia	[FŌ-bē-ă]	Irrational or obsessive fear of something.
pica	[PĪ-kă]	Eating disorder in which the patient compulsively eats nonnutritive substances, such as clay and paint.
post-traumatic stress disorder (PTSD)		Condition of extreme traumatic stress that may occur and last for years after a traumatic time or incident.
psychiatry	[sĭ-KĪ-ă-trē]	Medical specialty concerned with the diagnosis and treatment of mental disorders.
psychology	[sĭ-KŎL-ō-jē]	Profession that studies human behavior and treats mental disorders.
psychosis	[sĭ-KŌ-sĭs]	Extreme disordered thinking.
psychotherapy	[sĭ-kō-THĀR-ă-pē]	Treatment of mental disorders with verbal and non-verbal communication.
schizophrenia	[skĭz-ō-FRĔ-nē-ă]	Condition with recurring psychosis, often with hallucinations.
social worker		Nonmedical professional who is trained as an advocate for people (such as the elderly or children) and may also be trained in treatment of mental disorders.
sociopathy	[SŌ-sē-ō-păth-ē]	Extreme callous disregard for others.
somatoform disorders	[SŌ-mă-tō-fŏrm]	Mental disorders including physical symptoms that have a psychological base.
therapist	[THĀR-ă-pĭst]	Nonmedical professional trained in the treatment of mental disorders through talk therapy.

CASE STUDY

Seeking Treatment

Alfred Willett has returned to the Drug Treatment Center (DTC) at a local hospital. Alfred, 50 years old, has been an inpatient for alcoholism at the DTC two times in the past. He had been sober for four years, but recently he started using both alcohol and cocaine.

Since returning to his addictions, Alfred's health has declined. The DTC has Alfred see the in-house physician for a check-up and one of the staff psychologists for an evaluation. His health history reveals that he is diabetic and has a smoker's cough. The current check-up finds a slight loss of hearing, but nothing else that is significant since his last inpatient admission four years ago.

Before Alfred can take advantage of the group and individual therapies available at DTC, he must first stay in the detoxification unit where he will be helped to rid his system of alcohol and cocaine. Often this withdrawal period is painful. A total withdrawal from alcohol can cause DT (delirium tremens).

 Critical Thinking

1. What is the medical term for Alfred's behavior?

2. Why would both a physical and psychological evaluation be necessary?

Psychiatric Disorders Exercises

Match the definition on the right with the term on the left.

3. defensiveness   a. obsessive fear of something

4. paranoia   b. abnormal restlessness

5. phobia   c. abnormal forcefulness

6. agitation   d. abnormal worry

7. ambivalence   e. psychological process that enables one to deny, displace, or repress something

8. catalepsy   f. abnormal distrust of others

9. delusional   g. feeling of conflicting emotions about the same person or issue

10. aggressiveness   h. mental confusion often with hallucinations

11. anxiety   i. trancelike state with holding of one pose for a long time

12. delirious   j. having false beliefs resulting from disordered thinking

Spell It Correctly

For each of the following words, write C if the spelling is correct. If it is not, write the correct spelling.

13. psychiotrist _____

14. paranoia _____

15. ankxiety _____

16. boulimia _____

17. schitzophrenia _____

18. hypochondria _____

19. catolepsy _____

20. dementia _____

Combining Forms and Abbreviations

The lists below include combining forms, suffixes, and abbreviations that relate specifically to psychiatry. Pronunciations are provided for the examples.

Combining Form	Meaning	Example
hypn(o)	sleep	*hypnosis* [hǐp-NŌ-sǐs], artificially induced trancelike state
neur(o), neuri	nerve, nervous system	*neurosis* [nū-RŌ-sǐs], psychological condition with abnormal anxiety
psych(o), psyche	mind, mental	*psychosocial* [sī-kō-SŌ-shǎl], pertaining to both the psychological and social aspects
schiz(o)	split, schizophrenia	*schizophasia* [skǐz-ō-FĀ-zē-ǎ], disordered speech of some schizophrenics

Suffix	Meaning	Example
-mania	abnormal impulse toward	*hypermania* [HĪ-pěr-MĀ-nē-ǎ], extreme impulsivity toward someone or something
-philia	craving for, affinity for	*necrophilia* [něk-rō-FĬL-ē-ǎ], abnormal affinity for the dead
-phobia	abnormal fear of	*claustrophobia* [klǎw-strō-FŌ-bē-ǎ], abnormal fear of confined spaces
-phoria	feeling	*euphoria* [yū-FŌR-ē-ǎ], feeling of well-being

Abbreviation	Meaning	Abbreviation	Meaning
AA	Alcoholics Anonymous	NAMH	National Association of Mental Health
AAMR	American Association on Mental Retardation	NARC	National Association for Retarded Children
APA	American Psychiatric Association	NIMH	National Institute of Mental Health
DSM	*Diagnostic and Statistical Manual of Mental Disorders*	OCD	obsessive-compulsive disorder
DT	delirium tremens	PTSD	post-traumatic stress disorder
ECT	electroconvulsive therapy	TAT	Thematic Apperception Test
EQ	emotional "intelligence" quotient	TDM	therapeutic drug monitoring
EST	electroshock therapy	WAIS	Wechsler Adult Intelligence Scale
IQ	intelligence quotient	WISC	Wechsler Intelligence Scale for Children
MHA	Mental Health Association	WPPSI	Wechsler Preschool and Primary Scale of Intelligence
MMPI	Minnesota Multiphasic Personality Inventory		

C A S E S T U D Y

Moving on in Treatment

DTC's patients come from all age and social groups. Once Alfred is released from the detoxification unit, he starts at Level 1, the level with the least personal freedom and with the most intensive scrutiny. All of Alfred's visitors and any packages he receives are examined for drugs. Alfred is given daily urine tests. He is encouraged to participate in a self-help organization such as AA, which holds meetings once a week at DTC.

Critical Thinking

21. Many people drink alcohol in moderation. Do you think Alfred can learn to be a moderate drinker?

22. How is drug monitoring being applied in Alfred's case?

Combining Forms and Abbreviations Exercises

Build Your Medical Vocabulary

Add one of the following suffixes to complete the term: -mania, -philia, -phobia.

23. Unnatural attraction to dead people: necro_____

24. Disorder with intense desire to steal: klepto_____

25. Unnatural fear of public places: agora_____

26. Unnatural attraction to children: pedo_____

Write the abbreviation(s) that best fits the description for each item below.

27. Self-help organization: _____

28. Intelligence test for children: _____

29. Type of therapy: _____

30. Type of mental disorder: _____

31. Official diagnostic manual: _____

Many businesses use personality trait tests to make sure that a potential employee will fit into the corporate culture.

Psychiatric Treatment Terms

Usually before treatment starts, either a clear diagnosis is made or the patient is put through a series of psychological tests designed to reveal intellectual ability and social functioning, along with an analysis of personality traits. Tests such as the *Stanford-Binet IQ Test* (testing intellectual ability) and the *Thematic Apperception Test* (testing personality traits) are widely used. The *Rorschach Test* asks patients to interpret an ink blot thereby revealing certain personality traits. The *Minnesota Multiphasic Personality Inventory* is a test of personality traits used at many stages of diagnosis and treatment.

Treatment of mental disorders is often based on a combination of psychopharmacology, the science that deals with medications to treat mental disorders, and psychotherapy. Psychotherapists have developed a number of techniques for changing patterns of thought and behavior. For children, **play therapy,** having a child reveal feelings through play, can provide a guide to treatment. Some therapists use **biofeedback,** a method of measuring physical responses (blood pressure or brain waves, for example) to emotional issues, and then use these responses to retrain the client to better recognize and deal with these stressors. Others use **hypnosis,** a state of semiconsciousness in which the patient may be able to reveal hidden thoughts and may be open to suggestions from the person performing the hypnosis. **Psychoanalysis** attempts to have the patient bring unconscious emotions to the surface to deal with them. **Behavior therapy** is the changing of a destructive pattern of behavior by substitution of a beneficial pattern of behavior. **Group therapy** involves a small group of people led by a trained psychotherapist who guides discussions among the participants in an attempt to get them to be open and to change personality problems in long discussions with others.

Various treatment centers around the country treat drug and alcohol addiction as well as eating disorders and many other mental disorders. Most use medications, behavior therapy or **behavior modification,** and individual talk as well as group therapy.

M O R E A B O U T...
EQ

In recent years, a number of experiments have been done to prove that emotional "intelligence" (EQ) may be more valuable than the traditional intelligence quotient (IQ). One such experiment followed a class of an Ivy League college for ten years. At first, the class was given a personality test that revealed what the researchers thought would be the most important factors for success in life. Over the ten years, it was found that the people with the highest IQ and the lowest EQ were the most unsuccessful, while the people with the lowest IQ and the highest EQ did very well in their lives and in their interpersonal relationships. The statistical results indicate that the bottom third of the class led the most successful lives in terms of careers and personal relationships.

Electroshock therapy (EST) or electroconvulsive therapy (ECT) is the use of electric current to a specific area of the brain that changes the brain's electrical activity or "scrambles" the communication from that area to the thought processes. This is only used for very severe cases that have failed to respond to medication and/or therapy. This treatment has made some drastic changes over the years. In the past, patients receiving this treatment were literally strapped to a table and electrodes were placed on their head. Patients would often have grand mal seizures as the current flowed through the brain. A piece of rubber was usually placed in the mouth to prevent them from biting their tongue. Today, EST patients receive a general anesthetic. They also have milder or fewer seizures since the current is now controlled by more sophisticated equipment.

Vocabulary Review

In the previous section, you learned terms relating to psychiatric treatment. Before going on to the exercises, review the terms below and refer to the previous section if you have any questions.

Term	Word Analysis	Definition
behavior modification		Substitution of a beneficial behavior pattern for a destructive behavior pattern.
behavior therapy		Therapy that includes the use of behavior modification.
biofeedback	[bī-ō-FĒD-băk]	Method of measuring physical responses to emotional issues.
electroconvulsive therapy (ECT)	[ē-LĔK-trō-kŏn-VŬL-sĭv]	See electroshock therapy.
electroshock therapy (EST)	[ē-LĔK-trō-shŏk] electro-, electrical + shock	Passing of electric current through a specific area of the brain to change or "scramble" communication from that area to the thought processes.
group therapy		Talk therapy under the leadership of a psychotherapist in which the participants discuss their feelings and try to help each other improve.
hypnosis	[hĭp-NŌ-sĭs] Greek hypnos, sleep + -osis, condition	State of semiconsciousness.
play therapy		Revealing of feelings through play with a trained therapist.
psychoanalysis	[sī-kō-ă-NĂL-ĭ-sĭs] psycho-, psychological + -osis, condition	Therapy that attempts to have patients bring unconscious emotions to the surface to deal with them.

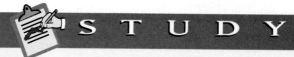

CASE STUDY

Dealing with Life Changes

Alfred's psychological evaluation reveals that he started abusing alcohol and drugs again about three months after his wife left him. He is the superintendent of a large apartment building and relations with the tenants have worsened. The psychologist observes that Alfred is having trouble dealing with the recent changes in his life. She also feels that counseling to help him deal with these changes would benefit him. At the moment, she suspects that he is depressed, but she does not speak to the staff psychiatrist about prescribing medication until he has been reevaluated after detoxification.

Critical Thinking

32. Why might it be easier to determine if Alfred suffers from depression after the process of detoxification?

33. Why is counseling used in combination with medications?

Psychiatric Treatment Terms Exercises

Explain the type of therapy and when and/or with whom it would be useful.

34. play therapy_____

35. biofeedback_____

36. hypnosis_____

37. behavior therapy_____

38. group therapy_____

39. electroshock therapy_____

Pharmacological Terms

Psychopharmacology is the science that deals with medications that affect the emotions. *Pharmacokinetics* is the study of the action of drugs on the body. Many beneficial drugs have been developed that stop or slow the progress of neurotic and psychotic behavior. **Antianxiety agents** generally calm anyone with moderate anxiety. **Antipsychotic agents** relieve the agitation and, sometimes, the disordered thinking of psychotics. **Antidepressants** control the effects of clinical depression on a patient. **Ataractics** and **tranquilizers** relieve anxiety. Many of these psychopharmaceuticals have possible harmful side effects, such as impaired liver or kidney function. For that reason, many patients on such drugs need to have **therapeutic drug monitoring (TDM)**, the regular measurement of blood for levels and effectiveness of prescribed medicines. Drug monitoring is also used to detect illegal substances in the blood or urine of addicts in treatment. Table 20-1 lists common psychopharmaceuticals used in treatment.

Illegal drugs can have a negative effect on emotions. *Mind-altering substances, psychedelics,* or *hallucinogens* are illegal substances that produce disturbed thoughts and illusions in a normal person. Most illegal substances are mind-altering to a greater or lesser degree. Because illegal drugs are not monitored, many addicts die each year after an **overdose,** a toxic dose of a substance. The well-publicized "war on drugs" is an attempt to limit access to such drugs while dissuading addicts from using drugs.

Table 20-1 Some Agents Used in Psychopharmacology

Drug Class	Purpose	Generic	Trade Name
antianxiety agent, ataractic, tranquilizer, sedative	to relieve anxiety	clorazapate alprazolam diazepam	Tranxene Xanax Valium
antidepressant	to relieve clinical depression	clomipramine fluoxetine sertraline	Anafranil Prozac Zoloft
antipsychotic	to relieve agitation and some psychoses	clozapine haloperidol	Clozaril Haldol

Vocabulary Review

In the previous section, you learned terms about pharmacology. Before going on to the exercises, review the terms below and refer to the previous section if you have any questions.

Term	Word Analysis	Definition
antianxiety agent		Tranquilizer.
antidepressant	[ĂN-tē-dē-PRĔS-ănt]	Agent that controls the effects of clinical depression.
antipsychotic agent	[ĂN-tē-sī-KŎT-ĭk]	Agent that relieves agitation and some psychoses.
ataractic	[ă-tă-RĂK-tĭk]	Tranquilizer.
overdose	[Ō-vĕr-dōs]	Toxic dose of a substance.
psychopharmacology	[sī-kō-FĂR-mă-KŎL-ō-jē]	Science that deals with medications that affect the emotions.
therapeutic drug monitoring (TDM)		Taking of regular blood or urine tests to track drug use and effectiveness of medication.
tranquilizer	[TRĂNG-kwĭ-lī-zĕr]	Medication used to relieve anxiety.

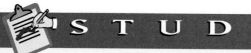
Talking to a Therapist

After three weeks, Alfred seems quite depressed. He is having trouble relating to the other patients. Alfred's psychologist prescribes therapy sessions three times a week, but does not ask the psychiatrist for antidepressant medications at this time. The psychologist encourages Alfred to express his feelings about his children and his ex-wife, while also encouraging him to understand why his marriage broke up.

 Critical Thinking

40. Medication for mental disorders is often regarded as a quick fix. What does it NOT accomplish?

41. The circumstances in Alfred's life could certainly depress someone, but Alfred is not being diagnosed with the mental disorder *depression*. Why did the psychologist prescribe psychotherapy?

Pharmacological Terms Exercises

Fill in the blanks.

42. An ataractic is a type of _____.

43. A medication used to relieve agitation and some psychoses is a(n) _____.

44. A mind-altering substance is a(n) _____.

45. The science that studies the actions of drugs on the body is _____.

USING THE INTERNET

Go to the American Psychological Association's web site (http://www.apa.org/). Find information about a mental disorder and describe it in a paragraph.

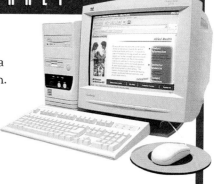

CHAPTER REVIEW

Definitions

Define the following terms and combining forms. Review the chapter before starting. Make sure you know how to pronounce each term as you define it.

Term	Definition
addict [ĂD-ĭkt]	
aggressiveness [ă-GRĔS-ĭv-nĕs]	
agitation [ă-jĭ-TĀ-shŭn]	
ambivalence [ăm-BĬV-ă-lĕns]	
anorexia nervosa [ăn-ō-RĔK-sē-ă nĕr-VŌ-să]	
antianxiety agent	
antidepressant [ĂN-tē-dē-PRĔS-ănt]	
antipsychotic [ĂN-tē-sī-KŎT-ĭk] agent	
anxiety [ănks-ZĪ-ĕ-tē]	
ataractic [ă-tă-RĂK-tĭk]	
autism [ĂW-tĭzm]	
behavior modification	
behavior therapy	
biofeedback [bī-ō-FĒD-băk]	
bipolar [bī-PŌ-lĕr] disorder	
bulimia nervosa [BŪ-lēm-ē-ă, BŪ-lĭm-ē-ă nĕr-VŌ-să]	
catalepsy [KĂT-ă-lĕp-sē]	
deliriousness [dē-LĬR-ē-ŭs-nĕs]	
delusional [dē-LŪ-zhŭn-ăl]	
dementia [dē-MĔN-shē-ă]	
depression [dē-PRĔSH-ŭn]	
dissociative [dĭ-sō-sē-Ă-tĭv] disorder	
electroconvulsive [ē-LĔK-trō-kŏn-VŬL-sĭv] therapy (ECT)	

Term	Definition
electroshock [ē-LĔK-trō-shŏk] therapy (EST)	
group therapy	
hypn(o)	
hypnosis [hĭp-NŌ-sĭs]	
hypochondria [hī-pō-KŎN-drē-ă]	
-mania	
manic [MĂN-ĭk]	
manic-depressive [MĂN-ĭk dē-PRĔ-sĭv] disorder	
mental retardation	
mixed-episode disorder	
neur(o), neuri	
neurosis [nū-RŌ-sĭs]	
obsessive-compulsive disorder	
overdose [Ō-vĕr-dōs]	
paranoia [păr-ă-NŎY-ă]	
-philia	
phobia [FŌ-bē-ă]	
-phobia	
-phoria	
pica [PĪ-kă]	
play therapy	
post-traumatic stress disorder (PTSD)	
psych(o), psyche	
psychiatry [sī-KĪ-ă-trē]	
psychoanalysis [sī-kō-ă-NĂL-ĭ-sĭs]	
psychology [sī-KŎL-ō-jē]	
psychopharmacology [sī-kō-FĂR-mă-KŎL-ō-jē]	
psychosis [sī-KŌ-sĭs]	
psychotherapy [sī-kō-THĀR-ă-pē]	
schiz(o)	
schizophrenia [skĭz-ō-FRĔ-nē-ă]	

Term	Definition
social worker	_____
sociopathy [SŌ-sē-ō-păth-ē]	_____
somatoform [SŌ-mă-tō-fŏrm] disorders	_____
therapeutic drug monitoring (TDM)	_____
therapist [THĀR-ă-pĭst]	_____
tranquilizer [TRĂNG-kwĭ-lĭ-zĕr]	_____

Abbreviations

Write the full meaning of each abbreviation

AA _____

AAMR _____

APA _____

DSM _____

DT _____

ECT _____

EQ _____

EST _____

IQ _____

MHA _____

MMPI _____

NAMH _____

NARC _____

NIMH _____

OCD _____

PTSD _____

TAT _____

TDM _____

WAIS _____

WISC _____

WPPSI _____

Answers to Chapter Exercises

1. alcohol/substance abuse, addiction
2. to see if a physical problem or another mental disorder is causing some of Alfred's problems
3. e
4. f
5. a
6. b
7. g
8. i
9. j
10. c
11. d
12. h
13. psychiatrist
14. C
15. anxiety
16. bulimia
17. schizophrenia
18. C
19. catalepsy
20. C
21. sample answer: No, addiction is a mental disorder; addicts do not usually have enough control.
22. daily urine tests and checking all packages and visitors
23. necrophilia
24. kleptomania
25. agoraphobia
26. pedophilia
27. AA
28. WISC
29. ECT or EST
30. PTSD
31. DSM
32. Drugs and alcohol can produce symptoms of other mental disorders.
33. Alfred needs to talk about his problems. Talk therapy can help a patient deal realistically with the actual stressors in his or her life.
34. observing and talking through play—children
35. measuring physical responses to psychological situations—for individuals who can be retrained to deal with stressors
36. state of semiconsciousness in which the patient may be able to reveal hidden thoughts and may be open to suggestions from the person performing the hypnosis
37. retraining of behavior—for anyone with destructive patterns of behavior that cause severe problems
38. talking out problems to a group of people with similar difficulties—for anyone needing psychological and social support
39. use of electric current to affect the brain—for anyone whose serious mental disorder has not responded to all other types of treatment
40. dealing with issues underlying the mental disorder
41. Alfred's depression was due to situations in his life, not to the mental disorder.
42. tranquilizer
43. antipsychotic
44. psychedelic or hallucinogen
45. pharmacokinetics
46. did not know his father, divorce
47. alcohol/substance abuse

CHAPTER 21

Terms in Dental Practice

After studying this chapter, you will be able to:

- Name the parts of the body treated in dentistry

- Describe the function of each body part treated in dentistry

- Define combining forms used in building words that relate to dental practice

- Identify the meaning of related abbreviations

- Name the common diagnostic, pathological, and treatment terms related to dental practice

- Recognize common pharmacological agents used in dental practice

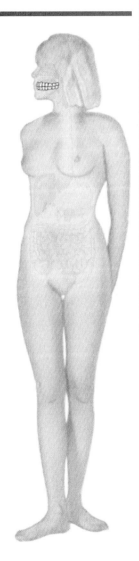

Terms in Dental Care

Dental practice (also known as *dentistry* or *odontology*) is the profession that studies, diagnoses, and treats the teeth and gums and any other parts of the oral cavity and facial structure that interact with teeth and gums. Dental practice includes prevention, diagnosis, and treatment, including both reconstructive and cosmetic surgery. **Dentists** are trained practitioners generally assisted by *dental hygienists*, trained technicians who clean teeth and gums, and by *dental technicians* or *assistants* who take x-rays, assist the dentist who is providing treatment, and perform general office tasks.

The oral cavity is part of the digestive system. Teeth and gums help masticate or chew food in the beginning of the digestive process. They are also important to speech and general appearance. The gums or **gingivae** surround the **sockets** that hold the teeth. Gums are dense fibrous tissue that form a protective covering around the sockets of the teeth and the part of the jawline inside the oral cavity. Infants are born with no visible teeth. **Primary teeth** or **deciduous teeth** begin to erupt through the gums at regular intervals at about six months old. The twenty primary teeth, ten in the upper jaw and ten in the lower jaw, are usually all in place by age four. **Pedodontists** are dentists who specialize in treating children. Then, at about age six, the **secondary** or **permanent teeth** begin to develop and push the primary teeth out of their sockets at regular intervals. Ultimately, by as late as the mid-twenties, most people have gone through the teething process, and all thirty-two permanent teeth have developed. Permanent teeth are not replaced by the body if they are lost.

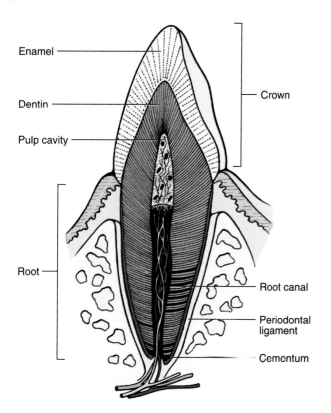

Enamel

Dentin

Pulp cavity

Crown

Root

Root canal

Periodontal ligament

Cemontum

Figure 21-1 A bicuspid tooth has a pointed crown.

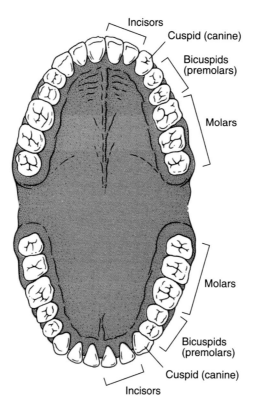

Incisors

Cuspid (canine)

Bicuspids (premolars)

Molars

Molars

Bicuspids (premolars)

Cuspid (canine)

Incisors

Figure 21-2 Genetics and good dental care usually determine if teeth will last a long time.

Each tooth has a **crown,** the part projecting above the jawline, and a **root,** the part below the jawline. The crown consists of an outer layer of glossy, white **enamel,** and an inner layer of hard bony substance called **dentin,** which surrounds the central portion of the tooth, the **pulp cavity.** The pulp cavity contains connective tissue, blood vessels, and nerves called the **pulp.** The pulp extends down into the root of the tooth. **Root canals** are tubular structures that carry the blood vessels and nerves from the bottom of the jaw up into the pulp cavity. The root of the tooth is held in place by **cementum,** a bony material surrounding the root, and a *periodontal ligament,* fibrous material that connects the cementum to the jaw. Figure 21-1 shows a cross-section of a tooth.

The average human has three types of primary teeth and four types of secondary teeth. Primary teeth include **incisors, cuspids,** and **molars** (sometimes called **premolars**). Incisors are the cutting teeth on either side of the center line of the jaw. The **central incisors** are the teeth on either side of the center line—two on top and two on bottom. Next, the **lateral incisors** or second incisors sit next to the cuspid, a tooth with a sharp-pointed projection called a **cusp.** Cuspids are also known as **canines** or **eyeteeth.** The **first molar** sits next to the cuspid, and the **second molar** sits at the back of a child's jaw. The types of secondary teeth include incisors, cuspids, and molars, as well as **bicuspids.** The secondary teeth also have central and lateral incisors, followed by one cuspid tooth. Next to each cuspid tooth is a **first bicuspid,** followed by a **second bicuspid.** Bicuspids are so named because they each have two cusps. Permanent teeth include a first, second, and **third molar** on each side of the jaw, both top and bottom. The third molar is popularly known as a *wisdom tooth,* because it usually appears after a person is fully grown. Figure 21-2 shows the arrangement of secondary teeth in the upper and lower jaws.

In dental care, the outer surfaces of teeth are referred to in special terms. The *labial* surfaces are the parts of the teeth that meet when the mouth is closed. The *buccal* surface is on the side of teeth nearest the cheek. The *lingual* surface is the inside surface of teeth nearest the tongue. The *mesial* surface is the short side of the tooth nearest the median of the jawline, and the *distal* surface is the short side of the tooth farthest from the median of the jawline. Figure 21-3 shows the names used for the surfaces of teeth.

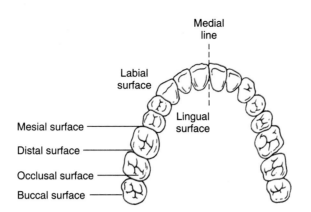

Figure 21-3 Dental work on tooth surfaces is usually labeled by the name of the tooth surface.

Vocabulary Review

In the previous section, you learned terms related to dental care. Before going on to the exercises, review the terms below and refer to the previous section if you have any questions.

Term	Word Analysis	Definition
bicuspid	[bī-KŬS-pĭd] bi-, two + Latin *cuspis*, point	Fourth and fifth tooth from the median of the jawline with two cusps.
canine	[KĀ-nīn]	Cuspid.
cementum	[sĕ-MĔN-tŭm] Latin *caementum*, quarry stone	Bony material surrounding the root of the tooth.
central incisor		Tooth on either side of the center jawline.
crown	[krŏwn]	Part of the tooth projecting above the jawline.
cusp	[kŭsp] Latin *cuspis*, tooth	Sharp-pointed tooth projection.
cuspid	[KŬS-pĭd]	Third tooth from the median of the jawline with a cusp.
deciduous	[dĕ-SĬD-yū-ŭs] tēēth Latin *deciduus*, falling off	Primary teeth.
dentin	[DĔN-tĭn] Latin *dens*, tooth	Inner bony layer of the crown of a tooth.
dentist	[DĔN-tĭst]	Practitioner trained in dentistry.
enamel	[ē-NĂM-ĕl]	Glossy, white outer covering of teeth.
eyetooth	[Ī-tūth]	Cuspid.

Term	Word Analysis	Definition
first bicuspid		Fourth tooth from the median of the jawline.
first molar		Sixth tooth from the median of the jawline.
gingivae	[JĬN-jĭ-vē]	Gums.
incisor	[ĭn-SĪ-zhūr]	First and second tooth next to the median of the jawline.
lateral incisor		Second tooth from the median of the jawline.
molar	[MŌ-lăr]	Any of the three teeth at the back of the mouth furthest from the median of the jawline.
pedodontist	[pē-dō-DŎN-tĭst] ped-, child + odont-, tooth	Dentist specializing in the treatment of children's teeth.
permanent teeth		Second set of teeth that erupt at regular intervals starting at age six.
premolar	[prē-MŌ-lăr] pre-, before + molar	Molar in primary teeth.
primary teeth		First set of teeth that erupt at regular intervals between six months and age four.
pulp	[pŭlp]	Connective tissue, blood vessels, and nerves that fill the pulp cavity.
pulp cavity		Center portion of a tooth.
root	[rūt]	Portion of the tooth that lies below the jawline.
root canal		Tubular structure holding blood vessels and nerves between the pulp cavity and the jawline.
second bicuspid		Fifth tooth from the median of the jawline.
second molar		Second to last tooth at the back of the mouth.
secondary teeth		Permanent teeth.
socket		Space in the jawline out of which teeth erupt above the gumline.
third molar		Molar furthest from the median of the jawline.

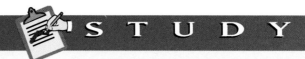

CASE STUDY

Getting a Check-up

Leila Secor made an appointment for a dental cleaning and check-up. Leila, a 42-year-old mother of two, had lost several teeth after the birth of her youngest child 8 years ago. During pregnancy, the mother's calcium is used first for fetal development. Her own teeth and gums may weaken as a result.

Leila now goes to the dentist regularly, and her teeth and gums have improved. Her dentist, Dr. Jack, examined her teeth and gums and pronounced everything in order. The hygienist then cleaned Leila's teeth carefully, and instructed her on a few areas Leila might want to floss more thoroughly.

Critical Thinking

1. Are gums important to teeth?

2. Why is diet particularly important for pregnant women's dental health?

Terms in Dental Care Exercises

Check Your Knowledge

Circle T for true or F for false.

3. Wisdom teeth are only secondary teeth. T F

4. The pulp of a tooth is the gum. T F

5. Primary teeth erupt through the gums all at once. T F

6. The outer layer of a tooth is the enamel. T F

7. The buccal surface is the side nearest the lip. T F

Combining Forms and Abbreviations

The lists below include combining forms, suffixes, and abbreviations that relate specifically to dentistry. Pronunciations are provided for the examples.

Combining Form	Meaning	Example
dent(o), denti	tooth	*dentilabial* [DĔN-tĭ-LĀ-bē-ăl], relating to both teeth and lips
gingiv(o)	gum	*gingivitis* [jĭn-jĭ-VĪ-tĭs], inflammation of the gums
odont(o)	tooth	*odontorrhagia* [ō-dŏn-tō-RĀ-jē-ă], profuse bleeding after a tooth extraction

Abbreviation	Meaning
DDS	doctor of dental surgery
def	decayed, extracted, or filled (primary teeth)
DEF	decayed, extracted, or filled (permanent teeth)
dmf	decayed, missing, or filled (primary teeth)
DMF	decayed, missing, or filled (permanent teeth)
RDH	registered dental hygienist
TMJ	temporomandibular joint

C A S E S T U D Y

Replacing Fillings

Leila's dentist updated her chart by putting in the date and type of service. He noticed that six teeth were marked DMF, but she has not needed further extractions or fillings in over eight years. Leila has two fillings that are over 20 years old. Her dentist made a note on the chart to take x-rays on the next visit to check the condition of those two fillings.

Critical Thinking

8. Why is it important to date a particular type of dental service?

9. Does Leila have two old fillings in her primary teeth?

Combining Forms and Abbreviations Exercises

Find a Match

Match the definition on the right with the correct term on the left.

10. dentiform   a. tooth disease

11. odontopathy   b. tooth-shaped

12. dentalgia   c. dentistry

13 gingivectomy   d. toothache

14. odontology   e. surgical resectioning of the gums

Diagnostic, Pathological, and Treatment Terms

Most dental work begins with *prevention* of *tooth decay,* **cavities,** or **caries,** gradual decay and disintegration of teeth, and **gingivitis** or *gum disease.* Preventive measures include cleaning of teeth and gums on a regular basis to remove **plaque,** microorganisms that grow on the crowns and along the roots of teeth causing decay of teeth and breakdown of gums. They also may include a **fluoride** treatment, washing of the mouth with a fluoride solution to prevent dental caries.

Once tooth decay has begun, the earlier it is caught the better the outcome. Dental x-rays reveal the beginnings of decay at and below the surface of teeth (Figure 21-4). They can also reveal any problems with the normal growth of permanent teeth, such as an *impacted wisdom tooth,* a third molar so tightly wedged into the jaw bone that it is unable to erupt or break through the surface of the gums thoroughly. Tooth decay can cause toothaches or **odontalgia,** which can be quite painful. Early tooth decay that has not invaded the central portion of the tooth usually receives a **filling,** a dental restoration. Filling includes **drilling,** cutting away some of the tooth including the decayed area, and placing into the space an **amalgam,** a mixture of metals or other substances that are designed to prevent further tooth erosion. If decay is deeper within the tooth, an **abscess,** infection and swelling of the soft tissue of the jaw, may result. In some cases, the tooth must be removed partially or totally and root canal work must be performed. *Root canal* work is the removal of affected nerves in the root canals and closing off of affected canals. **Endodontists** are dentists who specialize in root canal work.

When teeth are damaged by trauma or decayed so thoroughly that they cannot be filled, replacement "teeth" are used. **Dentures** are dental prostheses that can be permanently held in place or can be removable. Dentures are either **partial,** replacing one or more but not all teeth, or **full,** replacing a whole set of teeth. Partials that are attached to other teeth are called **bridges.** Dentists use a process of molding, shaping, and color-matching substances that are then made into dentures in a dental laboratory before being placed into the patient's mouth. A missing tooth may also be replaced with a dental **implant,** an artificial tooth that has an extension set into bone. An alternative to a partially damaged tooth is to cover it with a new, permanently placed artificial crown.

Gum disease or gingivitis can result from too much plaque, other medical conditions, or general poor dental hygiene and health. **Periodontists** are specialists who treat gum disease, often by cutting into the gums and removing diseased tissue and plaque in a process called *scaling.* Gingivitis is inflammation of the gums, usually with bleeding and swelling. Medication is sometimes necessary to reduce the inflammation before gums can be thoroughly treated.

Orthodontists are dentists who specialize in **orthodontics,** the correction and prevention of irregularities in the placement and appearance of teeth. They can correct **malocclusions,** abnormal closure of the top teeth in relation to the bottom teeth such as an overbite. Malocclusions may be corrected with surgical removal of any teeth that are crowding other teeth or with **braces,** appliances that put pressure on the teeth to move them slowly into place (Figure 21-5).

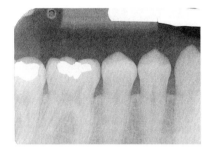

Figure 21-4 Dental x-rays can show decay as well as existing fillings.

Gold is sometimes used to fill teeth. It is considered a permanent filling and rarely allows decay to enter the internal portion of the tooth.

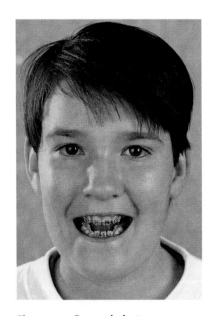

Figure 21-5 Braces help to straighten or align teeth.

Teeth can be stained by smoking. New products, *whiteners,* bleach teeth to a sparkling white.

Some dentists also treat **temporomandibular joint (TMJ) dysfunction,** pain in the jawline due to dislocation of the joint. Others perform cosmetic surgery by replacing and manipulating broken, discolored, or disfigured teeth. Still others treat discolored teeth with bleaching products to whiten them.

Vocabulary Review

In the previous section, you learned terms relating to dental diagnosis, pathology, and treatment. Before going on to the exercises, review the terms below and refer to the previous section if you have any questions.

Term	Word Analysis	Definition
abscess	[ĂB-sĕs]	Infection and swelling of the soft tissue of the jaw.
amalgam	[ă-MĂL-găm]	Mixture of metals or other substances used in fillings.
braces	[BRĀ-sĕz]	Appliances that straighten teeth slowly.
bridge	[brĭdj]	Partial that is attached to other teeth.
caries	[KĀR-ēz]	Tooth decay.
cavity	[KĂV-ĭ-tē]	Tooth decay.
dentures	[DĔN-tyūrs]	Artificial replacement teeth.
drilling		Cutting of a decayed area out of a tooth with a small dental drill.
endodontist	[ĕn-dō-DŎN-tĭst]	Dentist who specializes in root canal work.
filling		An amalgam placed into a drilled space to prevent further tooth decay.
fluoride	[FLŪR-ĭd]	Substance given as a mouth wash to prevent tooth decay.
full	[fŭl]	Complete (set of dentures).
gingivitis	[jĭn-jĭ-VĪ-tĭs]	Inflammation of the gums.
implant		Artificial replacement tooth that has an extension set into bone.
malocclusions	[măl-ō-KLŪ-zhŭns]	Abnormal closures of the top teeth in relation to the bottom teeth.
odontalgia	[ō-dŏn-TĂL-jē-ă]	Tooth pain.

Term	Word Analysis	Definition
orthodontics	[ōr-thō-DŎN-tĭks]	Dental specialty concerned with the correction and prevention of irregularities in the placement and appearance of teeth.
partial		One or more artificial replacement teeth.
periodontist	[PĔR-ē-ō-DŎN-tĭst]	Dentist who specializes in the treatment of gum disease.
plaque	[plăk]	Microorganisms that grow on the crowns and along the roots of teeth causing decay of teeth and breakdown of gums.
temporomandibular joint (TMJ) dysfunction	[TĔM-pŏ-rō-măn-DĬB-yū-lăr]	Pain in the jawline due to dislocation of the joint.

C A S E   S T U D Y

Feeling Pain

Leila was pleased with the results of her dental visit. She asked the receptionist to remind her when her next six-month appointment was needed. The reminder postcards keep Leila on track.

Two months after her visit, Leila felt a slight pain in one of her teeth. She thought she felt some food stuck between her teeth, so she flossed and the pain went away. A few days later, on a Saturday, Leila felt queasy and noticed a dull ache in the same tooth that had hurt a couple of days ago. Leila called the dentist's office and got an appointment for Monday morning. By Monday morning, the dull ache had become a painful toothache. The dentist took x-rays and saw that an abscess had formed under one of the old fillings. He explained to Leila that her tooth could be extracted totally (requiring a partial denture or a dental implant) or could be partially removed and an artificial crown put in its place. Leila chose to have the crown, thereby saving as much of her tooth as possible. In either case, because the abscess is an infection, root canal work would have to be performed. If the crown was just cosmetic, no root canal work would be needed.

 Critical Thinking

15. What type of specialist is Leila likely to have to see before the crown is put in place?

16. Will Leila have to remove the crown daily for cleaning?

Review the Information

Fill in the blanks.

17. Two types of dental prostheses are _____ and _____.

18. Amalgam is a material used to _____ teeth.

19. Abnormal closure of the top teeth in relation to the bottom teeth is called a _____.

20. Microorganisms that cause decay form _____ around the teeth and gums.

21. A specialist in the treatment of gum disease is a _____.

Pharmacological Terms

Dentists provide local anesthetics during certain treatments, such as drilling. The most commonly used are **Novocaine,** which is injected near the site being treated, and **nitrous oxide,** a gas inhaled by the patient. Nitrous oxide is also known as laughing gas because it produces laughing in some patients. If a dentist needs to prescribe antibiotics or pain killers after a procedure, there are limitations to the number and strengths they can prescribe.

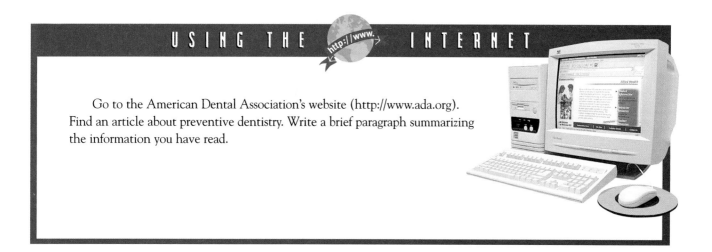

USING THE INTERNET

Go to the American Dental Association's website (http://www.ada.org). Find an article about preventive dentistry. Write a brief paragraph summarizing the information you have read.

CHAPTER REVIEW

Definitions

Define the following terms and combining forms. Review the chapter before starting. Make sure you know how to pronounce each term as you define it.

Term	Definition
abscess [ĂB-sĕs]	
amalgam [ă-MĂL-găm]	
bicuspid [bī-KŬS-pĭd]	
braces [BRĀ-sĕz]	
bridge [brĭdj]	
canine [KĀ-nīn]	
caries [KĀR-ēz]	
cavity [KĂV-ĭ-tē]	
cementum [sĕ-MĔN-tŭm]	
central incisor	
crown [krŏwn]	
cusp [kŭsp]	
cuspid [KŬS-pĭd]	
deciduous [dĕ-SĬD-yū-ŭs] teeth	
dent(o), denti	
dentin [DĔN-tĭn]	
dentist [DĔN-tĭst]	
dentures [DĔN-tyūrs]	
drilling	
enamel [ē-NĂM-ĕl]	
endodontist [ĕn-dō-DŎN-tĭst]	
eyetooth [Ī-tūth]	
filling	
first bicuspid	
first molar	
fluoride [FLŪR-ĭd]	
full [fŭl]	
gingiv(o)	

Term	Definition
gingivae [JĬN-jĭ-vē]	
gingivitis [jĭn-jĭ-VĪ-tĭs]	
implant	
incisor [ĭn-SĪ-zhŭr]	
lateral incisor	
malocclusions [măl-ō-KLŪ-zhŭns]	
molar [MŌ-lăr]	
nitrous oxide [NĪ-trŭs ŎK-sīd]	
Novocaine [NŌ-vă-kān]	
odont(o)	
odontalgia [ō-dŏn-TĂL-jē-ă]	
orthodontics [ōr-thō-DŎN-tĭks]	
partial	
pedodontist [pē-dō-DŎN-tĭst]	
periodontist [PĔR-ē-ō-DŎN-tĭst]	
permanent teeth	
plaque [plăk]	
premolar [prē-MŌ-lăr]	
primary teeth	
pulp [pŭlp]	
pulp cavity	
root [rūt]	
root canal	
second bicuspid	
second molar	
secondary teeth	
socket	
temporomandibulat [TĔM-pō-rō-măn-DĬB-yū-lăr] joint (TMJ) dysfunction	
third molar	
tooth decay	

1. Yes, they hold the teeth in place.
2. Teeth need calcium to remain healthy, and the embryo needs calcium to grow inside the womb. A pregnant woman usually requires a diet rich in calcium as well as other nutrients.
3. T

4. F
5. F
6. T
7. F
8. to know how old fillings are and to know when cleanings are needed
9. No, her primary teeth fell out long ago.
10. b
11. a

12. d
13. e
14. c
15. an endodontist
16. No, a crown is permanent.
17. dentures, implants
18. fill
19. malocclusion
20. plaque
21. periodontist

Terms in Pharmacology

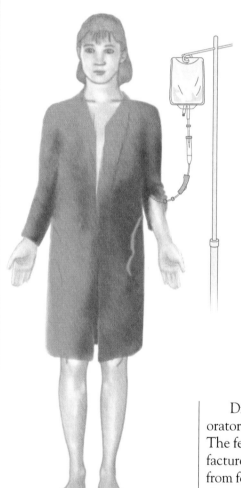

After studying this chapter, you will be able to

- Describe the source and types of drugs
- List various generic and trade names for common drugs
- Identify the various ways drugs are administered
- Describe some of the ways in which drugs affect the body
- Identify the meaning of related abbreviations

Drug Sources, Types, Function, and Administration

Drugs are biological or chemical agents. They are *therapeutic* when they are used to cure, alleviate, diagnose, treat, or prevent illness. They are *addictive* or habit-forming when they are used in unregulated and excessive quantities to stimulate or depress someone's moods. Therapeutic drugs are also called **medicines** or **medications.**

Drugs come from plants, animals, or through chemical synthesis in a laboratory. **Vitamins,** organic substances found in food, are also a form of drugs. The federal *Food and Drug Administration (FDA)* regulates the testing, manufacture, content, and distribution of all drugs that are not part of or derived from food. The FDA has an approval process that is intended to exclude drugs that may cause more harm than they can cure. They evaluate data submitted by pharmaceutical companies to determine the safety or harmful effects of a drug, and to ensure the drug provides effective treatment. The standards for approval are set by an independent committee in publications collected and published as the *United States Pharmacopeia (U.S.P.).* When the letters U.S.P. follow a drug name on the package, it means that the drug has met the stringent standards set by the committee.

Aside from the Pharmacopeia, doctors generally use one of two references in gathering drug information. The first, the *Hospital Formulary,* lists drugs that are approved for patient care in that particular facility. The use of formularies grew out of the need to control health care costs under managed care systems. The second, the *Physician's Desk Reference (PDR),* is a widely used reference for physicians. The PDR lists drugs by their drug class, and includes information such as indication for use, known side effects, appropriate dosages, and routes of administration. Figure 22-1 shows the PDR entry for aspirin.

Pharmacology is the science that studies, develops, and tests drugs. Some of the scientists who work in pharmacology specialize in the various subdivisions of the field. For example, *medicinal chemistry* is the study of new drugs, their structure, and how they work. **Pharmacodynamics** is the study of how drugs affect the body. **Toxicology** is the study of harmful effects of drugs on the body and of **antidotes,** substances able to cancel out unwanted effects. **Pharmacokinetics** is the study of how drugs are **absorbed, metabolized** (chemically changed so it can be used in the body), and **excreted** over time.

Some drugs are available **over-the-counter (OTC)**, sold without a doctor's **prescription,** which is an order for medication with the dosages, directions, route, and timing of administration included. Prescription drugs are dispensed by a **pharmacist** or druggist in a *pharmacy* or *drug store*. Drugs are also available from mail-order companies and from companies on the Internet.

Drugs can have several different names. First is a chemical name that describes the chemical formula of the drug. Second is a **generic** name that is a shortened or simpler version of the chemical name for legal purposes. Third is a **trade, brand, or proprietary name** that is given and copyrighted by the manufacturer for a specific drug. Each drug has only one chemical name and only one generic name, but it may have many trade names. For example, *acetylsalicylic acid* is the chemical name for *aspirin*, the generic name packaged under various trade names, such as Bayer aspirin. Table 22-1 lists some generic and trade names of drugs according to their function. Dosages of drugs vary depending on the age, size, severity of symptoms, and other medications in use. Some drugs are *tapered*; that is, they are given at a higher dose initially and then the dose is gradually reduced as the symptoms subside.

Ecotrin®   OTC
Enteric-Coated Aspirin
Antiarthritic, Antiplatelet

DESCRIPTION
"Ecotrin" is enteric-coated aspirin (acetylsalicylic acid, ASA) available in tablet form in 81 mg., 325 mg., and 500 mg. dosage units.
The enteric coating covers a core of aspirin and is designed to resist disintegration in the stomach, dissolving in the more neutral-to-alkaline environment of the duodenum. Such action helps to protect the stomach from injury that may result from ingestion of plain, buffered or highly buffered aspirin (see SAFETY).

INDICATIONS
'Ecotrin' is indicated for:
• Conditions requiring chronic or long-term aspirin therapy for pain and/or inflammation, e.g., rheumatoid arthritis, juvenile rheumatoid arthritis, systemic lupus

Figure 22-1. The entry for aspirin in the PDR lists uses or indications, side effects, and other important items.

The symbol Rx stands for Latin recipe, (a command to) take.

Table 22-1 Pharmacological agents, their functions, and examples.

Drug Class	Purpose	Generic	Trade Name
analgesic	relieves pain without causing loss of consciousness	acetaminophen acetylsalicylic acid ibuprofen	Tylenol aspirin (as Bayer) Advil, Motrin
anesthetic	produces a lack of feeling either locally or generally throughout the body	lidocaine HCL procaine HCL	Xylocaine Novacaine
antacid	neutralizes stomach acid	ranitidine cimetidine bismuth salicylate magaldrate	Zantac Tagamet Pepto-Bismol Riopan

(continued on next page)

Table 22-1 (continued)

Drug Class	Purpose	Generic	Trade Name
antianemic	replaces iron	ferrous sulfate	Imferon
antianginal	dilates coronary arteries to increase blood flow and reduce angina	nitroglycerine	Nitro-Bid
antianxiety	relieves anxiety	diazepam chlordiazepoxide HCL alprazolam	Valium Librium Xanax
antiarrhythmic	controls cardiac arrhythmias	propranolol HCL	Inderal
antibiotic, anti-infective, antibacterial	destroys or inhibits the growth of harmful microorganisms	penicillin cefaclor erythromycin ofloxacin	various Ceclor Ery-Tab, E-Micin Floxin
anticholinergic	blocks certain nerve impulses and muscular reactions, as in the movements of Parkinson's disease, or in cases of nausea	atropine scopolamine	Atropair Triptol
anticoagulant	prevents blood clotting	warfarin sodium heparin calcium	Coumadin Calciparine
anticonvulsant	inhibits convulsions	phenytoin carbamazepine	Dilantin Tegetrol
antidepressant	prevents or relieves symptoms of depression	amitriptyline HCL fluoxentine sertraline	Elavil Prozac Zoloft
antidiabetic	lowers blood sugar or increases insulin sensitivity	insulin	Humulin N
antidiarrheal	prevents or slows diarrhea	loperamide	Imodium, Kaopectate
antiemetic	prevents or relieves nausea and vomiting	dimenhydrinate trimethobenzamide	Dramamine Tigan
antifungal	destroys or inhibits fungal growth	fluconazole	Diflucan
antihistamine	slows allergic reactions by counteracting histamines	diphenhydramine clemastine	Benadryl Tavist
antihypertensive	controls high blood pressure	clonidine metoprolol	Catapres Lopressor
anti-inflammatory, nonsteroidal anti-inflammatory drug (NSAID)	counteracts inflammations	naproxed also aspirin and ibuprofen (see analgesics)	Naprosyn

(continued on next page)

Table 22-1 (continued)

Drug Class	Purpose	Generic	Trade Name
antineoplastic	destroys malignant cells	methotrexate cyclophosphamide busulfan	Folex Cytoxan Myleran
antiparkinson	controls symptoms of Parkinson's disease	levodopa	L-Dopa
antipsychotic	controls symptoms of schizophrenia and some psychoses	chlorpromazine haloperidol clozapine	Thorazine Haldol Clozaril
antipyretic	reduces fever	aspirin acetaminophen	various various
antitubercular	decreases growth of microorganisms that cause tuberculosis	ethambutol	Myambutol
antitussive, expectorant	prevents or relieves coughing	dextromethropan	Robitussin
antiulcer	relieves and heals ulcers	cimetidine ranitidine	Tagamet Zantac
antiviral	controls the growth of viral microorganisms	acyclovir didanosine zidovudine	Zorvirax Videx AZT, Retrovir
barbiturate	controls epileptic seizures	phenobarbital	Barbita, Luminal
bronchodilator	dilates bronchial passages	albuterol	Ventolin
decongestant	reduces nasal congestion and/or swelling	oxymetazoline phenylephrine pseudoephedrine	Afrin Neo-Synephrine Sudafed
diuretic	increases excretion of urine	chlorothiazide furosemide mannitol	Diuril Lasix Osmitrol
hemostatic	controls or stops bleeding	phytonadione	vitamin K_1
hypnotic, sedative	produces sleep or a hypnotic state	chloral hydrate secobarbital	Noctec Seconal
hypoglycemic	lowers blood glucose levels	insulin chlorpropamide	Semitard Diabinese
laxative	loosens stool and promotes normal bowel elimination	psyllium bisacodyl	Metamucil Dulcolax
vasodilator	decreases blood pressure by relaxing blood vessels	nitroglycerin isorbide dinitrate	Nitro-Bid Isordil
vasopressor	increases blood pressure by contracting muscles of arteries and capillaries	metaraminol norepinephrine	Aramine Levophed

Many drugs are synthesized to perform like substances in the body. For example, manufactured **hormones** (chemical substance in the body that forms in one organ and has an effect on another organ or part) are widely used in *hormone replacement therapy*. Many drugs are derived from plant material. Many drugs have been in use for centuries, such as aloe vera for infections. Today there are many people who prefer to use plant-based remedies instead of certain drugs. For example, St. John's Wort (a plant derivative) is widely used for cases of mild depression. The use of alternative drug therapies should always be checked with a physician. Herbal remedies can have side effects and can be contraindicated in certain cases, such as drug interaction with other prescription drugs.

Drugs are classified by their use in the body. For example, **antibiotics** or **anti-infectives** stop or slow the growth of harmful microorganisms, such as bacteria, fungi, or parasites. Subclassifications of antibiotics include the more specific purposes of the drug, as an **antifungal** is an antibiotic that kills fungi. Table 22-1 lists the major drug classes, their functions, and generic and trade name examples for each class.

Drugs come in many forms—pills, liquids, semiliquids, suppositories, foams, lotions, creams, powders, transdermal patches, sprays, or gases—depending on how the drug is to be administered to the patient. Pills or tablets (usually stored in a small bottle called a **vial**) may be available as the standard solid small tablet or they may be in the form of capsules, a tablet with a gelatin covering encasing a powder or a liquid. They may also be coated (**enteric-coated** capsules dissolve slowly in the intestine so as not to irritate the stomach) or delayed- or timed-release (as with a transdermal patch), which spreads the dosage of the medicine gradually over a period of hours. Pills may also be in the form of lozenges, tablets meant to be dissolved slowly in the mouth, not swallowed. Tablets and some liquids can also be placed **sublingually,** under the tongue, or **buccally,** inside the cheek, where they are left to dissolve. **Oral administration** is the most common method for giving pills and some liquids.

Liquid and semiliquid drugs may come in various forms, such as syrups, heavy solutions of sugar, flavoring, and water added to the medication, and emulsions, suspensions of oil and fat in water. Liquids can be swallowed, sprayed (as on a wound or in an inhalant form), or injected. They may also be released directly into the body from an implantable drug pump controlled by the patient. This method is usually used to administer pain control medication to chronically ill patients. Patients with diabetes can use a pump to release amounts of insulin as needed rather than in a specific dose.

Suppositories, drugs mixed with a semi-solid melting substance, are inserted into the vagina, rectum, or urethra. Foams are generally inserted into the vagina. Lotions and creams are applied **topically** to the surface of the skin. Powders may be inserted into a gelatin capsule or mixed with a liquid. Liquids or gases can be administered in **inhalation** form in which tiny droplets are inhaled through an inhaler, nebulizer, or spray. Sprays can be applied topically to the skin, into the nose (*intranasal*), or into the mouth.

Injection of a drug is called **parenteral administration.** Parenteral administration may be done by health care professionals. **Intradermal** or **intracutaneous** administration is the injection of a needle or **syringe** just beneath the outer layer of skin. **Subcutaneous** administration is injection of the substance into the fatty layer of tissue below the outer portion of the skin. **Intramuscular** administration is the injection of drugs deep into the muscles. Intravenous administration is the injection of drugs through an **intravenous (IV)** tube. Generally the liquid drugs are *titrated,* put into solution in a specific volume.

Inhalant therapy may soon replace parenteral administration for some commonly used medications. For example, an inhalant insulin is expected to be used widely.

An IV **infusion** is the slow intravenous administration of a drug so that fluid is added to the bloodstream at a slow and steady rate. IV tubes can also be put into a pump system controlled by the patient. Figure 22-2 shows the methods of parenteral administration. There are other types of parenteral injection that can only be performed by a physician. These types of injection are: **intracardiac** (directly into heart muscle), **intra-arterial** (directly into an artery), **intraspinal** or **intrathecal** (directly into spinal spaces as in a case of severe pain or cancer), and **intraosseus** (directly into bone).

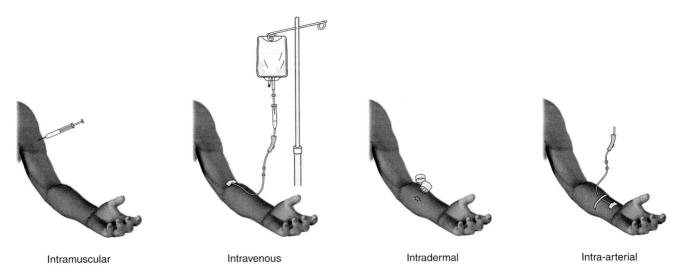

Intramuscular   Intravenous   Intradermal   Intra-arterial

Figure 22-2. Parenteral administration is the general term for administration by injection. These are only some types of parenteral administration.

Vocabulary Review

In the previous section, you learned terms relating to pharmacology. Before going on to the exercises, review the terms below and refer to the previous section if you have any questions.

Term	Word Analysis	Definition
absorb	[ăb-SŎRB]	To take into.
analgesic	[ăn-ăl-JĒ-zĭk] From Greek *analgesia*, insensibility	Drug that lessens or blocks pain.

Term	Word Analysis	Definition
anesthetic	[ăn-ĕs-THĔT-ĭk]	Drug that causes temporary loss of ability to perceive sensations at a conscious level.
antacid	[ănt-ĂS-ĭd] ant-, against + acid	Drug that lessens or neutralizes acidity.
antibacterial	[ĂN-tē-băk-TĒR-ē-ăl] anti-, against + bacterial	Drug that stops or slows bacterial growth.
antibiotic	[ĂN-tē-bī-ŎT-ĭk] anti- + Greek *biosis*, life	Drug that stops or slows the growth of harmful microorganisms.
antidiabetic	[ĂN-tē-dī-ă-BĔT-ĭk] anti- + diabetic	Drug that lowers blood sugar or increases insulin sensitivity.
antidote	[ĂN-tē-dŏt] Greek *antidotos*, given against	Substance able to cancel out unwanted effects of another substance.
antifungal	[ĂN-tē-FŬNG-găl] anti- + fungal	Drug that stops or slows the growth of fungus.
antihistamine	[ĂN-tē-HĬS-tă-mēn] anti- + histamine	Drug that reduces the action of histamines; used in allergy treatments.
anti-infective	[ĂN-tē-ĭn-FĔK-tĭv]	*See* antibiotic.
antitubercular	[ĂN-tē-tū-BĔR-kyū-lăr] anti- + tubercular	Drug that stops the spread of tuberculosis.
antiviral	[ăn-tē-VĬ-răl] anti- + viral	Drug that stops or slows the spread of a virus.
brand name		*See* trade name.
buccally	[BŬK-ăl-lē] Latin *bucca*, cheek	Inside the cheek.
contraindicated	[kŏn-tră-ĭn-dĭ-KĀ-tĕd] contra- + indicated	Inadvisable to use; said especially of a drug that might cause complications when used in combination with other drugs or when used on a patient with a particular set of symptoms.
drug	[drŭg]	Biological or chemical agents that can aid or alter body functions.
enteric-coated		Having a coating (as on a capsule) that prevents stomach irritation.

Term	Word Analysis	Definition
excrete	[ĕks-KRĒT]	To separate out and expel.
generic	[jĕ-NĀR-ĭk]	Shortened version of a chemical name.
hormone	[HŌR-mōn]	Chemical substance in the body that forms in one organ and moves to another organ or part on which the substance has an effect; manufactured version of that chemical substance.
infusion	[ĭn-FYŪ-zhŭn]	Administration of a fluid through an intravenous tube at a slow and steady rate.
inhalation	[ĭn-hă-LĀ-shŭn]	Taking in of drugs in a fine spray of droplets.
intra-arterial	[ĬN-tră-ăr-TĒ-rē-ăl]	Injected directly into an artery.
intracardiac	[ĬN-tră-KĂR-dē-ăk] intra-, within + cardiac	Injected directly into heart muscle.
intracutaneous	[ĬN-tră-kyū-TĀ-nē-ŭs] intra- + (sub)cutaneous	Injected just beneath the outer layer of skin.
intradermal	[ĬN-tră-DĔR-măl] intra- + dermal	*See* intracutaneous.
intramuscular	[ĬN-tră-MŬS-kyū-lăr] intra- + muscular	Injected deep into muscle tissue.
intraosseus	[ĬN-tră-ŎS-ē-ŭs] intra- + Latin *os*, bone	Injected directly into bone.
intraspinal	[ĬN-tră-SPĪ-năl] intra- + spinal	Injected directly into spinal spaces.
intrathecal	[ĬN-tră-THĒ-kăl] intra- + Greek *theke*, box	*See* intraspinal.
intravenous (IV)	[ĬN-tră-VĒ-nŭs] intra- + venous	Administered through a tube into a vein.
medication, medicine	[mĕd-ĭ-KĀ-shŭn, MĔD-ĭ-sĭn]	Drug that serves a therapeutic purpose.
metabolize	[mĕ-TĂB-ō-līz]	To change chemically or physically so as to make useful.

Term	Word Analysis	Definition
nonsteroidal anti-inflammatory drug (NSAID)		Anti-inflammatory drug that does not include steroids.
oral administration		Swallowing of pills or liquids via the mouth.
over-the-counter (OTC)		Available for sale without a doctor's prescription.
parenteral administration	[pă-RĔN-tĕr-ăl]	Administration of a drug by injection.
pharmacist	[FĂR-mă-sĭst]	Person licensed to dispense medications.
pharmacodynamics	[FĂR-mă-kō-dī-NĂM-ĭks] pharmaco-, drugs + dynamics	Study of how drugs affect the body.
pharmacokinetics	[FĂR-mă-kō-kĭ-NĔT-ĭks] pharmaco- + kinetics	Study of how the body absorbs, metabolizes, and excretes drugs.
pharmacology	[făr-mă-KŎL-ō-jē] pharmaco- + -logy, study	Science that studies, develops, and tests new drugs.
prescription	[prē-SKRĬP-shŭn]	Order given by a doctor for medication dosage, route, and timing of administration.
proprietary name	[prō-PRĪ-ĕ-tār-ē]	See trade name.
subcutaneous	[sŭb-kyū-TĀ-nē-ŭs] sub-, under + Latin cutis, skin	Injected into the fatty layer of tissue beneath the outer layer of skin.
sublingually	[sŭb-LĬNG-gwă-lē] sub- + Latin lingua, tongue	Under the tongue.
suppository	[sū-PŎZ-ĭ-tōr-ē] Latin suppositorium, placed underneath	Drug mixed with a semi-solid melting substance, meant for administration by insertion into the vagina, rectum, or urethra.
syringe	[sĭ-RĬNJ] Greek syrinx, tube	Instrument used for injection or withdrawal of fluids.
topically	[TŎP-ĭ-căl-lē]	On the surface of the skin.
toxicology	[tŏk-sĭ-KŎL-ō-jē] toxico-, poison + -logy	Study of harmful effects of drugs.

Term	Word Analysis	Definition
trade name		Name copyrighted by the manufacturer for a particular version of a drug.
vial	[VĪ-ăl] Greek *phiale*, drinking cup	A small receptacle for holding liquid or pill medications.
vitamin	[VĪT-ĭ-mĭn] Latin *vita*, life + amine	Organic substance found in food.

CASE STUDY

Getting an Evaluation

Many elderly people go to different doctors for different ailments without being monitored by one regular physician. Some people take so many medications that it affects their health adversely. Helen Metrone is an 86-year-old woman with high blood pressure, a tendency to retain water, skin allergies, and minor heart disease. Her preferred provider organization (PPO) allows her to see different doctors. Helen likes to go to various doctors. She almost always gets new prescriptions because of her symptoms. Often, she neglects to tell each doctor what medications she is already taking. When asked to list her medications, Helen will put one or two that she can remember. Also, Helen sometimes forgets which pills she has already taken in one day. This has led to several instances of fainting, disorientation, and dizziness. Helen's family is very concerned. They are looking into an assisted living arrangement where a nurse would give Helen her medication. They have also made an appointment with a gerontologist to review Helen's medications, outlook, and general health.

 Critical Thinking

1. Why is it important for the patient to inform their physician of all medications they are taking?

2. Why is it important for Helen to understand the instructions that come with her medication?

Drug Sources, Types, Function, and Administration Exercises

Follow the Route

Name the route of drug administration or type of drug from its description.

3. Drug is administered via a semi-solid into the rectum: _____

4. Drug is administered via vapor or gas into the nose or mouth: _____

5. Drug is administered under the tongue: _____

6. Drug is applied locally on skin or mucous membrane: _____

7. Drug is injected through a syringe under the skin, into a vein, into a muscle, or into a body cavity:

   _____

8. Drug is given by mouth and absorbed through the stomach or intestinal wall: _____

Find the Class

Give the *class* (not the name) of a drug that does the following. For example: stops diarrhea = antidiarrheal.

9. prevents/stops angina: _____

10. increases excretion of urine: _____

11. reduces blood pressure: _____

12. corrects abnormal heart rhythms: _____

13. relieves symptoms of depression: _____

14. prevents blood clotting: _____

15. promotes vomiting: _____

16. relieves pain: _____

17. neutralizes stomach acid: _____

Combining Forms and Abbreviations

The lists below include combining forms and abbreviations that relate specifically to pharmacology. Pronunciations are provided for the examples.

Combining Form	Meaning	Example
chem(o)	chemical	*chemotherapy* [KĒ-mō-thār-ă-pē], treatment of disease with chemical substances
pyret(o)	fever	*pyretogenous* [pī-rĕ-TŎJ-ĕ-nŭs], causing fever
tox(o), toxi, toxico	poison	*toxicogenic* [TŎK-sĭ-kō-JĔN-ĭk], caused by a poison

Abbreviation	Meaning		Abbreviation	Meaning
aa, a̅a̅	of each		H	hypodermic
a.c.	before meals (Latin *ante cibum*), usually one-half hour preceding a meal		h.	every hour (Latin *hora*)
			h.s.	hour of sleep (Latin *hora somni*)
ad	up to		IM	intramuscular
a.d., AD	right ear (Latin *auris dexter*)		inj	injection
ad lib	freely (Latin *ad libitum*), as often as desired		IV	intravenous
			mcg	microgram
AM, a.m., A	morning (Latin *ante meridiem*)		mEq	milliequivalent
a.s., AS	left ear (Latin *auris sinister*)		mg	milligram
a.u., AU	each ear (Latin *auris uterque*)		ml	milliliter
BID, b.i.d.	twice a day (Latin *bis in die*)		n., noct.	night (Latin, *nocte*)
c, c̅	with		non rep.	do not repeat
cap., caps.	capsule		NPO	nothing by mouth
cc., cc	cubic centimeter		NPO p MN	nothing by mouth after midnight
comp.	compound		N.S., NS	normal saline
cx	contraindicated		NSAID	nonsteroidal anti-inflammatory drug
DAW	dispense as written		N&V	nausea and vomiting
dil.	dilute		o.d., OD	right eye
disc, DC, dc	discontinue		oint., ung.	ointment, unguent
disp.	dispense		o.l.	left eye
div.	divide		o.s.	left eye
DW	distilled water		OTC	over the counter
D₅W	dextrose 5% in water		o.u.	each eye
dx, Dx	diagnosis		oz.	ounce
elix.	elixir		p	post, after
e.m.p.	as directed		p.c.	after meals (Latin *post cibum*), one-half hour after a meal
ex aq.	in water			
ext.	extract		PDR	Physician's Desk Reference
FDA	Food and Drug Administration		PM, p.m., P	afternoon (Latin *post meridiem*)
fld. ext.	fluid extract		p.o.	by mouth (Latin *per os*)
FUO	fever of unknown origin		PRN, p.r.n.	repeat as needed (Latin *pro re nata*)
g, gm	gram		pulv., pwdr	powder
gr	grain, gram		qam	every morning
gtt	drop		q.d.	every day (Latin *quaque dies*)

Abbreviation	Meaning	Abbreviation	Meaning
q.h.	every hour	subc, subq, s.c.	subcutaneously
q.i.d.	four times a day	supp., suppos	suppository
QNS	quantity not sufficient	susp.	suspension
q.o.d.	every other day	sym, Sym, Sx	symptom
q. s.	sufficient quantity	syr.	syrup
R	rectal	tab.	tablet
Rx	prescription	tbsp.	tablespoonful
s, s̄	without	t.i.d.	three times a day
Sig.	patient directions such as route and timing of medication (Latin *signa*, inscription)	tinct., tr.	tincture
		TPN	total parenteral nutrition
		TPR	temperature, pulse, respirations
SL	sublingual	tsp.	teaspoonful
sol., soln.	solution	U, u	unit
s.o.s.	if there is need	u.d.	as directed
sp.	spirit	ung.	ointment
ss, s̄s̄	one-half	U.S.P.	United States Pharmacopeia
stat	immediately		

C A S E S T U D Y

Visiting a Specialist

Helen finally did go to a gerontologist—this time with her niece. Her niece brought along a list of all her medications. The doctor advised coming off several of the medications over the next few weeks. The gerontologist also asked Helen to see her in three weeks for a medication evaluation. She asked Helen to bring in the prescription vials.

 Critical Thinking

18. How many times a day does Helen take Synthroid?

19. How many milligrams of Digoxin does Helen take daily?

NDC 0075-1505-43

Nasacort®
(triamcinolone acetonide) U.S. Pat. No. 49999999999

Black's Pharmacy   #3333 ph. 879-000-0000
36 Main St.
Norfolk, VA 34444

Rx: **666777**   Dr. Esteves, Marion D.
                St: B3456789

Use 2 sprays in each nostril once daily.

Nasacort Nasal inhaler RHO

You may refill this script 10 times before 4/26/XXXX.

Combining Forms and Abbreviations Exercises

Check Your Knowledge

Give abbreviations for the following.

20. three times a day _____

21. before meals _____

22. intramuscular _____

23. two times a day_____

24. intravenous_____

25. nothing by mouth_____

26. after meals_____

27. every hour_____

28. every morning_____

29. at bedtime_____

30. four times a day_____

31. when requested_____

32. every day_____

33. drops_____

Find the Root

Add the combining form to complete the word.

34. Resistance to the effects of chemicals: _____resistance

35. Treatment of fever: _____therapy

36. Study of poisons: _____logy

USING THE http://www. INTERNET

Go to the FDA's new site (http://www.fda.gov/opacom/hpnews.html) and find information about the approval of at least one drug. Explain what the medication is for.

CHAPTER REVIEW

Definitions

Define the following terms and combining forms. Review the chapter before starting. Make sure you know how to pronounce each term as you define it.

Term	Definition
absorb [ăb-SŎRB]	
analgesic [ăn-ăl-JĒ-zĭk]	
anesthetic [ăn-ĕs-THĔT-ĭk]	
antacid [ănt-ĂS-ĭd]	
antibacterial [ĂN-tē-băk-TĒR-ē-ăl]	
antibiotic [ĂN-tē-bī-ŎT-ĭk]	
antidiabetic [ĂN-tē-dī-ă-BĔT-ĭk]	
antidote [ĂN-tē-dŏt]	
antifungal [ĂN-tē-FŬNG-găl]	
antihistamine [ĂN-tē-HĬS-tă-mēn]	
anti-infective [ĂN-tē-ĭn-FĔK-tĭv]	
antitubercular [ăn-tē-tū-BĔR-kyū-lăr]	
antiviral [ăn-tē-VĬ-răl]	
brand name	
buccally [BŬK-ăl-lē]	
chem(o)	
contraindicated [kŏn-tră-ĭn-dĭ-KĀ-tĕd]	
drug [drŭg]	
druggist [DRŬG-ĭst]	
enteric-coated	
excrete [ĕks-KRĒT]	
generic [jĕ-NĂR-ĭk]	
hormone [HŌR-mōn]	
infusion [ĭn-FYŪ-zhŭn]	
inhalation [ĭn-hă-LĀ-shŭn]	
intra-arterial [ĬN-tră-ăr-TĒ-rē-ăl]	

Term	Definition
intracardiac [ĬN-tră-KĂR-dē-ăk]	
intracutaneous [ĬN-tră-kyū-TĀ-nē-ŭs]	
intradermal [ĬN-tră-DĔR-măl]	
intramuscular [ĬN-tră-MŬS-kyū-lăr]	
intraosseus [ĬN-tră-ŎS-ē-ŭs]	
intraspinal [ĬN-tră-SPĪ-năl]	
intrathecal [ĬN-tră-THĒ-kăl]	
intravenous (IV) [ĬN-tră-VĒ-nŭs]	
medication, medicine [měd-ĭ-KĀ-shŭn, MĔD-ĭ-sĭn]	
metabolize [mě-TĂB-ō-līz]	
nonsteroidal anti-inflammatory drug (NSAID)	
oral administration	
over-the-counter (OTC)	
parenteral [pă-RĔN-tĕr-ăl] administration	
pharmacist [FĂR-mă-sĭst]	
pharmacodynamics [FĂR-mă-kō-dī-NĂM-ĭks]	
pharmacokinetics [FĂR-mă-kō-kĭ-NĔT-ĭks]	
pharmacology [făr-mă-KŎL-ō-jē]	
prescription [prē-SKRĬP-shŭn]	
proprietary [prō-PRĪ-ĕ-tār-ē] name	
pyret(o)	
subcutaneous [sŭb-kyū-TĀ-nē-ŭs]	
sublingually [sŭb-LĬNG-gwă-lē]	
suppository [sū-PŎZ-ĭ-tōr-ē]	
syringe [sĭ-RĬNJ]	
topically [TŎP-ĭ-căl-lĕ]	
tox(o), toxi, toxico	
toxicology [tŏk-sĭ-KŎL-ō-jē]	
trade name	
vial [VĪ-ăl]	
vitamin [VĪT-ĭ-mĭn]	

Answers to Chapter Exercises

1. Medications can cause interactions or side effects.
2. Instructions, such as "take with food," can help avoid side effects.
3. suppository
4. inhalation
5. sublingually
6. topically
7. parenteral
8. oral administration
9. antianginal
10. diuretic
11. antihypertensive, vasodilator
12. antiarrhythmic
13. antidepressant
14. anticoagulant
15. antiemetic
16. analgesic
17. antacid
18. once
19. 250 mg
20. t.i.d.
21. a. c.
22. IM
23. b.i.d.
24. IV
25. NPO
26. p.c.
27. q.h.
28. qam
29. h.s.
30. q.i.d.
31. ad lib
32. q.d.
33. gtt
34. chemoresistance
35. pyretotherapy
36. toxicology
37. four
38. prednisone

APPENDIX

A

Combining Forms, Prefixes, and Suffixes

Listed below are the word parts that appear throughout this textbook. You can find examples of their use by looking in the index. The page numbers given indicate those pages on which the parts are defined and used in an example of a medical term. When a combining form ends in a vowel, the vowel is surrounded with parentheses only in those cases where the term may also appear used in words without the vowel. For example: abdomin(o) represents the combining form used both in *abdominoskeletal* and in *abdominal*.

a-, without, 21
ab-, abs-, away from, 21
abdomin(o), abdomen, 50
acanth(o), spiny; thorny, 13
acetabul(o), cup-shaped hip socket, 50, 126
acromi(o), end point of the scapula, 126
actin(o), light, 13
-ad, toward, 24
ad-, toward, to, 21
aden(o), gland, 50, 454, 525
adenoid(o), adenoid, gland, 233
adip(o), fat, 50, 78
adren(o), adrenal glands, 50, 525
aer(o), air; gas, 13
agglutin(o), agglutinin, 422
alge, algesi, algio, algo, pain, 13
-algia, pain, 24
alveol(o), air sac, alveolus, 50, 233
ambi-, both, around, 21
amni(o), amnion, 361
amyl(o), starch, 13
an-, without, 21
an(o), anus, 484
ana-, up, toward, 21
andr(o), masculine, 13, 392
angi(o), vessel, 50, 178
ankyl(o), bent, crooked, 126
ante-, before, 21
anti-, against, 21
aort(o), aorta, 50, 178
apo-, derived, separate, 21

append(o), appendic(o), appendix, 51, 484
arteri(o), artery, 51, 178
arteriol(o), arteriole, 51
arthr(o), joint, articulation, 51, 126
-asthenia, weakness, 25
ather(o), plaque; fatty substance, 13, 178
atri(o), atrium, 178
audi(o), audit(o), hearing, 559
aur(i), aur(o), auricul(o), ear, hearing, 51, 559
aut(o)-, self, 21

bacill(i), bacilli; bacteria, 13
bacteri(o), bacteria, 13
balan(o), glans penis, 392
bar(o), weight; pressure, 13
bas(o), basi(o), base, 13
bi-, twice, double, 21
bil(o), bili, bile, 484
bio, life, 13
-blast, immature, forming, 25, 603
blast(o), immature cells, 14, 603
blephar(o), eyelid, 51, 559
brachi(o), arm, 51, 126
brachy-, short, 22
brady-, slow, 22
bronch(o), bronchi, bronchus, 51, 233
bronchiol(o), bronchiole, 234
bucc(o), cheek, 51, 484
burs(o), bursa, 51, 126

cac(o), bad; ill, 14
calc(o), calci(o), calcium, 14, 126
calcane(o), heel bone, 51, 126
cali(o), calic(o), calix, 317
capn(o), carbon dioxide, 234
carcin(o), cancer, 14, 603
cardi(o), heart; esophageal opening of the stomach, 51, 178
carp(o), wrist bones, 51, 127
cata-, down, 22
cec(o), cecum, 484
-cele, hernia, 25
celi(o), abdomen, 51, 484
-centesis, puncture, 633
cephal(o), head, 51, 127
cerebell(o), cerebellum, 51, 281
cerebr(o), cerebrum, 51, 281
cerumin(o), wax, 559
cervic(o), neck; cervix, 51, 127, 361
cheil(o), chil(o), lip, 51
chem(o), chemical, 14, 682
chir(o), hand, 52
chlor(o), chlorine, green, 14
chol(e), cholo, bile, 52, 484
cholangi(o), bile vessel, 484
cholecyst(o), gallbladder, 484
choledoch(o), common bile duct, 484
chondri(o), chondr(o), cartilage, 14, 52, 127
chore(o), dance, 14
chrom, chromat, chromo, color, 14
chrono, time, 14

chyl(o), chyle, a digestive juice, 14
chym(o), chyme, semifluid present during digestion, 14
-cidal, destroying, killing, 25
-cide, destroying, killing, 25
cine(o), movement, 14, 633
circum-, around, 22
-clasis, breaking, 25, 633
-clast, breaking, 25, 633
co-, col-, com-, con-, cor-, together, 22
cochle(o), cochlea, 559
col(o), colon(o), colon, 52, 484
colp(o), vagina, 52, 361
condyl(o), knob, knuckle, 127
coni(o), dust, 14
conjunctiv(o), conjunctiva, 559
contra-, against, 22
cor(o), core(o), pupil, 52, 559
corne(o), cornea, 559
cortic(o), cortex, 52
costi, costo, rib, 52, 127
crani(o), cranium, 52, 127, 281
crin(o), secrete, 14
-crine, secreting, 25
-crit, separate, 25
cry(o), cold, 14
crypt(o), hidden; obscure, 14
cyan(o), blue , 14
cycl(o), circle; cycle; ciliary body, 15, 559
cyst(o), cysti, bladder, cyst, cystic duct, 15, 317
cyt(o), cell, 15, 52
-cyte, cell, 25
-cytosis, condition of cells, 25

dacry(o), tears, 559
dactyl(o), fingers, toes, 52, 127
de-, away from, 22
dent(i) , dento, tooth, 52, 663
derm(o), derma, dermat(o), skin, 52, 78
-derma, skin, 25
-desis, binding, 25
dextr(o), right, toward the right, 15
di-, dif-, dir-, dis-, not, separated, 22
dia-, through, 22
dips(o), thirst, 15
dors(o), dorsi, back, 15
duoden(o), duodenum , 52, 484
dynamo, force; energy, 15
-dynia, pain, 25
dys-, abnormal; difficult, 22

echo, reflected sound, 15
ect(o)-, outside, 22
-ectasia, expansion; dilation, 25
-ectasis, expanding; dilating, 25
-ectomy, removal of, 25, 633
-edema, swelling, 25
electr(o), electricity; electric, 15, 633

-ema, condition, 25
-emesis, vomiting, 26
-emia, blood, 26
-emic, relating to blood, 26
encephal(o), brain, 52, 281
end(o)-, within, 22
enter(o), intestines, 52, 484
eosin(o), red; rosy, 15, 422
epi-, over, 22
epididym(o), epididymis, 392
epiglott(o), epiglottis, 234
episi(o), vulva, 52, 361
ergo, work, 15
erythr(o), red, redness, 15, 422
esophag(o), esophagus, 485
-esthesia, sensation, 26
esthesio, sensation, perception, 15
ethmo, ethmoid bone, 15
etio, cause, 15
eu-, well, good, normal, 22
ex-, out of, away from, 22
exo-, external, on the outside, 22
extra-, without, outside of, 22

fasci(o), fascia, 127
femor(o), femur, 127
fibr(o), fiber, 15, 127
fluor(o), light; luminous; fluorine, 15, 633
-form, in the shape of, 26
fungi, fungus, 15

galact(o), milk, 16, 361
gangli(o), ganglion, 281
gastr(o), stomach, 52, 485
-gen, producing, coming to be, 26
gen(o), producing; being born, 16
-genesis, production of, 26
-genic, producing, 26
gero, geront(o), old age, 16
gingiv(o), gum, 53, 663
gli(o), neuroglia, 281
-globin, protein, 26
-globulin, protein, 26
glomerul(o), glomerulus, 317
gloss(o), tongue, 53, 485
gluc(o), glucose, 16, 485, 525
glyc(o), sugars, 16, 485, 525
glycogen(o), glycogen, 485
gnath(o), jaw, 53
gonad(o), sex glands, 53, 525
gonio, angle, 16
-gram, a recording, 26, 633
granulo, granular, 16
-graph, recording instrument, 26, 633
-graphy, process of recording, 26, 633
gyn(o), gyne, gyneco, women, 16, 361

hem(a), hemat(o), hemo, blood, 53, 422
hemangi(o), blood vessel, 178

hemi-, half, 22
hepat(o), hepatic(o), liver, 53, 485
hidr(o), sweat, 53, 78
histi(o), histo, tissue, 53
home(o), homo, same; constant, 16
humer(o), humerus, 127
hydr(o), hydrogen, water, 16
hyper-, above normal; overly, 22
hypn(o), sleep, 16, 648
hypo-, below normal, 22
hyster(o), uterus, hysteria, 53, 361

-iasis, pathological condition or state, 26
iatr(o), physician; treatment, 16
-ic, pertaining to, 26
ichthy(o), dry; scaly; fish, 16, 78
-ics, treatment, practice, body of knowledge, 26
idio, distinct; unknown, 16
ile(o), ileum, 53, 485
ili(o), ilium, 53, 127
immun(o), safe; immune, 16, 154
infra-, positioned beneath, 23
inguin(o), groin, 53
inter-, between, 23
intra-, within, 23
ir(o), irid(o), iris, 53, 559
ischi(o), ischium, 53, 127
-ism, condition, disease, doctrine, 26
iso-, equal, same, 23
-itis (pl. -itides), inflammation, 26

jejun(o), jejunum, 485

kal(i), potassium, 16
karyo, nucleus, 16, 53
kerat(o), cornea, 53, 78, 559
ket(o); keton(o), ketone; acetone, 16
kin(o), kine, movement, 16
kinesi(o), kineso, motion, 17
-kinesia, movement, 27
-kinesis, movement, 17
kyph(o), humpback, 17, 127

labi(o), lip, 53, 485
lacrim(o), tears, 559
lact(o), lacti, milk, 17, 361
lamin(o), lamina, 53, 127
lapar(o), abdominal wall, 53
laryng(o), larynx, 54, 234
latero, lateral, to one side, 17
leiomy(o), smooth muscle, 127
-lepsy, condition of having seizures, 27
-leptic, having seizures, 27
lepto, light, frail, thin, 17
leuk(o), white, 17, 422
lingu(o), tongue, 54, 485
lip(o), fat, 17, 54, 78
lith(o), stone, 17
lob(o), lobe of the lung, 234

log(o), speech, words, thought, 17
-logist, one who practices, 27
-logy, study, practice, 27
lumb(o), lumbar, 127
lymph(o), lymph, 54, 454
lymphaden(o), lymph nodes, 454
lymphangi(o), lymphatic vessels, 454
lys(o), dissolution, 17
-lysis, destruction of, 27
-lytic, destroying, 27

macr(o), large; long, 17
mal-, bad; inadequate, 23
-malacia, softening, 27
mamm(o), breast, 361
-mania, obsession, 27, 648
mast(o), breast, 54, 361
mastoid(o), mastoid process, 559
maxill(o), maxilla, 54, 127
meato, meatus, 317
medi(o), middle; medial plane, 17
mediastin(o), mediastinum, 234
medull(o), medulla, 54
meg(a), megal(o), large; million, 17
meg(a)-, megal(o)-, large, 23
-megaly, enlargement, 27
melan(o), black; dark, 17, 79
mening(o), meninges, 54, 281
men(o), menstruation, 361
mes(o), middle; median, 17
mes(o)-, middle, median, 23
meta-, after, 23
metacarp(o), metacarpal, 128
-meter, measuring device, 27
metr(o), uterus, 361
-metry, measurement, 27
micr(o), small; one-millionth; tiny,
    17
micro-, small, microscopic, 23, 633
mio, smaller; less, 17
mon(o)-, single, 23
morph(o), structure; shape, 17
muc(o), mucus, 54
multi-, many, 23
muta, genetic change, 603
mutagen(o), genetic change, 603
my(o), muscle, 54, 128
myc(o), fungus, 79
myel(o), spinal cord; bone marrow,
    54, 128, 281
myring(o), eardrum, middle ear,
    559

narco, sleep; numbness, 17
nas(o), nose, 234, 559
necr(o), death; dying, 17
nephr(o), kidney, 54, 317
neur(i), neuro, nerve, 54, 281, 648
noct(i), night, 18
normo, normal, 18
nucle(o), nucleus, 18
nyct(o), night, 18

ocul(o), eye, 54, 559
odont(o), tooth, 54, 663
-oid, like, resembling, 27
olig(o)-, few; little; scanty, 23
-oma (pl. -omata), tumor, neoplasm,
    27, 603
oncho, onc(o), tumor, 18, 603
onych(o), nail, 54, 79
oo, egg, 54, 361
oophor(o), ovary, 54, 361
ophthalm(o), eye, 54, 559
-opia, vision, 27
-opsia, vision, 27
-opsy, view of, 27, 634
opt(o), optic(o), eye; sight, 55, 560
or(o), mouth, 55, 234, 485
orch(o), orchi(o), orchido, testis, 55,
    392
orth(o), straight; normal, 18
-osis (pl. -oses), condition, state,
    process, 27
osseo, ossi, bone, 55
ossicul(o), ossicle, 560
ost(e), osteo, bone, 55, 128
-ostomy, opening, 28, 634
ot(o), ear, 55
ov(i), ovo, egg; ova, 55, 361
ovari(o), ovary, 55, 361
ox(o), oxi, oxygen, 234
-oxia, oxygen, 28
oxy, sharp; acute; oxygen, 18

pachy, thick, 18
pan-, pant(o)-, all, entire, 23
pancreat(o), pancreas, 485, 525
par(a)-, beside; abnormal; involving
    two parts, 23
-para, bearing, 28
parathyroid(o), parathyroid, 525
-paresis, slight paralysis, 28
-parous, producing; bearing, 28
patell(o), knee, 128
path(o), disease, 18
-pathy, disease, 28
ped(o), pedi, foot; child, 55, 128
pelvi(o), pelvo, pelvic bone; hip, 55,
    128
-penia, deficiency, 28
-pepsia, digestion, 28
per-, through, intensely, 23
peri-, around, about, near, 23
pericardi(o), pericardium, 178
perine(o), perineum, 361
peritone(o), peritoneum, 485
-pexy, fixation, usually done surgi-
    cally, 28, 634
phac(o), phak(o), lens, 560
-phage, -phagia, -phagy, eating,
    devouring, 28
phag(o), eating; devouring; swallow-
    ing, 18, 422
phalang(o), finger or toe bone, 128

pharmaco, drugs; medicine, 18
pharyng(o), pharynx, 55, 234, 485
-phasia, speaking, 28
-pheresis, removal, 28
-phil, attraction; affinity for, 28
-philia, attraction; affinity for, 28,
    648
phleb(o), vein, 55, 178
-phobia, fear, 28, 648
phon(o), sound; voice; speech, 18,
    234
-phonia, sound, 28
-phoresis, carrying, 28
-phoria, feeling; carrying, 28, 648
phot(o), light, 18
phren(o), phreni, phrenico, mind;
    diaphragm, 55, 234
-phrenia, of the mind, 28
-phthisis, wasting away, 28
-phylaxis, protection, 29
physi, physio, physical; natural, 18
-physis, growing, 29
physo, air; gas; growing, 18
phyt(o), plant, 18
pil(o), hair, 55, 79
-plakia, plaque, 29
-plasia, formation, 29, 603
-plasm, formation, 29, 603
plasma, plasmo, plasmat(o), plasma,
    18, 55
-plastic, forming, 29, 603
-plasty, surgical repair, 29, 634
-plegia, paralysis, 29
-plegic, one who is paralyzed, 29
pleur(o), pleura, rib; side; pleura, 55,
    234
pluri-, several, more, 23
-pnea, breath, 29
pneum(a), pneumat(o), pneumo,
    pneumon(o), lungs; air; breathing,
    55, 234
pod(o), foot, 55, 128
-poiesis, formation, 29
-poietic, forming, 29
-poietin, one that forms
poikilo, varied; irregular, 18
poly-, many, 23
-porosis, lessening in density, 29
post-, after, following, 23
pre-, before, 23
pro-, before, forward, 24
proct(o), anus, 55, 485
prostat(o), prostate gland, 392
pseud(o), false, 18
psych(o), psyche, mind, 56, 648
-ptosis, falling down; drooping, 29
pub(o), pubis, 128
pulmon(o), lung, 56
pupill(o), pupil, 560
pyel(o), renal pelvis, 56, 317
pylor(o), pylorus, 485
pyo, pus, 18

pyret(o), fever, 19, 682
pyro, fever; fire; heat, 19, 682

quadra-, quadri-, four, 24

rachi(o), spine, 56, 128
radi(o), radiation; x-ray; radius, 19, 128, 603, 633
re-, again, backward, 24
rect(o), rectum, 56, 485
ren(i), reno, kidney, 56, 317
retin(o), retina, 560
retro-, behind, backward, 24
rhabd(o), rod-shaped, 128
rhabdomy(o), striated muscle, 128
rhin(o), nose, 56, 234
-rrhage, discharging heavily, 29
-rrhagia, heavy discharge, 29
-rrhaphy, surgical suturing, 29, 634
-rrhea, a flowing, a flux, 29
-rrhexis, rupture, 30

sacr(o), sacrum, 56
salping(o), tube, 19, 362
sarco, fleshy tissue; muscle, 56
scapul(o), scapula, 128
-schisis, splitting, 30
schisto, split, 19
schiz(o), split; division, 19, 648
scler(o), sclera, hardness; hardening, white of the eye, 19, 56, 560
scoli(o), crooked; bent, 19, 128
-scope, instrument for observing, 30, 634
-scopy, use of an instrument for observing, 30, 634
scot(o), darkness, 19, 559
seb(o), fat, 79
semi-, half, 24
sial(o), salivary glands; saliva, 56, 485
sialaden(o), salivary gland, 486
sidero, iron, 19
sigmoid(o), sigmoid colon, 56, 486
sito, food; grain, 19
somat(o), body, 19, 56
somn(o), somni, sleep, 19
-somnia, sleep, 30
son(o), sound, 19, 633
-spasm, contraction, 30
spasmo, spasm, 19
sperm(a), spermato, spermo, semen; spermatozoa, 56, 392

spher(o), round; spherical, 19
sphygm(o), pulse, 179
spin(o), spine, 281
spir(o), breath; breathe, 19, 234
splanchn(o), splanchni, viscera, 56
splen(o), spleen, 56, 454
spondyl(o), vertebra, 56, 128
squamo, scale; squamous, 19
-stalsis, contraction, 30
staphyl(o), grapelike clusters, 19
-stasis, stopping; constant, 30
-stat, agent to maintain a state, 30
-static, maintaining a state, 30
steat(o), fat, 79, 486
steno, narrowness, 19
-stenosis, narrowing, 30
stere(o), three-dimensional, 20
stern(o), sternum, 56, 128
steth(o), chest, 56, 234
stom(a), stomat(o), mouth, 57, 486
-stomy, opening, 30, 634
strepto, twisted chains; streptococci, 20
styl(o), peg-shaped, 20
sub-, less than, under, inferior, 24
super-, more than, above, superior, 24
supra-, above, over, 24
syl-, sym-, syn-, sys-, together, 24
synov(o), synovial membrane, 128
syring(o), tube, 20

tachy-, fast, 24
tars(o), tarsus, 129
tel(o), tele(o), distant; end; complete, 20
ten(o), tendin(o), tendo, tenon(o), tendon, 57, 129
terato, monster (as a malformed fetus), 20
test(o), testis, 57
thalam(o), thalamus, 282
therm(o), heat, 20
thorac(o), thoracico, thorax, chest, 57, 129, 234
thromb(o), blood clot, 179, 422
thym(o), thymus gland, 57, 454
thyr(o), thyroid gland, 57, 525
tibi(o), tibia, 129
-tome, cutting instrument, segment, 30, 634
-tomy, cutting operation, 30, 634
tono, tension; pressure, 20

tonsill(o), tonsils, 235
top(o), place; topical, 20
tox(i), toxico, toxo, poison; toxin, 20, 454, 682
trache(o), trachea, 57, 235
trachel(o), neck
trans-, across, through, 24
trich(o), trichi, hair, 79
trigon(o), trigone, 317
-trophic, nutritional, 30
tropho, food; nutrition, 20
-trophy, nutrition, 30
-tropia, turning, 30
-tropic, turning toward, 30
-tropy, condition of turning toward, 30
tympan(o), eardrum, middle ear, 560

uln(o), ulna, 129
ultra-, beyond, excessive, 24, 633
un-, not, 24
uni-, one, 24
ur(o), urin(o), urine, 317
ureter(o), ureter, 317
urethr(o), urethra, 317
-uria, urine, 31
uter(o), uterus, 362
uve(o), uvea, 560

vag(o), vagus nerve, 282
vagin(o), vagina, 362
varico, varicosity, 57
vas(o), blood vessel, duct, 57, 179
vasculo, blood vessel, 57
veni, ven(o), vein, 57, 179
ventricul(o), ventricle, 57, 282
-version, turning, 31
vertebr(o), vertebra, 57, 129
vesic(o), bladder, 57, 317
vivi, life, 20
vulv(o), vulva, 362

xanth(o), yellow, 20, 79
xeno, stranger, 20
xer(o), dry, 20, 79
xiph(o), sword; xiphoid, 20

zo(o), life, 20
zym(o), fermentation; enzyme, 20

B

Abbreviations

Listed below are the medical abbreviations that appear throughout this textbook.

Abbreviation	Meaning
-	minus/concave
+	plus/convex
aa, $\overline{aa}$	of each
AA	Alcoholics Anonymous
AAMR	American Association on Mental Retardation
AB	abortion
ABG	arterial blood gases
a.c.	before meals (Latin *ante cibum*), usually one-half hour preceding
acc.	accommodation
AcG	accelerator globulin
Ach	acetylcholine
ACTH	adrenocorticotropic hormone
ad	up to
a. d., AD	right ear (Latin *auris dexter*)
ad lib	freely (Latin *ad libitum*), as often as desired
ADH	antidiuretic hormone
AF	atrial fibrillation
AFB	acid-fast bacillus (causes tuberculosis)
AFP	alpha-fetoprotein
A/G	albumin/globulin
AGN	acute glomerulonephritis
AH	abdominal hysterectomy
AIDS	acquired immunodeficiency syndrome
AIH	artificial insemination homologous
A-K	above the knee
ALL	acute lymphocytic leukemia
ALS	amyotrophic lateral sclerosis
AM, a.m., A	morning (Latin *ante meridiem*)
AML	acute myelogenous leukemia
AP	anteroposterior
A&P	auscultation and percussion
APA	American Psychiatric Association
APTT	activated partial thromboplastin time
ARD	acute respiratory disease
ARDS	adult respiratory distress syndrome
ARF	acute respiratory failure, acute renal failure
ARMD	age-related macular degeneration
a. s., AS	left ear (Latin *auris sinister*)

Abbreviation	Meaning
AS	aortic stenosis
ASCVD	arteriosclerotic cardiovascular disease
ASD	atrial septal defect
ASHD	arteriosclerotic heart disease
ATN	acute tubular necrosis
a. u., AU	each ear (Latin *auris uterque*)
AV	atrioventricular
AZT	Azidothymidine
B-K	below the knee
Ba	barium
BaE	barium enema
baso	basophil
BBB	blood-brain barrier
BCP	biochemistry panel
BID, b.i.d.	twice a day (Latin *bis in die*)
BID, b.i.d.	twice a day (Latin *bis in die*)
BMT	bone marrow transplant
BNO	bladder neck obstruction
BP	blood pressure
BPH	benign prostatic hypertrophy
BS	breath sounds
BUN	blood urea nitrogen
bx	biopsy
c, $\overline{c}$	with
C-section	caesarean section
C-spine	cervical spine (film)
C1	first cervical vertebra
ca	calcium
CA	carcinoma
CABG	coronary artery bypass graft
CAD	coronary artery disease
cap., caps.	capsule
CAPD	continuous ambulatory peritoneal dialysis
CAT	computerized axial tomography
cath	catheter
CBC	complete blood count
cc., cc	cubic centimeter
CCU	coronary care unit
CEA	carcinogenic embryonic antigen

Abbreviation	Meaning
CHD	coronary heart disease
chemo	chemotherapy
CHF	congestive heart failure
CIS	carcinoma in situ
Cl	chlorine
CLL	chronic lymphocytic leukemia
CML	chronic myelogenous leukemia
CMV	cytomegalovirus
CNS	central nervous system
CO	cardiac output
COLD	chronic obstructive lung disease
comp.	compound
COPD	chronic obstructive pulmonary disease
CP	cerebral palsy
CPK	creatine phosphokinase
CPR	cardiopulmonary resuscitation
CRF	chronic renal failure
CRH	corticotropin-releasing hormone
CS	caesarean section
CSF	cerebrospinal fluid
CT	computed tomography
CT or CAT scan	computerized (axial) tomography
CTA	clear to auscultation
CTS	carpal tunnel syndrome
CVA	cerebrovascular accident
CVD	cerebrovascular disease
cx	contraindicated
Cx	cervix
CXR	chest x-ray
cysto	cystoscopy
D	diopter
D & C	dilation and curettage
d.t.d.	give of such doses
D_5W	dextrose 5% in water
DAW	dispense as written
dB	decibel
DDS	doctor of dental surgery
def	decayed, extracted, or filled (primary teeth)
DEF	decayed, extracted, or filled (permanent teeth)
DES	diethylstilbestrol
diff	differential blood count
dil.	dilute
disc, D. C.	discontinue
disp.	dispense
div.	divide
DJD	degenerative joint disease
DLE	discoid lupus erythematosus
DM	diabetes mellitus
dmf	decayed, missing, or filled (primary teeth)
DMF	decayed, missing, or filled (permanent teeth)
DNA	deoxyribonucleic acid
DOE	dyspnea on exertion
DPT	diphtheria, pertussis, tetanus (combined vaccination)
DRE	digital rectal exam
DSA	digital subtraction angiography
DSM	*Diagnostic and Statistical Manual of Mental Disorders*
DT	delirium tremens

Abbreviation	Meaning
DTR	deep tendon reflex
DUB	dysfunctional uterine bleeding
DVA	distance visual acuity
DVT	deep venous thrombosis
DW	distilled water
dx, Dx	diagnosis
e.m.p.	as directed
EBV	Epstein-Barr virus
ECC	endocervical curettage
ECC	extracapsular cataract extraction
ECG, EKG	electrocardiogram
ECHO	echocardiogram
ECT	electroconvulsive therapy
EDC	expected date of confinement
EEG	electroencephalogram
EENT	eye, ear, nose, and throat
EIA, ELISA	Enzyme-linked immunosorbent assay
elix.	elixir
EMB	endometrial biopsy
EMG	electromyogram
ENT	ear, nose, and throat
eos	eosinophils
EQ	emotional "intelligence" quotient
ER	estrogen receptor
ERCP	endoscopic retrograde cholangiopancrea-tography
ERT	estrogen replacement therapy
ESR	erythrocyte sedimentation rate
ESRD	end-stage renal disease
EST	electroshock therapy
ESWL	extracorporeal shock wave lithotripsy
ET tube	endotracheal intubation tube
ETT	exercise tolerance test
ex aq.	in water
ext.	extract
FDA	Food and Drug Administration
FEF	forced expiratory flow
FEV	forced expiratory volume
FHT	fetal heart tones
fld. ext.	fluid extract
FSH	follicle-stimulating hormone
FUO	fever of unknown origin
FVC	forced vital capacity
fx	fracture
Fx	fracture
g, gm	gram
G	gravida (pregnancy)
G-CSF	granulocyte colony-stimulating factor
GH	growth hormone
GM-CSF	granulocyte macrophage colony-stimulating factor
GOT	glutamic oxaloacetic transaminase
gr	grain, gram
gtt	drop
GTT	glucose tolerance test
Gy	unit of radiation equal to 100 rads
gyn	gynecology
H	hypodermic
h.	every hour (Latin *hora*)
h.s.	hour of sleep (Latin *hora somni*)
HBOT	hyperbaric oxygen therapy

Abbreviation	Meaning
HCG	human chorionic gonadotropin
HCT, Hct	hematocrit
HD	hemodialysis
HDL	high-density lipoprotein
HGB, Hgb, HB	hemoglobin
HIV	human immunodeficiency virus
HRT	hormone replacement therapy
HSG	hysterosalpingography
HSO	hysterosalpingoophorectomy
HSV	herpes simplex virus
ICCE	intracapsular cataract cryoextraction
ICP	intracranial pressure
IDDM	insulin-dependent diabetes mellitus
IgA	immunoglobulin A
IgD	immunoglobulin D
IgE	immunoglobulin E
IgG	immunoglobulin G
IgM	immunoglobulin M
IM	intramuscular
IMV	intermittent mandatory ventilation
inj	injection
IOL	intraocular lens
IOP	intraocular pressure
IPPB	intermittent positive pressure breathing
IQ	intelligence quotient
IRDS	infant respiratory distress syndrome
IRV	inspiratory reserve volume
IUD	intrauterine device
IV	intravenous
IVC	intravenous cholangiography
IVP	intravenous pyelogram
IVU	intravenous urography
K+	potassium
KUB	kidney, ureter, bladder
L_1	first lumbar vertebra
LDH	lactate dehydrogenase
LDL	low-density lipoprotein
LH	luteinizing hormone
LLL	left lower lobe [of the lungs]
LMP	last menstrual period
LP	lumbar puncture
LUL	left upper lobe [of the lungs]
LV	left ventricle
LVH	left ventricular hypertrophy
M.	mix
MBC	maximal breathing capacity
mcg	microgram
MCH	mean corpuscular hemoglobin
MCHC	mean corpuscular hemoglobin concentration
MCP	metacarpophalangeal
MCV	mean corpuscular volume
MDI	metered dose inhaler
mEq	milliequivalent
METS, mets	metastases
mg	milligram
MHA	Mental Health Association
MI	mitral insufficiency; myocardial infarction
ml	milliliter
MMPI	Minnesota Multiphasic Personality Inventory

Abbreviation	Meaning
mono	monocyte
MR	mitral regurgitation
MRA	magnetic resonance angiography
MRI	magnetic resonance imaging
MS	multiple sclerosis
MS	mitral stenosis
MSH	melanocyte-stimulating hormone
MUGA	multiple-gated acquisition scan
multip	multiparous
MVP	mitral valve prolapse
n., noct.	night (Latin, *nocte*)
N.S., NS	normal saline
N&V	nausea and vomiting
Na+	sodium
NAMH	National Association of Mental Health
NARC	National Association for Retarded Children
NHL	non-Hodgkin's lymphoma
NIDDM	noninsulin-dependent diabetes mellitus
NIMH	National Institute of Mental Health
NMR	nuclear magnetic resonance (imaging)
non rep.	do not repeat
NPO	nothing by mouth
NPO p MN	nothing by mouth after midnight
NSAID	nonsteroidal anti-inflammatory drug
NVA	near visual acuity
OB	obstetrics
OCD	obsessive-compulsive disorder
OCP	oral contraceptive pill
o.d., OD	right eye
oint., ung.	ointment, unguent
o.l., OL	left eye
OM	otitis media
o.s., OS	left eye
OTC	over the counter
o.u., OU	each eye
oz.	ounce
p	post, after
P	para (live births)
P	phosphorus
p.c.	after meals (Latin *post cibum*), one-half hour after a meal
p.o.	by mouth (Latin *per os*)
PA	posteroanterior
Pap smear	Papanicolaou smear
PCP	*Pneumocystis carinii* pneumonia
PCV	packed cell volume
PDR	Physician's Desk Reference
PE tube	polyethylene ventilating tube (placed in the eardrum)
PED	penile erectile dysfunction
PEEP	positive end expiratory pressure
PERRLA	pupils equal, round, reactive to light and accommodation
PET	positron emission tomography
PFT	pulmonary function tests
pH	power of hydrogen concentration
PID	pelvic inflammatory disease
PIP	proximal interphalangeal joint
PKU	phenylketonuria
PLT	platelet count

Abbreviation	Meaning
PM, p.m., P	afternoon (Latin *post meridiem*)
PMN, poly	polymorphonuclear neutrophil
PMP	previous menstrual period
PMS	premenstrual syndrome
PND	paroxysmal nocturnal dyspnea; postnasal drip
PPD	purified protein derivative
primip	primiparous
PRL	prolactin
PRN, p.r.n.	repeat as needed (Latin *pro re nata*)
PSA	prostate-specific antigen
PT	prothrombin time
PTCA	percutaneous transluminal coronary angioplasty
PTH	parathyroid hormone, parathormone
PTSD	post-traumatic stress disorder
PTT	partial thromboplastin time
pulv.	powder
PUVA	psoralen—ultraviolet A light therapy
PVC	premature ventricular contraction
q. s.	sufficient quantity
q.d.	every day (Latin *quaque dies*)
q.h.	every hour
q.i.d.	four times a day
q.o.d.	every other day
qam	every morning
QNS	quantity not sufficient
r	roentgen
R	rectal
Ra	radium
rad	radiation absorbed dose
RAI	radioactive iodine
RBC	red blood cell count
RD	respiratory disease
RDH	registered dental hygienist
RDS	respiratory distress syndrome
RIA	radioimmunoassay
RLL	right lower lobe [of the lungs]
RNA	ribonucleic acid
ROM	range of motion
RP	retrograde pyelogram
RT	radiation therapy
RUL	right upper lobe [of the lungs]
Rx	prescription
s, s̄	without
s.o.s.	if there is need
SA	sinoatrial
SAH	subarachnoid hemorrhage
seg	segmented mature white blood cells
SG	specific gravity
SIDS	sudden infant death syndrome
Sig.	patient directions such as route and timing of medication (Latin *signa*, inscription)
SL	sublingual
SLE	systemic lupus erythematosus
SOB	shortness of breath
sol., soln.	solution
SOM	serious otitis media
sp.	spirit
SPECT	single photon emission computed tomography
SPP	suprapubic prostatectomy
SR; sed. rate	sedimentation rate
ss, s̄s̄	one-half

Abbreviation	Meaning
stat	immediately
STH	somatotropin hormone
subc, subq, s.c.	subcutaneously
sup., supp.	suppository
susp.	suspension
SV	stroke volume
Sx	symptoms
syr.	syrup
t.i.d.	three times a day
T&A	tonsillectomy and adenoidectomy
T1	first thoracic verterbra
tab.	tablet
TAH-BSO	total abdominal hysterectomy with bilateral salpingo-oophorectomy
tal.	such
tal. dos.	such doses
TAT	Thematic Apperception Test
TB	tuberculosis
tbsp.	tablespoonful
TDM	therapeutic drug monitoring
TIA	transient ischemic attack
tinct., tr.	tincture
TLC	total lung capacity
TMJ	temporomandibular joint
TNM	tumor, nodes, metastasis
tPA, TPA	tissue plasminogen activator
TPN	total parenteral nutrition
TPR	temperature, pulse, and respiration
TSH	thyroid-stimulating hormone
tsp.	teaspoonful
TSS	toxic shock syndrome
TURP	transurethral resection of the prostate
Tx	treatment
U, u	unit
U/S	ultrasound
u.d.	as directed
U.S.P.	United States Pharmacopeia
UA	urinalysis
UC	uterine contractions
ung.	ointment
URI	upper respiratory infection
UTI	urinary tract infection
V/Q, V/Q scan	ventilation/perfusion scan
VA	visual acuity
VC	vital capacity
VCU, VCUG	voiding cystourethrogram
VF	visual field
VLDL	very low-density lipoprotein
VSD	ventricular septal defect
VT	ventricular tachycardia
WAIS	Wechsler Adult Intelligence Scale
WBC	white blood cell count
WISC	Wechsler Intelligence Scale for Children
WPPSI	Wechsler Preschool and Primary Scale of Intelligence
XRT	x-ray or radiation therapy
ZDV	Zidovudine

Index
with Key Terms Highlighted

The following index includes key terms highlighted in boldface type. This listing serves as a guide to the location of the definitions of all key terms in the text. At the end of the course, most of the key terms should be familiar to the student. This index may serve as a useful study guide by locating any key terms that the student has not yet mastered.

albumin, 410, 416
albuminuria, 330
alcohol abuse, 543,
aldosterone, 519, 520
alimentary canal, 472, 478
allergen, 459, 460
allergy, 458, 460
allograft, 96, 97
alopecia, 72, 74, 624
alopecia areata, 88
alpha cells, 518, 520
alphafetoprotein (AFP) test, 605
alpha-hydroxy acid, 99, 100
alpha rays, 621, 625
alveolar, 606, 607
alveolus, 227, 228
Alzheimer's disease, 288, 290
amalgam, 665, 666
ambivalence, 642, 645
amenorrhea, 368, 370
amino acid, 472, 478
amnesia, 288, 290
amniocentesis, 373, 374
amnion, 354
amniotic fluid, 354
amphiarthrosis, 116, 118
amylase, 474, 478
amyotrophic lateral sclerosis (ALS), 288, 290
anabolic steroids, 402
anacusis, 567, 568
anal canal, 472, 478
anal fistula, 493, 494
anal fistulectomy, 500, 501
analgesic, 148, 149, 298, 299, **673, 677**
anaphylactic shock, 459
anaphylaxis, 459, 460
anaplasia, 599, 600
anaplastic, 606, 607
anastomosis, 201, 202, **500, 501**
androgen, 518, 520
anemia, 430, 432
anesthetic, 99, 100, 288, 290, **673, 678**
aneurysm, 190, 192, 289, 290
angina, 191, 193
angina pectoris, 191 193
angiocardiogram, 183
angiocardiography, 183, 186
angiogram, 183
angiography, 183, 186, 622
angioplasty, 201, 202
angioscopy, 201, 202
angiotensin converting enzyme inhibitor, 206, 209
anisocytosis, 431, 432

ankle, 116, 118
ankyloglossia, 491, 494
ankylosis, 136, 138
anorchism, anorchia, 396, 397
anorexia, 491, 494
anorexia nervosa, 643, 645
anovulation, 368, 370
antacid, 503, 504, **673, 678**
anteflexion, 368, 370
anterior, 43, 47
anterior chamber, 550
anterior-posterior, 625
anthracosis, 243, 244
antianginal, 206, 210
antianxiety agent, 652, 653
antiarrhythmic, 208, 210
antibacterial, 674, 678
antibiotic, 676, 678
antibody, 447, 451
anticlotting, 209 210
anticoagulant, 209, 210, **436, 437**
anticonvulsant, 298, 299
antidepressant, 652, 653
antidiabetic, 674, 678
antidiuretic hormone (ADH), 518, 520
antidote, 673, 678
antifungal, 676, 678
antigen, 448, 451
antiglobulin test, 426, 428
antihistamine, 674, 678
antihyperglycemic, 537, 538
antihypertensive, 207, 210, 674
antihypoglycemic, 537, 538
anti-infective, 676, 678
anti-inflammatory, 99, 100, 148, 149
anti-inflammatory nonsteroidal drug, 674
antibacterial, 99, 100
antibiotic, 99, 100
antidiarrheal, 503, 504
antiemetic, 503, 504
antifungal, 99, 100
antihistamine, 99, 100
antipruritic, 99, 100
antipsychotic agent, 652, 653
antiseptic, 99, 100
antispasmodic, 503, 505, 338
antitoxin, 450, 451
antitubercular, 675, 678
antitussive, 255, 675
antiulcer, 675
antiviral, 675, 678
anuresis, 329, 330
anuria, 329, 330
anus, 472, 478
anxiety, 642, 645

cystitis, 329, 330
cystocele, 329, 331
cystolith, 329, 331
cystopexy, 334, 335
cystoplasty, 334, 335
cystorrhaphy, 334, 335
cystoscope, 323, 326
cystoscopy, 323, 326
cytoplasm, 37, 600
cytotoxic cell, 450, 451

dacryoadenitis, 567, 569
dacryocystectomy, 573, 574
dacryocystitis, 567, 569
deafness, 567, 569
death, 588, 590, 593, 594
debridement, 96, 97
decibel, 552, 554
deciduous, 659, 661
decubitus ulcer, 85, 89
dedifferentiated, 599, 600
deep, 43, 47
deep vein thrombosis, 190, 194
defecation, 476, 479
defensiveness, 642
degenerative arthritis, 137, 139
deglutition, 473, 479
deliriousness, 642, 645
delusional, 642, 645
dementia, 288, 291, 642, 645
demyelination, 288, 291
dendrite, 268, 276
densitometer, 133
dentin, 660, 661
dentist, 659, 661
dentistry, 659
dentures, 665, 666
deoxygenated blood, 168
deoxyribonucleic acid (DNA), 37, 599–600
depigmentation, 86, 89
depolarization, 170, 173
depression, 642, 645
dermabrasion, 96, 97
dermatitis, 85, 89
dermatochalasis, 567, 569
dermatology, 81, 82
dermis, 71, 72, 74
descending colon, 477
diabetes, 530, 531
diabetes insipidus, 529, 531
diabetes mellitus, 529, 531
diabetic nephropathy, 531
diabetic neuropathy, 531, 532

diabetic retinopathy, 531, 532
diagnostic, 629, 630
Diagnostic and Statistical Manual of Mental Disorders, 642
diagnostic imaging, 620, 625
dialysis, 324, 326
diaphoresis, 73, 74
diaphragm, 39, 40, 227, 229, 352, 355
diaphysis, 112, 119
diarrhea, 493, 495
diarthroses, 116, 119
diastole, 169, 173
diastolic pressure, 169
diencephalon, 272, 276
differentiated, 599, 600
diffuse, 606, 607
digestion, 472, 479
digestive system, 39, 40, 472–506
digestive tract, 472
digital rectal exam (DRE), 605
digital subtraction angiography, 183, 186, 622
dilation and curettage (D&C), 373
dilator, 629, 630
diopter, 563, 564
diphtheria, 242, 245
diplopia, 566, 569
directional terms, 43
discoid lupus erythematosus (DLE), 90
disk, disc, 115, 119
diskography, 132, 134
dislocation, 136, 139
dissociative disorder, 643, 645
distal, 43, 47, 661
diuretic, 206, 210, 338
diverticula, 493, 495
diverticulitis, 493, 495
diverticulosis, 493, 495
dopamine, 288, 291
Doppler ultrasound, 183, 187
dorsal, 43, 47
dorsal cavity, 39, 40
dorsal vertebrae, 115, 119
double pneumonia, 243
drilling, 665, 666
drug, 672,
ductless gland, 515, 521
ductus arteriosus, 171, 173
ductus venosus, 171, 173
duodenal ulcer, 492, 495
duodenum, 476, 479
dura matere, 272, 276
duritis, 289, 291
dwarfism, 529, 532
dyscrasia, 430, 432

hemostatic, 436, 437
hemothorax, 244, 246
heparin, 209, 210, **411**, 418
hepatic duct, 478
hepatic lobectomy, 500, 502
hepatic portal system, 477
hepatitis, 492, 496
hepatomegaly, 492, 496
hepatopathy, 492, 496
hernia, 396, 398
herniated disk, 136, 140
herpes, 86, 90
herpes simplex virus Type 1, 86, 90
herpes simplex virus Type 2, 86, 90
herpes zoster, 86, 90
heterograft, 96, 97
heteroplasia, 599, 600
hiatal hernia, 492, 496
high blood pressure, 190, 195
hilum, 227, 229, **311**, 314
Hippocrates, 1
Hippocratic Oath, 1–2
hirsutism, 530, 532
histamine, **413**, 418
histiocytic lymphoma, 459, 460
HIV, **458**, 461
hives, 85, 91
Hodgkin's disease, 459, 460, 610
Hodgkin's lymphoma, 459, 460
Holter monitor, 182, 187
homeostasis, 599
homograft, 96, 97
hordeolum, 567, 569
hormone, 352, 356, **515**, 521, **676**, 679
hormone replacement therapy (HRT), 377, 537, 538
hospice, 590
Hospital Formulary, 672
human development, 587–594
human chorionic gonadotropin (HCG), 605
human growth hormone, 537, 538
human immunodeficiency virus, **458**, 461
human papilloma virus, 369
humerus, **116**, 120
humoral immunity, **449**, 451
Huntington's chorea, 288, 292
hyaline membrane disease, 243
hydrocapnia, 242, 246
hydrocele, 396, 398
hydrocephalus, 282, 292
hydrochloric acid, 475,
hydronephrosis, 329, 331
hymen, 351, 356
hyperadrenalism, 530, 532
hyperbilirubinemia, 492, 496

hyperchromatic, 606, 607
hypernephroma, 610
hyperopia, 566, 570
hyperparathyroidism, 530, 532
hyperplastic, 606, 607
hyperpnea, 242, 246
hypersecretion, 529, 532
hypersensitivity, 459, 461
hypersplenism, 459, 461
hypertension, 190, 195
hypertensive heart disease, 190, 195
hyperthyroidism, 529, 532
hypertrophy, 136, 140
hyperventilation, 242, 246
hypnosis, 650, 651
hypoadrenalism, 530, 533
hypochondria, 644 645
hypochondriac regions, 45, 47
hypodermis, 70, 72, 75
hypogastric region, 46, 48
hypoglycemia, 530, 533
hypoglycemic, 537, 538
hypoparathyroidism, 530, 533
hypophysectomy, 535
hypophysis, **516**, 521
hypoplastic, 606, 607
hyposecretion, 529, 533
hypospadias, 396, 398
hypotension, 190, 195
hypothalamus, **516**, 521
hypothyroidism, 529, 533
hypotonia, 136, 140
hypoxemia, 242, 246
hypoxia, 242, 246
hysterectomy, 373, 375
hysterosalpingography, 366, 622
hysteroscopy, 365, 366

icterus, 492, 497
identical twins, 389
ileostomy, 500, 502
ileum, 476, 480
ileus, 492, 497
iliac regions, 46, 48
ilium, 116, 120
imaging, 620 625
immunity, **449**, 451
immunoglobulin, 450, 451
immunosuppressive disease, **458**, 461
impacted fracture, 136, 140
impetigo, 85, 91
implant, 588, 591, **665**, 666
impotence, 396, 398
incisor, 660, 661

mastectomy, 374, 375
mastication, 473, 481
mastitis, 369, 371
mastoiditis, 567, 570
mastoid process, 113, 121
mastopexy, 374, 375
maxillary bone, 114, 121
maxillary sinus, 114, 121
meatotomy, 334, 335
meatus, 310, 314
medial, 43, 48
medial plane, 43, 48
mediastinoscopy, 238, 239
mediastinum, 226, 230
medical records, 8–9
medication, 672, 679
medicine, 672, 679
medulla, 311, 314
medulla oblongata, 272, 277
medullary cavity, 112, 121
medulloblastoma, 610
megakaryocyte, 414, 418
melanin, 71, 75
melanocyte, 71, 75
melanocyte-stimulating hormone (MSH),
    518, 522
melanoma, 610
melatonin, 516, 522
melena, 493, 497
membranous labyrinth, 552, 556
menarche, 350, 357
Meniere's disease, 567, 570
meninges, 272, 277
meningioma, 289, 292
meningitis, 288, 292
meningocele, 287, 292
meningomyelocele, 287, 292
menometrorrhagia, 368, 371
menopause, 350, 357
menorrhagia, 368, 371
menstruation, 350, 357
mental retardation, 643, 645
mesentery, 476, 481
mesial, 660
mesothelioma, 244, 246
metabolized, 673, 679
metacarpal, 116, 121
metaphysis, 112, 121
metastasis, 459, 461, 599, 601, 605
metatarsal bones, 116, 121
metrorrhagia, 368, 371
microcytosis, 431, 433
microglia, 270, 277
midbrain, 272, 277
middle age, 590

middle adulthood, 588, 593, 594
middle ear, 551
middle lobe, 227, 230
midsagittal plane, 43, 48
mineralcorticoid, 519, 522
minimally-invasive, 629, 630
miotic, 575, 576
miscarriage, 368, 371
mitosis, 599, 601
mitral insufficiency, reflux, 192, 195
mitral stenosis, 192, 196
mitral valve, 166, 174
mitral valve prolapse, 192, 196
mixed-episode disorder, 644, 645
mixed-tissue tumor, 599
modality, 614
Moh's surgery, 96, 97, 629, 631
molar, 660, 662
monocyte, 413, 418
mons pubis, 351, 357
mood disorders, 643
morning-after pill, 376, 377
mouth, 472, 473–474, 481
mucus, 475,
multiple-gated acquisition angiography, 184,
    187
multiple myeloma, 432, 433, 610
multiple sclerosis, 288, 292
murmur, 182, 190, 196
muscle, 111, 121
muscle relaxant, 148, 149
muscle tissue, 38, 40
muscular dystrophy, 137, 140
musculoskeletal system, 38, 41, 111, 121
mutation, 600, 601
myalgia, 136, 140
myasthenia gravis, 288, 292
myelin sheath, 268, 277
myelitis, 289, 292
myeloblast, 431, 433
myelogram, 284, 285
myelography, 132, 134, 622
myeloma, 138, 141
myocardial infarction, 191, 196
myocarditis, 192, 196
myocardium, 165, 174
myodynia, 136, 141
myoma, 138, 141
myomectomy, 373, 375
myometrium, 351, 357
myopia, 566, 570
myoplasty, 145, 146
myositis, 137, 141
mydriatic, 575. 576
myringitis, 567, 570

patch, 84, 92
patch test, 81, 82
patella, 116, 122
patent ductus arteriosus, 192, 196
pathogen, 449, 452
pathological fracture, 136, 141
Patient's Bill of Rights, 6–7
peak flow meter, 238, 240
pediatrician, 589
pediatrics, 589, 591
pediculated polyp, 85, 92
pediculosis, 87, 92
pedodontist, 659, 662
pelvic cavity, 39, 41, 122
pelvic girdle, 115, 122
pelvic inflammatory disease, 369
pelvimetry, 366, 367
pelvis, 115, 122
pemphigus, 85, 92
penile erectile dysfunction, 396
penile prosthesis, 394
penis, 388, 390
pepsin, 475, 481
peptic ulcer, 492, 497
percussion, 237, 240
percutaneous transluminal coronary
    angioplasty, 200, 204
perfusion deficit, 191, 196
perfusion study, 623
pericarditis, 192, 196
pericardium, 165, 174
perilymph, 552, 556
perimenopause, 350, 358
perimetrium, 351, 358
perineum, 351, 358, 388, 390
periodontist, 665, 667
periosteum, 112, 122
peripheral vascular disease, 190, 196
peristalsis, 472, 481
peritoneal dialysis, 324, 326
peritoneoscopy, 488, 490
permanent teeth, 659, 662
pernicious anemia, 430
personality disorders, 643
pertussis, 243, 247
petechia, 85, 92, 191, 196
petit mal seizure, 288, 293
Peyronie's disease, 396, 398
pH, 323, 326
phacoemulsification, 573, 574
phagocytosis, 449, 452
phalanges, 116, 122
phantom limb, phantom pain, 142
pharmacist, 673, 680
pharmacodynamics, 673, 680

pharmacokinetics, 673, 680
pharmacology, 673, 680
pharyngeal tonsils, 225, 230
pharyngitis, 242, 247
pharynx, 472, 474, 481
phenylketones, 323, 326
phimosis, 396, 398
phlebitis, 190, 196
phlebogram, 183
phlebography, 183, 187
phlebotomy, 201, 204, 424, 428
phobia, 642, 646
phosphorus, 111, 122
photophobia, 566, 571
physical therapy, 138, 142
Physician's Desk Reference (PDR), 672
pia mater, 273, 278
pica, 643, 646
pilonidal cyst, 85, 92
pineal gland, 516, 523
pinkeye, 567, 571
pinna, 551, 556
pituitary gland, 516, 523
placenta, 350, 358
placenta previa, 368, 371
planes of the body, 43
plantar wart, 86, 92
plaque, 84, 92, 190, 197, 665, 667
plasma, 409, 418
plasma cell, 449, 452
plasmapheresis, 411, 418
plastic surgery, 96 97
platelet, 409, 418
platelet count (PLT), 425, 428
play therapy, 650, 651
pleomorphic, 606, 607
pleura, 227, 230
pleural cavity, 227, 230
pleural effusion, 244, 247
pleuritis, pleurisy, 242, 247
pleurocentesis, 251, 252
pleuropexy, 252, B252
plurals, 4
pneumobronchotomy, 251, 252
pneumoconiosis, 243, 247
pneumocystis carinii pneumonia, 243
pneumonectomy, 250, 252
pneumonia, 243, 247
pneumonitis, 242, 247
pneumonthorax, 244, 247
podagra, 137, 142
podiatrist, 132, 134
poikilocytosis, 431, 433
polarization, 170, 174
polycystic kidney disease, 329, 332

spinal nerves, 273, 278
spinous process, 115, 123
spirometer, 238, 240
spleen, 448, 452
splenectomy, 463
splenomegaly, 459, 461
splinting, 145, 147
split lamp ocular device, 563
spondylolisthesis, 138, 142
spondylolysis, 138. 143
spondylosyndesis, 145, 147
sponge, 352, 358
spongy bone, 112, 123
sprain, 136, 143
spur, 136, 143
sputum sample, culture, 238, 240
squamous cell carcinoma, 87, 93
squamous epithelium, 71, 76
stage, 605, 608
standard precautions, 629, 631
stapedectomy, 573, 574
stapes, 551, 557
staples, 629, 631
steatorrhea, 493, 498
stem cell, 411, 419
stenosis, 191, 197
stent, 201, 204
stereotactic frame, 624, 626
stereotactic surgery, stereotaxy, 296, 297
sternum, 115, 123
steroid, 537, 538
stimulus, 270, 278
stomach, 472, 482
stool, 477, 482
strabismus, 566, 571
strain, 136, 143
stratified squamous epithelium, 71, 76
stratum, 71, 76
stratum corneum, 71, 76
stratum germativum, 71, 76
stress incontinence, 329
stress test, 182, 187
striae, 72, 76
striated muscle, 116, 123
stridor, 242, 248
stroke, 289, 293
sty, 567, 571
styloid process, 113, 123
subcutaneous, 676, 680
subcutaneous layer, 71, 72, 76
subdural space, 273, 278
sublingually, 676, 680
subluxation, 136, 143
substance abuse, 643
sudden infant death syndrome (SIDS), 593,

594
suffix, 12, 24
sulcus, 112, 123, 272, 278
superficial, 43, 48
superior, 43, 48
superior lobe, 227, 231
superior vena cava, 169, 175
supine, 43, 48
suppository, 676, 680
suppressor cell, 450, 452
suprarenal gland, 517, 523
surgery, 629, 631
surgical scissors, 629, 631
surgical margin, 612
suture, 113, 123
suture needles, 629, 630
sweat glands, 70, 76
sweat test, 239, 240
sympathetic nervous system, 274, 278
sympathomimetic, 517, 523
symphysis, 116, 123
synapse, 268, 279
synarthrosis, 116, 123
syncope, 289, 293
syndrome of inappropriate ADH (SIADH),
  529, 533
synovectomy, 145, 147
synovial fluid, 116, 124
synovial joint, 116, 124
synovial membrane, 116, 124
syphilis, 369, 372
syringe, 676, 680
system, 37, 38–39, 41
systemic lupus erythematosus (SLE), 93
systolic pressure, 169

tachycardia, 190, 197
tachypnea, 242, 248
talipes calcaneus, 136, 143
talipes valgus, 136, 143
talipes varus, 136, 143
target cell, 515, 523
tarsus, tarsal bones, 116, 124
taste, 548, 557
taste buds, 553, 557
taste cells, 554, 557
Tay-Sachs disease, 287, 293
T cell, 448, 452
tear, 551, 557
tear duct, 551
temporal bone, 113, 124
temporal lobe, 272, 279
temporomandibular joint, 113, 124
temporomandibular joint (TMJ) dysfunction,

true ribs, 115, 124
tubercle, 112, 124
tuberculosis, 243, 248
tuberosity, 112, 124
tumor, 85, 93, 598, 599, 601
tuning fork, 563
tympanic cavity, 551
tympanic membrane, 551, 557
tympanitis, 567, 572
tympanoplasty, 573, 574
Type I diabetes, 530, 534
Type II diabetes, 530, 534

ulcer, 85, 93
ulcerating, 606, 608
ulcerative colitis, 492, 498
ultrasonography, 183, 622, 627
ultrasound, 183, 622, 627
ultraviolet light, 99, 101
umbilical cord, 354, 358
umbilical region, 45, 48
undescended testicle, 396
undifferentiated, 599, 606, 608
United States Pharmacopeia
    (U. S. P.), 672
universal donor, 415
universal recipient, 415
upper respiratory infection, 242, 248
uptake, 623, 627
urea, 311, 314
uremia, 329, 332
ureter, 310, 315
ureterectomy, 334, 336
ureteritis, 329
ureteroplasty, 334, 336
ureterorrhaphy, 334, 336
urethra, 310, 315
urethritis, 329
urethrocystitis, 329
urethrogram, 394, 395
urethropexy, 334, 336
urethroplasty, 334, 336
urethrorrhaphy, 334, 336
urethrostomy, 334, 336
urethrotomy, 334, 336
uric acid, 311, 315
uric acid test, 133, 134
urinalysis, 322, 327
urinary bladder, 312, 315
urinary catheterization, 322
urinary incontinence, 329
urinary system, 39, 41, 310, 315
urinary tract infection (UTI), 328, 332
urine, 312, 315

urine sugar, 527, 528
urologist, 334
urology, 334, 336
urostomy, 334, 336
urticaria, 85, 93
uterine tube, 348, 358
uterus, 348, 358
uvea, 550, 557
uvula, 474, 482

vaccination, vaccine, 449, 452
vagina, 348, 358
vaginitis, 369, 372
vagotomy, 296, 297
valve, 166, 175
valve replacement, 201, 204
valvotomy, 201, 204
valvulitis, 192, 198
valvuloplasty, 201, 204
varicella, 85, 94
varicocele, 396, 398
varicose veins, 191, 198
vascular lesion, 84, 94
vas deferens, 387, 391
vasectomy, 400, 401
vasoconstrictor, 206, 210
vasodilator, 206, 210
vasopressin, 518, 523
vasovasostomy, 400, 401
vegetation, 192, 198
vein, 166, 175
vena cava, 169, 175
venipuncture, 201, 204, 424, 428
venogram, 183
venography, 183, 188
ventilation study, 623
ventilator, 254, 256
ventral, 43, 48
ventral cavity, 39, 41
ventral thalamus, 272, 279
ventricle, 165, 175, 272, 279
ventriculogram, 183, 188
venule, 168, 175
vermiform appendix, 477
verruca, 86, 94
verrucous, 606, 608
vertebra, 115, 124
vertebral body, 115, 124
vertebral column, 115, 124
vertigo, 567, 572
vesicle, 85, 94
vestibule, 552, 557
vial, 673, 681
villi, 476, 482